The Western Medical Tradition

The Western Medical Tradition, 1800–2000 gives an account of the last two centuries of the development of 'Western' medicine, a traditon now important worldwide. It is a new account, written by leading experts who not only describe the most important people, events, and transformations, but give explanations for why medicine developed as it did, becoming as important as it has in the modern world. It contains one of the first historical summaries of the development of medicine after the Second World War. It is an authoritative source of new information as well as a synthesis of the current state of knowledge on this fascinating subject.

The Western Medical Tradition, 1800–2000 is a companion volume to *The Western Medical Tradition, 800 BC to AD 1800*.

W. F. Bynum is Professor Emeritus of the History of Medicine at University College London. He is the co-editor (with Roy Porter) of *Medicine and the Five Senses* (Cambridge, 1993), and *William Hunter and the 18th Century Medical World* (Cambridge, 1985), and author of *Science and the Practice of Medicine* (Cambridge, 1994).

Anne Hardy is Reader in the History of Medicine at the Wellcome Trust Centre for the History of Medicine at University College London. She is the author of *The Epidemic Streets: Infectious Disease and the Rise of Preventive Medicine, 1856–1900* (1993), and *Health and Medicine in Britain since 1860* (2001). She is the co-editor of *Women and Modern Medicine* (2001) and *The Road to Medical Statistics* (2002).

Stephen Jacyna is Senior Lecturer at the Wellcome Trust Centre for the History of Medicine at University College London. He is the co-author (with Edwin Clarke) of *Nineteenth-Century Origins of Neuroscientific Concepts* (1987), *Philosophic Whigs: Science, Medicine and Citizenship in Edinburgh, 1789–1848* (1994), and *Lost Words: Narratives of Language and the Brain, 1825–1926* (2000).

Christopher Lawrence is Professor of the History of Medicine at the Wellcome Trust Centre for the History of Medicine at University College London. He is the author of *Medicine in the Making of Modern Britain* (1994), and *Rockefeller Money, the Laboratory and Medicine in Edinburgh, 1919–1930: New Science in an Old Country* (2005).

E. M. (Tilli) Tansey is Reader in the History of Modern Medical Sciences at the Wellcome Trust Centre at University College London, and convenor of the Wellcome Trust's History of Twentieth Century Medicine Group, which organises and publishes the highly successful *Wellcome Witnesses to Twentieth Century Medicine* series (1997–present). She has published widely in scientific, medical, and historical journals and is the co-editor of *Women Physiologists* (1993), *Ashes to Ashes: The History of Smoking and Health* (1998), and *Biographies of Remedies* (2002).

The Western Medical Tradition

1800 to 2000

W. F. BYNUM

ANNE HARDY

STEPHEN JACYNA

CHRISTOPHER LAWRENCE

E. M. TANSEY

University College London

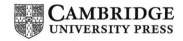
CAMBRIDGE
UNIVERSITY PRESS

CAMBRIDGE UNIVERSITY PRESS
Cambridge, New York, Melbourne, Madrid, Cape Town, Singapore, São Paulo

Cambridge University Press
40 West 20th Street, New York, NY 10011-4211, USA

www.cambridge.org
Information on this title: www.cambridge.org/9780521475242

First published 2006

Printed in the United States of America

A catalog record for this publication is available from the British Library.

Library of Congress Cataloging in Publication Data

The western medical tradition : 1800 to 2000 / W. F. Bynum . . . [et al.].
p.   cm.
Includes bibliographical references and index.
ISBN-13: 978-0-521-47524-2 (hardback)
ISBN-10: 0-521-47524-4 (hardback)
ISBN-13: 978-0-521-47565-5 (pbk.)
ISBN-10: 0-521-47565-1 (pbk.)
1. Medicine – History.   I. Bynum, W. F. (William F.), 1943–   II. Title.
R131.W472   2006
610 – dc22   2005022914

ISBN-13   978-0-521-47524-2 hardback
ISBN-10   0-521-47524-4 hardback

ISBN-13   978-0-521-47565-5 paperback
ISBN-10   0-521-47565-1 paperback

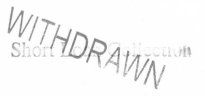

Contents

Contents

Chronological table for chapter 4

List of Illustrations

vii

Tables

xi

Acknowledgements

The authors would like to thank their editor at Cambridge University Press, Frank Smith, for his patience with this project. In early 2000, Roy Porter reinvigorated the plans for this volume; from the autumn of 2000, Harold J. Cook coordinated the efforts of the authors and subsequently wrote the introduction. Caroline Overy provided crucial research assistance, especially in the compilation of the tables and charts, timelines, and illustrations. Carole Reeves read the final versions of all the chapters and edited them for voice and consistency. The authors owe a special thanks to the Wellcome Trust, whose continuing support for the history of medicine has made this and many other projects possible.

Introduction

This work is the companion to *The Western Medical Tradition, 800 BC to AD 1800*. Like the former work, it is written by members of the academic staff of The Wellcome Trust Centre for the History of Medicine at University College London (successor to the Academic Unit of the Wellcome Institute). In its planning, it was also decided to devote a chapter to the half century just past, resulting in one of the first extensive historical overviews of medicine's most recent past published anywhere. The collective aims of the authors are similar to those of the first volume: to examine the Western medical tradition as broadly as possible within the space allowed. They deal not only with medicine as a set of intellectual and material resources used to treat the ill, often in negotiation with patients, but the power of science within medicine, the legal and institutional faces of medicine within the state, and the medical relationships developed beyond the nation, including international frameworks and commerce. Many of these subjects have become of greater importance in the last two centuries than anytime before, making the recent history of medicine different in a number of ways from the Western medical tradition described in the first volume.

What then is this 'Western medical tradition'? Or perhaps we should even ask 'is there a Western medical tradition'? The authors recognize that not only historians, but health care professionals of many kinds are constantly inventing medical 'traditions' – common sets of values, memories, and icons – to support their own views of the present. The past is often described as pointing to matters in the present and an imagined future to convince others about how things are meant to be. For instance, when, early in the twentieth century, the influential physician Sir William Osler was working to bring 'science to the bedside', as the slogan had it, he commissioned a young historian, Charles Singer, to write about the history of science and the history of science in medicine to make one vision of medicine's path appear to be 'natural'. In this sense, the authors acknowledge that the 'Western medical tradition', too, is an invented tradition, and that it may not mean quite the same thing when applied to the last two centuries that it does when applied to the period before 1800. Indeed, the introduction

1

to the companion volume even declared its 'demise' in the nineteenth century.

Yet the idea of a Western medical tradition not only helps to shape the book that follows, but points to the confluence of several long-term developments. What do we mean by it? The first point of definition is the word 'Western'. We all recognize that the kind of medicine now sometimes called 'Western' has spread across the globe, and that some of the most important changes in it are emerging in countries far from Europe and North America. Our authors refer to many other places (most especially the former Soviet Union), but they focus mainly on Northwestern Europe and North America as the regions in which a certain kind of nation-state, with particular social and economic forms, medical organizations, and intellectual culture first generated the widespread view that science in medicine would benefit not only some individuals but all citizens. This focus is not meant to denigrate other medical traditions in the West or elsewhere, only to enable the authors to discuss within the compass of one book the major developments in the medical tradition that have come to dominate the thinking of most governmental and non-governmental organizations (NGOs) of the early twenty-first century.

The second point to note is that the Western medical tradition is often seen to be based on a set of concepts. Indeed, the introduction to our companion volume referred to it as a 'system of medical ideas' and 'systems of explanation'. Evident in the last two centuries is the further development of an analytical and largely materialist endeavour to study the body and those things that affect it. This kind of thinking, long practised at the bedside and in the dissecting theatre, has had the power of the laboratory added to it over the course of the last 200 years. These endeavours are ordinarily treated under the rubric of 'science in medicine' (as William Bynum has it). The meanings of that term have varied widely, however. The studies that go under the label of 'medical science' from about 1800 have ranged from investigations into the kinds of tissues that made up bodily organs, to the development of cell theory and germ theory, to the discovery of hormones, vitamins, and genes, to molecular biology. It might be said that in this strand of medicine, the investigations into living bodies have focused their attention on smaller and smaller structures; it has been accompanied by the assumption that by examining complex systems in light of the relationships between the simplest components, information becomes available that in turn can be used to affect change. There have, of course, also been many movements within medicine that have opposed materialism and reductionism, such as the early-nineteenth-century physicians who were suspicious about the extent of the claims of morbid anatomists, the opposition to Koch's ideas on the grounds that disease could not be reduced merely to the presence of germs in the body, and a variety of holistic movements in the early and late twentieth century (a point particularly stressed by Christopher Lawrence) emerging within orthodox medicine. Other forms of protest have been voiced by religious groups, animal rights advocates, and patients' organizations, among others. Perhaps more importantly, scientific reductionism does little to capture the complexities and ambiguities of clinical knowledge nor the varieties of change in patient experience. Nevertheless, there has been a constant stream of investigators who have, by examining the smallest structures possible, tried to find out how living things work and how disturbances of their normal function come about. Over the years, tools of investigation of greater and greater precision have been created to aid their work. Very powerful intellectual claims have resulted, and are embodied in such matters as reproductive technology. The story of how this strand of thinking has developed can be built into a coherent historical narrative about how one thing leads to another.

Yet concepts also affect social relationships. Those who know certain things often distinguish themselves from others who do not or who hold other views, thus creating self-defined communities. In medicine, many of these groups, most notably doctors, have attempted, often successfully, to give their knowledge public authority through the law. In unregulated practice, the power of even the most knowledgeable practitioners over their clients and patients is seldom great because patients can take their custom elsewhere and often have their own ideas about what they want from the practitioners they consult. At its most simple, then, the doctor-patient relationship is one of negotiation and persuasion between almost equal partners. The development of the modern nation-state has altered this, however. On the argument that the public needs protection from the incompetent or malign, legislation has been used to suppress practitioners who do not conform to particular rules, so that, for instance, only those approved of by certain medical bodies are able to practise openly, in turn limiting the options of those seeking medical assistance. Even more easily policed rules have been developed in other settings: associations of practitioners decide who can belong to their groups; universities, hospitals, armed forces, and government departments regulate the appointment of members of their institutions; and health insurance companies or state payment systems limit recompense for treatment to certain kinds of practitioners. Very often, the ability to gain entry to an institution, to join a group, or to be remuner-ated is made conditional on the possession of knowledge of a certain kind, especially where clearly defined concepts and information make assess-ment easy. In this sense, scientific medicine has been a bureaucratic tool that allows some groups to flourish and others to be handicapped. How various medical groups have claimed authority and tried to institute it is, then, another theme that runs throughout these chapters.

Medicine is, however, more than a way of creating concepts or social dis-tinctions. It also affects bodies. To prove that any particular kind of knowl-edge has benefits in practice is very difficult. There are many examples of enthusiasm for apparently well-grounded practices that are now con-sidered inappropriate: 'preventive' appendectomies, excessive transorbital lobotomies and electro-convulsive therapy, or the prescription of thalido-mide as a sedative, all on a very widespread basis, suggest the power of scientific medicine to harm as well as to help. Yet, without a doubt, from the point of view of both patients and governments, there have been enor-mous improvements to the human condition that result from medicine. As any observer of the modern media is aware, one of the most obvious signs of human progress to most people lies in medical improvements, particularly in surgery and pharmacy. These include the development of anaesthesia, aseptic and antiseptic procedures, organ transplants and keyhole surgeries, and the production of antibiotics and other 'miracle drugs'. It is also notable that, compared to previous centuries, the burden of communicable disease has been remarkably lessened and life expectancy lengthened. Many alter-ations in the conditions of life have affected such morbidity and mortality patterns, from better nutrition and housing to less daily hard labour. But medicine has also contributed its share to these demographic changes, often by identifying ways to better prevent disease, such as by improving sanita-tion or introducing vaccination, although the extent of its contribution is much contested.

Governments and other parties have, therefore, invested large amounts of political and financial capital in encouraging certain kinds of medicine, claiming that it would yield positive results in the struggle against disease and disability. Their aims have sometimes been far from humanitarian: to increase the population and the number of fit productive workers paying taxes rather than drawing on them, to reduce the financial burden on pow-erful business interests or to favour certain kinds of economic development, to return soldiers to the battlefield as quickly as possible, or to recruit more souls to a religious movement or more voters to a political party. At other times, especially at moments of widespread political representation and commitment, politicians and civil servants have found it possible to move against established interests for the improvement of the public's health. Whatever the mixture of causes, despite horrific setbacks and continuing challenges, there have been clearly measurable improvements in human health in the West over the last centuries because governments have supported certain kinds of interventions to prevent disease. It is less easy to say whether the results have created greater happiness because the modern world has also developed, sometimes with the aid of medicine, new methods for controlling behaviour and even for enabling mass murder. Yet, if matters such as the development of powerful analgesics, reconstructive surgery, and better methods to help women control their fertility are taken into consideration, perhaps medicine can even be said to have contributed some share to human happiness as well as to material betterment. The Western medical tradition's association with the growing apparatus of the nation-state has therefore not only helped it gain authority over patients and publics, it has also, at least in some kinds of political systems, yielded benefits.

The Western medical tradition is not bounded by the nation-state, however. Beyond the nation lies the world of international organizations and of global corporations and financial capital. Several international bodies have given medical matters top priority in efforts to improve human health by coordinating the work of the member governments, among them the Red Cross, the League of Nations Health Organization, and more recently the World Health Organization (WHO). It is, for instance, hard to imagine how the eradication of smallpox as a communicable disease could have been achieved without the collaboration of medical personnel in many countries, even if local authorities and individuals sometimes resented their efforts. The authors are also aware that many important medical relationships occur outside the system of nations. The Rockefeller Foundation, for instance, used its private resources to promote science in medicine throughout the world in the twentieth century. Based in the United States, it was not a government agency, and although its work generally also helped to advance U.S. interests, it could do things that a government agency could not. The support for scientific medicine within religious institutions, NGOs, and other charities has also helped to disseminate it widely. Moreover, global financial interests have affected health and disease. Among such interests are medical corporations, the most visible of which are the pharmaceutical companies, which have in their harvesting of resources, production methods, and distribution and remuneration systems, affected people the world over for good and ill in ways that national governments can sometimes not control even when they try.

Yet not even a combination of ideas, social relations, and political economy fully captures the complexity of the Western medical tradition. Medical schools and hospitals, philanthropic associations, and many individual persons also figure in the story. For instance, the authors have noted changes in the techniques of microscopy and imaging; in the organization of medical schools, hospitals, and research centres; in the entry of women into medicine; in changes in surgery and childbirth practices; in the movement to professionalize nursing; in the ways in which race and class have affected medicine; in war and medicine, and colonization; in the commodification of medicine; and in public opinion and the media. Clearly, the Western medical tradition has many strands, for it has never existed as anything but the cumulative effect of the efforts of countless people. The past points to no fixed future, and promises nothing certain. It does, however, provide an important legacy on which we and our successors will be able to draw as we feel our way onward.

Harold J. Cook
Professor of the History of Medicine and
Director of the Wellcome Trust Centre
for the History of Medicine,
University College London

Chronological table for chapter 1:
1800–1849

Year	Medical events	Contemporary events
1800	Xavier Bichat studies post mortem changes in human organs; chlorine used to purify water; Benjamin Waterhouse is first U.S. physician to use smallpox vaccine; College of Surgeons of London founded	Electric battery introduced by A. Volta
1801	Philippe Pinel advocates more humane treatment of the insane; Thomas Young discovers the cause of astigmatism	First census of population in England and Wales
1802		Peace of Amiens ends European war
1803	Percival publishes code of medical ethics	Louisiana Purchase
1804		Napoleon Bonaparte crowned Emperor of France; steam railway locomotive developed by R. Trevithick
1805	Morphine isolated from laudanum by Frederick Setürner	Resumption of Napoleonic Wars; Battle of Austerlitz; Battle of Trafalgar
1806		End of Holy Roman Empire
1807		Slave trade abolished within British Empire
1808		Start of the Peninsular War
1809	Franz Gall publishes the first volume of his treatise on the nervous system, *Recherches sur le système nerveux en général, et sur celui du cerveau en particulier*; first successful ovariotomy	
1810	Samuel Friedrich Hahnemann introduces homeopathy	
1811	Charles Bell's *New Anatomy of the Brain*	Luddite riots in Britain; George (later IV) becomes Prince Regent due to George III's insanity

Year	Medical events	Contemporary events
1812	Benjamin Rush's *Medical Inquiries and Observations upon the Diseases of the Mind*	
1813		Berzelius develops system of chemical symbols
1814		Treaty of Ghent ends War of 1812 between Britain and the United States; end of the Peninsular War
1815		Battle of Waterloo; German Confederation; giant eruption of Tanbora volcano in Indonesia
1816		
1817	Cholera pandemic spreads from India; James Parkinson publishes *Essay on the Shaking Palsy*	
1818		Mary Shelley's *Frankenstein*
1819	Laennec publishes *De l'auscultation médiate*	
1820		British and Russian expeditions explore Antarctic Peninsula; George III dies, George IV crowned
1821	Charles Bell describes facial paralysis	
1822		J-F Champollion deciphers hieroglyphic writing; Brazil declared independent of Portugal; first permanent photograph made
1823	William Prout discovers hydrochloric acid in stomach secretions; *the Lancet* first published	Monroe Doctrine
1824	Henry Hickman uses carbon dioxide as a general anaesthetic on animals; second cholera pandemic begins	Death of Louis XVIII of France, succeeded by Charles X. Carnot's second Law of Thermodynamics
1825	First successful tracheotomy performed by Pierre Bretonneau	First railway from Stockton to Darlington
1826	Bretonneau describes symptoms of diphtheria	
1827	Richard Bright describes disease of the kidney	
1828	Friedrich Wöhler synthesizes urea	
1829	Johann Schönlein describes haemophilia; Burke and Hare scandal	

Year	Medical events	Contemporary events
1830		
1831	Cholera epidemics spread across Europe from Asia; Samuel Guthrie discovers chloroform	Charles Darwin joins crew of HMS Beagle
1832	Thomas Hodgkin describes cancer of the lymph nodes; Pierre-Jean Robiquet isolates codeine; sale of bodies for dissection legalised by Warburton Anatomy Act	Reform Bill in England
1833		Abolition of Slavery Act
1834	Amalgam first used for filling teeth; Pierre Louis' *Essay on Clinical Instruction*	New Poor Law in England
1835		
1836	Heinrich Gottfried von Waldeyer-Hartz notes that the nervous system is built from separate cells; Influenza pandemic	
1837		Victoria accedes to British throne
1838		Registration Act (births, deaths, and marriages) in England
1839	Third cholera pandemic begins; Theodor Schwann defines the cell as the basic unit of animal structure	Photography introduced by Daguerre
1840	Elizabeth Fry founds Institute of Nursing in London	First Opium War between China and Britain; Penny post introduced in the United Kingdom
1841	F. G. J. Henle publishes treatise on microscopic anatomy	
1842	Edwin Chadwick's *Report on the Sanitary Conditions of the Labouring Population of Great Britain*; ether first used as an anaesthetic by C. W. Long	
1843	E. H. du Bois-Reymond shows electricity is used by the nervous system	
1844	Connection established between dirt and epidemic disease in England by the Commission for Enquiring into the State of Large Towns; first use of nitrous oxide as an anaesthetic in dentistry by H. Wells	

Year	Medical events	Contemporary events
1845	First description of Leukaemia by R. Virchow	Failure of Irish potato crop
1846	W. T. Morton uses ether as an anaesthetic at the Massachusetts General Hospital	Smithsonian Institution established in Washington, DC (opened in 1855)
1847	James Young Simpson uses chloroform to relieve pain of childbirth; Karl Ludwig invents kymograph; Ignaz Semmelweis discovers contagiousness of puerperal fever; American Medical Association founded	
1848	Semmelweis introduces antiseptic methods in Vienna; First Public Health Act in Britain sets up General Board of health; cholera epidemic and influenza pandemic	Republic restored in France; K. Marx and F. Engels write the *Communist Manifesto*
1849	In the United States, Elizabeth Blackwell becomes first woman to qualify as a doctor; Thomas Addison describes pernicious anaemia	Gold Rush in California

1 Medicine in transformation, 1800–1849

STEPHEN JACYNA

Introduction

REVOLUTION AND INDUSTRIALIZATION

When applied to the period after 1800, the notion of the Western Medical
Tradition raises a number of problems. Perhaps the most obvious of these
is discerning a single tradition encompassing the vast regional, national,
and local diversity of Europe and its assorted satellites. The first half of the
nineteenth century was, moreover, a period of far-reaching political, social,
and economic change. Medicine was not exempt from these transformations. Continuity with the past is a less salient feature of the epoch than
revolution in medical doctrine, practice, and institutions.

In 1800, the hub 'West' lay in northwestern Europe. The economic
and cultural predominance that the Mediterranean countries had enjoyed
throughout the medieval and Renaissance eras was long past. The eighteenth century had, moreover, witnessed the decline of the Netherlands as
a major commercial and colonial power. The dynamic centre now lay in
the Atlantic powers of Britain and France. It was in these countries that the
characteristic signs of economic and political modernity first manifested.
In the words of one historian, during the period 1789–1848, 'the world
was transformed from a . . . Franco-British, base' (Hobsbawm, 2002, p. 11).

Before 1870, 'Germany' consisted of a patchwork of states. This very
condition of disunity was, as we shall see, to have a significant effect on the
impact of this region on developments in medicine. East of the Elbe, political
reaction and economic backwardness were the rule. Despite the considerable power it wielded in the aftermath of the Napoleonic Wars, Russia
remained a marginal and equivocal part of the Western world. The Haps-
burg Empire was stagnant and reactionary. Joseph II's experiment with
Enlightened Despotism had, however, created the conditions for Vienna
to become a significant medical centre. Indeed, during the first half of the
nineteenth century it was second only to Paris.

Some of the European powers had established outposts on the North American continent. Through a succession of wars during the eighteenth century, the British deprived the French of their American empire. France exacted a measure of revenge by supporting the thirteen colonies in their successful rebellion against the mother country between 1775 and 1783. The new United States of America retained close economic ties with Britain in addition to a cultural affinity with France. These were in part manifested by a flow of American medical students to French medical schools in the years following 1815. The control that the Iberian states exerted over their Latin American empires was fatally weakened by the upheavals of the late eighteenth and early nineteenth centuries. By the 1820s these colonies had attained political independence, though at the price of economic dependency on Britain.

European imperial powers had, in previous centuries, also established outposts in Asia, chiefly to facilitate trade. The most significant of these was the British presence in the Indian subcontinent. After 1800, the region increased in economic importance as British industry sought an outlet for manufactured goods. By the 1840s, the Indian territory under direct British control had greatly expanded as a result of conquest facilitating the exploitation of this market. British rule in India, which was to endure until the mid-twentieth century, created a site where Western medicine was forced to confront native beliefs about health and disease.

Britain and France may therefore be regarded as the leaders of the Western world during this period. In particular, the twin revolutions that convulsed these two nations at the turn of the nineteenth century were to have global consequences. The French Revolution that commenced in 1789 set the political agenda for the following decades. It was also a *social* revolution that permanently undermined some of the most fundamental features of the old regime and allowed new structures and modes of interaction to arise.

Among the most important of these transformations was the revolution's subversion of the traditional organization of society into 'orders'. Such arbitrary classification of men (the condition of women did not figure prominently in this discourse) into hierarchical systems based on birth or occupation was deemed irrational by the liberal ideology of the revolutionary era. There was a novel focus upon the individual, conceived as a natural, self-contained entity, as the atom of a rational polity. This individual was endowed with certain inalienable rights, of which self-determination – the prime good of 'liberty' – was the most significant. These principles had been adumbrated by the American revolutionaries. It was the French Revolution, however, that was to disseminate them throughout Europe and, indeed, to project them as far afield as the West Indies and Bengal.

Another legacy of the Enlightenment reorientation in Western thought should be noted. One consequence of the increasingly secular cast of the European mind was an emphasis on the well-being of the body as a focus of interest and care. Health vied with liberty for the title of the greatest good. Indeed, the two might be seen as inseparable. What good was political freedom to an individual incapacitated by illness, who could not exercise it? Moreover, it became persuasive to maintain that bodily health was in large part dependent on the salubrity of civic society. A complex web of metaphor bound the two realms together. Political radicals, for instance, would depict themselves as 'doctors to society', ready to administer a purge that would cure a diseased constitution. Conversely, medicine assumed a new cultural prominence as a means of enhancing and prolonging what was the only life in which credence was still placed.

The prime dogma of liberalism was, of course, largely fictive. When severed from one form of association, individuals were soon assimilated into other groupings derived from class, religious, and national difference. 'Professions' in the modern sense also became an increasingly prominent feature of Western societies after 1800. Although deformed and subverted, the ideal of individualism remained, however, potent throughout the nineteenth century.

The social upheavals and ideological currents flowing from the revolution impinged on medicine in a variety of ways. The impact on the organization and practice of medicine in France of the innovations of the revolutionary era will be discussed in some detail in the following text because these were to have an import that far exceeded their immediate context. The medical revolution that took place in France after 1794 was, indeed, among the most significant events in the history of Western medicine.

The early, destructive phase of the revolution was characterized by an almost fanatical commitment to the principle of individual liberty and by hostility to what was construed as corporate privilege. This prejudice was pursued even to the extent of creating, for a brief time, an unregulated market in the provision of medical services. In the later stages of the revolution, however, the rights of the individual were held to include certain provisions from the state, including a right to medical treatment in times of sickness. Acting out of recognition of this responsibility, French governments laid the foundations of a system of public assistance that may be seen as the forerunner of later state-funded healthcare systems.

The ideals of the revolution also influenced nineteenth-century medicine in other more diffuse, but no less significant, ways. The political views of individual medical men, of course, covered the widest range of orientations. In the case of Britain, for instance, for every John Allen or William Lawrence who sympathised with the ideals of the revolution, there was a staunchly Tory James Gregory or John Abernethy. But in France and the German states, in particular, there was a marked medical alignment with what might be broadly described as liberal and self-consciously progressive causes.

The reasons for this are evident. Medical men were in many respects typical representatives of the social cadres that identified with the principles of liberalism. They were self-made professionals whose claims for status and remuneration rested not on birth or connection, but on ability, learning, and personal endeavour. Medicine was thus preeminently a 'career open to the talents'. Even within medicine there were, of course, elements of the 'old corruption' that remained a reproach to these ideals; but such backward elements served only to sharpen the sense of identity of those who saw themselves at the forefront of professional improvement and progress. Moreover, the medical profession rested its claims to authority on secular, natural knowledge, something that further identified it with the movement of modernity.

All these generalizations have to be qualified by a due appreciation of the social diversity of what may loosely be described as the 'medical profession' even within a single national context. In post-revolutionary France, for example, the professors of the medical faculties may be numbered among the *haute bourgeoisie*. They, therefore, had a vested interest in the maintenance of order. It is notable, however, that some of the leading figures of the early-nineteenth-century Paris medical school retained sympathy for republican and Bonapartist causes. At the other end of the scale, the typical rural *officier de santé* was perhaps on a par with the local *curé*. In Britain, many of the general practitioners struggling to survive in urban practice were scarcely elevated above the proletariat among whom they lived. These medical 'little men', whose education and aspirations were so incongruous to their circumstances, were often drawn to 'Jacobin' or, in the case of Britain, 'radical' causes. Medical students, too, constituted a politically volatile element. In both France and the Central European states, they played a prominent role in the revolutions of 1848. In Britain, the stereotype of medical student was of a less politicized, but no less disruptive, individual.

Liberalism was not, however, merely an ideology that placed the self-governing individual at the centre of politics. Through the doctrines of political economy, it was both a putative description of and prescription for human nature and conduct. Political economy vies with medicine for the title of the first human science. We shall see that there were close links between the two fields during this period. The counterpart of the autonomous citizen exercising his right to liberty was *homo economicus*, a being who planned his every move by reference to a calculus of profit and loss. This conception of human nature was in part a post facto legitimation of the encroachments that capitalism had already made within Western societies. Political economy also served to recommend and justify the removal of such obstacles to further capitalist development that still remained. The degree of that encroachment varied from region to region: in 1800 Britain was undoubtedly the most advanced capitalist economy. While it had escaped the political revolution that had engulfed so much of Europe at the end of the eighteenth century, Britain had undergone a transformation that was in its own way still more profound and portentous, not only for this small island, but for the entire world. There is much debate about when this 'Industrial Revolution' may be said to have commenced. Indeed, some historians have argued that industrialization was so protracted a process that the term 'revolution' is inapplicable. Even in the first half of the nineteenth century, preindustrial forms of production and intermediate types coexisted with capitalist modes even in the most advanced Western economy (Hudson, 1992; Daunton, 1995). Whatever time frame is adopted, however, the rise of an industrial society involved fundamental and extensive change. In the first place, labour had to be mobilized to serve in the new centres of industry. This involved a transfer of population from the countryside to burgeoning urban centres. This shift was especially marked in the case of Britain where, in the course of the eighteenth century, commercial and industrial centres such as Manchester, Birmingham, and Leeds came to outstrip established urban centres such as Norwich. The conditions for this shift had been created by the commercialization of British agriculture in the eighteenth century.

For complex reasons, the factory became, in the first half of the nineteenth century, the preferred site for industrial production. Those employed in these factories were expected to learn new rhythms and disciplines that were foreign to the rural or even proto-industrial labourer. Some manufacturers 'attempted to take charge of the whole life of the worker and his family . . .' (Daunton, 1995, p. 181). They were, moreover, subject to the periodic phases of boom and bust of the business cycle, a phenomenon that was only dimly recognised during this period.

The sum of these changes created social strains of an unprecedented nature. The unplanned growth of towns created conditions in which disease flourished. The authoritarian industrial regime imposed severe pressure upon factory workers. The imperative of maximising profit led employers to drive wages down to a minimum, creating a population that, even in relatively good times, existed at a subsistence level. During periods of economic downturn, these workers and their families could be pauperized. These were circumstances in which social resentment and political radicalism could flourish; during the 1830s and 1840s a British revolution seemed a real possibility. The alliance of bourgeois and landed interests that by now controlled the state machinery was confronted with the challenge of averting this catastrophe. In France in addition to Britain, the burgeoning urban centres became the focus of special anxiety: they were the lairs of 'dangerous classes' that formed the chief threat to stability and the existing social order.

The 'Social Question' of the early nineteenth century possessed an obvious medical aspect. Rampant disease was seen as among the leading consequences of the rise of industrial society, although the exact nature of the relationship between poverty and morbidity was contentious. The question of public health was highlighted by epidemics, notably the cholera outbreak that swept through Europe before spreading to North America between 1831 and 1833. The contagion claimed no fewer than 52,000 lives in Britain alone. The close connection between disease and social order was highlighted by the fact that the outbreaks of cholera led to riots in several European cities. Further outbreaks followed between 1836 and 1842. The impotence of both government and the medical profession in the face of this terrifying disease threatened to undermine the authority of both. Medical men could not even agree on the causes – and in some instances, even on the existence – of the disease. Under these circumstances, resort to prayer rather than physic seemed a reasonable choice (Lawrence, 1994, p. 42).

Although cholera was the most lurid of the epidemics of the period, it was by no means the only one. Influenza, typhus, and scarlet fever also took a heavy toll among both the rural and urban populations. In 1848, the year of European revolutions, several of these diseases combined with a new outbreak of cholera in Britain to decimate entire communities.

Tuberculosis (TB), or 'consumption' (also known as 'phthisis'), was an endemic source of illness and death. The annual death rate from tuberculosis in Paris, for instance, rose steadily in the course of the first half of the nineteenth century (Barnes, 1995, p. 6). Crowding in the new industrial and commercial centres promoted the spread of these diseases. In the case of consumption, other more psychological explanations were invoked. 'Sorrowful passions' were widely recognized as a cause of the disease, and these were held to be more frequently evoked by an urban environment than elsewhere. Masturbation and other vices were also cited as contributory causes.

Contemporaries also noted a correlation between rates of mortality and such economic factors as levels of unemployment and the price of food. Mortality figures in the poorer boroughs of London could be twice as high as those in more affluent areas of the city. When cholera struck New York in 1832, mortality was again concentrated in the slums of the city, leading some to conclude that the epidemic was a judgment on the drunken and debauched habits of the poor. As in the case of tuberculosis, there was thus a readiness to confuse 'moral' and physical aetiological factors.

The same ideologues that struggled with questions of administration, public order, and poor relief were therefore obliged also to address the looming issue of 'public health'. The urban poor were 'dangerous' because they posed a threat not only to the property, but also to the health of the ruling classes. Put another way, the social question was, from an early stage, seen to be in large part about the proper management of *bodies* to ensure the mutually reinforcing goals of economic efficiency, political stability, and salubriousness.

We shall see that the medical profession was not necessarily considered the best-equipped section of society to pursue the last of these goals. Yet medical men, narrowly defined, could not escape the consequences of the momentous changes convulsing early-nineteenth-century society. The triumph of capitalism brought with it the ascendancy of what the social commentator Thomas Carlyle (1795–1881), in his 1839 essay on 'Chartism' called the 'cash nexus'. In his critique of modern society, Carlyle lamented the passing of an era when: '*Cash Payment* had not then grown to be the universal sole nexus of man to man.' He maintained that in the past, notions of mutual dependence and obligation, which had no pecuniary basis, had regulated social relations: 'Not as buyer and seller alone, of land or what else it might be, but in many senses still as soldier and captain, as clansman and head, as loyal subject and guiding king, was the low related to the high.' Carlyle was especially concerned with the relations between the aristocracy and the working class. His insights may, however, be applied to other sections of society, including the medical profession.

DOCTORS AND SOCIETY

Whereas in earlier centuries, a wide range of codes had been available to medical men, including those involving gentlemanly and or scholarly values, by the end of the eighteenth century the demands of the market had become paramount. Thus the provincial papers (*affiches*) of eighteenth-century France abounded with advertisements for a range of medical goods and services. Indeed, medicine and health lay 'at the very heart of the commercializing, publicizing project of the Affiches' (Jones, 1996, p. 27). Nor was it merely quacks and nostrum-mongers who availed themselves of this resource; medical entrepreneurship was no less evident among members of the professional establishment.

What is as significant, however, is that the older forms of identity were not abandoned or rendered altogether obsolete. Instead, they were adapted to the new context of medical practice, in large part to mask the stark, and sometimes unpalatable, realities of professional life in an increasingly market-driven society. Perhaps the most perplexing of the antinomies that medical men were forced to confront was that between the collegiality that was supposed to exist between them and the increasingly fractious and competitive environment in which they were obliged to conduct their professional affairs.

Such evasions do not conceal the rampant medical entrepreneurship of the period. Medical men strove to maximise their own position by offering an ever-expanding range of services to an assortment of customers. Among the most interesting results of this competitive and acquisitive state of affairs was the incentive it provided for innovation of various kinds. It is natural to think of doctors as primarily concerned with serving the needs of patients, although how these needs were defined was a matter of negotiation. In this context, medical men vied with one another to produce new theories of and treatments for disease that would distinguish them from their competitors. They fashioned personae for themselves calculated to bring the most (and most lucrative) patients to the doors of their consulting rooms. In many cases, they sought a foothold within the public hospitals, leading to a gradual medicalization of these institutions.

Some medical entrepreneurs sought to enhance their market position by developing new specialist hospitals where particular kinds of disease were treated and novel techniques employed. In Britain, the prototype for such developments was the Royal Ophthalmic Hospital established at Moorfields, London, in 1804. The founder, John Cunningham Saunders (1773–1810), was prompted to launch this initiative by his inability to advance his career through the existing voluntary hospitals. So great was the success of Saunders's establishment that it spawned numerous emulators in other British, European, and North American urban centres. After 1830, many more specialized hospitals were opened, some devoted to specific kinds of illness (e.g., diseases of the nervous system), others to particular medical interventions (e.g., orthopaedics), while yet others catered to the needs of special classes of patient (e.g., children) (Granshaw, 1993, p. 1189).

The personal qualities deemed to constitute an eligible medical practitioner varied widely between national and local contexts, and with the kind of patient they were designed to attract. Manners and deportment remained important: a London consultant, for instance, was expected to visit patients in a 'chariot' as a sign of his status. Some practitioners, such as the surgeon John Abernethy (1764–1831), flourished by adopting a contrarian approach and affecting a bluff, even rude, manner when dealing with the most socially distinguished patients. A doctor's religious and political posture might also attract certain patients – while repelling others. What is perhaps more noteworthy, however, is that patients were in some instances drawn to a particular practitioner because of his reputation for specialized knowledge in some particular department of medicine. In other words, *functional* criteria were beginning to supplement, but not supplant, those drawn from social status. This standing might rest on publications or on the fact that he taught a particular topic at a medical school: thus, scholarly or scientific distinction too could yield some market advantage. There were, however, also risks in identifying oneself too strongly as a 'scientific' doctor. In both Britain and the United States, such claims might lead prospective clients to conclude that the practitioner concerned was too theoretically minded and insufficiently concerned with the needs of the patient.

The 'patient-doctor' relationship, as usually conceived, does not, however, exhaust the range of interactions in which early-nineteenth-century doctors were involved. In addition to selling clinical services to individual clients, a growing number of practitioners derived income directly or indirectly from a range of corporate patrons. Thus, especially during the war years of 1792–1815, many medical men spent part of their career in the service of the Crown. To perform this function they were obliged to acquire skills and aptitudes that were not necessarily demanded in civilian practice. This military experience led to various technical innovations. Through a combination of ingenuity and necessity, military surgeons during the revolutionary and Napoleonic wars did much to simplify the treatment of wounds and to improve techniques for amputation of limbs (Vess, 1975, pp. 102–22, 131–2).

This lengthy exposure to military medicine had, however, a more extensive and profound effect. Doctors became increasingly accustomed to thinking and dealing in terms of patients and potential patients in the aggregate. These attitudes and methods were to prove serviceable when dealing with the particular problems posed by civilian populations. There were obvious analogies between the environment of an army camp or naval ship and that of a workhouse or prison. There was even continuity between the populations of these various establishments: many impressed seamen came directly from jails. Indeed, the tightly packed tenements of a nineteenth-century city had much in common with the lower decks of a man-of-war; typhus and pulmonary consumption flourished in both spaces.

Put another way, competences acquired in the military service of the state helped persuade sometimes sceptical governments that medical men were equipped to contribute to the management of the civilian population, especially that of the burgeoning cities. It should be noted, however, that some of the preventive measures that proved effective in the disciplined and relatively confined domains of military and naval medicine proved far more difficult to implement among civilian populations. European governments also employed growing numbers of medical men in other capacities: for instance, to staff asylums or to help administer workhouses and similar public-assistance establishments. Hospitals, as we have seen, were a further source of employment. In some countries these, too, were run by the state, although in Britain voluntary establishments predominated during this period.

MEDICAL SCHOOLS AND MEDICAL TEACHING

Another important market for medical enterprise lay in the field of medical education and training. By the first half of the nineteenth century most European nations possessed university medical schools staffed by professors who devoted a considerable amount of their time to academic duties. England was something of an exception. The ancient universities of Oxford and Cambridge were not active centres for medical education. The Scottish medical schools at Edinburgh and Glasgow were more dynamic; from the eighteenth century, many English students accordingly went north of the border to take advantage of their facilities. Most medical teaching in England was done by other kinds of institution, such as the private anatomy schools that flourished in eighteenth-century London. The best known of these was the Great Windmill Street School established in 1767 by William Hunter (1718–83). In 1812, the Scottish anatomist Charles Bell (1774–1842) became the proprietor of the school. In addition to anatomy, courses of chemistry, surgery, and medicine were also taught at Great Windmill Street and similar institutions.

In the course of the first half of the nineteenth century, these establishments were supplanted by medical schools attached to hospitals. The Council of the Royal College of Surgeons of London had a financial interest in promoting this shift. By 1830, after its professors had moved to hospital teaching posts, the Great Windmill Street School effectively ceased to operate. Some of the other private schools managed, however, to survive for some decades, the last of them closing in 1863 (Cope, 1966, p. 105). The hospital medical schools had the advantage of affording facilities for clinical training to supplement lectures and demonstrations. A number of provincial medical schools were also set up in the first half of the nineteenth century. The first of these was established in Manchester by Thomas Turner (1793–1873) in 1824 (Anning, 1966, p. 121).

The establishment, in 1826, of the University of London, later renamed University College London (UCL), added a further dimension to medical education in Britain. The new university was notable for a number of its features. It was differentiated from the ancient English universities by being a secular – or in the words of its detractors, an 'infidel' – establishment. In other words, it did not impose some form of religious test on those who wished to study there. The kind of training that medical students received at UCL was also distinguished by a greater emphasis on the importance of basic sciences, such as physiology, than was the case in the more clinically orientated hospital schools.

To provide its students with adequate facilities for clinical instruction, the new university constructed a new hospital, which in 1837 was renamed University College Hospital (UCH). This institution is noteworthy because it was to become a site at which crucial issues of the content of orthodox medical knowledge and of the locus of medical authority were contested and decided. John Elliotson (1791–1868), who was appointed Professor of Medicine at UCL, was in many respects an orthodox, indeed progressive, practitioner. His status within the profession was signified by his presidency of the Medico-Chirurgical Society of London. Elliotson was, moreover, one of the first British doctors to make use of the stethoscope.

Elliotson was, however, also an enthusiast for the possible medical applications of mesmerism, or 'animal magnetism' as it was sometimes known. This doctrine maintained that it was possible for one individual to alter the mental state of another by means of some form of poorly defined 'influence' flowing from the one to the other. If sustained, these claims had major implications for medicine: notably, mesmerism might be used as a form of anaesthesia to relieve patients of the pain involved in surgical procedures. The mesmeric experiments that Elliotson conducted on the wards of UCH were, however, also designed to explore the alleged diagnostic and therapeutic possibilities of the technique.

Elliotson's activities attracted considerable attention both within and outside the medical profession. The novelists Charles Dickens (1812–70) and George Cruickshank (1792–1878) were among the eminent members of society who visited UCH to witness these happenings. Dickens was convinced by what he saw and began to practice mesmerism. Mesmerism possessed a special appeal for middle-class women. For instance, the author Harriet Martineau (1802–76) employed it to treat her own complaints, which orthodox medical men tended to dismiss (Cooter, 1991). The growing popularity of mesmerism, however, excited increasing concern within University College and among the medical establishment more generally. This anxiety arose in part from the fact that laymen were apparently as capable of employing mesmerism as the trained professional.

But what ultimately decided Elliotson's fate was that he allowed lay *women* to exercise an active role within the wards of the hospital – that bastion of male supremacy – and this was considered deeply subversive. Among his experimental subjects were two young domestic servants, Elizabeth and Jane O'Key. When in a mesmeric trance, these women were supposedly endowed with extraordinary powers, including the ability to provide diagnoses and prognoses of the state of their fellow patients. By allowing the O'Keys to arrogate this status to themselves, Elliotson violated various boundaries and seemed to open the way to a reversal of the social hierarchy. Thanks to mesmerism, patients were assuming the role of the physician. Moreover, these were *hospital* patients – objects of charity drawn from the lower, and supposedly subordinate, classes. Finally, not only were the O'Keys female, they were also Irish, and thus, by the prejudices of the time, members of an inferior race (Winter, 1998, pp. 68–9).

The council of the University College medical school eventually decided that it was imperative to end these transgressions. They ordered the expulsion of Elizabeth O'Key and other mesmeric subjects from UCH. Much to their satisfaction, Elliotson resigned in protest. William Sharpey (1802–80), Professor of Physiology and one of the foremost proponents of medical science at UCL, wrote with satisfaction to a colleague: 'You will see we have done away with [animal] magnetism at the sacrifice of Elliotson.'

He continued to practice and profess mesmerism, but now outside the boundaries of the medical establishment. Elliotson's departure, and the subsequent vilification he received as the gullible dupe of his social inferiors, marked an important point in the self-definition of medical orthodoxy. In addition to heroes, the Western Medical Tradition has a need for fools and knaves.

University College Hospital was also the site of another notable medical experiment. In December 1846, the surgeon Robert Liston (1794–1847) undertook the first operation in Britain where the patient was anaesthetized using ether. The technique had previously been pioneered in the United States. The mind-numbing properties of ether had been known for some time. Before the 1840s, however, its chief application for doctors was as a means of intoxication much favoured by medical students.

It will be recalled that anaesthesia had been one of the medical uses ascribed to mesmerism. In a well-publicised case in 1842, mesmerism was used for this purpose during the amputation of the leg of James Wombell. The patient evinced no signs of pain other than a low moaning (Winter, 1998, p. 165). The use of mesmerism in surgery proved to be especially popular in India where it was, in particular, used during operations to remove scrotal hydroceles. It might be surmised that the medical profession would welcome this innovation as a means to alleviate the suffering of their patients. The actual reaction was, however, much more equivocal. Medical men felt reservations and expressed scepticism about the claims of mesmerism, in part because they enjoyed no monopoly over the employment of the technique. For instance, in the case of Wombell, the mesmerist was a barrister. Anxiety was also expressed about the morality of rendering another person unconscious and, thus, at the mercy of another.

A number of influential movements in the early-nineteenth-century Britain and America, however, encouraged a novel interest in the alleviation of pain. Both evangelical Christians and secular-minded utilitarians were, for different reasons, attracted to the ideal (Lawrence, 1997). An alternative method of anaesthesia, therefore, became a desideratum. Chemically induced trances proved to be far more acceptable to the ruling ideology of Western medicine. As Liston put it at the end of his well-publicized pioneering operation: 'this Yankee dodge beats mesmerism hollow.' It is instructive to contrast the iconic status bestowed upon Liston and other pioneers of chemical anaesthesia with the neglect and indeed contempt accorded to Elliotson and his mesmerist brethren.

Almost all of those who taught at European medical schools supplemented the income derived from these duties with private practice and other forms of paid employment. A synergy sometimes obtained between these activities: holding a chair in the Edinburgh medical school could, for instance, enhance a doctor's reputation and public visibility and, therefore, boost the number of patients seeking his advice. Payment for teaching came in various forms. University professors at continental medical schools might receive a substantial stipend, insulating them from the rigours of the market. This could lead to complacency and conservatism. The German poet and satirist, Heinrich Heine (1797–1856) captured something of this immobility when in 1826 he wrote: 'In a university town like this [Göttingen] there is an incessant coming and going, and a new generation of students is found every three years; it is a ceaseless stream of humanity, in which one term's wave supplants another, and only the old professors remain standing amid this general flux, firm and immovable, like the pyramids of Egypt – except that these academic pyramids contain no hidden wisdom.' Many teachers relied, however, on capitation fees: in other words, their income was dependent on the number of students their classes attracted. In both Britain and Germany, medical students enjoyed considerable discretion in deciding which courses to attend (p. 136ff). Something akin to a free market in medical education obtained, with lecturers vying with one another to attract students.

In France, too, numerous private lecture courses outside the official curriculum were available to medical students. Major figures within the Paris medical school, such as Xavier Bichat (1771–1802) and François Magendie (1783–1855), offered such courses. It should be noted that, in addition to providing additional income and the possibility of advancement to those who taught them, these private courses often provided a setting for the development of disciplines, such as experimental physiology, neglected by the faculty (Lesch, 1984, pp. 55–6). This synergy between professional self-interest and technical, disciplinary, and cognitive innovation, is a theme to which we will return.

Those operating in these extramural schools thus possessed many of the characteristics of entrepreneurs. Lacking the *rentier* status of the salaried university professor, they were obliged to exert themselves to devise forms of instruction that would attract a discerning clientele of paying customers. As in other businesses of the time, such entrepreneurial activity was a rich source of innovation: new techniques, forms of representation, and, indeed, bodies of knowledge issued from the activities of independent teachers. The more successful of these entrepreneurs were rewarded by an appointment to the faculty where the incentives for originality and effort were considerably less. Their place was, however, taken by a new generation of hungry, ambitious men.

HISTORIOGRAPHIC TRANSITIONS: MARX AND FOUCAULT

It is evident from the preceding review that the history of Western medicine cannot be separated from an understanding of the social, political, and economic transformations that occurred in the first half of the nineteenth century. Two major historiographic transitions have dominated discussion of this period. The first, Marxist interpretations, were contemporaneous with the events. Karl Marx (1818–83) and his collaborator Friedrich Engels (1820–95) described and sought to understand the changes taking place around them. In particular, Engels's *The Condition of the Working-Class in England* (1844) provided a graphic account of the loathsome and insalubrious environment in which the new industrial proletariat was forced to live. Such, he wrote: 'is the Old Town of Manchester, and on re-reading my description, I am forced to admit that instead of being exaggerated, it is far from black enough to convey a true impression of the filth, ruin, and uninhabitableness, the defiance of all considerations of cleanliness, ventilation, and health which characterize the construction of this single district, containing at least twenty to thirty thousand inhabitants. And such a district exists in the heart of the second city of England, the first manufacturing city of the world. If any one wishes to see in how little space a human being can move, how little air – and *such* air! – he can breathe, how little of civilization he may share and yet live, it is only necessary to travel hither. True, this is the *Old* Town, and the people of Manchester emphasise the fact whenever any one mentions to them the frightful condition of this Hell upon Earth; but what does that prove? Everything which here arouses horror and indignation is of recent origin, belongs to the *industrial epoch*.'

We will see that many such polemical accounts, combining in equal measure horror and fascination at the state of the urban proletariat, appeared in the first half of the nineteenth century as the lineaments of the 'social question' began to take form in the minds of middle-class commentators. Others, such as the novelist Honoré de Balzac (1799–1850), seemed simply to delight in describing in lurid detail the 'tattered filth' inhabiting the nineteenth-century city. What distinguished Marx (who was an avid reader of Balzac) and Engels's commentary, however, was the rigour and depth of the analysis they provided of what was occurring in Western society. Marx drew attention to the basal nature of economic change: political power flowed to those who controlled the means of production. Cultural productions, such as religion, political theory, and even the sciences, were merely ideologies designed to mask the realities of inequality and exploitation that underpinned the emerging capitalist order.

These insights have been refined and elaborated by later historians. Of particular significance for present purposes is the work that has been undertaken on the ideological content of the systems of knowledge that emerged during this period. Theories of the causes of and remedies for disease, for example, tended to reflect the political interests of those who articulated them. At the institutional level, much medical work in hospitals and poorhouses will be seen to have depended upon the exploitation of the bodies of the poor, and especially of those members of the working class who were no longer fit for labour. The public hospital served in part to try to restore the sick poor to health so that they could resume work. At the same time, however, they were pressed into service to train future medical practitioners who could then apply their skills to paying patients.

Should the hospital patient succumb to their illness, their usefulness was not at an end; they could still be anatomized and autopsied. These operations evinced what Marx might have called the characteristic thriftiness of the bourgeoisie: they were reluctant to let anything go to waste, even the bodies of those they had harried to an early grave. Charles Babbage (1792–1871), who celebrated rather than criticized the new capitalist order, regarded the ingenious 'employment of materials of little value' as one of its greatest virtues. He singled out for special praise the establishments for slaughtering horses too old or decrepit for work, at Montfaucon near Paris. By extracting the last scintilla of value from the carcasses, 'the dead horse . . . which can be purchased at from 8s. 6d. to 12s. produces from £2.9s. to £4.14s.' Babbage provided a table showing how much each part of the dismembered horse contributed to this total. The anatomists who purchased cadavers from the morgue of the Hôtel-Dieu of Paris, or from the grave robbers of Edinburgh and London, would have been able to provide as precise an account of the monetary value of each cadaver and body part they procured (Richardson, 1988, p. 57).

The second historiographic strand that must be taken into consideration derives from the work of Michel Foucault (1926–84). His work is often seen as a challenge to or correction of Marxian historiography. In particular, Foucault's concept of power differs significantly from Marx's. Moreover, while Marxist history tends to be written on a broad canvas, a defining characteristic of Foucault's method is to focus tightly on some particular location over a relatively short period of time. He is especially concerned with the way in which bodies are distributed and controlled within these spaces. Foucault's relevance to the history of medicine partly derives from the fact that some of the spaces he has discussed include hospitals and asylums. However, his focus on the disciplining of the body in modern social systems provides insights into various themes that will be considered in this chapter: for instance, the inculcation of professional skills through regimes of training. His supposed localism notwithstanding, Foucault also offers important insights, which are fully compatible with Marxian thinking, about how issues of health and disease fit into larger strategies for the governance of industrial societies.

Neither Marx nor Foucault showed any great awareness of the question of how gender difference and identity impinged upon the historical issues that they addressed. This lacuna has been corrected by a large corpus of subsequent literature, which has yielded important insights for the history of medicine. One of the most striking characteristics of the 'Western Medical Tradition', however the term is construed, has been its misogyny and phallocentrism. Working-class women were subjected to distinctive forms of economic exploitation. Indeed, the exploitation of their labour was often seen as a cheap alternative to mechanization, especially in the sweated trades (Berg, 1985, pp. 146–7). Similarly, women of all classes found themselves the object of specialized medical discourses that helped to maintain their positions of dependence and inferiority. Put another way, women's bodies were increasingly seen as raw material upon which medical men could undertake ever more skilled forms of labour.

As for medical practice, by 1800, medical men had largely succeeded in supplanting women in areas, such as midwifery, where they had previously been dominant. Lying-in hospitals were, during the eighteenth century, established in London and elsewhere for the care of pregnant women unable to pay for medical attention. But these establishments also served to train medical students in obstetrics. This was, however, seen by the élite of the profession as a somewhat distasteful and demeaning form of practice. The idea of admitting women to the medical profession was, throughout the first half of the nineteenth century – and beyond – anathema to most doctors.

The remainder of this chapter develops these themes more fully. First, however, some of the ambiguities and perplexities involved in the use of the concept of 'tradition' require exploration.

Inventing medical tradition

PYRAMID PRACTICE: PROFESSIONAL HIERARCHY

Cultural historians have shown the extent to which communities manufacture the traditions celebrated in particular times and places to meet immediate concerns. In the introduction to the seminal collection of essays on *The Invention of Tradition*, Eric Hobsbawm has discussed the complex and often deliberately mystifying processes whereby various groups have, since 1800, actively reshaped their relations with an imagined past. He notes that these invented traditions have certain characteristics in common: they normally involve an element of repetitive ritual designed to affirm the values and identity of a group. While there is an insistence on an unbroken connection with the historic past, 'the peculiarity of "invented traditions", is that the continuity with it is largely factitious. In short, they are responses to novel situations which take the form of reference to old situations, or which establish their own past by quasi-obligatory repetition' (Hobsbawm, 1983, p. 2).

Such traditions manifest themselves in various forms and settings. They are, however, most manifest in 'officially instituted and planned ceremonials' (Hobsbawm, 1983, p. 4). Hobsbawm gives the example of the symbolism and ritual accompanying Nazi rallies in the 1930s. There is a clear analogy between these and the practices of the Colleges of Surgeons and Physicians considered in the following text. In addition to being ceremonial, it might be added that such strategies often involve the generation of representative texts, or bodies of texts, designed to commemorate, amplify, and propagate the messages inhering in the ritual. Thus, the ceremonial of both the College of Physicians and of Surgeons was accompanied by the delivery of orations expounding certain historical claims that were subsequently published. William Macmichael's book, *The Gold-Headed Cane* (1827), which is discussed in the following text, constituted a similar ancillary effort.

Hobsbawm notes that the invention of tradition is most prevalent 'when a rapid transformation of society weakens or destroys the social patterns for which "old" traditions had been designed' (Hobsbawm, 1983, p. 4). The past is shaped and re-imagined to meet the needs of the present and to promote an envisaged future. This generalization applies to the case of medical men in the first half of the nineteenth century. They were confronted with novel threats and challenges, in addition to new opportunities. In response to the upheavals facing them, the early nineteenth century saw many attempts by medical men to look to history for resources that might lend them identity, authority, and legitimacy.

In 1800, the formal organization of medicine in Britain still complied with a venerable model. It is misleading to speak of a 'medical profession' during this period. There were instead at least three legally recognized medical professions, each with its own corporate representation, mode of training, and assigned area of competence. Clear hierarchical relations were, moreover, held to obtain between these branches of medicine.

At the pinnacle of the pyramid were the physicians. Their corporate body was the Royal College of Physicians of London established in 1518. The physicians' corporate privilege was embodied in legislation stipulating that, excepting graduates of Oxford and Cambridge, no one should be allowed to practice as a physician unless examined and licensed by the college. The number of practitioners thus licensed was small: in 1800 the total membership of the college numbered only 179 (Waddington, 1984, p. 2). This number was, moreover, further subdivided into fellows, licentiates, and extra-licentiates. Fellows and licentiates were entitled to practice in and around London; extra-licentiates were supposed to work only away from the capital. Only fellows could occupy offices within the college and thus determined policy.

The privileges enjoyed by the College of Physicians, and in particular by its fellows, had long seemed anomalous and controversial. As early as 1703, physicians' purported monopoly over the prescription of medicines had been successfully challenged in the courts. Nonetheless, in the first half of the nineteenth century the college retained considerable prestige and authority. This was in large part because its fellowship, at least, was deemed to consist of *gentlemen*. They qualified for this rank partly because of their education: the archetypal physician was a graduate of the same ancient universities at which sons of the ruling class were educated. The education that the aspirant physician would receive at these seminaries of the oligarchy was predominantly literary in character, concentrating on the study of classical texts rather than on the inculcation of practical skills. He would, moreover, learn how to behave like a gentleman. The physician could also claim gentle status because, in theory, he did not work with his hands, delegating the more manual aspects of medical practice to the lower orders of the medical economy. The prerogatives enjoyed by the higher orders of the college, therefore, could be and were justified on the grounds that it redounded to the general credit of medicine to have among its practitioners an élite of individuals who were on a par with the most elevated members of society.

Surgeons, as the very etymology of the word suggested, were, in contrast, the manual workers of medicine. They had for centuries been trained by apprenticeship rather than in an academic setting. Book learning was deemed to be of less importance to the trainee surgeon than acquaintance with such practical skills as venesection and applying a blister. Surgery was, in short, a *craft* on a par with such trades as leather working or candle making. Indeed, for much of their history, British surgeons were coupled with barbers: it was only in 1745 that a separate Company of Surgeons was established. Even after that date some surgeons offered a range of services, which might include making wigs in addition to letting blood.

The appellation 'company' for the surgeons' corporate body was an indication of their artisanal status. In 1800, however, they were granted a new charter establishing a Royal College of Surgeons of London, a grant that potentially revolutionized the status of surgery. It might, for instance, be taken to imply that surgeons should enjoy a status as elevated as that of the members of the more venerable College of Physicians. The new title also suggested that surgery rested in part upon academic in addition to practical accomplishments. In the course of the first half of the nineteenth century, much effort was expended in asserting and contesting these claims in different contexts and through a variety of media. The symbolic resources deployed in the contestation of the new status for surgeons will be considered more fully in the following text.

The third traditional medical order was by far the least interesting. The 'Worshipful Society of Apothecaries' had been established in 1617; previously the apothecaries had been affiliated with the Grocers' Company. Apothecaries were also expected to learn their business by apprenticeship. If physicians were the gentlemen and surgeons the artisans of medicine, apothecaries were its tradesmen. As such, they were the lowest of the low; they were unclean. Originally, they were expected to confine themselves to filling prescriptions written by a physician. By the early eighteenth century, however, apothecaries had won the right to prescribe. Nonetheless, in the early decades of the nineteenth century, the constitution of the society was 'more typical of a city trading company than of a professional organisation' (Waddington, 1984, p. 5).

The formal organization of medicine in Britain at the beginning of the nineteenth century thus closely mirrored the typical structure of prein-dustrial society. This was characterized by 'a classless hierarchy' (Perkin, 1969, p. 17). Class was, of course, latent in eighteenth-century British soci-ety, but it had not yet attained the dominance over social relations it was later to acquire. Occupational groups were distributed into various 'orders', to which appertained different forms of status. The most crucial division was between those deemed 'gentle' and the rest. Another significant fea-ture of this hierarchy was that status was dissociated from considerations of skill and utility. Thus, physicians justified their position at the pinna-cle of the medical economy by reference to their associations and cultural attainments, not by claims to professional competence.

A similar hierarchy had existed in France. The revolution, however, effec-tively demolished it. Even during the period of reaction that followed the fall of Napoleon, attempts to return to the medical *ancien régime* were half-hearted and ineffectual. The British case is of particular interest because, in the absence of a political revolution, overtly the old order persisted. Indeed, the Royal Colleges of Physicians and Surgeons survive as impor-tant institutions to this day. In the first half of the nineteenth century, the medical corporations continued to serve as centres for homosociability and performed various ceremonial functions. They were not merely decorative institutions; they exercised important duties in respect of the examination and licensing of practitioners.

The apparent continuity with the past is, however, misleading. Medical practice in Britain had for some time diverged from the neat allocation of roles ascribed by the hierarchy described in the preceding text. By the eighteenth century, most medical men were de facto general practitioners who took on, in various combinations, the work of physician, surgeon, and apothecary. This trend became more marked after 1800: general practition-ers increasingly coalesced as a self-conscious group. With the founding of the *Lancet* by Thomas Wakley (1795–1862) in 1823, they gained an official organ.

Although the most numerous group within the medical economy, gen-eral practitioners were excluded from the offices that wielded most power within the profession. Superimposed upon the old tripartite division, a new and rancorous schism developed between those engaged in general practice and an élite of 'consultants', who claimed to confine themselves to 'pure' physic or surgery. Although their numbers were small, consultants exercised a disproportionate power within medicine; they also enjoyed levels of remuneration far in excess of what most practitioners could anticipate. An eminent surgeon, such as James Paget (1814–99), or a society physician, such as Sir Henry Halford (1828–97), could earn £10,000 a year.

While the official hierarchy reflected the structure of traditional society, the reality of medical politics in early-nineteenth-century Britain thus represented a microcosm of the class conflict that defined industrial society. A plutocratic élite, in command of the instruments of government, fought to preserve its privileges at all costs, at the expense of a repressed and sometimes impoverished medical proletariat.

The consultants occupied two chief power bases. They held posts at the major voluntary hospitals that provided them with income from students in addition to the opportunity to cultivate valuable patronage among the lay governors. Secondly, they controlled the councils of both the Royal Colleges. One of the *Lancet*'s most bitter reproaches against this crew was that they exploited the latter advantage to enhance their dominant position within medical education. In particular, the consultants manipulated the regulations of the Royal College of Surgeons to force students wishing to enter for its diploma to attend the classes they gave in the hospital schools. They were, in effect, seeking to secure a monopoly over medical education in the capital at the expense of teachers who lacked a hospital appointment.

Control of the colleges was thus of great strategic value in enhancing the market position of the consultant clique. But these institutions also did important symbolic work. At the same time as they acted with a rapacity, at which the most ruthless Lancashire mill owner might balk, in pursuit of their self-interest (even if this meant the extirpation of long-established and respected institutions), the leadership of the Royal Colleges presented themselves as guardians of a venerable medical tradition. The legitimacy of the medical élite was seen to depend in large measure upon the credibility of these claims. The fabrication of such historical lineages served also to divert attention from the exploitative relations underpinning the current medical polity. There emerged elaborate rituals, centred upon the colleges, which were designed to further these ends.

Hobsbawm identifies three overlapping types of invented tradition: (1) those establishing or symbolizing social cohesion or the membership of groups, real or artificial communities; (2) those establishing or legitimizing institutions, status, or relations of authority; and (3) those whose main purpose was socialization, the inculcation of beliefs, value systems, and conventions of behaviour (Hobsbawm, 1983, p. 9).

The medical traditions of the first half of the nineteenth century may be seen to conform to all of these types. The rituals and official discourses of the colleges were, in the first place, an affirmation of corporate identity. They were also implicit or explicit affirmations of the status of particular sets of medical practitioners – an attempt to distinguish them from and elevate them above rivals in the medical economy. Hobsbawm's comment that invented traditions tend to serve to 'foster the corporate sense of *superiority* of élites' (Hobsbawm, 1983, p. 10), such as the Fellowship of the Royal College of Physicians, is particularly germane here. The implied audience for both these purposes would be extensive. These practices, in addition, served to inculcate certain values and norms into cadet members of the relevant medical communities.

MAKING MEDICAL HEROES

These endeavours were sometimes focused upon trying to find a single figure in the past that might serve some polemical purpose. One instance of this is found in the efforts of British surgeons after 1800 to bestow an iconic status upon one of their forebears. John Hunter (1728–93) was chosen to fill this role. Hunter was fitted to the part because he was, in many ways, untypical and seemed to contradict many of the extant presumptions about surgery. He was not noted as an operator: indeed, he regarded resort to the knife as a last resort, preferring to rely on conservative medical treatment of surgical conditions. Although successful as a metropolitan practitioner and teacher, Hunter did not indulge in conspicuous consumption or seek to ape the manners and lifestyle of the upper class – indeed, he was known for his plain, if not blunt, speech and unaffected deportment.

Hunter was, nonetheless, deemed to have made British surgeons 'gentlemen' through his intellectual activities and attainments. Thus, while he eschewed the manual skills conventionally associated with the accomplished surgeon, Hunter sought to understand the basic pathological processes at work in inflammation. This knowledge would allegedly equip surgeons to treat patients in a more rational fashion. He also engaged in a wide variety of what might somewhat anachronistically be called 'biological' researches. For instance, Hunter studied such topics as the organ of hearing in fish and undertook transplant experiments. He was as interested in the distribution of the feathers on the body of a bird as he was in the pathophysiology of inflammation. Investigations earned Hunter the

Fellowship of the Royal Society in 1767. The most obvious monument to these researches was a collection of 14,000 specimens, which passed to the newly formed College of Surgeons after Hunter's death.

The early leadership of the College of Surgeons appropriated Hunter's name in addition to his collection to create an icon that served a range of linked interests. Hunter served to refute the reproach that surgeons were mere hand-workers and, therefore, of inferior status to the physician. He had instead demonstrated the essentially intellectual foundation of the surgical profession. The lack of any practical point to many of his researches was a token of a kind of gentlemanly indifference to considerations of mere utility. The freedom with which Hunter had spent money in the pursuit of these interests, leaving his widow with major debts, had something of the aristocratic about it. These themes were endlessly reiterated in the annual Hunterian Oration delivered at the college. There was an obvious irony, not lost on commentators, such as Thomas Wakley, in the contrast between the ideal surgeon limned in this representation of Hunter – one who was indifferent to personal gain and saw money merely as the means to facilitate scientific endeavour – and the grasping behaviour of the surgical élite that now purported to wear his mantle.

The surgeons' attempt to finesse their transition from artisan to gentle-man occurred in a complex dialectic with an older narrative, which was at once an inspiration and a challenge to the champions of the Hunterian legacy. The physicians had long possessed an exemplary figure in the shape of William Harvey (1578–1657), discoverer of the circulation of the blood (p. 318). The advocates of scientific surgery had no wish to belittle Harvey's legend: they did, however, insist that surgery now possessed as imposing a figure in its history.

At much the same time, the physicians were, for reasons of their own, engaged in redefining the relationship of past to present in their own history. During the 1820s, the Royal College of Physicians of London was in the process of seeking to reassert its authority and to refurbish its image. Prominent in this endeavour was Sir Henry Halford, who was President of the College between 1820 and 1844. Under Halford's guidance, the college moved to new premises in Pall Mall where a series of evening meetings was held. These meetings were intended not only for medical men, but also for members of the general public; the subject matter of papers presented was adapted accordingly. There was, in short, a concerted effort by the college to present a new face to the world. Integral to this project, however, was an emphasis on the physicians' historical relationships.

Halford was seconded in these efforts by his colleague, William Macmichael (1783–1839), who maintained that there was no better way to awaken 'renewed interest in the venerable College than by directing attention to its past history and to the achievements of the illustrious men who had connected with it' (Macmichael, 1925, pp. xvii-xviii). The most tangible result of this urge to consolidate the college's future by representing its past was a book entitled *The Gold-Headed Cane* published in 1827. The work revolves around a curious conceit: it is purportedly narrated by the walking stick of the title, one that has enjoyed an unusually interesting and distinguished career. The cane is steeped in symbolism. Originally, such items had been a functional part of the physician's accoutrements. The hollow head was filled with aromatic spices that were supposed to protect the doctor from the contagious airs he might encounter in the course of his work. Subsequently, such canes became a token of the physician's identity and status, among other things distinguishing him from the multitude of other healers in the medical marketplace.

The eponymous cane had, over a period of 150 years, been owned by a succession of distinguished physicians. When Matthew Baillie (1761–1823), the last of these, died, his widow donated it to Halford who, in turn, put it on display in the library of the college. The cane thus came to possess, to use anthropological terminology, the attributes of a *fetish*, an inanimate object in which special virtue was deemed to inhere. In this instance, this potency derived from the fact that it had been handled by practitioners whom nineteenth-century physicians wished to feature among their ancestors. The cane also possesses an obvious phallic symbolism, signifying the potency of the physician who bears it. The transfer of the same cane to successive generations amounts to an attempt to perpetuate the mana inherent in especially charismatic individuals, and to make it part of the enduring endowment of energy belonging to the community they helped to constitute.

Macmichael's book begins with an account of the cane's arrival at its new home. Its initial depression at being consigned to a corner of the library is mitigated: 'by my overhearing the elegant oration of the President of the College; and an occasional glance I had of scarlet dresses recalled the decorum and propriety of the days of yore, when, on solemn occasions of public meeting, the Fellows appeared habited in the doctors' robes of their respective universities' (Macmichael, 1925, p. 2).

The historical continuity expressed by the college's ceremonial is thus emphasized. Within this setting, the cane comes to discern a future for itself on the grounds that: 'I had . . . been closely connected with medicine for a century and a half; and might consequently . . . look upon myself as the depository of many important secrets, in which the dignity of the profession was nearly concerned' (pp. 3–4).

The subsequent memoirs are therefore intended to complement the physicians' other efforts at commemoration. The device of the cane as narrator makes it possible, for instance, to claim posthumous approval from famed physicians of the past for the college's current strategies. Thus the cane 'listened with increased attention when I heard him [the President of the College] speak of the donation of the Radcliffe Trustee's, and every fibre thrilled within me at the consciousness of the heartfelt delight with which first kind master would have grasped me, could he have foreseen the liberal spirit of the future guardians of his princely fortune' (pp. 2–3). John Radcliffe (1650–1714) had been the cane's first owner and it was, therefore, in a position to speak authoritatively about his views.

Although Radcliffe was the first physician the cane served, its narrative made clear that the tradition to which its owners had contributed, and which the college now perpetuated, reached far into the past. Thus it recalled that Radcliffe, during a consultation at Kensington House, paused to gaze 'for a moment on the likeness of the Founder of the College of Physicians, Dr. Linacre, painted by Holbein, which was hanging in one of the rooms, amongst the royal portraits of Henrys, and several other of the Kings and Queens of England and Scotland' (pp. 6–7). The fact that the image of the founder of the college, painted by a distinguished artist, was hung among those of royalty clearly enhances his status. Nineteenth-century physicians could bask in this reflected glory.

Thomas Linacre's (c. 1460–1524) reputation as a renowned literary figure introduces another important theme in the cane's narrative: British physicians' honourable tradition as men of letters and patrons of the fine arts. This theme is most fully developed in the cane's recollection of a dialogue between the eighteenth-century physician Richard Mead (1673–1754) and a number of other physicians, intended to rebut imputations levelled against the profession. Mead begins by demanding: 'What class of men have deserved better of the public than physicians?' Various names, including those of Linacre and John Caius (1510–73), are mentioned to demonstrate the contribution of physicians to the arts. Mention of Caius's name, however, leads Mead in a different direction: 'The zeal displayed by Caius in the cause of literature deserves every commendation, but it is perhaps more to our purpose to dwell upon the claim he has upon our grateful remembrance as the founder of the Science of Anatomy in England . . . let it never be forgotten that Caius, on his return from Italy, imbued with the spirit of inquiry and enlightened by the lamp of science lately kindled in that country, taught Anatomy to the Surgeons in their own Hall. Here, beyond the precincts of the College of Physicians, reflecting great honour upon that body, adding to his own reputation and conferring no small advantage on the Surgeons, he laid that solid foundation for the study of Anatomy, to which may easily be traced the glory and after discoveries of Harvey' (Macmichael, 1925, p. 87).

The ostensible point of this passage is to draw attention to the role of physicians in propagating and developing the scientific side of their profession. Yet, by alluding to the role of Caius and others in teaching *surgeons* the anatomy of the human body, additional polemical work is done. This reminder of historical dependency upon physicians for instruction in the theoretical bases of their art was a corrective to the surgeons' current overweening pretensions. Nor had this relation of tutelage been confined to the time of Caius. Mead recalled that: 'When I was appointed by the Company of Surgeons to read Anatomical Lectures in their Hall, which I did for six or seven years, I always insisted strongly upon the obligations their branch of the profession was under to the early Fellows of the College of Physicians, and I hope, as information becomes more diffused, and scientific attainments more universal, the Surgeons themselves will not be so ungrateful as to forget or disown it' (Macmichael, 1925, p. 100).

Given their pride in the achievements of Hunter, there was, of course, every danger that the surgeons would show such forgetfulness and ingratitude.

'PARIS MEDICINE'

The French, too, felt a need for medical heroes who embodied values and aspirations that were deemed to demand promotion. While the British might make much of the Hunterian school, Paris was generally acknowledged as the centre of the Western medical world in the first half of the nineteenth century. There was thus no shortage of candidates for elevation to the pantheon. These reputations were, however, fashioned over a number of decades – as was the myth of 'Paris Medicine' – in response to changing context and contingencies.

The French Revolution was, as already mentioned, as much a social as a political upheaval. It involved not merely a change in system of government and regime but also far-reaching changes in the fabric of French society.

Medical institutions did not escape these sweeping transformations. Pre-revolutionary French medicine was organized upon broadly similar lines to the hierarchy that, at least formally, obtained in Britain. If anything, the hierarchy was even more pronounced and rigid in France, although the last decades of the Bourbon monarchy did see significant innovation. The French counterpart of the College of Physicians of London was the Faculty of Medicine of Paris. This was, in effect, a physicians' guild that controlled medical licensing and practice in the city. It also claimed a wider jurisdiction throughout France and sought to ensure that its graduates enjoyed wide-ranging privileges. As in Britain, there was a wide discrepancy between the official tripartite division of medicine and the realities of practice. In the French countryside, barber-surgeons dealt indiscriminately with complaints of all kinds.

The very extent of the faculty's pretensions limited the support on which it could call. In particular, the Crown developed a strategy of fostering rival medical institutions as counterweights to these preening Parisian physicians (Gelfand, 1993, p. 1127). During the eighteenth century, successive French governments supported the efforts of surgeons to elevate themselves from the status of artisans and to claim a place among the liberal professions. Thus, in the first half of the eighteenth century, a Royal College and, later, an Academy of Surgery were established. In 1743, surgeons were freed from their medieval union with barbers and their effective independence from the Paris Faculty was asserted. The Crown also favoured apothecaries, the pariahs of medical practice, notwithstanding the stigma that attached to them.

The reasons for the French state's patronage of surgeons in the eighteenth century were complex. But they derived in part from the government's desire to ensure a supply of competent practitioners for the armed forces. The empirically minded surgeons were more likely to meet this need than the hidebound physicians. Surgeons were in the forefront of developing hospitals as centres for medical education. Especially significant for future developments was Pierre Joseph Desault's (1744–95) clinic at the Hôtel Dieu of Paris. This trend was to be extended and reinforced following the revolution.

The privileges of all medical corporations, whether as ancient as the Faculty of Medicine, or relatively new creations, such as the Academy of Surgeons, came under increasing scrutiny and criticism in the latter decades of the eighteenth century. Such prerogatives were inimical to the liberal economic and social doctrines that were increasingly gaining support among those with other grievances against the polity of France. This discontent was often articulated in terms of the *laissez-faire* economic theory favoured by the bourgeoisie. The ideas were most fully formulated by a group of economic writers known as the 'Physiocrats'. Licensing regulations, together with restrictions on the right to teach and practice, were depicted as iniquitous trammels upon the workings of the medical market.

With the coming of the revolution, these concerns were addressed in a remarkably doctrinaire fashion. It demands a tremendous effort of imagination to recapture something of the mentality of this first generation of revolutionaries. They stood on the threshold of a new era for humanity – indeed they hoped to remake humanity anew. Their optimism was not clouded by recollection of previous revolutions that had faltered and failed, or of heroes who had betrayed the trust of millions. Beethoven had not yet, with angry strokes, erased the name of Bonaparte from the score of the *Eroica*.

Such men could aspire to abolish not only doctors, but also disease itself. In a society ordered according to nature, each man would live to his due term. Such men had little time for the arcane rigmarole of the old medical regime. Nor did they distinguish between the ancient rights of the physician and the privileges that the surgeon had more recently wheedled from the monarch. All were equally pernicious: all were to be consigned to the cesspit of history.

In regard to medicine, the revolutionaries were indeed astonishing in their faithfulness to the physiocratic dogmas they preached. In March 1791, the old corporations were swept away to be replaced by a virtual free market in medical practice. Everyone could, on payment of a fee, be not only his or her own physician, but provide medical services to whomever chose to consult them. The commercial, market-driven side of medicine, which had already begun to bloom in the final decades of the *ancien régime*, was now allowed to luxuriate (Brockliss and Jones, 1997, pp. 807–8).

Conversely, the patient had an unprecedented choice of medical attendant. Formal medical training, in so far as it was still available, was not a prerequisite. Much of the apparatus of medical education was in fact dismantled; one of the few courses to survive was Desault's surgical clinic at the Hôtel Dieu. Some revolutionaries argued that public opinion was a sufficient guide to the competence of a practitioner, rendering all other forms of regulation otiose.

If the Girondin wing of the revolutionary movement thus took liberalism to new extremes, other tendencies were also evident. Some called for greater state involvement in medicine through some form of 'medical police', a term borrowed from the German-speaking world. Those bourgeois reformers whose ear was attuned to the word on the *sans culottes* street, argued that the role of the state was not restricted to the abolition of ancient abuses and removal of irrational checks upon personal liberty. The great nation must also take responsibility for the welfare of its citizens, especially when they were incapacitated by age and illness. These views were especially strongly represented on the *Comité de mendicité* that sought to address what were seen as the conjoined problems of ill health and poverty. Efforts to realize these ideals led to the creation of a system of public assistance that involved far-reaching reorganization of the hospitals.

The medical utopia of the early years of the revolution was not to last. How could it? Within a few years the surviving old regimes of Europe had banded together to crush what they rightly regarded as a threat to the survival of all they represented. Funded by a seemingly endless stream of British gold, the monarchist armies advanced upon the borders of France and seemed, at one stage, to be on the brink of overthrowing the republic. To throw back this malevolent tide, the revolutionary regime mobilized an unprecedented number of men: it was a *levée en masse* – the first citizen army, numbering more than a million men, a harbinger of modern warfare. They also mobilized such savants as had survived the Terror to contribute their expertise to the struggle for national survival.

To care for the needs of this host, bind its wounds, and tend its sick, the republic had need of a medical corps on which it could rely. Medical men were, indeed, summoned to the cause even before the general conscription had begun. There was also massive investment in the military-medical infrastructure: while hospitals had been viewed with suspicion in the early years of the revolution, they were now considered indispensable to the war effort.

One early medical recruit to the revolutionary cause was Dominique-Jean Larrey (1766–1842) who, after studying surgery with Desault, joined the French army of the Rhine in 1792. In the following year he introduced the *ambulance volante*, a service of doctors and nurses who provided medical attention near to the battlefront. The need for such trained and resourceful attendants was, moreover, insatiable, for these doctors readily fell victim to the perils of war: of the 2,700 medical officers in service in 1793, nearly 1,000 had fallen by the following spring (Ramsey, 1988, p. 75).

Largely driven by these needs, moves to create a new system of medical education commenced in 1794. Schools of health were established in Paris,

Montpellier, and Strasbourg in the following year, to create a supply of competent medical men. No distinction was made between the training of physicians and surgeons. Indeed, the kind of clinically based training pioneered by surgeons, such as Desault, before the revolution, was now to provide the model for the education of all doctors. Conversely, surgeons who served in the military were often required to perform duties that required forms of expertise previously regarded as the reserve of the physician. Antoine-François de Fourcroy (1755–1809), one of the authors of the scheme, summed up the ethic of the new school of medicine in the aphorism: 'Reading little, seeing and doing much: this will be the basis of the new teaching.' Fourcroy contrasted the emphasis upon utility apparent in the curricula of the new *écoles de santé* with the 'sterile definitions' that characterized the teaching of the old faculties (Brockliss, in Hannaway and La Berge, 1998, p. 72). The main site at which this seeing and doing was to occur was in the hospitals. These became, in effect, manufactories of medical practitioners to serve the civil and military needs of the state. The new system of medical education was, in 1803, consolidated under the Napoleonic regime.

Of the three schools that were founded in the 1790s, Paris was by far the most distinguished. Indeed, the name 'Paris Medicine' is used generically to describe the most salient features of Western medicine in the first half of the nineteenth century. In brief, the Paris school possessed three defining characteristics. First, detailed observations of the patient during life were made. This might include physical examination using instruments, such as the newly invented stethoscope. When the case ended in death, these case histories were supplemented by routine autopsy designed to reveal the organic lesions associated with particular clinical presentations. Finally, statistics were used to ascertain with unprecedented precision, such issues as the efficacy, or otherwise, of particular treatments. While these general characteristics were recognized by most commentators, the precise content and import of Paris Medicine has, however, always been subject to negotiation.

The Paris School of the early nineteenth century spawned many iconic figures, including Xavier Bichat (1771–1802) and Gaspard-Laurent Bayle (1774–1817). Bichat's heroic status was enhanced by the fact that he died from an infection contracted while dissecting cadavers; he thus became a martyr to medical science. By the beginning of the twentieth century, however, the archetypal representative of Paris Medicine was deemed to be René Théophile Laennec (1781–1826). He was one of the first students trained at the new Paris School of Medicine. After a period as a surgeon in the military hospitals of Nantes, Laennec had come to Paris as a student in 1801. He attended the course of Bichat, one of the founders of pathological anatomy. He became a friend of Bayle, another important figure in the establishment of the discipline. Laennec also attended the lessons of Jean-Nicholas Corvisart (1755–1821), who was, among other things, Napoleon's personal physician.

After graduating, Laennec gained a reputation as an expert in pathological anatomy. He also developed a fashionable practice among the élite of Parisian society. A staunch Catholic and royalist, Laennec fared well after the restoration of the Bourbons. In 1816, he was appointed physician to the Necker Hospital in Paris, a position that gave him access to a wide range of patients and the opportunity to make numerous postmortem examinations. It was during this period that Laennec introduced the innovation for which he is chiefly remembered: mediate auscultation. Legend has it that he stumbled on the technique by accident when he used a rolled up paper to listen to the chest of a woman patient and discovered that the medium improved acoustic quality.

Laennec came to embody the definitive features of the Paris school: he thus epitomized the contribution of this historical epoch to the Western Medical Tradition. This reputation rested on two main achievements. Laennec was among the first and most assiduous of those to take advantage of the favourable circumstances for the pursuit of pathological anatomy afforded by the post-revolutionary French hospital system. In this he was not unique – Gaspard-Laurent Bayle's credentials, for instance, might seem as impressive. Bayle played a prominent part in establishing the pathological anatomy of the clinical condition known as phthisis and, therefore, in creating the nosological entity of tuberculosis. Indeed it was Bayle who coined the term.

But what distinguished Laennec was that he devised a means of applying the theoretical resources emerging from the morgues of Paris to medical practice. He developed the technique of auscultation as a means of gaining access to morbid changes occurring in the body while the patient was still alive. These findings could then be correlated with lesions discovered postmortem (Fig. 1.1). In his pursuit of this project, Laennec developed a new medical instrument, the stethoscope (Fig. 1.2), which was to become emblematic of the medical profession, playing much the same function as the gold-headed cane had for previous generations.

Some were quick to seize on its significance. John Forbes, Laennec's English translator, asserted in his preface to Laennec's work, *Treatise on*

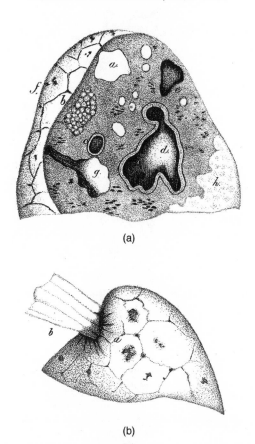

(a)

(b)

Fig. 1.1. Sections of lung showing the cavities and lesions of tuberculosis. *Source*: Rene Laennec, *A Treatise on Diseases of the Chest*, London, Underwood, 1821. Wellcome Library Early Printed Books. *Credit*: Wellcome Library, London (L0003982).

Mediate Auscultation, '(if his [Laennec's] new diagnostics are as certain as he affirms) he may be said to have realized the wish of the antient [sic] philosopher, and to have placed a window in the breast through which we can see the precise state of things within.' However, the fully developed version of Laennec's place in the history of medicine took several decades to emerge. Even Forbes appeared to think that the diagnostic technique Laennec had devised was separable from his work in pathological anatomy. Laennec's immediate posthumous reputation was equivocal. He was denied the customary *éloge* at the Royal Academy of Medicine; nor was his death marked in any notable way by the Paris Faculty of Medicine. A number of reasons can be advanced for this neglect. Laennec died in Brittany where he had retired due to ill health; he was thus removed from the centre of attention. His reputation was, moreover, tarnished by his association with a politically

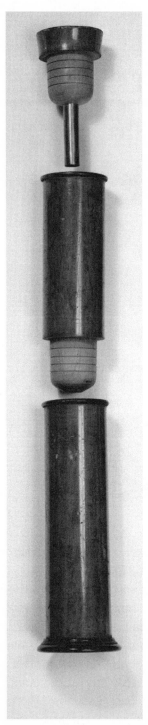

Fig. 1.2. Monaural stethoscope made of cedar wood with a 2 cm hollow core, designed by Laennec. *Source*: Wellcome Historical Medical Museum. *Credit*: Wellcome Library, London (M0014325EC).

44

motivated purge of the medical faculty in 1822. In a predominantly liberal and secular medical milieu, Laennec's Catholicism and monarchism did not play well. Even those favourably disposed to him, however, tended to see Laennec more as a *primus inter pares* rather than as a towering figure in the Paris school. As for mediate auscultation, this was widely seen as an important innovation (although *im*mediate auscultation long continued to have its supporters); but this technique was not regarded as marking a new epoch in medical history. Indeed, for a time, Laennec appeared as a somewhat old-fashioned figure.

His contemporary, François-Joseph-Victor Broussais (1772–1838), champion of a revolutionary 'physiological medicine', seemed of far greater importance to the future of medicine (Weisz, 1987). Broussais was not content to concentrate upon the diagnostic and pathological aspects of medicine. He also laid great stress upon therapeutics, recommending wholesale use of bleeding as a remedy for almost all ills. In the course of the nineteenth century, the relative reputation of the two men was reversed: Broussais now figures as, at most, a minor, somewhat eccentric, figure in canonical medical history (Ackerknecht, 1953a). This rehabilitation of Laennec's memory – or, more properly, invention of new memories – was, in part, the result of the increased institutionalization of pathological anatomy in France during the 1830s. In 1836, a chair devoted to the subject was created at the Paris Faculty of Medicine. As the discipline came to have an autonomous institutional existence, so did pathological anatomists seek ancestral figures to provide legitimacy and stature to their science. By demanding recognition for Laennec's achievements, pathological anatomists were, in effect, demanding credit for their own field. Laennec thus became a metonym for the discipline that appropriated him.

There were alternative candidates that might have served this purpose. Laennec was uniquely qualified, however, because his work in auscultation underlined the intimate links between pathological anatomy and clinical medicine. As pathological anatomy became more institutionally and intellectually distinct, so there was a danger that its relevance to medical practice would become problematic. Laennec could be presented as a reminder of the interdependence of the two fields: auscultation was both dependent on a grounding in pathological anatomy and supplied new data to that science.

It was only in the second half of the nineteenth century that Laennec's status as an 'emblematic hero of medical science' was consolidated (Weisz, 1987, p. 555). This move was dependent upon the professional and broader national preoccupations of the period. There was, in the first instance, a growing rivalry between France and the emergent power of Germany. Because this competition included disputes over the relative scientific achievements of the two countries, a need arose to identify an outstanding French figure: Laennec was to be this superhero. The medical profession in France was keen to foster such endeavours because of its own efforts to raise its national influence and status. In terms of appeals to a wider public, Laennec possessed an edge over possible rivals. His invention of the stethoscope provided a concrete achievement of evident relevance to the patient, around which to construct an image of the physician. Thanks to these impulses, Laennec was transformed from the mentor of one medical specialty, to a representative figure of French medicine.

Recent scholarship has drawn attention to certain aspects of Laennec's work that were effectively suppressed or ignored in the various representations of him fashioned after his death. For instance, his aspirations to the status of a physiologist, manifested most clearly in the lectures he delivered at the Collège de France, have only lately been recovered. Various reasons may be advanced for this neglect. But among the most salient was that pathological anatomists had little interest in commemorating this aspect of Laennec's work: indeed, they found his aspirations to go beyond a solidist and localizationist view of disease somewhat embarrassing. Physiologists, on the other hand, were increasingly wedded to an interventionist experimental methodology that found Laennec's ideas either irrelevant or inimical (Duffin, 1998, pp. 291–4).

The fate of Laennec's reputation was, to an extent, reflected in the moulding of the memory of Paris Medicine more generally during the nineteenth century. The process of memorialization and contextualization began contemporaneously with the events: there were references to the 'Paris School' as early as the second decade of the century. The term was meant to have a wider connotation than the institutions for the training of medical students that had been established in the aftermath of the reforms of 1794. It referred rather to a general orientation to medical theory and practice (Hannaway and La Berge, 1998, p. 6).

Certain key elements of the representation of Paris Medicine were to prove stable: for instance, the insistence on hospital experience as essential to medical training, on physical diagnosis coupled with routine autopsy, and, somewhat less prominently, on the utility of medical statistics. Basic historiographic assumptions also tended to persist; there was general agreement that the history of the Paris School was essentially the chronicle of the contributions of a series of great men. This emphasis did not, however, entirely exclude a recognition of institutional and wider social and political factors. In other respects, however, the most salient features, events, and personalities that made up the tradition were subject to extensive revision and reinterpretation over time.

Early histories of the Paris School, such as that of Jean-Baptiste Bouillaud, were notable for their cosmopolitan perspective. While proud of the recent achievements in medicine of his countrymen, Bouillaud was ready to admit that the foundations of the Paris method had been laid elsewhere in Europe in the latter part of the eighteenth century. Indeed, Bouillaud was anxious to establish a still more venerable lineage for the Paris School: he traced its roots to Hippocrates.

But Bouillaud was also decidedly modernist in his insistence that medicine should model its methodology upon the physical sciences. He thus passed over a strand of early-nineteenth-century French medicine upon which other commentators were to insist: the vitalism of such major figures as Xavier Bichat. Later accounts of the Paris School sought to rehabilitate this tradition. These efforts were to have only limited success. While French vitalism has attracted some scholarly attention (Haigh, 1975, 1984), this aspect of the tradition has been largely elided from the received depiction of the Paris School.

Later in the nineteenth century, the received view of the historical significance of Paris Medicine was subjected to a number of revisions. In the 1840s, a 'Young Paris School', which numbered among its members such figures as Paul Broca (1824–80), argued that new techniques must be added to the traditional methodology. It insisted, in particular, on the importance of the microscope to future medical progress (La Berge, 1994). This polemic may be seen as the precursor to more wide-ranging calls for the closer integration of clinical and laboratory medicine. Claude Bernard (1813–78), for instance, was anxious to expand the extension of Paris Medicine to include the experimental tradition typified by François Magendie (Hannaway and La Berge, 1998, pp. 20–1).

After 1871, French representations of the Paris medical tradition assumed an increasingly nationalistic, indeed Chauvinist, aspect. In the aftermath of defeat in the Franco-Prussian War (1870–1), French commentators felt obliged to wrestle with questions of national decline. Germany appeared to have seized preeminence in science in addition to the economic and military fields. French medical historians increasingly looked back for inspiration and guidance on what appeared as a golden age in the early decades of the nineteenth century. Thus, the fact that the efflorescence of Paris Medicine had occurred immediately after an earlier military defeat, was seen as cause for hope that French science might yet rejuvenate itself despite the current adverse circumstances (Hannaway and La Berge, 1998, pp. 24–7). Under these conditions, tradition, a sense of continuity, and analogy between past and present became a source of comfort and inspiration.

The content and meaning of this period of French medicine was also negotiated outside the borders of France. Any discussion of the formulation and perpetuation of the traditions surrounding what came to be known as Paris Medicine must recognize its international character. In the first half of the nineteenth century, medical practitioners came to Paris from throughout the Western world to study in what was generally regarded as the world's foremost centre of research and practice. British and American doctors figured prominently among these visitors (Warner, 1985; Maulitz, 1987). These travellers, however, came to Paris with diverse aims; and they derived different benefits and impressions from their time there. Moreover, the memories of Paris that they recorded, which became elaborated into national traditions of the historical significance of Paris Medicine, differed in important respects.

So prominent was this French episode in collective memory that the period between the 1820s and the 1850s came to be known as the 'Paris period' in American medicine. The process of memorializing Paris began while these American visitors were still embarked upon their French adventures. They seemed to feel 'a duty to remember what they had witnessed and tell about it' (Warner, 1991, p. 302). These memories were not merely elaborated, but significantly altered when these travellers returned to their native lands. The elaboration of these narratives was in part a matter of selection and refinement, processes common to all forms of memorialization. But there was also a deliberate shaping of the recalled French experience to meet immediate polemical needs. From the outset, even the most apparently personal accounts, in the form of letters and diaries, were written with some audience in mind.

Early American accounts tended to stress what the visitor saw and did; this accorded well with the empiricist ideology of the Paris school. While impressed by the scale of the facilities available for teaching and research in Paris, not all reports of these experiences were favourable. There was, in particular, criticism of an alleged French emphasis on the research role of the clinic at the expense of patient care. Even at this stage, therefore, American practitioners were striving to forge a distinctive identity for themselves through their French experience – one that was, among other things, adapted to the realities of professional life they would face when they returned home. There was from the outset, a dialectic between perceptions of the foreign and the domestic: in important respects, these visitors brought memories of their native land to their perception of Paris as much as they modified their view of American medicine through what they witnessed abroad.

There was, therefore, no pure or primitive experience that was later modified or distorted. Memories of Paris did, however, assume different form and significance after travellers returned home. There was, in the first place, an effort to give those memories concrete form in the native context by making use of such facilities as American hospitals afforded for clinical investigation. A telling example of this yearning to maintain continuity between memory of the exotic and immediate experience is found in William Wood Gerhard's (1809–72) use of the same journal he had used in Paris to record cases he later encountered at the 'Hôpital de Pennsylvanie' (Warner, 1991, p. 310). We see here an instance of an intensely *practical* tradition.

Such emulation of a foreign model was not, however, universally welcomed and celebrated. It met resistance from practitioners who saw themselves as defenders of an indigenous American medical tradition. Such competition between traditions provides a valuable vantage point from which to survey divergent notions of expertise, authenticity, and authority. It may also display different understandings of the priorities of medicine. In this instance, the native American school claimed superiority over the Parisians because it allegedly paid more attention to the care of the patient.

As we have seen, this was a reproach that the advocates of French Medicine had anticipated. Lest they should seem to yield ground to their opponents, however, their own criticisms now became more muted. But they retained their emphasis on empiricism as the chief virtue of the Paris School. In the domestic context, this possessed novel resonance, appealing to a culture that was suspicious of dogma and mystification, and where professional authority was increasingly questioned.

The American advocates of French medicine adopted familiar techniques to generate and to propagate their vision of past, present, and future. Introductory lectures at the opening of medical school sessions were a favoured method of seeking to expose new generations of practitioners to a particular vision of medical history. Such addresses were often an opportunity for personal reminiscence. With time, however, as the individuals concerned died, the memory of Paris became more an aspect of the collective memory of American medicine. As in France, *éloges* and obituaries provided an occasion for the perpetuation of these recollections. Warner notes that the experience of many American medical visitors in the later nineteenth century was shaped by their familiarity with this tradition (Warner, 1991, p. 317).

By the middle of the nineteenth century, the glamour of Paris was being ever more challenged in America, as elsewhere, by the appeal of the German medical schools. An imperative then arose to reconcile these two competing foci of inspiration. By the last decade of the nineteenth century, the Paris tradition had become a resource for those wishing to resist, or at least mitigate, the growing encroachments of experimental medicine on the clinical domain.

The British case differed in interesting respects. Representations of 'Paris Medicine' did figure prominently in the medical polemics of the first half of the nineteenth century; but it was a rather different Paris from that recalled and regaled in the United States. Rather than attempting to perpetuate a French-inspired tradition in their native land, 'Paris' served as a model for the criticism and reform of established British customs and institutions. This rhetoric therefore involved a whole-scale discounting of British medical traditions.

The main champions of the French model were spokesmen for general practitioners, an oppressed and parvenu segment within the medical polity, whose numerical superiority, as explained in the preceding text, was not reflected in the influence they enjoyed. These agitators were especially incensed by the power and prerogatives of the élite metropolitan physicians and surgeons who dominated the governance of the Royal Colleges. They also exerted an undue influence over appointments to the London teaching hospitals and controlled student access to the wards. They allegedly exercised these prerogatives with an eye to personal gain and the promotion of private interest. In the radical rhetoric of the period, they were thus deemed aspects of the 'Old Corruption' (Desmond, 1989, Ch. 3).

'Paris' served as a rebuke and alternative model to this tainted system. The French had, it was argued, in the aftermath of the revolution, reformed their medical establishments to ensure that they were both efficient and equitable. Thus, appointment to hospital positions was determined by an open competition ensuring that the best candidate was appointed, regardless of personal influence. Accredited students had free access to the hospital wards independent of the favour of the medical staff. In contrast to Britain, there was, moreover, a plentiful supply of bodies for dissection and autopsy through legal channels. French science was, moreover, vastly superior to

British efforts. The Scottish anatomist Robert Knox (1791–1862) insisted (*pace* the Hunterian Orators) that John Hunter was a mere dabbler in comparative anatomy compared to Georges Cuvier (1769–1832). This was, of course, a somewhat idealized representation of the state of affairs in France. But such simplification and exaggeration suited the polemical ends of the British reformers (Warner, 1991).

In the aftermath of the Revolutionary and Napoleonic wars, the expression of a preference for French over established British institutions carried a marked political charge. The London surgeon William Lawrence (1783–1867) provoked a storm of controversy when he favourably noticed developments in French physiology in lectures at the Royal College of Surgeons. Lawrence's chief antagonist in this dispute, John Abernethy, retorted by invoking the memory of John Hunter, who was represented as the spokesman of a distinctively British physiology of a vitalist hue, free of the shortcomings and materialist taint of the French school.

There was a comparable response to the invocation of French institutional practices as templates for the reform of British medicine. Defenders of the established order condemned the 'Gallomaniacs' for exaggerating the merits of foreigners while ignoring the virtues of tried and tested native ways. In particular, even if the French were in some respects superior in medical science, the British excelled in medical practice. In the words of Benjamin Brodie (1783–1862): 'I assert that ours is the better method with a view to the education of those who wish to become *not mere philosophers, but skilful and useful practitioners*' (Warner, 1991, p. 141).

These controversies rehearse tropes familiar from the political debates that followed the revolution in France. On the one hand, there was a Burkean defence of the embodied wisdom of tradition. This was coupled to dire warnings of the folly of recklessly meddling with institutions that had stood the test of time. On the other hand, was a readiness to judge established customs against first principles: if they were found wanting, radical reform was indicated.

British polemics surrounding the significance of Paris Medicine, therefore, show how the subversion of tradition can help to constitute collective identity: in this case, that of the increasingly self-conscious general practitioners. This process involved, of course, the erection of something of a straw man representation of the state of British medicine. In this instance, tradition was invented to be vilified.

Reiterating on themes familiar in contemporary political debates, reformers depicted the ruling medical institutions as mired in sloth, obscurantism, and corruption. France, in contrast, presented a system that had escaped the chains of centuries of ad hoc customary accretion, and refashioned the medical policy according to rational principles. The major social upheaval that had accompanied this reorganization did not figure prominently in reformist rhetoric. Presumably, the British were thought capable of taking the best aspects of French practice while avoiding the excesses.

These professed radicals were to a degree, however, traditionalist. Even the most ardent Gallomaniac conceded that, while the French might excel at science, the British were preeminent in matters of practice. A familiar stereotype of the French doctor as zealous in the pursuit of the seat of disease while largely indifferent to its cure was contrasted to the image of the more balanced British paragon. Because the general practitioner was dependent on patient goodwill for his income, this reservation about alleged French priorities was understandable (Warner, 1991, p. 147). There is some irony in the fact that, while the received understanding of Paris Medicine is of a radical departure in the history of medicine, many of the actors involved stressed its affinity to medical tradition. The *idéologue*, Pierre Jean Georges Cabanis (1757–1808), who supplied a theoretical underpinning for the Paris school, claimed Hippocrates as a forerunner of the method that he recommended (Rosen, 1946, p. 335). This putative ancestry was taken up by a number of the clinicians associated with Paris Medicine. It was also perpetuated by such American Parisians as Elisha Bartlett (1804–55; Warner, 1991, p. 316).

Thus, Laennec chose to write his doctoral thesis on Hippocrates. Despite his show of philological erudition, Laennec depicted the Father of Medicine as remarkably modern; as, in fact, a precursor of organicism and critic of nosological essentialism. In this and in comparable instances, an ancient figure of irreproachable stature was made to fight contemporary causes by proxy (Duffin, 1998, pp. 49–50). Laennec's interest in Hippocrates did not end with the successful defence of his thesis. To a remarkable degree, he continued throughout his career to regard Hippocratic doctrines as of immediate relevance to his own researches. Such engagement with the past reveals an attitude to medical history that disappeared during the second half of the nineteenth century (p. 405).

The notion of medical tradition is not, therefore, without interpretative value. It can provide insights into the construction of corporate and individual medical identities, and serve to highlight the processes whereby current preoccupations are inscribed upon the past. An uncritical reliance on tradition, as conventionally understood, as an approach to the history of medicine is, however, liable to a number of objections. There is a more or less explicit celebratory or triumphalist tone to such accounts of Western medicine. The narrative comprises an account of the achievements of a series of notable individuals whose contribution to the cumulative sum of knowledge earns them a place in some version of the medical 'pantheon'. This may be complemented by the compilation of a canon of classical texts, which constitute key moments in the unfolding of the tradition.

While there may be value in such exercises, there is a danger of divorcing medicine from its context. In particular, the entire political economy of the history of medical doctrine and practice is, perhaps conveniently, overlooked. The remainder of this chapter will examine, with particular reference to the period between 1800 and 1850, historiographic strategies that give due weight to the social relations of medicine.

Sociologies of nineteenth-century medicine

HOSPITAL MEDICINE

In 1967, Erwin H. Ackerknecht published a book entitled *Medicine at the Paris Hospital*. This was, in many ways, a very traditional account: indeed, it has been noted that Ackerknecht's approach owes much to Bouillaud's 1836 history of the Paris School (Hannaway and La Berge, 1998, p. 11). In this work, however, Ackerknecht offered a classification of the major stages in the history of Western medicine that proved to be remarkably influential.

In Ackerknecht's view, 'Paris Medicine' represented a distinct historical type. It was neither ancient 'bedside medicine' nor modern 'laboratory' medicine. It was moreover, wrong to see it as a transitional, intermediate type. Instead, Paris Medicine was to be understood as the dominant form of medical practice in the period following the upheavals of the 1790s. Although its centre was situated in France, its influence spread throughout Western Europe, to Russian, the Americas, and Asia. According to Ackerknecht, this period of dominance ended around 1848, when laboratory medicine, represented in France by such figures as Claude Bernard, began to come to the fore (Ackerknecht, 1967, pp. xi, xiii).

Ackerknecht was anxious to avoid the obvious objections any such sweeping generalization invited. He recognised that 'at all times, doctors of all possible persuasions were practising in Paris and that the medicines of the past, present, and future were coexisting there' (Ackerknecht, 1967, p. xiii). Nonetheless, it was, in his view, possible to identify the dominance of a particular persuasion in the first half of the nineteenth century. The defining characteristics of Paris Medicine were, as we have seen, an emphasis on physical examination, routine autopsy, and the use of statistics. It was also notable for its emphasis on clinical training, sometimes seemingly to the exclusion of other forms of instruction. The techniques could only be pursued properly in a hospital setting. Hence the system could also be designated 'hospital medicine'. The latter appellation is preferable because it loosens the links between a technology that was to attain global application and the site at which it first became dominant. Ackerknecht held that the events that occurred in Paris during the aftermath of the 1789 Revolution marked the beginning of medical modernity, or, as he put it, 'the closing hour of medical medievalism', a characterization that the authors of these reforms would surely have embraced (Ackerknecht, 1967, p. 33).

One aspect of this transformation was the abolition of the long-standing separation of medical and surgical training. Paradoxically, however, this reform was portrayed as a return to the primitive unity of medicine. Owsei Temkin had, in a 1951 paper, drawn attention to the importance of the surgical perspective on the development of modern medical thinking. Temkin sought, however, to place the reforms of post-revolutionary France in the context of a much longer history of interaction between surgery and physic (Temkin, 1951).

In a 1973 paper, Ivan Waddington took up Ackerknecht's distinction between hospital and bedside medicine to seek to illuminate the power relations and underlay modern medical regimes. Once again, events in post-revolutionary France were seen as crucial to understanding the transitions in status and authority involved. As the subtitle to his paper – 'A Sociological Analysis' – implies, while using Ackerkencht's categories as a starting point, Waddington was far more concerned with analyzing the shifting social relations implicated in the creation of new systems of medical thought and practice.

Above all, the move toward hospital-based medicine had profound implications for the patient/doctor relationship. The eighteenth century had been characterized by a type of clinical encounter in which the relation between patient and doctor was structured by a patronage model. Under such circumstances, 'client [i.e., patient] control was maximised, and the technically-based authority of the doctor minimized' (Waddington, 1973, p. 213). The patient was the chief arbiter of the priorities inherent in the clinical encounter; this led to an emphasis upon therapy. The patient was also the judge of the requisite qualities of a practitioner. Social graces and cultural interests were as, if not more, important as technical accomplishment.

Under such a regime, there was little incentive for doctors to engage in research. Indeed, the power the patient wielded militated against the trial of potentially risky new treatments.

What changed with the reorganization of medicine in Paris following the revolution was a fundamental shift in the balance of power between patient and practitioner. In the reformed hospital setting, the doctor was in a dominant position, one that enabled him to set the clinical agenda in accord with a new set of priorities, and that encouraged various forms of diagnostic and therapeutic innovation. In brief, the patient ceased to be a *person*, with whom the practitioner was obliged to negotiate and to whom he was obliged to defer, and became a *body* upon which an ever-increasing repertoire of procedures might be performed.

Waddington sought to explain this transformation by pointing to the difference in social status between patient and doctor in the hospital setting. Hospital consultants, he maintains, comprised the highest echelon of the medical profession: they would thus rank among the *haute bourgeoisie*. Patients, on the other hand, were drawn from the lower classes; they were, indeed, among the most destitute members of society. Hospital doctors were, therefore, able to assume an attitude of superiority to their patients. The latter, on the other hand, were in no position to dispute or challenge the practitioner's determinations. They were expected to defer to his judgment and to submit to whatever he demanded. If they protested or resisted, they would be expelled from an institution they would only enter as a last resort (Waddington, 1973, pp. 215–16).

A stark illustration of the relative status of practitioner and hospital patient is supplied by an account of Mark Akenside's bedside manner at St. Thomas's Hospital in London: 'If the poor affrighted patient did not return a direct answer to his queries, he would often instantly discharge them from the hospital. He evinced a particular disgust for females & generally treated them with harshness . . . .' On one occasion, Akenside ordered the expulsion of a patient who was unable to swallow a prescribed pill, declaring: '"he shall not die under my care". As the sister was removing him in obedience to the doctor, the patient expired' (Lawrence and Macdonald, 2003, p. 23).

Because of this lack of patient power, the hospital provided an ideal location for the introduction of new methods of examination in addition to treatment. Hence the possibility arose to develop forms of physical diagnosis, such as auscultation. Other forms of examination involved even more intrusive procedures upon the body of the patient, allowing the exposure of the 'private' parts to the gaze of the physician, and often to a crowd of inquisitive students. The hospital patient's submissive role made it impossible for them to decline to be used for pedagogic purposes.

Waddington suggests, however, that it was not simply inequalities in power that permitted these innovations to be implemented. Cultural differences between hospital patients and those encountered in private practice were also significant. Notions of the body and its boundaries are not natural and immutable: they vary between and within cultures and over time. Norbert Elias has drawn attention to a secular tendency in the history of Western societies towards the formation of the notion of the body as a private self-enclosed entity. Strict limitations were imposed upon exposure of parts of the body and upon the performance of certain functions. These codes were first instituted among the upper echelons of society and gradually percolated downwards (Elias, 1994, pp. 110–12). As late as the nineteenth century, however, these protocols had not yet been established among the urban and rural poor of a country, such as France. There was, in other words, a much higher tolerance for public nudity and less embarrassment about bodily functions among the class from which the typical hospital patient was drawn. This relative lack of modesty also facilitated the institution of new, more intrusive medical practices. Paris was, for instance, regarded as an especially advantageous place to study midwifery because lower-class women were, in the words of one observer, 'callous to exposure' (Waddington, 1973, p. 220).

This interpretation of the social foundations of early-nineteenth-century medicine was considerably elaborated by N. D. Jewson. Like Waddington, Jewson took as his starting point a somewhat idealized vision of eighteenth-century medicine, which he designated 'bedside medicine'. Under this regime, the patient was conceptualized as 'a conscious human totality'. The physician's primary task was to seek to grasp this totality and produce treatment and regimen adapted to the maintenance of health and cure of disease. The patient's phenomenological account of his or her bodily states was essential to this process (Jewson, 1974).

The advent of hospital medicine represented a move from this person-orientated to an object-orientated medical cosmology. The patient came to be increasingly understood as a diseased body, which was in turn analyzed into a series of anatomical sites in which disease could become immanent. The truth of disease was to be uncovered through physical manipulation and probing, coupled with postmortem examination. The patient's voice was marginalized, if not suppressed. These tendencies were reinforced by the succeeding cosmology of laboratory medicine. Under this regime, the doctor was no longer even dealing with the entirety of the diseased body: diagnoses could be made on the basis of samples transported from the hospital ward to the laboratory.

All these cosmologies, however, possessed certain common structural characteristics. In each case, a 'patron' can be distinguished. This was a class of individual or institution that exerted effective economic control over the clinical environment. In the case of bedside medicine, patronage took the form of fees paid by the patient to the doctor. Under hospital medicine, patronage was dispensed by the career structure of the medical profession. Laboratory medicine saw a shift to a scientific career structure centred on university rather than hospital appointments (Jewson, 1976, p. 228).

Jewson's analysis shows a clear Marxist, or at least Marxian, influence. He is concerned with the 'modes of production' of medical knowledge. In other words, he sees the cognitive aspect of medical cosmologies as the result of material processes akin to those involved in the generation of other artefacts. His is thus an account of the economics, or perhaps more precisely, the political economy of medicine. The source of 'patronage' – best understood as control of the means of production broadly construed – in any given epoch, is crucial to the forms of clinical interaction and cognitive formations that will emerge. The development of ideas about health, disease, and the body is, therefore, no disembodied process, but the result of the power relations at work in any given historical setting.

Medical knowledge is, therefore, not discovered; it is *constructed* by means of a variety of work processes (Armstrong, 1994, p. 19). Jewson's account of the history of Western medicine can be viewed as a form of social constructivism. This form of analysis has, however, tended to offer less sweeping forms of explanation. Certain theoretical commitments in the early-nineteenth-century phrenology debates have, for instance, been linked to the social interests of their proponents (Shapin, 1979), while Adrian Desmond has tried to show how contrasting schools of comparative anatomy were intimately associated with conflicting political agendas (Desmond, 1989, *passim*). Jewson, on the other hand, operates at a more general level, that of the overall 'cosmology' predominant over a wide geographical expanse over a lengthy period of time.

Jewson's account of the trajectory of Western medicine since 1800 embodies an implicit humanist critique. His depiction of the ideal eighteenth-century clinical encounter emphasises the egalitarian relations between patient and practitioner; diagnosis and course of therapy were supposedly determined through negotiation and consensus. The 'sick man' was in a position to exert an influence upon how his case was conceptualized and on how he would be treated. The consultative relationship was based upon the personal empathy between the parties (Jewson, 1976, p. 233). Under the successor medical regimes, however, the patient is alienated from these processes. His or her body and complaint was no longer their own: 'the sick-man found himself unequivocally subordinated to the medical investigator' (ibid p. 234). In epistemological terms, while the clinical encounter under bedside medicine demanded hermeneutic understanding, both hospital and laboratory medicine imposed a subject/object relationship between practitioner and patient.

The character of medical authority undergoes a transformation concomitant with the reification of the patient. The conditions of bedside medicine obliged the doctor to cultivate the personal qualities needed to engage in a successful and meaningful interaction with the patient/patron. A practitioner unable to show sufficient empathy and powers of persuasion would not succeed in the prevalent medical marketplace. In short, medical authority was of a personal, charismatic variety. The ultimate arbiter of whether a doctor possessed the requisite qualities was the patient. Under hospital and laboratory medicine, in contrast, authority was derived from a practitioner's status within some institutional structure, be that clinical or academic; it was thus *ascribed*. The patient had no role in constructing authority of this kind. This increasing social distance between patient and practitioner was especially marked under laboratory medicine where the community of medical investigators appeared to inhabit 'an insulated intellectual cocoon' (Jewson, 1976, p. 238).

Jewson refers almost in passing to Michel Foucault's *The Birth of the Clinic* as a source of information on the transformations in early-nineteenth-century medicine with which he is also concerned. Compared with Jewson's sweeping scheme, Foucault's is an apparently much more narrowly focused discussion of the transformations in French medicine in the aftermath of the revolution. At first glance, Foucault's, Waddington's, Jewson's, and indeed Ackerknecht's interpretations of the significance of these events appear broadly similar. In each case, there is an insistence that these events in Paris mark a new epoch in the history of Western medicine. They all see the novel primacy of the hospital as central to this reorganization. There is a common recognition that the new modes of medical practice and knowledge that emerged during this period were dependent upon a shift in power relations within the medical economy.

It is important, however, to recognize the degree to which Foucault's analysis breaks new ground. His concept of power differs from the more familiar one employed by Jewson: the latter sees power as repressive and essentially negative. Changing power relations were instrumental in creating the conditions for medical revolution in the early nineteenth century by creating a passive class of patient over whom doctors exercised an unprecedented degree of control. Because of the economic dependency of the hospital population, practitioners were, for example, able to override any opposition to intrusive physical examination or to the appropriation of cadavers for autopsy.

For Foucault, power is, in contrast, positive and productive. It permeates, and indeed constitutes, a social field in which new discursive forms emerge. The creativity of power is not, however, confined to the creation of new ideas and forms of practice. New *bodies* were fabricated in the hospitals of early-nineteenth-century Europe to incorporate the anatomical and pathological entities that comprised medical discourse, and to suffer the diagnostic and therapeutic operations that discourse enjoined. What is sometimes overlooked is that not only a new kind of patient, but also a new doctor was also generated as part of this process. Patient and doctor were '"trapped" in a common, but non-reciprocal situation' (Foucault, 1973, p. xv). The dichotomy of empowered and powerless, victim and oppressor that lurks within Jewson's account thus loses much of its meaning.

Foucault himself defined his position relative to conventional sociological accounts of the 'patient-doctor relationship', poking fun at the 'feebly eroticized' undertones of the notion (Foucault, 1973, p. xiv). Fundamental to the difference between his approach and that of the likes of Waddington and Jewson, is that Foucault does not admit the existence of stable historical actors who assume the roles of patient and doctor in varying configurations of power in different epochs. There is, in short, no stable human subject to be objectified through the operations of an emergent medical regime. The techniques of observation and manipulation that arose at the turn of the nineteenth century engendered unprecedented bodies to be known in addition to producing new knowing, investigating bodies (Armstrong, 1994, pp. 20–1).

Thus, the Paris clinic of the early nineteenth century saw the constitution of a body composed of tissues disseminated through a variety of organs, engendering the paradox of the internal surface. These tissues 'are the elements of the organs, but they traverse them, relate them together, and constitute vast "systems" above them in which the human body finds the concrete forms of its unity' (Foucault, 1973, p. 128). The pathologist's analysis of these structures mirrored the process of decomposition wreaked within the body by disease itself.

Foucault's work is also noteworthy in that he places the changes taking place in medicine during the early nineteenth century in the context of reorganization that was occurring at a wide range of sites. Similar techniques, which Foucault encompasses under the rubric of 'disciplinary power', were being employed to survey bodies in factories, schools, prisons, and army barracks. The military exemplar is of particular significance given the fact that many medical men in the early decades of the nineteenth century spent part of their careers in the service of the army or navy.

The experience of dealing with large populations within a rigid, authoritarian framework created expertise and a problematic that was then transferred into medical intervention in the civilian sphere. This process of transfer was especially marked in the French case where 'many sociopolitical investigators of the post-Imperial era received their introduction to widespread and severe famine, social disruption, and desperate medical necessity in this hostile environment of battlefield and military hospital' (Coleman, 1982, p. 15).

Personal experience was not, however, a necessary condition for appreciating the potential value of military medicine to the problems of civilian populations. In 1833, William Pulteney Alison (1790–1859), Professor of the Institutes of Medicine at Edinburgh, remarked on the difficulty of isolating with any certainty the influences that engendered disease. He remarked on 'the very great variety of the circumstances, capable of affecting health, in which individuals are placed, and of the difficulty of varying these, so as to obtain such observations, in the way of induction, or exclusion, as shall be decisive as to the efficacy of each.' These difficulties highlighted 'the importance of the observations, intended to illustrate this matter, being as extensively multiplied as possible; and hence also the peculiar value, with a view to the investigation of the causes of diseases, of observations made on large and organized bodies of men, as in the experience of military and naval practitioners.' The conditions of military practice provided the medical observer with a body of subjects whose circumstances: 'are in many respects exactly alike; they are accurately known to the observer, and are indeed often to a certain degree at his disposal; they are often suddenly changed, and when changed as to one portion of the individuals under observation, they are often unchanged as to another; and therefore, the conditions necessary to obtaining an *experimentum crucis* as to the efficacy of an alleged cause of disease, are more frequently in the power of such an observer, than of one who is conversant only with civil life.' The military camp or naval ship is thus configured as a laboratory uniquely adapted to the study of the causes of disease.

The parallel between the clinic and the factory is also revealing. Foucault can be seen as promoting a form of social constructivism. In particular, he conceives scientific disciplines as 'apparatuses of power that function to produce knowledge about the human world they bring under control' (Golinski, 1998, p. 71). In other words, disciplinary power constructs novel subjects and objects through the application of a range of techniques. Thus, 'the various clinical techniques which doctors have used to study the body as an object are not merely the symbols of a repressive force but are components in the productive assembly line through which reality is created' (Armstrong, 1994, p. 23).

An instructive analogy can be developed between the clinic and an assembly line. Both rely upon a supply of raw materials: in the case of the clinic, the chief of these are students and the sick. The interior space of the clinic is structured to accommodate these materials in order to impose certain effects. The sick are classified and allocated to particular wards according to the outcome of a preliminary diagnosis. Here they are subject to a range of techniques that transform the sick man or woman into a *case*. Some of these techniques are physical or instrumental: the stethoscope or even the humble method of percussion may be viewed as progenitor of a vast range of diagnostic procedures. But it is also important to recognize the prominence of documentary technologies within this regime. Foucault has pointed out that a common characteristic of disciplinary systems is the generation of a vast and complex body of documentation. In the clinic, this took the form of the patient record that was regularly updated throughout the patient's stay in the hospital. These reports formed a crude resource that might subsequently be transformed by means of further processing into a published report or included in a monograph or textbook. Through these techniques, the amorphous mass of the sick was transformed into the serviceable materials of medical knowledge.

Most patients would, in due course, be discharged, whether as 'cured' or with some other label. When, however, they perished, their bodies were not discarded as mere waste product. Foucault has written of the new attitude to death that emerged at the turn of the nineteenth century. Far from being a point of absolute closure, death opened up a vast range of possibilities: 'The living light is dissipated in the brightness of death' (Foucault, 1973, p. 146).

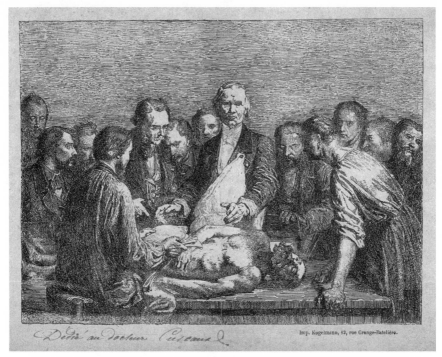

Imp. Kugelmann, 13, rue Grange-Batelière.

Fig. 1.3. The Parisian surgeon and anatomist, Alfred Velpeau (1795–1867) performing an anatomical dissection, 1864. *Source*: Etching after a painting by F. N. A. Feyen-Perrin, Paris. Wellcome Library Iconographic Collection. *Credit*: Wellcome Library, London (V0010456).

Autopsy was, of course, integral to the work of the clinic. The case record would routinely include a description of postmortem appearances when the patient died. But cadavers also provided an important resource for medical education. It was established doctrine that the best way to learn the structure of the body was for each student to conduct his own dissections. This demanded a large and steady supply of subjects. In Paris, in addition to the university dissection rooms, numerous private anatomy schools existed in the early nineteenth century. These were clustered around the exit from the morgue of the Hôtel Dieu, eloquent testimony to the source of their materials (Weiner, 1993, p. 183) (Fig. 1.3).

The students who entered the clinic were, themselves, subjected to a series of processes designed to transform them into serviceable elements within this system of production. The revived system of medical education in post-revolutionary France was overtly meritocratic; ability, rather than birth or connection was supposed to determine admission. This was a feature that particularly impressed British enthusiasts for the Paris model.

Once admitted, students were subjected to a process of appraisal intended to distinguish the future medical élite from the proletariat of the profession. Appointment to the coveted internship was on the basis of open competition. In France, in particular, examination was seen as the best method of determining the true value of an individual. The state's immediate goal of securing an adequate supply of qualified practitioners for military and civil use was thus secured at the same time as new cadres of medical investigators were refined from the raw material of the student body.

Foucault maintains that among the effects of disciplinary regimes is the production of new forms of subjectivity. In the case of the formation of the medical student, this would include an investigative posture – an investment in the advancement of scientific knowledge. It would also involve the inculcation of the competitive spirit required by a system that placed such emphasis on examination and grading. Also demanded, however, was a certain coarsening or numbing of affect. The point may be illustrated by means of the correspondence of an early-nineteenth-century British medical student. Hampton Weekes wrote, on September 24, 1801, to his surgeon father of an operation on a case of scrotal hernia he had witnessed at Guy's Hospital. He felt the need to allude to the question of his reaction to the surgery: 'Now for fainting Dr. Dick, dont [sic] suppose I was carried off as a dead man Dr, but I felt a something indescribable as I have heard you say & took myself off just as they had taken hold of the Artery with the Tenaculum & immediately recovered, I wont do so again for I will persue the means you recommend, I can dissect I know, & could have performed the operation myself' (Ford, 1987, p. 44).

Weeke's initial response to witnessing the operation was, therefore, one of an involuntary revulsion that threatened to overcome his self-possession. His frank admission of this anticipated reaction is coupled with a defensive insistence that such a show of weakness would not recur. Weekes insists, moreover, that *technically* he is already competent to perform the procedure. All that is lacking was the necessary callousness to do to a living body what he had already practised on cadavers.

Less than a month later, Weekes wrote once more to his father to inform him that: 'I have seen several operations since I wrote last & mind nothing about it, the more the poor devils cry ye. more I laugh with the rest of them . . .' (p. 49). He thus makes his newfound indifference to the suffering of the patient a point of pride. He stresses, moreover, how his reaction to the patient's screams conforms to that of his peers: 'I laugh with the rest of them.' There is, on the one hand, an alienation from the patient, who is reduced to the status of a more or less instructive subject matter. While, on the other hand, the aspirant doctor is assimilated into a sense of corporate identity. In addition to the acquisition of knowledge and skills, becoming a doctor thus involves a sense of separation from and superiority to the common run of humanity.

LABORATORY MEDICINE

Several commentators have drawn attention to Foucault's preoccupation with space. Indeed, his work has been compared with a form of cartography. He focuses upon such circumscribed spaces as the clinic and asylum. These are the sites at which particular forms of power/knowledge are articulated. But he is no less concerned with delimiting discursive boundaries. This concern complements Foucault's emphasis upon bodies as the focus of power and its concomitant discursive forms. It is through the localization of bodies within figured spaces that they are enabled to yield knowledge (Driver, 1994, pp. 115–16).

Such notions are applicable to sites of medical work other than the clinic. As Jewson's schema indicates, the laboratory became, in the course of the nineteenth century, an increasingly important locus within the Western medical economy. Initially, laboratory work was only for a tiny élite who aspired to enlarge the bounds of medical knowledge. By the middle of the nineteenth century, however, a tendency to make laboratory techniques part of the training and subsequent practice of every medical man was becoming apparent.

Any discussion of the emergence of laboratory medicine must be predicated on an understanding that the term connotes not only a set of specialized spaces, but also bodily and instrumental technologies, in addition to distinctive subjectivities. The variety of sites and diversity of the kinds of work undertaken in them must also be appreciated. There was a vast difference between a side room of a hospital ward where elementary blood and urine analysis might be undertaken, and the elaborate physiology laboratories that were appearing in Germany by the middle of the nineteenth century. A weakness of Jewson's account of laboratory medicine is that he fails to give due weight to this variety.

The rise of 'experimental medicine' in the first half of the nineteenth century is particularly associated with developments of France. We have seen the prominence of French institutions in the fields of clinical medicine and education. The predominance of the clinic is usually thought to have been an impediment to the development of laboratory science within the medical curriculum. Indeed, Ackerknecht argued that this bias explains the stagnancy of the Paris school by the middle of the century and its eventual overshadowing by the Germans.

John Lesch has, however, argued that certain features of the post-revolutionary medical regime were, in fact, of crucial importance to the development of experimental physiology in France. The abolition of the traditional distinction between the branches of medicine provided a supply of individuals trained in the techniques of surgery. These skills could be and were then applied in experimental procedures on animals. Perhaps the most notable of these surgeon-physiologists was François Magendie, who, along with his protégé Claude Bernard, is generally regarded as the founding father of French physiology (Lesch, 1984, p. 89).

Although he obtained an M.D. in 1808, Magendie was more noted for experimental research and the teaching of physiology than as a clinician. He brought to the science something of the self-conscious empiricism that was the trademark of the Paris clinical school. In addition to performing experiments on the respective functions of the spinal nerves, Magendie did original work in the field later known as experimental pharmacology. Because Magendie originally trained as a surgeon at the Hôtel-Dieu of Paris, Lesch's thesis can be seen as an extension of Temkin's claims for the centrality of the surgical contribution to modern medicine.

Lesch also perpetuates a historiographic tradition that focuses almost exclusively upon a handful of individuals who supposedly embody the grand tradition of experimental medicine, a tradition that can be traced at least as far back as Claude Bernard. As in the case of the histories of French clinical medicine discussed in the preceding text, insistence on this particular tradition no doubt served a range of polemical goals. In Bernard's case, there was an obvious nationalist agenda. This account of the history of physiology is, however, subject to serious objections. In particular, the French medical schools played little part in the establishment of experimental medicine before 1850; the Académie des Sciences was a far more important patron. The physiology professed in the medical faculties was far more clinical and anatomical than experimental in its character (Elliot, 1990).

It should be noted that central to the programme for the creation of an experimental medicine was the impulse to achieve control over the workings of the living body. This may be seen as an instance of the instrumental reasoning typical of modern Western societies (Marcuse, 1964). This value was especially celebrated in Bernard's *Introduction to the Study of Experimental Medicine* (1865). A determination to achieve control over the body was to become fundamental to the ethos of Western medicine. It is indicative of the growing absorption of medical doctrine by the ruling technological a priori that seeks cognitive and technical dominion over nature with a view to economic exploitation. This antagonistic attitude to nature contains the seeds of contemporary biotechnologies with all their extensive ramifications. Not the least of these is that whatever nominal distinctions were previously maintained between *human* bodies and the rest of nature, have been effectively eliminated. Humans are now as potentially available for manipulation and intervention as any nineteenth-century laboratory animal. The technologies of genetic engineering are the most obvious instance p. 412ff. Potent commercial interests promote the realization of these possibilities. Only the flimsy shield of 'bio-ethics' forefends.

The received notion of a grand experimental tradition relies, moreover, on unquestioned assumptions about unbroken continuities between key links in the chain. While it is justifiable to assume such a lineage between Magendie and Bernard, in the case of Bichat the question becomes much more problematic. Bichat figures chiefly in the history of medicine as a founder of pathological anatomy. But, in the course of his researches, he also performed experiments on live animals. It was, therefore, a facile step to represent him as a precursor of the physiological tradition that developed later in the nineteenth century. A Foucauldian analysis has, however, undermined these assumptions (Albury, 1977).

The conventional view is that experimental physiology developed more slowly in Britain than in France for a number of reasons. The strength of a native anatomical tradition that insisted on the need to maintain a link between structure and function has been adduced as one impediment (Geison, 1978, pp. 18–23). We have seen, however, that a similar bias persisted in French medical schools in the first half of the nineteenth century. There is also thought to have been a cultural difference in British and French tolerance to the infliction of pain on animals.

The Scottish anatomist, Charles Bell, summed up this scepticism about vivisection when he declared: 'experiments have never been the means of discovery; and a survey of what has been attempted of late years in physiology, will prove that the opening of living animals has done more to perpetuate error, than to confirm the just views taken from the study of anatomy and natural motions' (Bell, 1823, pp. 289–307). It should be noted, however, that even as staunch an advocate of the anatomical method as Bell was, he did on occasion perform experiments.

This resistance is further evinced by the horrified reaction of one British witness to one of Magendie's experimental demonstrations. William Sharpey recalled in 1875 that 'when I was a very young man studying in Paris, I went to the first of a series of lectures which Magendie gave upon experimental physiology, and I was so utterly repelled by what I witnessed that I never went back again. My objection in these experiments was two-fold. In the first place they were painful . . . and they were made without any sufficient object. As an example Magendie made incisions into the skin of rabbits to show that the skin is sensitive. Now surely all the world knows the skin is sensitive, no experiment painful or without pain is needed to prove that' (Sykes, 2001, p. 79).

But it is clear that some British medical men, including Sharpey, did engage in experiments upon living animals in the early nineteenth century. Thus, in 1836, Sharpey wrote to his friend and colleague Allen Thomson (1809–84) of a vivisectional experiment he performed that was designed to confirm the findings of a French physiologist. He showed no apparent concern for the suffering of the dog involved, but was chiefly preoccupied with the technical aspects of the experiment (Jacyna, 1989, p. 2). Sharpey also copied Magendie's practice of illustrating his lectures in London with experimental demonstrations, although he pointed out that these were 'more on *dead* than on *living* animals however' (p. 14). There may be an implicit distinction here between the forms of experimentation deemed suitable in public rather than private spaces.

The contention was that such procedures should only be undertaken when the potential scientific or pedagogical benefits were sufficiently impor-tant. British physiologists may have shown greater sensitivity by trying to minimize the pain inflicted on the subjects of these experiments. Such experimentation often took place in domestic, improvised settings. They are evidence that an experimental 'form of life' had taken root among certain classes of medical men in Britain early in the nineteenth century: that is, a commitment to the pursuit of scientific knowledge by means of certain agreed material, linguistic, and social technologies (Shapin and Schaffer, 1985, pp. 14–15).

A point of some interest is that this experimental social technology was viable independent of any obvious institutional base or career structure. The kind of experimental activity so far discussed was confined to a small group of (mainly) medical men. By the middle of the nineteenth century, however, the first steps had been taken to making laboratory experience of some kind part of the training of all doctors. In its early stages, this movement was particularly marked in the German-speaking states of Europe. In Germany, unlike both France and Britain, medical education remained based in the universities during the nineteenth century. German universities were among the first to develop a research culture – to insist that the primary responsibility of the academic was to produce new knowledge, and only secondarily to promulgate established truths through teaching. It thus became possible to pursue a career in science. The division of Germany into a number of independent states created a competitive environment in which governments vied with one another to secure the services of the most distinguished scientists. These researchers were, therefore, in a position to demand elaborate facilities for the conduct of their work. Novel collaborative forms of investigation developed as eminent figures, such as Johannes Müller (1801–58) based in Berlin, developed schools of researchers around them.

Perhaps the first such research school was established by Jan Evangelista Purkyně (1787–1869) at the University of Breslau. After graduating in medicine at the University of Prague in 1819, Purkyně undertook research into the physiology of sensation and is regarded as an early figure in the history of experimental psychology. He was also a leading histologist and embryologist who was among the first to make use of the microtome. Purkyně's aim was to create an environment at the Physiology Institute he founded in Breslau during the 1830s, where students would gain the skills to become original researchers. They would thus become what Foucault calls 'active bodies'. In this endeavour he was inspired by the work of the educational theorist Johann Heinrich Pestalozzi (1746–1827) who had stressed the importance of personal interaction with the world in the formation of character. While Pestalozzi and most of his followers were primarily concerned with primary education, Purkyně sought to apply these theories at the level of university education. Purkyně propounded a sensualist theory of knowledge somewhat reminiscent of the one favoured by the French medical reformers of the early nineteenth century. He was, in particular, highly critical of systems of education that relied exclusively on book learning. Instead, he insisted on the importance of hands-on training: certain students were expected to perform experiments rather than merely witnessing demonstrations performed by the professor (Coleman, 1988, p. 21).

For Purkyně and Müller, however, laboratory skills were appropriate only to a small élite, consisting of professors and a few chosen students who might one day aspire to an academic career. Both these professors were remarkably successful in forming a group of researchers, drawn from the larger student body around them, working on related subjects, notably in the new field of histology. But it was left to a later generation of professors to begin to disseminate these techniques to a wider audience.

The ruling ideology of, in particular, the Prussian educational system revolved around neohumanist notions of *Bildung*, or personal development. This bias might seem calculated to militate against practical training of any sort within the university curriculum, and there was, indeed, a tendency in the early nineteenth century for a distinction to be drawn between the forms of pedagogy appropriate in an academic setting and those suited to institutions devoted to technical training. This tendency to demarcate theoretical and practical instruction was, however, countered by a lively awareness on the part of ruling élites within Germany of the importance of meeting the needs of an industrializing society through the promotion of technological progress. It was generally acknowledged that the best means of acquiring the skills demanded by modern modes of production was for each student to have personal experience of these methods as part of his education (Tuchman, 1988, pp. 69–70).

These assumptions produced a context that fostered the introduction of laboratory training into the medical curriculum. At the vanguard of this movement was the introduction and dissemination of medical microscopy.

MEDICAL MICROSCOPY

The compound microscope had been employed as a tool of scientific research since the seventeenth century (Wilson, 1995). As late as the turn of the nineteenth century, however, substantial doubts persisted about the reliability of evidence derived by this means (Fig. 1.4). Such major figures as Bichat and Laennec shared this scepticism. Even Müller and Purkyně, who were eventually to play a leading role in the establishment of histology, tacitly acquiesced in this view of the unreliability of the compound microscope by restricting themselves to the use of simple lenses in their early investigations. A common criticism was that each observer saw what he wanted through the microscope. The collapse of the so-called 'Globule Theory', which postulated that all living matter was composed of minute spherical forms, seemed to confirm these doubts. Although described and depicted by seemingly reliable observers, these globules were eventually dismissed as, for the most part, mere artefacts and optical illusions.

By the late 1820s, however, new 'achromatic' microscopes were beginning to become available. These were constructed to avoid the

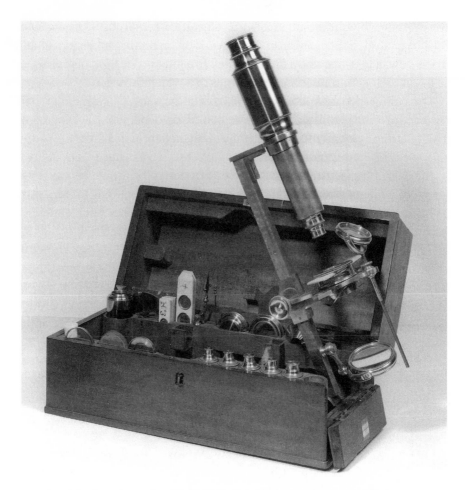

Fig. 1.4. Chest microscope made by 'Dolland, London', *c.* 1800. In 1758, John Dolland had corrected chromatic aberration by using a combination of crown glass (containing no lead or iron) and flint glass in lenses. *Source*: Wellcome Historical Medical Museum. *Credit*: Wellcome Library, London (M0017160).

optical defects that had characterized earlier instruments. These microscopes were at first very rare and expensive; in 1834, even the University of Berlin possessed only one such microscope. As late as 1846, Purkyně had only secured four achromatic instruments for his laboratory in Breslau. It was, therefore, often necessary for investigators to share a microscope, a circumstance that had the incidental effect of encouraging collaborative research. By the middle of the century, however, less elaborate and cheaper microscopes were being manufactured, making it possible to teach microscopic method to relatively large classes.

In addition to instruments, however, the establishment of laboratory medicine required the creation of social forms adequate to the inculcation of the skills involved in the manipulation of the microscope and of other instruments. Techniques were needed to produce bodies that were active, in the sense of being capable of performing certain operations, but also passive inasmuch as they were subject to disciplinary norms. The dilemma was resolved by ensuring that these norms were internalized by the student who became, in Foucauldian terms, self-disciplined. These needs became acute at the point where microscopy ceased to be a craft cultivated by individuals in loose associations, and became a skill inculcated through formalized systems of pedagogy.

Efforts to create a corps of disciplined microscopic observers occurred within the context of a more general reorganization of the conditions of seeing. This involved the reconstitution of the body as the subject of a range of institutional power and discursive formations. The appearance of the new observer was an aspect of the complex of changes associated with the consolidation of capitalist modernity (Crary, 1990, pp. 2–3). It has been noted that certain optical devices, such as the stereoscope, featured as foci for the operation of power on the body, producing (from some perspective) a disciplined functional observer. The microscope may be added to the list of such instruments. In this case, the utility served by training observers competent to the use of the instrument was the performance of forms of medico-scientific work.

All these techniques of the observer relied upon the existence of a discourse about the material conditions of seeing. Vision was corporealized – deemed a function – and as such, subject to physiological enquiry and exposition. Among the earliest exponents of such research was Johannes Müller. He propagated a doctrine of specific nerve energies that effectively deprived the act of seeing of its classical veridical status. Müller maintained, for instance, that the same stimulus could generate different sensations depending on the system of nerves on which it impinged. Conversely, different stimuli applied to the same nerves produced what was perceived as identical effects. The vagaries of vision revealed by the physiologist thus not only enabled, but *required* the invention of such techniques of control and normalization. In the first half of the nineteenth century, 'the body was becoming the site of both power and truth' (Crary, 1990, p. 79).

Among the first to generate such systems for the normalization of microscopic observation was Jacob Henle (1809–85), one of Müller's protégés. Henle was, in 1841, to publish his *Allgemeine Anatomie*, generally regarded as the first systematic work in the field of histology following the promulgation of the cell theory. While working with Müller in Berlin during the 1830s, Henle had already begun to provide students with classes in the use of the microscope, making the best use of makeshift facilities for the purpose. Albrecht Kölliker (1817–1905), one of Henle's early students, who himself became a notable histologist, recalled these early attempts at microscopical instruction: 'I still see the narrow, long hallway in the university building next to the auditorium where Henle, for lack of another room for demonstrations, showed us and explained the simplest things, so awe inspiring in their novelty, with scarcely five or six microscopes: epithelia, skin scales, cilia cells, blood corpuscles, pus cells, semen, then teased-out preparations from muscles, ligaments, nerves, sections from cartilage, cuts of bones, etc.' (Tuchman, 1988, p. 75).

This passage is notable for a number of reasons. In the first place, it reveals the excitement surrounding the achromatic microscope in the early days of its propagation. The instrument seemed to open a veritable new world to the eyes of young medical men, some of whom, such as Kölliker, were sufficiently inspired to devote their own lives to microscopic research. But Kölliker's recollections also reveal how marginal histological teaching was, at this stage, to the mainstream of medical education.

This novelty and marginality go far, however, to explain why those ambitious for distinction within academic medicine were drawn to the microscope. Competition for appointments within the German university system was intense: numerous *Privatdozenten* jostled to attain one of the relatively few professorial posts. This struggle for recognition encouraged junior teachers to explore new specialties, accomplishment in which would serve to distinguish them from the crowd (Turner, 1971, pp. 143–4). Expertise in a new field, such as microscopy, thus provided Henle with a competitive edge, which was to prove decisive to the progress of his career. French pioneers of medical microscopy, such as Alfred Donné (1801–78), were also drawn to the instrument as a means to attract notice and promotion within a highly competitive environment (La Berge, 1994, p. 301).

In 1840, Henle was appointed to the Chair of Anatomy at the University of Zurich. There he continued to develop practical histological training for medical students. The reputation he thus acquired prompted the University of Heidelberg to offer him a post in 1843. The authorities at Heidelberg were anxious to revive the fortunes of their medical school by attracting professors capable of teaching the most modern medical doctrines and techniques. Henle's reputations as a master of the microscope thus made him an attractive target (Tuchman, 1988, p. 81).

It is notable that in both Zurich and Heidelberg, Henle worked in close association with a clinical professor named Karl Pfeufer (1806–69) who was a noted German exponent of French clinical methods of percussion and auscultation, coupled with pathological anatomy. He was also convinced that future advance in medicine was dependent on progress in the basic sciences of anatomy and physiology. Pfeufer and Henle joined in advocating a new 'rational medicine' that would realize these ideals of fruitful interaction between the laboratory and the clinic. Synergies of this kind draw attention to the difficulties of sustaining any rigid distinction between bedside and laboratory medicine.

Interesting parallel developments occurred in France and Britain. During the 1840s, ambitious young French medical men took up the cause of the microscope. Among these was Paul Broca, who combined this interest with a commitment to the classic practices of Paris Medicine (Schiller, 1979; La Berge, 1994). As in Germany, these French advocates of the medical importance of the microscope tended to be 'progressive' in a broader sense. There was, in particular, in both countries a marked inclination towards political liberalism among these groups. Thus, Rudolf Virchow (1821–1902), another of Müller's students, combined microscopy with an active interest in the social and political role of the medical profession (McNeely, 2002, pp. 12–31). Henle was also marked as a radical. Because of his political activities as a young man, he was sentenced to a term of imprisonment although he never served his sentence.

A similar correlation between politically advanced ideas and the championing of new medical ideas and technologies was less obvious in Britain. However, George Eliot's fictional account of the progressive doctor, Tertius Lydgate, in her novel *Middlemarch* (1871–2), hints at similar connections. Lydgate is intellectually advanced: he has studied in Paris and is familiar, *inter alia*, with the doctrines of Broussais. He is portrayed as 'a spirited young adventurer' eager to expand on Bichat's epoch-making work in pathology. To this end he would make use, 'not only of the scalpel, but of the microscope . . . .' Despite these lofty scientific aims, Lydgate did not disdain medical practice in a provincial setting; his plan was 'to do good small work for Middlemarch, and great work for the world.' He is portrayed as an advocate of reform, calling, for instance, for the establishment of a new fever hospital (Eliot, 1986, pp. 121–2, 102).

There are, nonetheless, interesting similarities between the careers of some of the early British enthusiasts for the microscope and what was occurring on the Continent. Although British opticians had been among the pioneers of the achromatic lens, the medical applications of the new microscopes had to be imported from continental centres. This technological transfer was accomplished by a relatively small group of individuals. The typical pattern was to travel to the Continent relatively early in a medical career. France was usually the first port of call where, in addition to gaining clinical experience and taking advantage of the facilities for pathological anatomy, British doctors might gain some acquaintance with microscopy. This was often supplemented by trips to the various German centres where systematic instruction in histology was being developed.

Upon returning home, the skills and knowledge thus acquired were deployed in a range of domestic contexts. The career of one such figure, John Hughes Bennett (1812–75), in some respects parallels that of Henle. After acquiring histological skills in France and Germany, Bennett was able to employ these attainments to further his career as a teacher. During the early 1840s, he mounted a course in practical microscopy in the Edinburgh extramural school. This was the first such course to be offered in Britain. This extramural teaching helped Bennett gain the reputation that led to his appointment in 1848 as Professor of the Institutes of Medicine at the University of Edinburgh. There he continued to offer practical histology instruction. Moreover, as in Germany, histology provided the foundation for the introduction of a wider range of practical physiology training in the second half of the nineteenth century.

For Bennett, as for Henle, the microscope possessed an ideological function. Both men saw it as a symbol of what was variously described as 'rational', 'experimental', or 'scientific' medicine. The principal tenet of this doctrine was that advances on medical practice depended on sciences, such as physiology and pathology, that revealed the basic workings of the body in health and disease. This claim justified the place of these sciences within the medical curriculum in addition to the expenditure of ever-greater resources on providing the laboratories and other facilities that such research demanded. The ideology of scientific medicine also served to distinguish orthodox medical practitioners more clearly from other competitors in the medical marketplace.

By the turn of the twentieth century, these dogmas came to dominate Western medicine. In the first half of the nineteenth century, however, they elicited considerable scepticism and, indeed, opposition. This resistance to the idea of scientific medicine had a number of sources. Some medical men, especially in England, felt that the proper foundation of medical culture lay in classical and other humanistic studies rather than in science. Others were, with some justification, incredulous about the supposed relevance of laboratory science to medical practice; it was indeed difficult to point to any practical benefits that had been derived from this source. The best that Bennett could summon up to legitimate the medical relevance of the microscope was the discovery of the causative agent of scabies. It is noteworthy that the proponents of the various forms of 'alternative' medicines, such as homoeopathy, which arose in the first half of the nineteenth century, were especially scathing about the pretensions of laboratory science.

The introduction of practical histology teaching into the training of medical practitioners is amenable to a Foucauldian disciplinary analysis. Among the most interesting aspects of this case is that it involved a training of the *eye* in addition to a training of the hand. We have seen that a common criticism by those sceptical of the value of the microscope was that it led to solipsism: each observer exercised a unique microscopic vision. A prerequisite for the science of histology was the creation of a degree of perceptual consensus. Various pedagogic techniques were developed to meet this prerequisite. A favoured device among early histology teachers was to mount a microscope on a circular table and adjust the focus before allowing each student to look through the eyepiece. French lecturers, such as Magendie, also sought to circumvent the problem of the paucity of microscopes for student use by projecting magnified images on a wall (La Berge, 1994, p. 305). Microscopic observation was preceded and accompanied by verbal instruction by the teacher.

These mechanisms were also used in conjunction with schematic drawings designed as a further constraint upon the eye. Thus John Goodsir's (1814–67) class in practical histology at Edinburgh was accompanied by 'diagrams suspended on the wall' (Jacyna, 2001, p. 234). At a more advanced stage in his training, the microscopist was required to acquire a facility for drawing the microscopic structures observed (Fig. 1.5). These representations were subjected to the same scrutiny and critique as the student's verbal performances. The production of such drawings was also intended to address some of the problems of replicability confronting histology. It was, however, recognized that there was an irreducible subjective element in all such representations. From the 1840s, microphotography was hailed as a means of eliminating this human source of delusion and error (La Berge, 1994, p. 302–3).

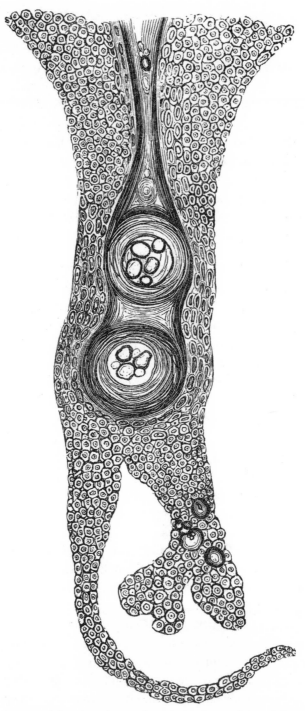

Fig. 1.5. Drawing of a histological section from Virchow's *Die Cellularpathologie* (1859), showing the cells of a cancerous epithelial tumour of the lip. *Source*: Rudolph Virchow, *Die Cellularpathologie*, Berlin, August Hirschwald, 1859. Wellcome Library Early Printed Books. *Credit*: Wellcome Library, London (L0031002).

The cases outlined in the preceding text also reveal the limitations of a purely Foucauldian approach. Foucault is noted for his 'antihumanism', that is, his determination to eschew the usual assumption that history is shaped by individuals or collections of individuals acting in accordance with some form of rationality. It is difficult, however, to write the history of the beginnings of laboratory medicine without reference to the entrepreneurial activities of, for example, Henle and Bennett who perceived the microscope as, among other things, an instrument for personal advancement. Put in more general terms, it is necessary to take account of the political economy of medicine and of individuals' efforts to adapt to the demands and to manipulate the possibilities of the particular market in which they seek to sell skills and services.

ENTREPRENEURIAL MEDICINE

The acknowledgment of these interpretative possibilities need not imply an essentialist view of human nature as inherently acquisitive or self-interested. Rather, the appearance of entrepreneurial activity in the medical sphere is symptomatic of a more general phenomenon in cultural formation during the nineteenth century, that is, a growing homogeneity in which economic rationality and market-driven behaviour became the norm in a multiplicity of contexts. Medical men were merely acquiescing in what was to become an all-encompassing tendency when they acted as if medical knowledge was a commodity to be made and traded like any other (Poovey, 1995, pp. 3–4).

These reflections give added significance to the activities of some of the medical 'firms' at work in the first half of the nineteenth century. These may be seen as analogous to forms of commercial organization typical of a relatively early stage of capitalist formation. A particularly interesting aspect of such entrepreneurship was that the search for competitive advantage often led to technological innovation. We have seen how this impacted upon the dissemination of microscopy. Market incentives also had an effect on the development of new forms of medical representation. Thus, in his efforts to consolidate his position as a lecturer within the relatively free market of the Edinburgh extramural school, John Thomson (1765–1846) pioneered the use of coloured depictions of disease to illustrate his lectures. One of his agents in this endeavour, (Sir) Robert Carswell (1793–1857), used an extensive collection of such illustrations to launch his own professorial career (Maulitz, 1987, pp. 219–23; Jacyna, 1994, pp. 132–3).

These illustrations purported to provide *typical* representations of particular conditions. As such, they claimed to supply a proxy for direct experience, or indeed a distillation of reality superior to direct contact with a pathology. These claims were by no means uncontroversial. The prominent anatomy teacher, Robert Knox, was scornful of what he called the 'Pictorial Anatomy School', which he maintained grossly misrepresented nature and which was no substitute for direct experience of the object concerned (Secord, 2002, p. 47). Such griping is indicative of the resentment and alarm these innovations provoked in those who lacked the expertise to compete directly with such techniques, or who had invested heavily in older forms of pedagogy.

The use of these images is exemplary of processes whereby knowledge claims and skills were translated into commodities possessing some market value. The ultimate source of these commodities was some version of the 'clinical encounter'. In the course of the transformations intervening between a bedside meeting in a Paris hospital and the display of an image at an Edinburgh or London lecture, the patient became a case, which was in turn rendered into a representative image. Individuality was progressively erased along with sovereignty over the body that was the original nidus of all these processes.

The activities of particular groups of doctors acting as entrepreneurs in the field of medical education, raises a number of more general considerations. In the first place, there is a need to take a more reflective stance to the popular notion of the 'medical marketplace'. There has been a tendency to take this as a given, reflecting certain irreducible aspects of medical practice. A more productive approach would be to ask when medical men in particular national and local contexts first began, primarily, to construct their identities in terms appropriated from the commercial sphere. That is, to see themselves as providers of clinical and other services within a cash nexus. It has been argued that entrepreneurial attitudes were widespread among British medical practitioners no later than the eighteenth century (Loudon, 1987, pp. 101–3). It is noteworthy that the period in which medical men become fully assimilated into the commercial sphere is also when they become increasingly concerned to retail images of themselves as scholars, scientists, and humanitarians. The ideological, mystifying function of such representations is obvious.

Resources for attempting such an analysis may be drawn from recent work in sociology of science that deals with the way in which identity is created through the active manipulation of various 'repertoires' available to actors in a particular setting (Lawrence and Shapin, 1998). This approach serves as a valuable corrective to a Foucauldian methodology that leaves little role for individual discretion and negotiation. A wide range of such repertoires was available to practitioners in the first half of the nineteenth century. These included philanthropic self-images, which often possessed some religious element. The incorporation of Quaker ideals into the persona of a practitioner, such as Thomas Hodgkin (1798–1866), provides an obvious example (Kass, 1988, *passim*). Civic humanist codes, as reinvigorated by the revolution in France, provided a more secular alternative within which to frame activity at least overtly directed to the benefit of some community, whether that be city, state, or nation. Such commitments shaded readily into political allegiances: there was, in particular, in several European countries during the first half of the nineteenth century, an association between medicine and radical and liberal causes.

The list could be extended. An especially significant repertoire, however, involved the assumption of a form of scientific persona. Any discussion of this topic must be prefaced by a recognition of the variety of activities that might be designated 'scientific' during this period. These include observational natural history in addition to experimental studies (Warner, 1985). All these forms of life, however, shared a common ethos: they demonstrated a commitment to the augmentation of knowledge. An important aspect of this scientific morality was that such investment of time and effort was purportedly *selfless* in the sense that it was not undertaken with a view to personal profit. In this respect, identification with the ideals of science was antithetical to the norms of the market. From a purely commercial viewpoint, time spent in scientific enquiry reduced potential earnings from clinical practice. When practitioners, such as John Hunter, sank a portion of their earnings into, for instance, the creation of extensive private museums, they were further reinforcing the ethos that subordinated the accumulation of wealth to higher ideals. Dedication to science was thus a token of a form of altruism. It bespoke a certain indifference, if not disdain, for material gain. It might be seen as gesturing towards the superiority of gentlemanly or scholarly codes over those of the mercantile classes.

Such identification may help to explain some of the ferocity of the priority disputes of the period, notably that between the Hunters and Alexander Monro (*secundus*, 1733–1817), and that between Charles Bell and Magendie. These were matters of *honour* in which personal reputation and *amour propre* was at stake. Such sensitivity to imputations about personal credit and credibility were critical to the representation of the natural philosopher as gentleman (Shapin, 1994, p. 407).

Analysis in terms of the adoption and adaptation by historical actors of the range of repertoires or identity envelopes available in a culture, yields valuable insights. But it also presents a number of possible pitfalls. Taken to the extreme, this interpretative mode leads to a free circulation of signifiers untrammelled by any material constraints. In other words, identity is simply a garment to be donned or exchanged at will, a view somewhat reminiscent of the philosophy of Herr Teufelsdröckh. It is, however, possible to combine these explanatory resources with more traditional historiographic approaches. Even in a postmodern world, there is, in particular, some merit in insisting on a distinction between base and superstructure.

Thus, the identity of an élite early-nineteenth-century practitioner, such as John Thomson, may be seen as composed of a number of repertoires. There is, for instance, an overtly political posture – he was pronounced in his allegiance to the Whig cause – in addition to being ostentatiously committed to the generation and promulgation of scientific knowledge. Important synergies can, moreover, be discerned between these different aspects of Thomson's persona: engagement in science was, in his context, endowed with political, as well as professional, significance. This was evinced by the patronage of these lectures by the members of the Whig literati. This complex of interrelated activities was constitutive of Thomson's public presentation of self. It is also possible to recover aspects of his more private persona as a husband and father.

A principle of subordination is, however, discernible within this network of identities. In particular, Thomson's efforts to strengthen his persona as a man of science served to further his reputation as a teacher. This had the immediate benefit of bolstering his position within the market for medical teaching in Edinburgh. In the longer term, it enhanced his chances of moving from the extramural school into the university medical faculty. His political allegiances were likewise crucial to professional advancement. Such concerns impinged even upon the domestic sphere. It is clear that Thomson regarded his sons as agents who, especially during their foreign travels, served his agenda through the accumulation of reports, representations, and artefacts that could enhance his academic standing. His sons were also clearly marked to inherit the material, political, and cultural capital that John Thomson had accumulated (Jacyna, 1994, pp. 148–54).

Disputes over priority of discovery may, as we have seen, manifest gentlemanly concern for personal honour and credibility. But they were no less disputes over *property* rights. Scientific investigation and achievement was of direct instrumental value to a medical teacher, such as Charles Bell. One of the advertised attractions of the lectures he offered to medical students was that they claimed to provide an exposition of new knowledge unavailable from any other source. Possession of a great discovery was, therefore, of direct advantage in a competitive pedagogic context. In Bell's case, the alleged discovery was of the distinct functions of the spinal nerve roots.

Again, these examples should not be construed as evidence for some necessary predominance of market rationality. They do indicate, however, that in the period in question it is possible to organize a wide range of presentations of self around a central entrepreneurial identity.

The social body

MEDICAL POLICE AND MEDICAL POLITICS

Attention has tended to centre upon the relatively small, specialized spaces, such as the hospital and the penitentiary, to which Foucault pays most attention. The localized nature of disciplinary power should not, however, obscure the fact that it serves, in aggregate, to govern populations *en masse*. Even in *The Birth of the Clinic*, Foucault discusses the subjection of wider social spaces to the medical gaze. A relatively neglected chapter of the book describes the creation of a new form of medical experience concerned with the health and sickness of populations.

A new medical consciousness emerged at the end of the eighteenth century that had as its object the comprehension and control of the epidemic and epizootic diseases that attacked large numbers of individuals and livestock. These outbreaks of disease were seen as unique historical events brought about by the intersection of a wide range of geographic, climactic, and demographic factors. This multiplicity demanded a collective effort – a 'multiple gaze' – to garner all the materials necessary to an understanding of the phenomenon (Foucault, 1973, p. 25). In the final years of the *ancien régime*, this gaze was institutionalized with the creation of the Société Royale de la Médecine, which superintended the activities of a corps of medical observers at work throughout the territory of the French Crown.

It is notable that in discussing these developments, Foucault pays more attention than usual to the role of the state in promoting medical interest in the health and disease of populations. He makes it clear, for instance, that the new medical experience that took form during this period was intended

81

to guide *interventions* of various kinds: 'A medicine of epidemics could exist only if supplemented by a police: to supervise the location of mines and cemeteries, to get as many corpses as possible cremated instead of buried, to control the sale of bread, wine, and meat, to supervise the running of abattoirs and dye works, and to prohibit unhealthy housing . . .' (p. 25). The doctors involved in this enterprise thus became servants of the state – a medical police.

An essential aspect of their activities was, moreover, to instil the population at large with an adequate understanding of the principles governing health and sickness. They were, in other words, obliged to assume an educational role. The efficacy of the new medical police was dependent upon the internalization by the population at large of certain hygienic doxa. Ultimately, each household and family member would become self-policing in matters of diet, dress, and manner of life.

Medicine thus acquired a political status inasmuch as it gained a new relevance to the interests of the state. These developments may be seen both as consequent upon some of the most prominent tropes of the Enlightenment thought, notably its interest in the well-being of the body, and as antecedent to the discourse of public health that flourished in the nineteenth century. Conversely, however, politics became medicalized. A novel interest in the bodily state of the nation emerged, a new sense that the state's responsibilities extended not only to the prevention of the causes and mitigation of the effects of disease, but also to maximising the health of the population; a responsibility that was increasingly seen to apply not only to the current generation, but to extend to future cohorts. Here were the seeds of later concerns with optimal motherhood and improvement of the racial stock that marked the nineteenth and twentieth centuries p. 327ff.

This discussion in *The Birth of the Clinic* of the growth of a medical police in late-eighteenth-century France shows the application of Foucauldian concepts to the history of what might loosely be called the *public sphere*. The medical gaze evolved during this period was intensely local, depending on representatives dispersed throughout the territory of the French Crown. However, channels of communication permitted the transmission of information accumulated by these sources to centres of reckoning. There was a tight relationship between knowledge and power inasmuch as information was sought as a prelude to intervention. But power was not manifest merely in the form of administrative action. The success of the strategies of hygiene was dependent on the internalization of certain rules of behaviour by the population at large.

Foucault elaborated on these themes in a later paper on 'The Politics of Health in the Eighteenth Century'. In particular, he qualified the centrality of the state to the rise of 'noso-politics'. The state was only one of a number of bodies active in developing strategies designed to address the increasingly exigent problematic of the health of the population. Rather than occurring as a result of a top-down directive, the new politics of health was manifest as 'the emergence at a multitude of sites in the social body of health and disease as problems requiring some form or other of collective control measures.' Lay and religious benevolent societies, in addition to learned societies and academies, were no less engaged in this enterprise; indeed, in some cases, it was the *raison d'être* of these bodies (Foucault, 1972, pp. 167–8).

In this essay, Foucault diverges from his customary reluctance to relate the institutional and intellectual developments with which he is concerned, to economic change. Noso-politics can only be understood as a response to the requirements of emergent capitalism. The demands of the labour market required a reevaluation of strategies for the management of poverty within society (Fig. 1.6). The immobilization of vast sums of

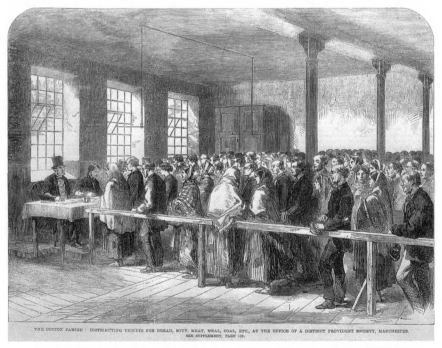

THE COTTON FAMINE : DISTRIBUTING TICKETS FOR BREAD, SOUP, MEAT, MEAL, COAL, ETC., AT THE OFFICE OF A DISTRICT PROVIDENT SOCIETY, MANCHESTER. SEE SUPPLEMENT, PAGE 556.

Fig. 1.6. Distributing tickets for food during the Lancashire cotton famine (1861–2) resulting from the American Civil War. There were 250,000 people supported by the rates and as many others helped by private charity. *Source*: *Illustrated London News*, 41 (1862), 541. *Credit*: Wellcome Library, London (L0004799).

capital in foundations designed to provide for the poor, was deemed to be economically wasteful. Instead, the poor should, as far as possible, be directed towards productive work. As part of this decomposition of traditional notions of poverty, the 'sick poor' acquired a novel identity and visibility.

The optimal management of the indigent sick for the purposes of the labour market was, however, not the most significant aspect of noso-politics. The maintenance and enhancement of the *health* of the population was the predominant concern. The state and its ancillary agencies were, in effect, expanding their traditional remit. No longer was the state merely concerned with the exercise of military force and the maintenance of civil order. In the course of the eighteenth century, 'we find a further function emerging, that of the disposition of society as a milieu of physical well-being, health and optimal longevity' (Foucault, 1972, p. 170). In short, by the end of the eighteenth century, the *body*, in all its material aspects, had become a politicized object.

Urban spaces were seen as especially in need of urgent scrutiny and intervention. Cities were at once most menacing as depositories of disorder of all kinds, including the disorder of chronic and epidemic disease. At the same time, they were, however, also perceived as more malleable than other environments. As man-made habitats they were amenable to correction through administrative interventions guided by enlightened principles. Systems of medical police elaborated earlier in the eighteenth century for the management of smaller, specialized spaces, such as ships and army camps, provided a template for these more ambitious strategies.

In the pursuit of this goal, systems of surveillance on a grand scale were instituted. The medical profession was uniquely placed to serve as the agents for elaborating the understanding of the conditions of health that power now demanded. This medical discourse was, however, inseparable from the concurrent wider analysis of the economics of assistance. Foucault calls this a 'medico-administrative' knowledge. The entire edifice of what in the nineteenth century came to be known as the *social* or *human sciences* rested on similar foundations.

With remarkable economy Foucault places the transformations that he described in *The Birth of the Clinic* within this larger context. He denied that the private, individualized clinical encounter possesses historical priority and that collective medicine somehow evolved from it. On the contrary, both the private and the public sphere of modern medicine emerged concurrently in response to imperatives that were at root economic.

The reform of the hospital that took place at the turn of the nineteenth century was thus intended to make these institutions more serviceable to the ends of noso-politics, especially in relation to the efficient management of the urban population. The hospital was expected to cease to be an instrument of assistance and to become a machine for restoring the sick poor to productive health. To this end, it was to articulate with other aspects of the health apparatus, such as dispensaries and domiciliary care. It was also charged with the development of more effective understanding and treatment of disease. The hospital was, moreover, through its educational function, to serve as the nidus for the production of new medical personnel adequate to the needs of society. These demands provide the true background to the birth of the clinic.

Foucault's work on governmentality provides important insights into medical interventions in public health in the first half of the nineteenth century. During this period, in the name of increased productivity and security, a distinctly 'social' space was configured, one that was deemed to be autonomous of the economic and political realms. The discourse constituting the social was peculiarly preoccupied with the physical characteristics of the population and, in particular, of the 'poor' who were conceptualized as an especially problematic group. While investigations into the social were thus focused upon the corporeal characteristics of the individuals forming certain segments of the population, it also displayed a marked tendency to abstraction. Concrete bodies were translated into aggregates and exemplary types through various forms of representation, notably through statistical analysis, and the deployment of tables, diagrams, and maps (Poovey, 1995, p. 31). This tendency might be compared to the movement discussed in the preceding text towards the transformation of the individual patient into a typical case by means of a battery of technologies of representation.

This movement can be characterized as medical in character because it mirrored the morphology of the clinical gaze. The development of technologies of surveillance, accounting, and numeration served to make the health of the poor *visible* and thus subject to governance. The strategy of abstraction was, however, characteristic of a wide range of discourses that appeared in the aftermath of the Scientific Revolution. These strategies emerged in parallel with the evolving needs of modern governments to conceptualize their domains in ways that would facilitate the collection of revenue and the maintenance of order (Olson, 1993, Ch. 5). Medicine was, in this, as in other areas, caught up in this disseminated rationality of domination. Its major contribution was to facilitate the naturalization of the abstract spaces that were in the process of formation.

SANITARIANISM

It is important to note that although doctors played a part in the elaboration and implementation of this strategy, medical qualifications were, at least in Britain, not a prerequisite in the first half of the nineteenth century. Edwin Chadwick (1800–90), whose *Sanitary Report* of 1842 was among the outstanding instances of sanitarianism, was not a doctor; he was, indeed, sceptical about the relevance of medicine, narrowly conceived, to the endeavour. Chadwick trained as a lawyer and worked for a time as a journalist. His political associations were of more importance than his professional qualifications for determining his impact on public life in Victorian Britain. He was a close associate of Jeremy Bentham (1748–1832) and other prominent advocates of philosophical radicalism. The school of political thinking to which Chadwick belonged was known as 'utilitarianism', the principal tenet of which was that society should be reorganized in a way that would maximise the general well-being while militating against the baleful effects of sectional interests. This political orientation was evinced by Chadwick's writings in the *Westminster Review* and his membership of the London Debating Society, a well-known gathering place for the devotees of utilitarianism. Less important than the direct involvement of medical personnel, however, was the growing prominence of the metaphor of the 'social body' – one that invited the application of quasi-clinical reasoning to the management of large populations (Poovey, 1995, pp. 37–8).

Sanitarianism became most fully developed in Britain in the first half of the nineteenth century. Britain was the first industrial nation and thus was in the forefront of dealing with the problems of maintaining the health of large, and growing, urban populations. These problems were at one level technical, involving the provision of adequate water and sewage facilities for city dwellers. But sanitarianism always possessed a more or less explicit political agenda. It formed part of a concerted effort by the governing classes to confront and manage the threats and challenges posed by the 'poor' and, in particular, by the urban working class. The more discursive aspects of these strategies were couched in a language of technical managerial rationality, of which utilitarianism constituted the type. This language served, among other purposes, to obscure the class interests at work in the social policy of the period.

Within the ruling discourse the proletariat was identified as a source of disorder. This might take the form of overt political and industrial unrest, a concern that became especially marked with the rise of the Chartist movement in the 1830s, which among other things demanded universal male suffrage. Parliamentary reform was, moreover, seen as the first step to thoroughgoing social and economic change. Some of the more extreme Chartists were advocates of 'physical force' as a means of gaining their ends; others expressed sophisticated socialist views. Chartism was strongest in towns and cities, including both old declining and new rising industrial centres. But the urban poor were also seen as a source of disorder within the social body because individually and collectively they engendered and spread disease.

Sanitarian views of the causes and transmission of disease may be characterized as strongly environmentalist. Thus, diseases, such as tuberculosis, which were endemic during the period, were linked to the living and working conditions of those most prone to the condition. 'Modern natural science,' Friedrich Engels wrote, 'has proved that the so-called "poor districts" in which the workers are crowded together are the breeding places of all those epidemics which from time to time afflict our towns. Cholera, typhus, typhoid fever, small-pox and other ravaging diseases spread their germs in the pestilential air and the poisoned water of these working-class quarters.' The remedy was, accordingly, to ensure that living and working spaces were clean, well lit, and properly ventilated. Fever was also a prominent concern of early-nineteenth-century sanitarians. In particular, the growing incidence of typhus appeared to be related to the condition of the new industrial centres, although it was at least as prevalent in parts of the countryside (Hamlin, 1998, pp. 63–4). Although predisposition to fever, and the origins of outbreaks were also seen to depend largely upon environmental factors, its contagious character was acknowledged.

The boundaries between locale and the bodies that occupied that space were, however, so weak as to sometimes be invisible. Thus, the dominant sanitarian theory of disease aetiology was miasmatist: that is, the theory that noxious air caused those who came into contact with it to fall sick. Much attention was accordingly devoted to the elimination of cesspits and accumulations of decaying organic matter that might poison the air of a neighbourhood. But, conversely, exhalations *from* a morbid body could infect a locale and spread disease to others. Thus, Bartholomew Parr (1750–1810) maintained that fever could be generated spontaneously where bodies were closely confined in insalubrious conditions, adding that:

'When the fever is actually formed, it is well known that it may be communicated by its effluvia' (p. 65).

Working-class neighbourhoods and their inhabitants were particularly liable to be pathogenic because of the poor's ignorance of sound hygienic principles. The squalid conditions in which they lived had a depressing effect on mind as well as body. Through the mediation of the nervous system, such mental 'depression' could also increase susceptibility to illness. The infections they produced could not, however, be confined to these areas: there was a risk if not a probability that they would spread to the respectable middle-class members of society. The prevalence of consumption, even among the most respectable sections of society, bore out this fear.

Previous generations might have assumed that as the rich and poor possessed different physiologies, so were they prone to divergent pathology. One of the outcomes of the dominant liberal ideology of the early nineteenth century was a greater sense of equality between members of society, whatever their social station. One unfortunate consequence of this human commonalty was that the humblest could potentially infect the loftiest citizen. The essentially ideological character of liberal notions was, however, registered through the widespread recognition that this putative equal right to disease was, in practice, modified by differential susceptibility dependent on income and living conditions.

The Sanitarians, therefore, felt obliged to police both the spaces inhabited by the poor and their bodies. The perceived need to address the first set of problems led to increased government involvement during the mid-nineteenth century in the field of public health. A series of Acts of Parliament were passed defining the responsibilities of local and central authorities to remove nuisances and other preventable causes of disease. This legislation was part of a wider programme of measures designed to address the perceived problem of poverty. These relationships were embodied in the person of Chadwick, the leading figure in the implementation of sanitary reform.

Chadwick began his career as a public servant in the capacity of an assistant commissioner appointed in 1832 by the Whig government to investigate the workings of the Poor Law. The enquiry was triggered by the 'Captain Swing' riots of 1830 in protest at high prices and lack of employment among rural labourers. In part, the impetus for a reform of the Poor Law arose from a desire to make the relief system a more effective instrument of social control that would prevent future disturbances of this kind. But a much wider range of considerations was also relevant to the measure that was to emerge from these deliberations.

POVERTY, DISEASE, AND POLITICAL ECONOMY

Early-nineteenth-century debates over the propriety of providing relief for the poor were overshadowed by the work of Thomas Malthus (1766–1834), who in his *Essay on Population* (first edition, 1798), had argued that there was an inexorable tendency for increase in population to outstrip growth in food supply. Indiscriminate distribution of relief to the lower classes would merely encourage them to produce more children, leading eventually to a demographic crisis. Disease, along with starvation, was the chief means by which 'nature' would reduce population to a level consistent with the supply of sustenance. The political economist David Ricardo (1772–1823) reinforced Malthus's argument against the poor laws, arguing that they served merely to divert money from the industrious to the idle.

The Poor Law Amendment Act of 1834 was, in part, intended to address such concerns. The legislation applied utilitarian reasoning to the question of poor relief in a doctrinaire fashion. It imposed much more stringent conditions for the receipt of relief from public funds than the system it replaced. Outdoor relief was abolished; paupers would have to enter a workhouse to receive aid. These were to be so unattractive as to ensure that the principle of 'least eligibility' would apply. In the words of the Royal Commission report, 'Every penny bestowed that tends to render the condition of the pauper more eligible than that of the independent labourer, is a bounty on indolence and vice.' Only those who truly had no other resort would seek assistance from this source. The new Poor Law was, above all, orientated towards ensuring that all but the most destitute would prefer the demands of the labour market to reliance on government relief. Chadwick was among the principal authors of the new legislation. He was largely responsible for the organization of Boards of Guardians throughout the country, each with its own medical officer.

The system of union workhouses established under the new poor law was to have important implications for medicine in Britain. Among those housed in these institutions were significant numbers who required medical attention; in the decades following the introduction of the act, the proportion of ill and infirm inmates grew. By mid-century, the rate of mortality in some workhouses had risen to an alarming level. Tuberculosis was, in particular, rampant in these institutions. It therefore became necessary for infirmaries to be attached to workhouses. Eventually, these infirmaries were to house more patients than the voluntary hospitals. The Poor Law infirmaries also created employment opportunities for a significant number of medical men drawn from the local population of general practitioners. Indirectly, the state thus became, for the first time, a major source of civilian employment for members of the medical profession.

Following outbreaks of influenza and typhoid in 1837 and 1838, Chadwick, again at the bidding of the government, turned his attention to questions of sanitation. He was drawn to the issue by sound utilitarian reasoning. Chadwick had observed that many of the destitute poor were driven to the poorhouse because of illness; sanitary measures should, therefore, serve to relieve demand upon the new system while maximising the number of fit workers available to the economy. To further this end, Chadwick appointed three doctors; Neil Arnott (1788–1874), James Philip Kay-Shuttleworth (1804–77), and Thomas Southwood-Smith (1788–1861) – political fellow travellers all – to investigate the causes of disease in the London districts. These enquiries were subsequently extended to other British cities. Chadwick's investigations pioneered technologies that were to become definitive of subsequent social investigations: notably, the house-to-house survey and compilations of statistics that purported to provide an objective representation of the state of the neighbourhoods surveyed. Chadwick was also instrumental in the introduction of the Registration Act in 1836. This called for the recording of the causes of death and thus provided an important additional resource for gaining knowledge of patterns of morbidity within the population.

Medical men played a prominent part in the development of these new techniques for knowing the social body. Indeed, this tradition might be traced back to the 'social anatomy' of the physician, William Petty, in the seventeenth century. In the nineteenth century it was, however, the Belgian mathematician and astronomer Adolphe Quetelet (1796–1874) who provided modern statistics with crucial techniques and concepts. In particular, Quetelet sought to establish the means of defining the 'average' or 'normal' human, which enabled authoritative statements about the incidence in a population of the abnormal and pathological.

Inspired by a visit by Quetelet to England to demonstrate his methods to members of the British Association for the Advancement of Science, Charles Babbage and others, in 1834, founded the London Statistical Society. Some medical men were prominent in the work of the society in its early years, exploring various aspects of morbidity and mortality. It should be noted, however, that these were medical men acting as individuals with their own particular concerns and agendas. The profession as a whole did not assume any collective role in the pursuit of public health.

Chadwick's 1842 report on 'The Sanitary Condition of the Labouring Population of Great Britain', which was published at his own expense, reaffirmed the sanitarian doctrine that environmental conditions were key to the health of the population. It is striking, however, how much of Chadwick's report is devoted to the character and mores of the proletariat, including worrying signs of an incipient class-consciousness. It must, therefore, be regarded as a 'political document' (Hamlin, 1998, p. 157). In particular, Chadwick's strategy was to redefine the problem of poverty in narrow technical terms that precluded any more radical consideration of the relations of social conditions and disease. Part of his hostility to the involvement of the medical profession in this field derived from the fact that some of its more radical members, such as Thomas Wakley, editor of the *Lancet*, had begun to ask probing questions about the impact of the draconian New Poor Law on the health of the poor. It has been noted that Chadwick's most effective means to accomplishing this strategy was not through an overt polemic against those whose views he wished to demolish, but by an ostentatious display of a laborious 'empiricism' that purported to be independent of any political presupposition or agenda.

Crucially, Chadwick maintained that disease was a cause of poverty. He denied the converse proposition with all its disturbing political implications. His position was challenged by the Scottish physician William Pulteney Alison, who was far more sensitive to the wider social conditions that fostered the incidence of disease and death among the deprived. Alison noted, for instance, that contagious fever was far more common among the destitute inhabitants of Scottish cities, who then proceeded to spread the affliction wherever they wandered. Alison also recognised that the distinction between the 'deserving' and 'undeserving' poor, often made during this period, was specious. Given the fluctuations of the market, workers could no more avoid unemployment than disease. Once deprived of an income, moreover, they fell easy prey to a variety of illnesses, which further reduced their ability to fend for themselves.

Alison refuted the conventional Malthusian view of the relationship between population growth and the generosity of public provision for the poor. In fact, the poor were most likely to produce children in environments where least was done to relieve their condition. Alison cited the dire state of the people of Ireland, where there was no state assistance for the poor, as the classic instance of this correlation. Alison was no revolutionary; he called for the establishment in Scotland of a somewhat more humane version of the English New Poor Law: workhouses were to be complemented by a network of fever hospitals. Housing the destitute in some central location would, among other things, limit the spread of fever. In what was a radical departure from the Scottish tradition of voluntary charitable provision for the poor, the new system was to be funded by the state. Nonetheless, his writings of the 1840s have been described as marking 'the epitome of a medical critique of industrialism and capitalism the like of which did not reappear until the twentieth century' (Hamlin, 1998, p. 81).

Chadwick's views can also be contrasted with the earlier investigations of Louis René Villermé (1782–1863), a French doctor who had, in the 1820s, addressed the question of differential mortality within the different districts of Paris. Villermé first attempted to explain these discrepancies by reference to such environmental factors as location, meteorological conditions, and population density. Eventually, however, none of these seemed to provide an adequate explanation. He concluded that mortality could be directly correlated to income; the wealthy enjoyed a far higher life expectancy than the poor inhabitants of a neighbouring *arrondissement*. Death, in short, was a 'social disease' (Coleman, 1982). In the United States, the bookseller and publisher, Lemuel Shattuck (1793–1859), undertook comparable studies in Boston, which linked mortality and the incidence of communicable diseases to living conditions.

Villermé did not, however, draw radical political conclusions from his observations, although his research into the conditions in the French cotton industry was instrumental in the introduction, in 1841, of legislation to regulate child labour. His work coincided with the beginnings of a socialist movement in France and was, in fact, orientated toward promoting solutions that would preserve the existing order (Barnes, 1995, p. 32). Villermé maintained that the best remedy for the high morbidity and mortality of the poor was for them to be trained by their social betters to higher standards of hygiene. Others preferred to continue to stress the decisive influence of the classic nonnaturals upon susceptibility to disease, and so direct attention away from economic considerations. As we shall see, this strategy was also favoured by the British sanitarians.

There were, however, dissidents from this characteristic bourgeois defensive posture; notably, the German doctor Rudolph Virchow's analysis of the causes and remedies of illness among the most impoverished sections of society. Virchow, another student of Johannes Müller, had, in 1848, been commissioned by the Prussian government to investigate an outbreak of typhus fever in Upper Silesia, a particularly deprived region. Virchow's report, which was in many respects modelled on earlier British and French surveys, concluded that the medical state of the Silesians could not be separated from their wider political, social, and even cultural circumstances. He declared, for instance, that 'the proletariat is the result, principally, of the introduction and improvement of machinery ... shall the triumph of human genius lead to nothing more than to make the human race miserable?' Virchow's prescription to improve the health of this oppressed population was to demand extensive social and political reform.

Despite these insights, and his avowedly progressive political posture, Virchow's account of the inhabitants of Upper Silesia displays a characteristic middle-class revulsion, even horror, at the mores and bodily condition of a people whom he clearly found profoundly alien. He deplored their lack of personal hygiene complaining that the Silesian left 'it to celestial providence to free his body occasionally by a heavy shower of rain from the crusts of dirt accumulated on it.' The Silesians' addiction to drink, 'canine subservience', and indifference to bourgeois values, such as thrift and accumulation, likewise provoked Virchow's incredulity and disgust (McNeeley, 2002, p. 14).

Special local circumstances coloured this account: Upper Silesia was a recent addition to the dominions of the Prussian state. Its inhabitants were of Polish stock and fervently Roman Catholic – the latter characteristic was particularly obnoxious to Virchow. However, a similar sense of the poor as utterly other, as a race apart, can be found in other contemporaneous accounts by middle-class visitors to the more deprived areas of cities such as London, Manchester, and Paris. In the British case, the Irish were similarly seen as an alien racial group that was deemed to pose special public health problems because of their atavistic habits and mentality. In Belgium, the Walloons entertained a similar opinion of the Flemings.

In Virchow's view, only thoroughgoing reform could remove the conditions that allowed disease to spread and claim so many lives. He maintained that the medical profession was the natural champion of such backward and oppressed sections of society. Virchow's forays into the realm of public health are further illustrations of the liberal leanings of some medical men during this period. Eight days after his return to Berlin from Silesia, Virchow further demonstrated those commitments by playing a modest part in the Revolution of March 1848. His contribution to the revolutionary cause was, however, constrained by his failure, despite strenuous efforts, to obtain a working firearm.

His recommendations may, however, also be viewed as heralding a technocratic rationality that sought to ameliorate social problems through the application of specialized skill and knowledge by suitably trained experts. Virchow's was, in other words, a 'political medicine'. In Britain, public health was no less political; in the first half of the nineteenth century, however, medical men, with some significant exceptions, were less prominent in this endeavour. There was no *professional* identification with the cause of reform and scientific management.

Chadwick's solution to the problems of public health was also essentially technocratic. However, he assigned far more importance to engineering than to medical expertise in this field on the grounds that 'filth' was the true source of disease. His recommendations led to the 1848 Public Health Act, which created a Central Board of Health responsible for such matters as sewage, water supply, and street cleaning. Local boards of health were also to be set up, with funding for improvements to come from the rates. The government of the time was prompted to implement these measures in part because of an outbreak of cholera in Britain in 1847–8 (Fig. 1.7). The

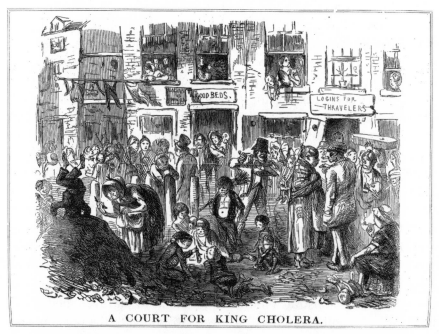

A COURT FOR KING CHOLERA.

Fig. 1.7. 'A Court for King Cholera'. Cartoon characterizing the sanitarian preoccupation with filth and muck in overcrowded city slums, to which the poor were often held to be indifferent. *Source*: Punch, 23 (1852), 139. *Credit*: Wellcome Library, London (L0003001).

act was, however, somewhat limited in its extent; London was, for example, excluded from its scope. Nonetheless, it provided the prototype for more inclusive legislation later.

At the same time as the state was seeking to ensure maximum productivity of the working-class population through reform of the system of poor relief, it thus sought to limit the disruption to economic activity caused by outbreaks of disease. Chadwick was, moreover, quite explicit that sanitary science also formed part of a wider strategy designed to contain social disorder.

To be fully effective, however, noso-politics, as Foucault pointed out, required the internalization of sound sanitary principles by the poor. In this campaign of health education, the state largely relied upon the efforts of private philanthropy. The discourse about the improvement of the poor that developed in conjunction with these efforts was characterized by a blurring of any distinction between moral and physical welfare. At the very least, bodily health was dependent upon a thorough reform of manners, habits, and attitudes. In the name of hygiene, sanitarianism thus sought to remake the minds of the poor.

The family, as Foucault pointed out, was the key site for these interventions. The state, in other words, did not disdain to notice what was occurring in each household; indeed, each body within that household became an object of government. What Mary Poovey calls the 'sanitary ideal' acted as an agent of normalization that ascribed roles to working-class people of both sexes, modelled upon idealized notions of middle-class behaviour. Women were seen as particularly susceptible to socialization of this kind. They were stereotyped as essentially domestic beings whose being was coextensive with motherhood and nurturing. This stereotype, of course, ignored the vital role played by women in industrial production. Because of this emphasis upon the corporeal, they depended on men for economic sustenance. While this vision confined women (at least notionally) to the household, it also constrained male roles in politically significant ways. The sanitary ideal stipulated that the workingman's primary attachment should be to the wife and family that depended upon him. It militated against forms of homosociability in which political associations and consciousness might be forged. Sanitarianism sought, in other words, to neuter any incipient working-class political culture (Poovey, 1995, pp. 123–5).

Efforts to extend a system of surveillance and police throughout a newly conceived social space were, however, never fully implemented. It is necessary to complement Foucauldian notions of the tendency to total control inherent in modern disciplinary regimes, with a recognition that local circumstances tended to impede and qualify the extension of the governmental gaze. In the case of medicine, older codes based, for instance, on forms of religious doctrine, were a hindrance to the dominance of this rationality. Vested interests, such as private water companies and landlords, mobilized opposition in Britain to the encroachments of a 'despotic' central government hindering the implementation of sanitarian measures. Indeed, Chadwick was soon forced out of office.

Moreover, the representation of society as a body in need of constant care created scope for a more extensive female role than an essentially patriarchal discourse could envisage or countenance. While the early-nineteenth-century movement for improvement in public health has received much attention from historians, the gendered politics of sanitarianism has, until recently, been overlooked. Such a perspective does, however, reveal some of the basic contradictions inherent in the discourse. In the words of Alison Bashford, 'in a range of ways, sanitary reform was never really settled as a masculine or feminine domain' (Bashford, 1998, p. 1). The most notable figures in the public health movement of this period were all men. Because of the centrality of the domestic in sanitarian programmes of improvement, women were, however, necessarily ascribed a key role in the implementation of sanitary measures. In the ideology of separate spheres that emerged in conjunction with capitalist modes of production, women were charged with the maintenance of the home. Crucially, this involved not only the upkeep of the domestic space, but also of the *bodies* within it. The boundary between these two responsibilities was, moreover, blurred: 'sanitary reformers wrote of bodies as houses to be kept clean and pure, and of houses as bodies to be purified and sanitized along the same hygienic principles' (Bashford, 1998, p. 2).

Working-class women were perhaps the most obvious agents of improvement, as the living spaces of the poor were viewed as, *par excellence*, both problem and solution. But 'respectable' women were also expected to play a role as educators; they were particularly well equipped to convey proper hygienic principles to the poor. They were, in effect, expected to impose middle-class standards of morality and cleanliness on those most in need of reformation. These women were, of course, supposed to perform this function under the supervision of men. In practice, however, they were able to assume a considerable degree of authority within the sanitarian movement, as they did within the charitable programmes of the period.

Conclusion

In his account of the defining characteristics of modernity, Jean Baudrillard has drawn attention to the novel mobility of signs and representations that followed the bourgeois revolution of the eighteenth century. The old society in which each person, at least all those who possessed personality, was attached to some fixed rank or order in society, was replaced by one where each individual was, in principle, equal and endowed with inalienable human rights. These rights inhered in the individual; they did not depend upon any particular social station. This transition led to an unprecedented social fluidity, one that was especially marked in the sphere of symbolic exchange. According to Baudrillard: 'There is no such thing as fashion in a society of caste and rank, since one is assigned a place irrevocably, and so class mobility is non-existent. An interdiction protects the signs and assures them a total clarity; each sign then refers unequivocally to a status . . . In caste societies, feudal or archaic, *cruel* societies, the signs are limited in number, and are not widely diffused, each one functions with its full value as interdiction, each is a reciprocal obligation between castes, clans or persons' (Baudrillard, 1983, p. 84).

Setting aside the characteristic hyperbole, this passage casts light on some of the principal themes of this chapter. In particular, it provides a vantage point from which to consider the apparent paradox that, at the same time as the medical profession, in common with the rest of Western society, was experiencing profound change and upheaval it manifested a novel preoccupation with tradition.

Baudrillard's remarks may be juxtaposed with a famous passage from the *Communist Manifesto* in which Marx sought to identify the essence of modern bourgeois society: 'All that is solid melts into air, all that is holy is profaned, and men at last are forced to face with sober senses the real conditions of their lives and their relations with their fellow men.' This passage has, with some plausibility been portrayed as an early example of a typically modernist vision (Berman, 1983, p. 89). But it also finds an echo in the sociologist Max Weber's (1864–1920) notion of *Entzauberung*, usually translated as 'disenchantment'. If the world was robbed of any numinous element, if social relations were simply a matter of human contrivance rather than divine decree, if all men were indeed equally endowed with rights, then why should any particular distribution of power and wealth be deemed legitimate and fated to endure?

The radical answer to this question was that established institutions were liable to be swept away in the name of reason and justice. Whatever arrangements failed to meet these criteria, or their second cousin 'utility', should be ruthlessly extirpated. For all its failures and disappointments, the French Revolution made it possible to think of society as historical and of even the most venerable regime as time-limited. The Industrial Revolution, for its part, notwithstanding the laments of nineteenth-century conservative organicists, facilitated the notion that societies were constructs, manufactured items, which were made, scrapped, and rebuilt according to immediate needs, demands, and even tastes.

We have seen that medical men were thrust willy-nilly into this world of flux and dissolution. They evinced its values when they created a market for medical services in which success depended upon entrepreneurial skill. By 1800, the old hierarchy of physicians, surgeons, and apothecaries, each with their place in a fixed cosmos, a 'society of caste and rank', had been overthrown. In Britain, it was replaced by a microcosm of the new world order, with an élite minority exploiting a medical proletariat. But the British example is also interesting because the Royal Colleges, the most visible representatives of the world that was lost, survived and flourished. Indeed, they served to further the processes of oppression and expropriation that sustained the medical political economy.

They were also the centres for the ritual celebration of the past: for a tireless, if sometimes tiresome, insistence on continuity and community. Thus, purportedly, all surgeons were bound together by a shared heritage, a common identity that transcended any immediate and local differences. The dignified opulence of the Hunterian Oration, the insistence that true surgeons worthy of that tradition were gentlemen and thus above the sordid concerns of the market, served to obscure the real conditions of contemporary medical labour. Thus, a representation of a world that was past and yet present, worked to restore something of the sacred to the profanity of a capitalist society.

As Baudrillard points out, however, another feature of modernity is that the exclusivity and paucity of signs that marked archaic societies is replaced by a 'proliferation of signs on demand'. It is no longer possible for any one élite to impose an exclusivity or monopoly in the symbolic real. Thus, multiple representations of the past are generated to suit different agendas.

A more radical stratagem was to disdain all reference to tradition. Current social arrangements were to be judged by other criteria, notably those of efficiency and function. By those standards it could, for instance, be asserted that a general practitioner was, due to his very versatility, a better, because more adaptable, doctor than a 'pure' physician or surgeon, however exalted their proffered pedigree. On *such* criteria he should, therefore, be entrusted with the government of the profession.

Although the terms can serve as serviceable shorthand, it is somewhat misleading to call the entrenched élites of nineteenth-century medicine 'conservative' or 'reactionary'. The traditionalist trappings they affected, notwithstanding, these cadres were distinctively modern in terms of the economic relations they embodied. Moreover, one of the most interesting features of the first half of the nineteenth century was the close association of sections of the medical profession with what may broadly be described as 'progressive' political causes. This correlation was especially marked in continental Europe. There were, of course, also medical radicals in Britain and North America. Thomas Wakley, for example, did not confine himself to inveighing against the abuses of the medical corporations – a cause, it should be noted, that he pursued even at the risk of personal injury from police truncheons. When, in 1835, he was elected Radical Member of Parliament for Finsbury, his maiden speech was a defence of the Tolpuddle Martyrs. Wakley also espoused the campaign for parliamentary reform and other Radical causes. He even defended the Chartist movement, although he did not agree with all its demands. Wakley's view on the utilitarian authors of the new Poor Law was that: 'they would have gone on and ground the bones of the poor, and used them for manure if they thought it would enrich the soil.' His associate, the surgeon Joseph Hume (1777–1855), was an even more avid Radical.

It was the peculiar conditions of the continental states, however, that provided the most favourable conditions for medical men to assume the role of champions of social and political progress. France lagged behind Britain in terms of industrialization for most of the nineteenth century. The revolution had, in fact, served to consolidate the position of the peasantry. Nonetheless, French society was most under the thrall of the cash nexus during this period; almost anything could be bought at the right price. In the German states, the landed interest continued to be politically predominant, though increasingly challenged by an urban bourgeoisie convinced that tomorrow belonged to them.

The position of the medical profession in these regions also differed in significant respects from the British case. There was, in particular, a greater dependence upon the state. In France, after a period of near anarchy in the 1790s, medical practitioners were licensed and regulated by the state. The French model was exported to several of the countries that were incorporated into Napoleon's empire. These included some of the German provinces where many doctors were employed as civil servants. In Prussia, there was a strong link between medicine and the military that was to prove remarkably persistent.

Despite these regional variations, certain common features are evident. In France and Germany, as in Britain, a binary division developed. A small élite occupied the commanding heights of the profession through its control of academic and hospital positions. This group, in effect, defined standards for the profession as a whole. Beneath them lay more numerous practitioners, but a less prestigious and more poorly remunerated corps of medical foot soldiers.

It is notable that medical liberals of the period, such as Paul Broca and Rudolf Virchow, aspired and eventually belonged to the élite of the profession in their respective nations. They saw no contradiction between this status and the progressive views they propounded. They could trace their lineage back to the prominent role medical men had played in the great French Revolution of 1789. As one physician-revolutionary had declared: 'Who then should denounce tyrants to mankind if not the doctors . . . who each day contemplate the human miseries that have no other origin but tyranny and slavery?' (Brockliss and Jones, 1997, p. 805). Also notable is the intimacy between their self-image as doctors and the political persona they assumed. Thus Virchow declared himself to be someone: 'whose medical beliefs fuse with his political and social ones. As a natural scientist I can be but a republican. The republic is the only form in which the claims, derived from the laws of nature and the nature of man, can be realized' (Ackerknecht, 1953, p. 16).

Also noteworthy is that Virchow took it for granted that being a doctor was synonymous with being a natural scientist. This implied that the medical liberal approached social issues with a distinct scientific perspective: one that was truly objective because purportedly free from class or factional bias. By virtue of this rationality, he was therefore uniquely equipped to contribute to political debate. In particular, the doctor was represented as a master of a form of *natural* knowledge. His understanding of the world could thus be opposed to the supernatural claims that still served to underpin archaic institutions, beliefs, and practices. This ideological antagonism was an especially marked feature of predominantly Roman Catholic countries where there was a long-standing association between established religion and political reaction.

The first half of the nineteenth century thus saw two apparently contradictory tendencies. On the one hand, the medical professions throughout Europe showed a growing concern to establish their place within a tradition that might reach back as far as Hippocrates. In terms of the great ideological divide that was the consequence of the revolution in France, they were thus firmly in the conservative Burkean camp. On the other hand, medical men were prominent in progressive movements that declared an avowed indifference, if not antipathy, to the legacy of the past. For them, 'tradition' was a dirty word.

The antinomy was more apparent than real. All these strategies should be viewed as attempts to adapt to, and perhaps even modify, the bewildering flux of events in which the medical profession was obliged to operate during these decades. A desire to assert continuity with the past amid this tumult served a range of interests. But another and, in the long run, perhaps more significant strategy, was for medical men to represent themselves as in the vanguard of progress – as the shock troops of the bourgeois revolution.

Chronological table for chapter 2:
1850–1913

Year	Medical events	Contemporary events	Nobel prize in physiology or medicine
1850			
1851	Ophthalmoscope invented by Hermann von Helmholtz; Pravaz introduces hypodermic syringe	Great Exhibition (London)	
1852	Antonius Mathijsen introduces plaster-of-paris bandages	Louis-Napoleon declares himself emperor Napoleon III	
1853	Smallpox vaccination made compulsory in England; John Snow administers chloroform to Queen Victoria for birth of Prince Leopold; first successful abdominal hysterectomy	Crimean War begins; David Livingstone begins explorations in Africa	
1854	John Snow closes the Broad Street Pump in London		
1855	Thomas Addison describes the hormone deficiency disease resulting from the malfunction of adrenal glands ('Addison's disease')		
1856	Introduction of the binaural stethoscope	End of Crimean War	

Year	Medical events	Contemporary events	Nobel prize in physiology or medicine
1857		Rebellion in British India	
1858	Medical Register and General Medical Council set up in Britain by Medical Reform Act; First Edition of *Gray's Anatomy*; Rudolf Virchow's *Cellularpathologie*		
1859		Publication of Charles Darwin's *Origin of Species*; first internal combustion engine	
1860	Etienne-Jules Marey introduces modern sphygmograph		
1861	Louis Pasteur discovers anaerobic bacteria	Outbreak of American Civil War; Italy unified under rule of Victor Emmanuel of Sardinia	
1862	Nightingale Nursing School founded at St. Thomas's Hospital, London		
1863	Fourth cholera pandemic begins	National Academy of Sciences founded in the United States	
1864	International Red Cross founded		
1865	Joseph Lister introduces phenol (carbolic acid) as a disinfectant in surgery; Jean-Antionne Villemin shows tuberculosis can be transferred by inoculation	End of American Civil War and of Slavery in the United States; Gregor Mendel's Plant Hybridity	
1866			

Year	Medical events	Contemporary events	Nobel prize in physiology or medicine
1867	First international medical congress in Paris	Russia sells Alaska to the United States; Dominion of Canada established; Karl Marx's *Das Kapital*	
1868	J. M. Charcot describes multiple sclerosis		
1869	Jacques Reverdin describes skin grafting; Sophia Jex-Blake matriculates in medicine at the University of Edinburgh (University reverses decision in 1873)	Suez Canal opens	
1870	Thomas Allbutt develops short clinical thermometer	Outbreak of Franco-Prussian War; Otto von Bismarck unifies Germany	
1871		Darwin's *Descent of Man*	
1872	Kaposi's sarcoma first described		
1873	William Osler writes on blood platelets		
1874	Louis Pasteur suggests sterilising instruments by placing in boiling water; Sophia Jex-Blake opens London School of Medicine for Women		
1875	Public Health Act passed in Britain		
1876	Robert Koch identifies anthrax bacillus; Cruelty to Animals Act passed in Britain; connection between the pancreas and sugar diabetes discovered	Alexander Graham Bell patents the telephone	

Year	Medical events	Contemporary events	Nobel prize in physiology or medicine
1877	Patrick Manson discovers that mosquitoes transmit filariasis	Zulu War (1877–8)	
1878	Koch's studies of wound infection published		
1879		Edison invents electric light bulb	
1880	Charles Laveran isolates blood parasite that causes malaria		
1881	Fifth cholera pandemic begins; Institute of Midwives established in London; Louis Pasteur devises a vaccine for anthrax		
1882	Robert Koch isolates the tubercle bacillus; operation for the removal of the gall bladder introduced; Paul Ehrlich introduces diazo reaction to diagnose typhoid fever	Eruption of Krakatoa in the Sunda Straits	
1883	Robert Koch discovers the cholera vibrio; Edwin Klebs and Friedrich Löffler identify the diphtheria bacillus; Francis Galton introduces the term 'eugenics'		
1884	Elie Metchnikoff describes phagocytosis; Nicolaier discovers tetanus bacillus		
1885	Louis Pasteur develops a rabies vaccine		

Year	Medical events	Contemporary events	Nobel prize in physiology or medicine
1886		Gold discovered in the Witwatersrand, South Africa	
1887	Introduction of Petri dish		
1888	The Pasteur Institute founded		
1889	Johns Hopkins Hospital opens in Baltimore; Infectious Diseases Act in England and Wales	Brazil ends Portuguese rule	
1890	Emil von Behring and Shibasabura Kitasato develop vaccines against tetanus and diphtheria; William Halsted develops surgical gloves		
1891	Association of American Medical Colleges established		
1892	William Osler's *Principles and Practice of Medicine*		
1893	Johns Hopkins Medical School opens		
1894	First use of diphtheria antitoxin in Britain	Nicholas II become last Tsar of Russia	
1895	Wilhelm Röntgen discovers X-rays	Marconi introduces wireless telegraphy	
1896	Antoine Becquerel discovers radiation; Scipione Riva-Rocci invents device for measuring blood pressure		
1897	Ronald Ross locates the malaria parasite in the Anopheles mosquito; first of seven volumes of Havelock Ellis' *Studies in the Psychology of Sex*		

Year	Medical events	Contemporary events	Nobel prize in physiology or medicine
1898	Patrick Manson's *Tropical Diseases*; Pierre and Marie Curie obtain radium from pitchblende		
1899	Sixth cholera pandemic; London School of Hygiene and Tropical Medicine founded; aspirin introduced	Boer War begins	
1900	Sigmund Freud's *Interpretation of Dreams*, Karl Landsteiner identifies the major blood groups; U.S. Army Yellow Fever Commission founded		
1901		Death of Queen Victoria	Emil Adolf von Behring 'for his work on serum therapy, especially its application against diphtheria, by which he has opened a new road in the domain of medical science and thereby placed in the hands of the physician a victorious weapon against illness and deaths'
1902	William Bayliss and Ernest Starling discover the hormone secretin; Registration of Midwives Act passed in Britain	Boer War ends	Ronald Ross 'for his work on malaria, by which he has shown how it enters the organism and thereby has laid the foundation for successful research on this disease and methods of combating it'

Year	Medical events	Contemporary events	Nobel prize in physiology or medicine
1903	Willem Einthoven describes the first electrocardiograph; Georg Perthes discovers that X-rays inhibit the growth of tumours	Wright brothers fly in petrol-powered aircraft	Niels Ryberg Finsen 'in recognition of his contribution to the treatment of diseases, especially lupus vulgaris, with concentrated light radiation, whereby he has opened a new avenue for medical science'
1904	Rockefeller Institute for Medical Research founded in New York	Work begins on Panama Canal	Ivan Pavlov 'in recognition of his work on the physiology of digestion, through which knowledge on vital aspects of the subject has been transformed and enlarged'
1905	James Mackenzie describes value of digitalis in cases of auricular fibrillation; Schaudinn and Hoffmann discover the causative agent of syphilis		Robert Koch 'for his investigations and discoveries in relation to tuberculosis'
1906	Jules Bordet discovers whooping cough bacillus; Frederick Gowland Hopkins starts experiments on 'accessory food factors' (vitamins); Charles Sherrington's *The Integrative Action of the Nervous System*	The tungsten-filament light bulb is introduced	Camillo Golgi, Santiago Ramón y Cajal 'in recognition of their work on the structure of the nervous system'
1907	Alois Alzheimer describes 'presenile dementia' (Alzheimer's disease)		Alphonse Lavaran 'in recognition of his work on the role played by protozoa in causing diseases'

Year	Medical events	Contemporary events	Nobel prize in physiology or medicine
1908			Ilya Mechnikov, Paul Ehrlich 'in recognition of their work on immunity'
1909	Archibald Garrod's *Inborn Errors of Metabolism*; Charles-Jules-Henri Nicolle discovers typhus fever transmitted by body louse	Industrial production of plastics begins with the development of Bakelite; Robert Peary and Matthew Hensen reach the North Pole	Emil Theodor Kocher 'for his work on the physiology, pathology and surgery of the thyroid gland'
1910	Paul Ehrlich announces the discovery of Salvarsan for syphilis		Albrecht Kossel 'in recognition of the contributions to our knowledge of cell chemistry made through his work on proteins, including the nucleic substances'
1911	National Insurance Act sets up first state medical insurance scheme in Britain	Roald Amundsen reaches the South Pole	Allvar Gullstrand 'for his work on the dioptrics of the eye'
1912	Harvey Cushing's *The Pituitary Gland and its Disorders*; Casimir Funk coins the term 'vitamin'	Titanic sinks on maiden voyage	Alexis Carrel 'in recognition of his work on vascular suture and the transplantation of blood vessels and organs'
1913	John Jacob Abel develops first artificial kidney; establishment of Medical Research Committee (Council from 1920) in Britain; A. Salomen develops mammography for diagnosing breast cancer		Charles Richet 'in recognition of his work on anaphylaxis'

2   The rise of science in medicine, 1₺

W. F. BYNUM

Medical science

Medicine in modern times has become so intertwined with science that it is taken for granted. More subtly, however, modern science has become so inextricably linked with technology that 'high-tech' rather than 'high-science' has become the more familiar adjective to describe the medicine that is practised in Western hospitals. The marriage of science and technology is largely a twentieth-century institution, but there was courtship in earlier decades. The visual images of late-nineteenth-century hospitals and consulting rooms often display the technological fruits and symbols of the period: electrical lighting, telephones, autoclaves, white coats, and X-ray machines. Before World War I (1914–18, also known as the 'Great War'), powerful hospital medical and surgical consultants would often arrive in their chauffeured automobiles. If general practitioners more often made their house calls on the bicycle, that too had been a technological innovation.

Technology had become important for daily life and, of course, medical practice shared in it. But science wrought more substantial changes for medicine than did technology during the period. Scientific discoveries altered the way medical students were trained, what doctors knew about health and disease, what they could do, and even (gradually) how some of them dressed. The principal differences between the structure of medical knowledge in 1850 and its equivalent in 1914 were largely the product of medical sciences, such as histology, physiology, biochemistry, pathology, microbiology, and immunology.

To be sure, not all doctors welcomed these developments. Worries about losing the art of medicine, not treating the whole patient, or jumping on every new scientific bandwagon were common enough. Science did not achieve its central position within medicine without a good deal of controversy, resistance, and negotiation. There are several reasons for this.

first, at some level, Western medicine since the Hippocratics had generally striven to be scientific. Galen (*c.* 129–200/216) certainly thought he was scientific; so did Vesalius (1514–64), William Harvey (1578–1657), and John Hunter (1728–93). The hospital medicine that French clinicians, such as R. T. H. Laennec (1781–1826) and Pierre Louis (1787–1872), perfected and exported widely through their foreign students during the first half of the nineteenth century, prided itself on being scientific (Ch. 1). The most systematic exposition of its underlying values, by an American product, Elisha Bartlett (1804–55), had the very word in its title: *An Essay on the Philosophy of Medical Science* (1844). Science in medicine was hardly new, but Bartlett's model reminds us of a second reason why late-nineteenth-century medical science was contested.

Second, for Bartlett, medical science consisted of bedside observations, repeated with care so many times that inductive laws of disease, diagnosis, and therapeutics would emerge. His science, like that of most of his Parisian teachers, was observational, not experimental. Bedside observation continued to feature within medicine and the clinico-pathological correlation so central to French hospital medicine remained central to the delineation of many new diagnoses later in the century. It remained important, but less cutting edge than the experimental medicine that came to maturity late in the century. 'Science' had different meanings for different factions within the wider medical community and individuals who believed they were marching behind the banner of science were often at odds with others who might be attracted to the same metaphor. 'Clinical science' and 'experimental medicine' sometimes had little to say to each other.

Third, this schism was grounded in another reason why science remained problematic: these two pursuits were practised increasingly by separate professional groups. Individuals who spent at least part of their time in clinical work had overwhelmingly produced the medical science of earlier times. Their contributions were based either on their clinical practice or on experimental research time stolen from the daily necessity to earn a living. In the emerging structures of medical education and research, medical scientists were more successful in carving out for themselves positions that were divorced from the grind of seeing patients. Those who produced scientific knowledge were not necessarily those who used it. This division of labour had its counterpart in the increasing specialization within clinical practice. But just as medical specialization was not greeted with acclaim by many generalists within the clinical sphere, so the separation of experimental medicine from the demands of the consulting room and clinic led many doctors to be suspicious of it.

To be sure, most medical scientists in the period had medical degrees, and many teachers of physiology, pathology, or medical chemistry combined teaching with clinical practice. But the trend, strongest in Germany, of devoting one's career to a single discipline, began to take root. When Michael Foster (1836–1907) obtained his chair in physiology at the University of Cambridge in 1883, he made it a stipulation that future holders of the chair would be barred from practising medicine. He had not practised for almost twenty years, and had been active in the constitutive foundations of an autonomous profession of physiology: the establishment of a specialist society and journal. Foster's activities had been duplicated by many medical scientists in countries throughout Europe and the Western world, and as the 'profession' of science matured, scientists increasingly talked to each other, rather than to their clinical colleagues.

Before the Great War, the Ph.D. was still a rare degree, and most professors of the medical sciences had qualified in medicine. But the most visible medical scientist of the whole century, Louis Pasteur (1822–95), had come into medicine through physics and chemistry, and his own career is highly significant for the role of science within medicine. Late in his life, he found his lack of a medical qualification a disadvantage, as medical colleagues had to administer his rabies vaccine to human patients. By the time he became an international medical superstar, in the 1880s, a stroke had limited his physical capacities, so physical as well as legal barriers stood in the way of his work with patients. Nevertheless, Pasteur stands as a potent symbol of medical science as something independent from, yet potentially linked to, clinical practice. He is the godfather of the many nonmedical Nobel Prize winners in physiology or medicine. He would have been a certain bet to have secured the first one, had he not died six years previously.

Medical science came to professional maturity during the second half of the nineteenth century. The remainder of this section examines the aspirations and achievements of the various sciences. Other sections will scrutinize aspects of this new knowledge base and rhetoric of medicine.

PHYSIOLOGY

Under the name 'Institutes of Medicine', physiology had been taught to medical students for generations. In Edinburgh, John Hughes Bennett (1812–75) was still teaching physiology at the Institutes in the 1850s. As its title suggests, it was considered as the basis of further medical knowledge, and, ultimately, of underlying medical practice. After all, doctors could not appreciate disease unless they first grasped the functions of the body in health. Function was also taught to medical students under the rubric of 'general anatomy' or teaching posts in anatomy and physiology were combined. Anatomical structure and physiological function had always been linked.

At one level, structure and function still seem natural together (the heart achieves its function of pumping blood by virtue of its structure), but from the mid-nineteenth century, these traditional bedfellows began to be separated. Gross anatomical dissection continued to be valued in medical education, but cutting-edge biomedicine became concerned with finer details of structure – the tissues and cells – and in aspects of organ (and cell) function that could not be deduced by structure–function considerations. In the German-speaking lands, especially, but elsewhere as well, physiologists began to assert that the proper goal of their discipline was to explain all living functions in terms of the physics and chemistry of organisms.

In 1847, four young physiologists, Carl Ludwig (1816–95), Emil Du Bois-Reymond (1818–96), Ernst Brücke (1819–92), and Hermann von Helmholtz (1821–94), published a clarion call for a new physiology based on physics and chemistry. It was a kind of declaration of independence from their teacher, Johannes Müller (1801–58), who had been central to much German scientific medicine from his post at the University of Berlin. Although Müller had been instrumental in the separation of anatomy from physiology (although his own chair was always jointly that of anatomy and physiology) and an active practitioner of the experimental ideal, his own worldview (*Weltanschauung*) was infused with the vitalism that had characterized the Romantic period in German medicine and natural science. His pupils absorbed his experimentalism, but rejected his vitalism. For them, physiology had to be rigorous and reductionist,that is, to reduce the functions of living organisms to the laws of physics and chemistry.

Each of these young Turks went on to distinguished careers in physiology. Ludwig was the most successful teacher. At his Physiological Institute in Leipzig, he trained dozens of young medical students in the art and science of precise physiological investigation. He invented the kymograph, essentially a revolving drum on which physiological phenomena, such as muscle contractions, could be recorded over time. The modern graphical method in the life sciences owes much to him. His research interests were wide, and included the mechanism of cardiac contraction and the elaboration of urine by the kidney. We shall examine his research establishment later.

Du Bois-Reymond inherited the physiological half of Müller's chair in Berlin, after the latter's death (probably from suicide) in 1858. His abiding fascination was in electrical phenomena in the body and he developed a good deal of sensitive apparatus to measure electrical currents in animals and to use external electricity to stimulate physiological actions, such as muscle contraction or gland secretion. He was powerful in Berlin scientific circles, although he made enemies with his resolute scientific positivism, which led him to disparage Goethe's romantic science. At the same time, he believed that there were questions that science cannot answer, including the origins of thought and free will, to which the only proper answer was *ignoramus* (we do not know) or *ignorabimus* (we will never know).

Brücke became professor in Vienna, where he trained a number of students, including Sigmund Freud. Like Ludwig, he wrote a successful physiology textbook and did original work on the physiology of speech and in linguistics. An expert microscopist, Brücke contributed to the development of cell theory and furthered the notion of 'protoplasm' as the unique substance within cells.

Helmholtz was the most brilliant of the quartet and eventually abandoned the medical sciences for experimental physics, although not before he had made his mark on physiology with fundamental work on the functions of the ear and the eye, and on practical medicine with his invention of the ophthalmoscope. He was also one of several natural philosophers who, during the 1840s, expounded the doctrine of the conservation of energy, that is, that energy is never created nor destroyed, but merely changes its various forms. Always insisting that living systems do not violate this fundamental law of nature, he applied its principles to his work on the special senses. Helmholtz first measured the transmission velocity of nervous impulses, demonstrating thereby that definite, material changes were involved in phenomena, such as movement and sensation. Much of his physiological work was done in Heidelberg, but he returned to Berlin late in his career, as professor of physics. He was a brilliant lecturer, and his general essays were collected and widely translated. They disseminated his gospel of science throughout the West.

Each of these four men worked in major centres of German research and education, the institutional forms of which we will examine later. Each came from training in medicine and understood its problems. But their careers were spent in laboratories and institutes removed from the daily demands of patient care. Although their philosophical commitments diverged later in their lives, each was in essence true to their collective youthful manifesto,

115

that the aim of physiology was to understand the functions of organisms in terms of the chemistry and physics of living systems. None of them, however, articulated the place of physiology within medicine as eloquently and subtly as their French colleague, Claude Bernard (1813–78), who was for many throughout the West *the* physiologist of the century.

Bernard was half a generation older than his German compeers, and that was important. More significant, however, was his nationality. Whereas the four younger physiologists reacted to the speculative excesses of Romanticism within German natural science and medicine, Bernard grew up within the solidly empirical tradition of French hospital medicine. His rebellion against the medical education of his youth was also firm, but he never embraced any thoroughgoing materialism, nor did he hold that physiology could ever become an incidental handmaiden of physics and chemistry. Rather, he held that physiology was, along with pathology and therapeutics, one of the three pillars of what he famously called 'experimental medicine'.

Bernard's early career was chequered. He went to Paris as a young man believing that he could make it as a playwright and man of letters. Showing his work to a literary critic, he was strongly advised to study medicine. Although he was an undistinguished student, he came to the attention of François Magendie, p. 65ff who encouraged his experimental bent. He qualified in medicine, but was saved from having to practise by marriage to a wealthy woman. The marriage proved unhappy, but his wife's dowry gave him the financial security to pursue an academic path. His M.D. thesis (1843), on gastric digestion and the fate of carbohydrates in animals, identified the problem that occupied him for the next few years. His work on the fate of ingested sugars, and the role of the liver and other digestive organs, provided a new model of animal metabolism. Bernard showed that animals are not simply the passive beneficiaries of foodstuffs synthesized by plants (as the German chemist Liebig had supposed); rather they are active biochemical systems in their own right, synthesizing and breaking down complex organic molecules. He showed that the liver is instrumental in producing glycogen from adsorbed dietary sugars, and that this compound is then broken down in such a way as to produce blood sugar as required by the animal.

Bernard's researches on sugar metabolism, and the functions of dietary organs, such as the stomach, liver, and pancreas, provided the basis for understanding both the ordinary nuances of digestion and metabolism, but also for explicating some of the factors in a common human disease:

diabetes. This research was facilitated by Bernard's gifts as an experimental animal surgeon: he worked mostly on dogs, and his investigations required him to perform delicate operations on his experimental animals, and to keep them alive afterwards. He applied these skills to a large number of other experimental problems, including the roles of motor and sensory nerves, the precise site of action of the poison curare, and the mechanism whereby carbon monoxide acts as a poison.

Bernard always had a philosophical turn of mind, and his lectures from the 1850s began to generalize the implications of his experimental results. This included his concept of the *milieu intérieur*, the notion that higher organisms have developed complicated mechanisms whereby the conditions of the blood and tissues are kept relatively constant, even in changing environmental conditions. In the twentieth century, Walter Bradford Cannon (1871–1945) further developed this insight into the modern principle of homeostasis p. 268. For Bernard, the constancy of the interior milieu provided the physiological basis of the capacity of warm-blooded animals (constancy of body temperature was one of Bernard's favourite examples) to thrive in a variety of external conditions.

Ill health limited the active experimentation of Bernard's later years and he wrote his physiological masterpiece, *An Introduction to the Study of Experimental Medicine* (1865), during convalescence from a serious disease. It is one of the most philosophically sophisticated accounts of a research career ever produced and provides a rationale for experimentation within medicine that still has resonance.

Bernard's *Introduction* is at once autobiographical and universal. He used his own laboratory life to erect a philosophy of discovery within the biomedical sciences. To be sure, his own laboratory notebooks reveal that his own research trajectory was not always so neat as portrayed in his later reconstructions. Nevertheless, his achievements within the laboratory offered scope for generalization.

French hospital medicine had been based on careful bedside observation. This was valuable, but only as a starting point. There were too many uncontrolled variables, and too much concern for the needs of the sick patient, to make knowledge gained at the bedside precise and reproducible. Hospitals, he insisted, are only 'the entrance to scientific medicine; they are the first field of observation which a physician enters; but the true sanctuary of medical science is the laboratory; only there can he seek explanations of life in normal and pathological states by means of experimental analysis' (Bernard, 1865, trans. 1957, p. 146). Only in the laboratory can

117

experimental conditions be mastered, so that the results can be interpreted unambiguously.

This certainty of experimental knowledge was the result of the one basic principle that Bernard insisted upon: determinacy. Under identical conditions, identical results always ensue. At the bedside, this could never happen, since conditions were far too messy, but in the laboratory the scientist was master. Knowledge gained there could then be applied in clinical situations. This knowledge was of three kinds, corresponding to Bernard's three experimental pillars. Experimentalists could teach doctors about normal functions, about abnormal ones, and about the mode and site of action of therapeutic agents, especially drugs. His own discoveries documented all three ways to greater medical power. Normal function was shown by the complex interactions of the abdominal organs to utilize sugar and to keep its concentration in the blood stream constant. Abnormal function could be seen when blood concentration of sugar was too high and the kidney secreted it into the urine. Bernard illustrated the actions of external substances, poisons as well as drugs, through his researches on curare and carbon monoxide. All medicinal substances, he believed, acted in specific ways, on specific sites within the body, and experimental pharmacology could elucidate these nuances.

The controlled conditions of the laboratory had other spin-offs. Unusual results were often the source of new experimental ideas, as when Bernard had noticed that the urine of his experimental rabbits turned acidic when they were fasted. Because rabbits' urine was normally alkaline, he reasoned that they were metabolizing their own bodily reserves, that is, their urine was like that of carnivores. This led him to investigate the dynamic balance between intake and output, and to appreciate the delicate balance of living organisms. Always, Bernard avowed, the experimentalist begins with an idea. He tests this idea with his experiment, and modifies it according to the experimental results. The experimental idea is like a hat he wears when he enters the laboratory. He takes it off when he comes in and simply observes the results of the experiment. On leaving the laboratory, he never forgets to put on his hat again to think about what he has seen. Philosophers call this the hypothetico-deductive method: deduce an experiment to test an hypothesis and then modify the hypothesis in the light of the experiment (if necessary). Many observers of science believe that this is how science should (and often does) work: Bernard offered a sophisticated programme of how this method operates, based on his own laboratory experiences.

118

The contrast that Bernard drew between the passive, observational medicine of the bedside and the active experimental one of the laboratory, found ready parallels in the life sciences more generally, where the older natural history tradition was being rendered quaintly antiquarian. The new biology was increasingly centred on the laboratory, even as the greatest of all natural historians, Charles Darwin (1809–82), had shown what important results there were to be had in the field. Darwin became in Britain what Bernard was in France: a national treasure. Bernard was the first French scientist to be accorded a state funeral when he died in 1878. Despite his controversial biological theories, Darwin was buried in the place of English national treasures: Westminster Abbey. Although evolutionary concerns had hardly touched Bernard's research, the reverse was not the case. Darwin was ever appreciative of the new experimental ethos in biology, and in the period after the publication of *On the Origin of Species* (1859), he became something of an experimentalist, turning rooms and greenhouses in his country retreat in Downe, Kent, into primitive laboratories. His own experimental work was mostly botanical in nature, but Darwin actively supported the emerging physiological community in Britain, signing petitions in support of the vivisection that the whole-animal physiology of the period required.

Darwin's 'bulldog', Thomas Henry Huxley (1825–95) was at the heart of this battle to place science centrally within human affairs, including medicine. One of Darwin's collaborators, John Scott Burdon-Sanderson (1818–1905), was professor of physiology successively at University College London and the University of Oxford. That he ended his career as Regius Professor of Medicine at Oxford says much for the way in which experimental medicine had become central to medical politics and medical ideals, even in Britain.

During the second half of the nineteenth century, experimental physiologists changed profoundly the way in which the functions of the human body were understood. It was primarily organ-centred, just as the pathology of the first half of the century had been. The functions of the major organs – heart, brain, liver, kidneys, stomach, pancreas – were elucidated, and those of the endocrine organs – thyroid, adrenals, ovaries, testes – brought into the open. We shall examine later the push-pull effect of this knowledge on the formation of clinical specialties, as well as the impact of experimental medicine upon medical education. One aspect of physiology influenced medical thinking from the 1860s and needs to be considered now: its impact on disease concepts.

The organ-based pathology of the early nineteenth century had been anatomical in its orientation. Laennec, Corvisart, Louis, and the high priests of French hospital medicine had defined disease largely in terms of the gross pathological changes that it produced. The lesion was the king of the hospital, the chief object of diagnostic enquiry. Physiology began to change this orientation, from the structures of diseases to their functions. In the hands of clinicians such as Carl A. Wunderlich (1815–77), physiological medicine came to the fore. Wunderlich pp. 165, 172 believed that the dynamics rather than the statics of disease were what mattered. He used in the clinical setting the graphical techniques that physiologists were applying in the laboratory to record the nuances of function over time. As we shall see, the fever chart was his forte, but his more general reflections on the nature of disease were just one example in which the approach of the physiologist found its place at the foot of the hospital bed. His plans to reform clinical medicine were helped by the fact that pathology, too, had become much more functional and dynamic in its approach.

PATHOLOGY

Experimental pathology was one of Bernard's pillars of experimental medicine, but most who called themselves pathologists during the second half of the century were less concerned with experimentation than with the dissection of dead bodies. Animals played a real, but minor, role in the discipline, with one important exception: bacteriology. The pathologist's 'laboratory' was generally the dead house, or morgue, of the hospital. The routine autopsy protocol was perfected by Karl Rokitanski (1804–78) in Vienna, who was said to have performed during his tenure as professor of pathology almost 40,000 post-mortem dissections. Rokitanski was systematic and thorough, describing several new pathological conditions, and providing firm pathological criteria for many more. He weighed the size of organs, carefully looked for signs of inflammation, abscesses, or tumour growth, noted congenital abnormalities of structure, and correlated all this with the clinical records that followed the patient on his or her final hospital journey.

Rokitanski enjoyed a deserved international reputation, and his massive textbook was widely translated and used, but the centre of pathological gravity had shifted from Vienna to Berlin, from Rokitanski to Virchow, a decade or two before the former died. Even if systematic autopsies became routine as important procedures in furthering medical knowledge, their very familiarity told against them. The autopsy was essential in defining disease, but it was relatively impotent in explaining it.

Cells rather than organs offered a more promising approach, and cellular pathology was above all associated with the dominant pathologist of the century, Rudolf Virchow (1821–1902). Virchow was a well-rounded individual, politically radical in his youth (active in the revolutions of 1848, p. 93, and liberal even in old age. His energy was legendary; he seemed to need only a few hours of sleep each night and packed into his long life several loosely connected careers: pathologist, politician, sanitary reformer, archaeologist, anthropologist, editor, teacher, even family man. These disparate activities were connected by Virchow's abiding belief in rationality and liberalism, and his conviction that science offered the best hope for human progress.

Pathology provided his bread-and-butter means of sustenance, and primary international reputation. The microscope was his constant research tool. He came to medical maturity when the cell theories of Schleiden and Schwann were still new. He accepted their statements that cells are the units of biological activity, in plants and animals, and systematically applied this to the realm of pathology. More importantly, he taught (he was not the first, but by far the most prominent) that there is a generational continuity of cells. *Omnis cellula e cellula*: all cells from cells. This was his rallying cry, and it explained much in microscopic pathology.

Following his political activity in the abortive revolution of 1848, the Prussian authorities disliked his continued presence in the Prussian capital, Berlin, and he was moved to a pathology chair in Würzburg. Among his colleagues there was the Swiss histologist, Rudolph von Kölliker (1817–1905), and Virchow's earlier penchant for microscopical analysis of pathological phenomena flourished. A steady stream of articles, mostly in the journal that Virchow had established in 1847, *Archiv für pathologische Anatomie und Physiologie und für klinische Medizin*, elucidated his ideas and explicated his researches. Seeing the cell as the basic unit of function, both normal and pathological, and stressing the fact that all cells, even abnormal ones, are derived from mother cells, produced a sea change in understanding disease processes.

Virchow had already described, independently from J. H. Bennett a cancer of the white blood cells. He named it 'leukaemia', literally, white blood, as patients suffering from the disease had the normal ratio of red and white blood cells in their blood streams reversed. It was one of the first truly microscopical diagnoses, and while Virchow and Bennett engaged in a rather undignified priority squabble, Virchow's label prevailed. (Bennett had called it 'leucocythaemia', literally, 'more white cells in the blood', ironically a more accurate name). Virchow continued to be interested in the microscopic dimensions of cancer, producing a classic multivolume work on the subject in the 1860s. Between them, Virchow and Kölliker put the medical faculty at Würzburg on the academic map. One of Johannes Müller's last achievements was to persuade the officials in Berlin to create a separate institute and chair in what was called 'pathological anatomy'. His political activities forgiven, Virchow (also a pupil of Müller) was appointed to this post in 1856 and remained there for the rest of his life.

A set of his early lectures there, consolidating and extending his previous work, was published in 1858 as *Cellular Pathology*. It went through three further German editions and was translated into the major European languages. It remains the classic text in nineteenth-century pathology. By urging doctors to think about disease in terms of cells, Virchow emphasized process rather than result. Looking at cell behaviour in diseases placed the pathological centre-of-gravity towards the beginning, rather than at the end stages of a disease. This in turn encouraged pathologists to think about functional issues, such as blood supply, nutrition, oxygenation, rate of cell division and like matters. In short, it led to a more dynamic pathology than the anatomical orientation of the French school earlier in the century. The anatomo-pathological definitions of many diseases remained pretty secure, but notions of cause and mechanisms also came to the fore.

Virchow peopled the Western pathological world with his pupils, and most of them continued to work within the boundaries he had set. The microscope as well as the dissecting scalpel became constant tools of the pathologist. Stains, microtomes, and fixation methods were developed, enabling thin sections of tissues to be cut and different kinds of cells to be more clearly differentiated. Carcinomas were distinguished from sarcomas on the basis of tissue of origin. Malignant cells were gradually shown to have intracellular characteristics that were useful in predicting the outcome of a tumour. By the end of the century, pathologists were sometimes examining sections removed by surgeons and giving advice on whether the tumour ought to be removed. Virchow was involved in a celebrated case, involving Frederick III, Emperor of Germany. Frederick was suffering from a growth on his larynx, which his German surgeons wanted to remove. An English surgeon, (Sir) Morrell Mackenzie (1853–1925) was called in consultation, removed a piece, and sent it to Virchow for examination. Virchow pronounced it benign and amenable to medical treatment. Frederick's painful death from cancer shortly afterwards showed that Virchow had been wrong.

By the century's end, pathological knowledge of most common disease was significantly different from what it had been when Virchow began his career half a century earlier. The discipline retained, throughout the period, much closer links with clinical problems than had physiology, and chairs in pathology had become common in medical schools throughout the West. Many of Virchow's most energetic students remained in the German-speaking lands, but students from all over Europe and North America came to his institute in Berlin. William Henry Welch (1850–1934), for instance, became the dominant figure in the most Germanic of American institutions, the Johns Hopkins University. Welch spent most of his initial period of study in Europe with one of Virchow's pupils, Julius Cohnheim, in Breslau, but his first major publication was in Virchow's *Archiv*. Ironically, perhaps, Welch's most lasting contributions to pathology followed from his second German sojourn, studying with another major Berlin figure, Robert Koch (1843–1910). The young Welch went to study cellular pathology and its physiological manifestations. In preparation for his chair in pathology at Johns Hopkins, the older Welch needed to learn about bacteriology.

BACTERIOLOGY

Most histories of medicine produced before the 1970s concluded that the germ theory of disease was the single most important discovery in medicine, in all times and all places. After all, infectious diseases were historically the most significant causes of mortality and morbidity, and their control in the developed world seemed pretty secure in the decades after World War II. The new emerging diseases, such as AIDS, the increased incidence of older diseases, such as tuberculosis (TB), and the widespread development of resistance to antibiotics and other antimicrobial drugs have punctured this cosy confidence pp. 444, 472. Awareness of the 'global village', the role of travel in the spread of disease, and the capacity of the media to bring the whole world into Western living rooms have further added to the anxiety. The contemporary concerns of both medical historians and health personnel are probably less insular than they were a generation or two ago. Their work has reminded people that infectious diseases never went away in many parts of the world.

None of this negates the considerable achievements of the principal architects of the germ theory, Louis Pasteur in France and Robert Koch in Germany. Nor is their permanent legacy abolished by the recognition that Pasteur and Koch had many predecessors and contemporaries who contributed to the microbiological revolution. Furthermore, the 'germ theory' that ultimately held sway was only one of many such theories put forth on the role of microorganisms in the cause of disease, and even so, the relationships between hosts and parasites turned out to be far more complicated than the early pioneers believed.

Pasteur was hardly the first to suggest that microorganisms could cause disease. Infection by worms had been widely noted by earlier workers, and those in search of precursors to Pasteur often go back as far as Fracastoro (c.1478–1533), who wrote about contagion and the 'seeds of disease'. There is an honourable list of other precursors between Fracastoro and the mid-nineteenth century, most immediately, perhaps, Jacob Henle (1809–1885), whose essay on *Miasma and Contagion* (1840) proved to be especially prescient. Inevitably, the increased use of the microscope in the middle decades of the century led to many sightings of bacteria and other microorganisms, and speculations about their relations to human beings and human diseases.

Nevertheless, Pasteur's work, from the early 1850s, stands out. This is partly because of his astonishing capacity to bet on the right horses, to elaborate hypotheses that turned out to have significant purchase even when his experimental evidence was less than conclusive. Pasteur's success also derived from his tenacious zeal to prove himself correct against all opponents. Finally, his central role in the elaboration of a germ theory of disease was linked to the fact that he approached it almost by accident, as a by-product of other phenomena associated with microorganisms.

Pasteur came to what became his life's work through chemistry and physics. Examining the curious capacity of certain organic compounds to rotate beams of light, he worked on issues of polarization for almost a decade, gradually realizing that isometric versions of a number of substances (i.e., compounds having identical chemical formulae but different crystalline structures) were intimately related to the activities of yeasts and other living agents. This convinced him that living organisms could do things that the chemist in his laboratory could not, for when he synthesized these organic acids in his laboratory, their dissolved crystals did not polarize light.

This interest in microorganisms led him to reexamine the old problem of spontaneous generation, the experimental procedure of which produced one of his lasting icons, the swan-necked flasks carefully designed to exclude dust particles from the air. This was the source, he believed, of contamination in traditional experiments that seemed to support the theory that simple organisms could be generated from nonliving matter.

These experiments, in the early 1860s, were the making of his international reputation. They were debated in public, in opposition to contrary results obtained by an older French naturalist, F-A. Pouchet (1800–72), whose advocacy of spontaneous generation was fuelled by his evolutionary fervour. The French Académie des Sciences judged in favour of Pasteur, after several public demonstrations and a good deal of heated debate. Modern historians have shown that Pasteur discarded experimental results that did not support his thesis, but that because he and Pouchet worked with a bacterium that produces heat-resistant spores, Pouchet's results (if not his interpretation) were sometimes more accurate.

From the late 1850s, Pasteur worked exclusively on his beloved microorganisms, developing methods of cultivating them in his famous flasks, studying their nutritional requirements and gradually implicating them in animal and human disease. His fully developed germ theory of disease emerged from his investigation of a devastating epidemic of silkworms, but he then extended it to the diseases of farm animals (e.g., 'cholera' in chickens – a disease unrelated to that of the same name in human beings) and a disease that humans share with their domesticated animals: anthrax. Ever aware of the economic in addition to the medical implications of understanding the lives of microorganisms, he had previously shown how common human activities, such as baking bread, brewing beer, and fermenting wine, could be more precisely controlled by appreciating the crucial roles that these microscopical beings played in the processes.

He also came to realize that the capacities of these organisms to cause disease were not an absolute property. 'Virulence', as he called it, could be augmented or diminished in the laboratory through a variety of procedures that he sometimes stumbled across accidentally. 'Chance favours the prepared mind', he famously said, and his discovery, after a weekend away from his laboratory, that the culture of chicken cholera bacilli, dried up in his absence, not only did not infect but actually protected, led him to the triumphal work of his later life, on vaccines, which is the general name he adopted in honour of Edward Jenner's smallpox vaccine. His public demonstration of his anthrax vaccine, in 1881, in a farmyard outside Paris, in Pouilly-le-Fort, was witnessed (by invitation) by newspaper reporters from several countries. The results were dramatic: the vaccinated sheep and goats stayed healthy, the unprotected ones died even as the reporters arrived. These observers quickly spread the word, in a way that resonates with modern methods of scientific communication of results deemed to be important.

His encore was even more audacious, because the disease he sought to treat (and not simply protect against) with vaccines, rabies, is caused (we now know) by a virus, which Pasteur could not see with the microscopes at his disposal. Despite not knowing what kind of infectious agent he was dealing with, he learned how to attenuate the virus through serial passage of infected material in the spinal cords of rabbits. Rabies has never been a common human disease, but it was (and is) much feared, because it kills painfully and inexorably. As always, it seems, the public Pasteur and the private one (as revealed in his laboratory notebooks) were not quite identical, and he hesitatingly tried his vaccine out privately in two cases (one lived and one died) before going public. The first public case involved a young boy, Joseph Meister, who had been bitten by a dog thought to be rabid. Meister survived his famous ordeal, and the rabies vaccine treatment became the subject of international wonderment. If Pasteur was venerated before rabies, he became a kind of scientific saint afterwards, with consequences we will examine later. His rabies vaccine was probably the apogee of nineteenth-century laboratory medicine, not just about cause (of which he remained ignorant) but about effective treatment of a horrible and universally fatal condition. Sceptics pointed out that it was impossible to judge its real efficacy because treatment had to be started before definite signs of clinical rabies began, so one could never be absolutely certain that the patient would have developed the disease (Fig. 2.1). Failures could always be attributed to the perennial medical excuse: treatment initiated too late. The problems associated with the rabies vaccine existed only at its margins. Its central core survived intact, with incalculable results for Pasteur's reputation, and biomedical research more generally.

Pasteur was a physical scientist who followed his nose into medicine, fascinated with what microorganisms could do. Koch, much younger, a doctor, and having grown up with the benefit of Pasteur's (and many others') two decades of experimental and microscopical work on this invisible world, was of a different stamp. He was a bacteriologist, not a microbiologist, more focused on the role of bacteria in the cause of human disease. He was introduced to bacteria and theories of contagion in medical school in Göttingen, and when he started to work with them, he sought out the advice of botanist Ferdinand Cohn (1828–98), who was actively studying these single-celled organisms that seemed to partake of characteristics of both plants and animals. Cohn brought a Germanic mentality to the problem, being especially concerned with their systematic classification as biological species, and in reforming scientific nomenclature in the field.

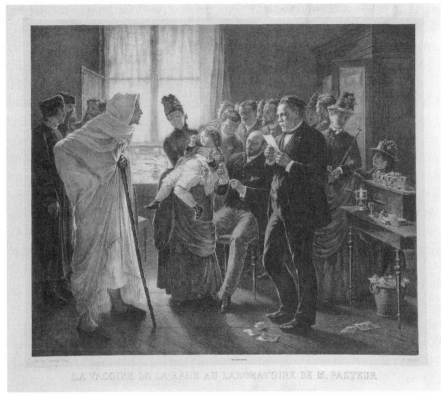

Fig. 2.1. Rabies vaccination in Pasteur's clinic in Paris. Pasteur stands in the foreground reading from a paper, 1887. *Source*: Lithograph by F. Pirodon after Laurent-Lucien Gsell; E. Desjobert, Paris. Wellcome Library Iconographic Collection. *Credit*: Wellcome Library, London (V0006860).

After graduation, Koch had military experience as a doctor in the Franco-Prussian War of 1870–1, following which he settled as a country medical practitioner. His first major scientific contribution dated from this period, when he elucidated the life cycle of the anthrax bacillus, showing that it had a spore form, which could live in the soil for many years and infect animals who tread in the mud. These spores were heat resistant and the anthrax bacillus, being closely related to the hay bacillus that Pasteur had used in his spontaneous generation experiments a decade earlier, Koch incidentally contributed to the resolution of the differences between Pasteur and Pouchet's experimental findings. More importantly, his work on the anthrax bacillus helped explain its pattern of infectivity and convinced Cohn that here was a researcher of rare gifts. He made laboratory facilities available to Koch, who in 1878 produced an important monograph on the bacteria responsible for wound infections. By this time, he was recognized as a leader in the field, and he followed his work on traumatic wound infections with two demonstrations that made his lasting reputation.

The tubercle bacillus was the first of these. Despite the fact that this disease had long been perceived as a chronic, constitutional one, its familial pattern being attributed to hereditary factors, a number of doctors from the 1860s began to suspect that some microbial agent might cause it. The French physician Jean Antoine Villemin (1827–92) had shown in 1868 that pus taken from the tuberculous lesions of patients autopsied with the condition could reproduce similar lesions in the lungs and other organs of guinea pigs, when injected. Finding an organism eluded several investigators, however, and most medical opinion in the 1870s would have polled against looking for a microorganism in the first place; phthisis, consumption, or whatever this chronic wasting disease of the lungs was called still being assumed to be utterly unlike the epidemic fevers that swept through communities.

The technical difficulties of identifying an organism associated with TB became understood only in retrospect, but Koch worked with what is now recognized as a slow-growing, fastidious bacterium. On the other hand, the tubercle bacillus is relatively easily recoverable from the sputum of tuberculous patients, or from the tubercles that were the hallmarks of the post-mortem findings. His search, from start to finish, took only eight months, a remarkable achievement given the obstacles. He triumphantly demonstrated the bacillus at a meeting of the Berlin Physiological Society on March 24, 1882. The process of convincing doctors that his bacillus was significant took longer. One of the historical ironies of this early chapter in TB research was that Koch's announcement, eight years later, that his killed bacterium treatment, tuberculin, could cure the disease, created an even greater international stir. The claims Koch made for tuberculin remain a telling example of medical hubris, or a demonstration that most new therapies 'work' for only a short time. We shall look briefly at Koch's later years below.

In the meantime, hard on the heels of the identification of the tubercle bacillus, Koch turned to cholera, the most frightening disease of the nineteenth century. Although it had not appeared in epidemic form in Western Europe since the 1860s, an epidemic in Egypt in the early 1880s led both German and French governments to send teams of experts there to study the disease and use the new tools of bacteriology to identify its causative organism. Infectious diseases of the intestines are exceptionally difficult to investigate, since a large number of bacteria live there normally: the gastrointestinal tract is, after all, open to the outside world at both ends. The contagiousness of cholera had been a subject of much international debate, in a series of international sanitary congresses dating from 1851. As we shall see, it was the first perceived international disease because the great pandemics that swept the nineteenth-century West had all originated in cholera's 'natural' homeland, India. By the 1870s, official policy of most European governments assumed that the disease was contagious, spread by some unknown agent along shipping routes. Quarantine was an obvious preventive strategy, resisted by the British government and its doctors. Because British interests controlled much of world shipping and quarantine was a costly and cumbersome nuisance to free trade, the extent to which economic considerations dictated British scientific policy was not lost on many at the time.

The Egyptian outbreak provided an opportunity to turn the new tools of bacteriology to account. It also offered French and German scientists the possibility of demonstrating to the scientific world the superiority of their differing approaches to infectious diseases. Pasteur was too infirm to go, but he orchestrated the composition of the French team of 'Pastorians', as they were already being called. Koch was the natural leader of the German team.

Egypt proved indecisive in identifying a causative organism, but the expedition was a disaster for the French, when one of their team died. He was Louis Thuillier (1856–83), a young Pastorian with much promise; his death was widely mourned in his fatherland. The German group at least all stayed healthy, and Koch believed that he had identified a bacterium that was consistently found in the guts of cholera victims, but not in those of the healthy. To pursue his investigations further, he went to India and, in late 1883, found in drinking water that was implicated as a possible source of local cholera, a curved bacterium that was also to be found in the stools of sufferers. He described this 'comma' bacillus, named after its shape, in a paper published in early 1884. His announcement was received in Germany with much more acclaim than it was in the rest of the Western world. French scientists had become suspicious of most things German, and the British were reluctant to attribute cholera to a microorganism that might be spread person-to-person because it cast doubt on decades of sanitary policy and gave substance to the disruptive strategy of quarantine. Ironically, Koch's findings were compatible with John Snow's (1813–58) demonstration, twenty-five years previously, that cholera was a waterborne disease p. 192.

The fact that each of these two new disease-causing organisms, the tubercle bacillus and the cholera bacillus, took years or decades to find general acceptance among practitioners and public health officials does not surprise us now. Doctors (and politicians) were being asked to change their modes of thought and to reconceptualize decades of cultural, clinical, and epidemiological experience. Phthisis had long been perceived as a familial, constitutional, and noncontagious affliction. The mode of spread of cholera was a puzzle (Snow's work had not significantly changed medical attitudes), but it was hardly a 'contagious' disease like smallpox, widely recognized as passing from person to person. Besides, Koch's two demonstrations occurred when new bacterial causes of diseases were beginning to come thick and fast. Germs were identified for cancer, various forms of heart disease, rheumatism, scurvy, beriberi, and insanity. Germs made the world a very scary place. We shall examine the wider cultural dissemination of the various germ theories below.

Sorting wheat from chaff is always a temporal process, and it is one of the perennial claims of science that it can eventually do this. But, however self-correcting science can be, it takes time. Bernard was within his rights to claim for scientists working in laboratories that they have greater control over the conditions of their world. Bedside observations are generally contaminated with the exigencies of therapeutic demands and human suffering. Koch recognized the essential logical conditions needed to show that some organism X is a cause of disease Y. These are now known as Koch's Postulates and, although Koch used them, they were more clearly enunciated by one of his colleagues, Friedrich Löffler (1852–1915), writing about diphtheria in 1883:

> 'If diphtheria is a disease caused by a micro-organism, it is essential that three postulates be fulfilled. The fulfilment of these postulates is necessary in order to demonstrate strictly the parasitic nature of a disease:
>
> 1. The organism must be shown to be constantly present in characteristic form and arrangement in the diseased tissue.
> 2. The organism, which, from its behaviour appears to be responsible for the disease, must be isolated and grown in pure culture.
> 3. The pure culture must be shown to induce the disease experimentally'
>   (Brock, 1988, p. 180).

These simple, logical steps had great purchase in many disorders, and in the last couple of decades of the century, many diseases were associated with specific microorganisms. Koch and his students contributed to the greater precision of bacteriology. They introduced the use of Petri dishes and agar-agar as the culture medium, the employment of photomicrography to make public the biological forms of the relevant microorganisms, and the identification of the varying conditions, such as temperature, nutritional requirements, and other essentials for the bacterium to grow readily. The use of vital stains in the preparation of microscope slides also helped differentiate the specific differences between the many bacteria that were investigated.

There were also many technical, perceptual, and practical difficulties. Bacteria were easy enough to identify, but many do not cause human disease, and the alimentary canal, skin, vagina, and naso-pharyngeal passages were never sterile, yet were subject to infectious diseases. Organisms that microbiologists associated specifically with diphtheria, typhoid fever, and other diseases could be cultivated from healthy individuals. Two people exposed to the same germ might have completely different responses, one falling ill and the other remaining completely healthy. A family exposed to the same bacteriological stimulus might fall ill of different conditions: the possible relation between typhoid fever and erysipelas puzzled many investigators, especially when the biological specificity of many microorganisms was still doubtful. The different morphological forms that bacteria could take (e.g., the spore form in anthrax) suggested to many doctors that these primitive creatures were pleomorphic, and therefore might under one set of environmental conditions cause one disease, but be implicated in another, completely different clinical disease under alternative circumstances. The doctrine of disease specificity, associated by later commentators with the germ theory, was hard fought at the time, and required an act of faith to believe in during the latter decades of the century.

These and a thousand other clinical, epidemiological, and scientific problems plagued bacteriology in its early decades. Koch contributed to one of these puzzles through his elaboration of the asymptomatic carrier state, most famously embodied in the case of 'Typhoid Mary', an Irish cook working in New York who serially infected families for whom she cooked, but remained well herself. Mary Mallon ended up being incarcerated, as an unwitting danger to the public. Her plight raised a host of ethical issues, and the carrier state created difficulties for public health officials and intensified racial and cultural suspicions of marginal groups.

We shall examine some of the social and public health ramifications of bacteriology and other facets of medical science later. Within medical science, however, these puzzles encouraged researchers to look at the interaction between the invading germ and receptive host more closely. Immunology was a science born out of this mire.

The consequences of what we now call immunity were noted long ago. That an attack of smallpox left its victim immune from subsequent risk was part of folk knowledge and had been the basis of inoculation (with the actual smallpox virus) in eighteenth-century England and elsewhere, and the further basis of Jenner's cowpox vaccination late in the century. Measles, chicken pox, and other diseases had the same lasting effect, and even diseases such as the plague and typhus seemed to have lesser potency the second time around. As Europeans colonized the tropical areas of the world, what was called the 'seasoning' process was seen in retrospect to involve immunity, among other physiological adaptations. At the time, it was more usually conceptualized in terms of bodily changes wrought by environmental factors, including heat, moisture, and dense air. The word 'immunity' was adopted into medicine from social politics, immune persons being excused from such public duties as taxes, military service, or public office.

Pasteur's work with chicken cholera and anthrax generalized both the concept of immunity and the use of the word 'vaccine', originally specific to smallpox. He assumed, quite reasonably, that immunity, relative or absolute, was related to the fact that nutrients essential for the microorganism's growth and reproduction were either wholly or partially exhausted in the host animal during the first attack. This followed naturally from his work on the varying nutritional requirements of microorganisms grown in the laboratory.

Towards the end of Pasteur's life, a gifted Russian biologist, Elie Metchnikoff (1845–1916) joined the group that was working in what was then the Institut Pasteur. Metchnikoff had famously observed in the early 1880s that a foreign body, such as a thorn, stuck into the transparent flesh of the starfish, stimulated cells to proliferate and attack the thorn, gradually digesting it. This was the basis of his theory of phagocytosis, literally 'eating cells'. He identified these cells with the white blood cells of mammals, including man, and spent the last decades of his life developing a theory of cellular immunity, whereby the main line of defence against invasion by a foreign organism resided in these blood cells, which attacked and killed disease-causing bacteria. His work (rewarded with a Nobel Prize in 1908) had much to recommend it. It provided an easy explanation of the origin of pus, which he perceived as collections of dead, brave warrior cells and their equally dead enemies. It explained why, in many infections, the number of white blood cells in the blood stream increased. (Cell counts of the various blood constituents, although laborious and not routinely done for several decades, became possible from the 1880s, with the development of the haemocytometer). And Metchnikoff's vision of the body and its defences legitimated the vocabulary of warfare that increasingly infused the way doctors described infection and its results. Metchnikoff's work was both immortalized and caricatured in George Bernard Shaw's play, *The Doctor's Dilemma* (1906), when a pompous, but scientific, surgeon sees it as his duty to his patients ever to 'stimulate the phagocytes'.

Metchnikoff's work showed that the white blood cell plays a central role in the body's response to infection. Colleagues at the Institut Pasteur, the centre of biomedical research in France, rallied round, and French immunology during the decades surrounding the turn of the nineteenth century was principally concerned with elucidating the mechanisms of cell-medicated immunity and defence.

At the same time, an alternative vision of immunity took root in Germany. It had equally persuasive experimental evidence to back it and its main architect was Paul Ehrlich (1854–1915). Ehrlich was a Jewish doctor in a time of rising anti-Semitism within Germany, which was one reason why his early medical career was dependent on the patronage of Friedrich von Frerichs, a powerful, scientifically minded clinician at the Charité, Berlin's main teaching hospital. After von Frerichs' sudden death in 1885, Ehrlich found himself at loose ends. His most important early research had dealt with the uptake of various organic dyes by cells, especially the various kinds of large cells in the blood, including the eosinophil, one of the 'white blood cells' that Ehrlich defined and named. He used this differential uptake of dyes to investigate the metabolic properties of living cells, but he also recognized that such dyes were also useful in identifying various bacteria implicated in disease. In 1888, tubercle bacilli were found in his sputum and he spent a year recovering in the warm, dry climate of Egypt. On his return, he received Koch's newly discovered tuberculin treatment and was convinced that it was instrumental in effecting a complete cure.

Although then without an academic appointment, he continued his research in a private laboratory. This led to important work on the staining (and therefore easier identification) of the 'acid fast' bacilli of TB, but also to a further appreciation of the chemical nature of many reactions between organisms and their environments. Work with Emil von Behring

(1854–1917) led to the internationally acclaimed development of an anti-toxin treatment for diphtheria, whereby the toxic substances produced by the diphtheria bacillus could be neutralized and the disease treated. This treatment built on work begun in France by one of Pasteur's disciples, Émile Roux (1853–1933). Diphtheria was one of those 'infectious' diseases that did not conform to the simple invasion paradigm for germs. The disease was not caused by the mere presence of the organism (which could be sometimes cultivated in healthy individuals), but by a toxic chemical that it secreted. The toxin rather than the mere germ caused this serious disease prevalent among young children. This toxin was an antigen and, there-fore, the disease could be treated by injecting the patient with appropriate antibodies.

Von Behring received the lion's share of the credit for introducing 'serum therapy', whereby antibodies generated in animals could be used in treating human disease. Ehrlich developed the scientific model in his famous 'lock and key' theory of the nature of the immune response. In this model, anti-gens, the molecules that identified the germ or its by-products as 'foreign' to the host, were neutralized and rendered harmless by antibodies, produced in the host and circulating in the bloodstream. Although Ehrlich had no idea of the actual molecular structures of either antigens or antibodies, this powerful model explained much about the nuances of what happens when an animal (including humans) was 'invaded' by a disease-causing germ.

Von Behring used horses to raise significant titres of antibodies against the diphtheria antitoxins and this proved dramatically effective in many cases of childhood diphtheria. There were also worrisome problems, as some patients reacted adversely to the other proteins in the horses' serum, producing what became a common 'iatrogenic' (i.e., produced by doctors) syndrome known as 'serum sickness'. The success of the diphtheria exam-ple stimulated much further research and, during the early decades of the twentieth century, serum therapy became common for a number of condi-tions. This episode, deserving of more historical study, provides an excellent example of the rewards and costs of scientific research. As serum therapy became fashionable, it was used for many disorders, including psychiatric and neurotic ones.

An early important discovery within the new science was Karl Land-steiner's (1868–1943) identification of the major human blood groups, which he initially called A, B and C, but which shortly became the famil-iar A, B, AB, and O types. (He was later involved in the discovery of the

Rhesus, Rh, factor.) Although the practical implications for blood transfusion of Landsteiner's work were not appreciated until later, his immunological ideas were part of the larger realization of what the scientific clinician Archibald Garrod called 'biochemical individuality'.

Ehrlich moved on from immunology to chemotherapy, applying his belief in the molecular specificity of biological reactions to search for chemical compounds that could react with invading parasites in such a way that the parasite was damaged, leaving the cells of the human host unaffected. His work on the trypanosomes, the causative organism of sleeping sickness, had relatively little European impact because it was for an exotic disease of little danger for Europeans in Africa. Syphilis was another matter, and the systematic study that Ehrlich and his team carried out on synthesized arsenical compounds ultimately resulted in compound 606, named 'Salvarsan'. This realized, albeit poorly, his dream of a 'magic bullet', a compound with selective properties of attacking and destroying the foreign invader without damaging the tissues of the host. A later compound, 'neo-salvarsan', helped redress the balance between toxicity and therapeutic effectiveness. Both compounds were more effective than alternative therapies (mostly mercurial compounds) for a common, dangerous, and stigmatizing disease.

Both serum therapies and the chemotherapies as represented by salvarsan, created public excitement, as well as problems. Each was the product of systematic laboratory research; each promised much and was eagerly sought by the afflicted and by the doctors who cared for them. Like the rabies vaccine, and vaccines for cholera, plague, typhoid, and other diseases produced before World War I, salvarsan and diphtheria antitoxin were part of the armamentarium of scientific medicine. Science and its attendant technologies had become part of the foundations of medicine.

Medical institutions

Science became inextricably linked to medical knowledge during the second half of the nineteenth century. Its influence on medical practice and on doctor-patient relationships will be examined later. Here, we look at the ways in which the findings and values of science were adapted in three institutional structures of medicine. Two of these institutions, medical schools and hospitals, were everyday components of the medical scene. The third, the independent research institute, was a more specific response to the scientific ethos of the period.

Most people, especially when they are well established in life, tend to resist change. A successful doctor (or lawyer, architect, or merchant) is unlikely to embrace new ideas, or new ways of doing things, if the old ones have worked. Institutions are even more resistant to change because many people are affected, and the institution itself has a kind of institutional drag that produces a resistance to radical transformation. Consequently, the ideas and discoveries coming from laboratories and research institutes in Europe (and, gradually, from North America) only slowly altered the shape and practices of the institutions of medicine. Older historians of medicine, and of medical ideas, naively assumed that a new discovery, especially one that has stood the test of time, was more or less instantly translated to universal acquiescence. It is as if individuals instantly recognize a new truth, or a better way of doing things. Modern historians of medicine and science have shown 'ideas' and practices take time to become assimilated, and that they are often adopted in ways that bear little relationship to their original formulation. We have learned to appreciate the fact that the clarion calls of Pasteur, Bernard, Ehrlich, and the other leaders of biomedical research, had a less immediate impact on ordinary medical structures and practice, than an older historiography naively assumed. For all that, the consciousness of living in societies undergoing rapid, even dramatic, change was part of the late-nineteenth-century worldview. Ours is not the first age of anxiety.

MEDICAL SCHOOLS: TYPES

Medical schools of one form or another are venerable institutions, hallowed by the Hippocratic tradition, in which the founding father of Western medicine took in pupils to initiate into the craft (i.e., art) of medicine. Although medical schools had assumed many forms by the mid-nineteenth century, a young man seeking a medical education within orthodox medicine might have found himself in one of five institutional settings, depending on his nationality, financial resources, and career ambitions.

The *apprenticeship* was the most basic form of medical training, and has sufficient historical importance to merit being called an institution. It had become more common among the less prestigious branches of the healing arts – surgeons, apothecaries, druggists, dentists, and general practitioners. Under the watchful eye and hand of a conscientious master, the apprenticeship had much to recommend it. The pupil learned all aspects of the 'business' of medicine (as its practice had often been called), including seeing the whole spectrum of patients, learning proper etiquette, compounding

medicines, keeping books, and encouraging patients to pay their bills. As
pupil became more experienced and independent, he might gain a valuable
local reputation, should he wish to stay in the area.

Often good on the practical dimensions of future practice, the apprenticeship was rarely ideal on more theoretical aspects of medicine, including
basic sciences such as anatomy and all of the experimental ones described
above. Further, the system was virtually impossible to police and too many
apprentices were exploited by their masters, given the drudging tasks of the
practice, and sent out on night calls with little preparation. As a medical
institution, it lost its hold by 1850, although its dying was prolonged and its
actual moment of death was imperceptible. It was not so much outlawed by
legislation as rendered obsolete by the new demands of medical knowledge
and the values of professionalism.

The apprenticeship was generally combined with a period of study at a
medical school to provide instruction in more formal aspects of medicine
and to satisfy the licensing requirements of the relevant medical corporations. There were four main types of medical school. Most basic was the
proprietary school, run by an individual or a group, offering instruction
in some medical subjects. They had become important throughout Europe
from the late eighteenth century, often as 'extramural' schools, situated
close to and supplementing more formally organized schools of the kinds
considered below. Anatomy was the most popular subject of proprietary
instruction, but ambitious or impecunious interns in France and *Privatdozenten* in the German-speaking areas often offered private classes on
a variety of topics to students willing to pay. In late-nineteenth-century
Europe, they maintained a kind of twilight existence, either as cramming
classes or, more often, as places where foreign students could obtain private
tuition in the students' native languages.

In *laissez-faire* America, proprietary schools dominated the medical
scene, not as an adjunct to supplement regular training but for total 'education'. Some of them were run by conscientious proprietors, aiming to
give good value for money and to instil a sense of professionalism in their
charges. Others were concerned primarily with profit, often achieved by low
fees and rapid throughput. Such schools also promulgated the ideological
beliefs of their founders, and in mid-century America, several medical sects
vied with 'orthodox' medicine for hegemony. Rothstein has commented
that in the 1850s regular (i.e., orthodox) doctors were under such threat
from practitioners espousing homeopathy, Thomsonianism, and medical
eclecticism, that it would have been a brave person who predicted that

137

come to dominate only a half century later (Rothstein,
schools of all stripes were perfectly legal and turned out
ter only a year or so of desultory instruction, complete
various degrees, including doctorates. Their profusion
surplus of doctors in the middle decades of the century,
putation that American medicine had abroad. Proprietary
the chief animus of Abraham Flexner's (1866–1959) late-
century campaign to reform American medical education.

A second type of medical school was common in continental Europe, but had no obvious counterpart in the English-speaking world. These were the practical, or secondary medical schools, which in Germany, France, and elsewhere produced a lower grade of medical man. The Germans called them *Wundaerzte*, the French called them *officiers de santé*, and these practitioners generally came from humble backgrounds and were destined to serve the poor and to work in areas where more formal medical help was unavailable. As the élite French physician and microscopist Alfred Donné (1801–78) put it, 'There are two categories of sick people, the rich and the poor: there must be two grades of doctors to meet the needs of the one and the other' (Bonner, 1995, p. 192). By mid-century, there were calls to abolish this two-tiered system of medical training. Virchow insisted in 1846 that the 'bread and butter studies' of the practical schools should be abolished: 'the training of future doctors must be given entirely to universities.' The practical schools started being phased out in the German-speaking areas in the 1850s, but the French did not abolish the *officier de santé* until 1892. The number of *officiers* had been declining steadily since mid-century, however, and efforts were made in the 1870s to improve the quality of clinical and scientific facilities and instruction available in these secondary schools.

A third kind of medical school was that associated with a hospital. Flexner described them as 'clinical schools' and identified this as a peculiarly English form of institution. Certainly it was common there. In a sense, however, the hospital medical school was also powerful in France during its golden period, when the medical schools were separate from the universities. Pasteur's post was at the École Normale and Bernard held chairs at the Sorbonne, Collège de France, and other institutions, not in the Paris medical school. Although some students took university courses in physiology, chemistry, or microscopy alongside their formal medical work, the relationship between French universities and medical schools remained distant until well into the nineteenth century. The Paris Medical School had, of course, its own faculty, publicly appointed, and it enjoyed the formal support of the state, including the right to grant degrees in medicine and surgery. It was not so much a hospital medical school, but a sprawling clinical faculty based in eight or ten of the major Parisian hospitals.

The hospital medical schools in England, especially as typified by the famous ones in London, were distinctive. By the 1860s, there were ten of them, of which St. Bartholomew's Hospital Medical School was the largest. Two other London schools, University College and King's College, London, had some features associated with a university. The hospital schools had proprietary elements because the teachers, generally on the clinical staff of the hospital, benefited from student fees. At the same time, the hospitals were nonprofit charities dependent on charitable giving to keep their doors open p. 216. Despite the fees that the teachers enjoyed, the hospital medical schools on the whole were financial liabilities to their parent institutions. It was difficult to generate the kind of charitable donations on which the hospitals depended for medical education (as opposed to patient care), and as the century progressed, the demands for new equipment, materials, space, and staff for the schools grew ever more persistent.

Because hospital medical school staff were mostly also engaged in medical practice, what was taught was generally of a practical nature. Hospital medical schools were in the business of preparing their charges for the realities of the medical marketplace. For many leaders of the profession (as it aspired to be), this was not enough.

For these individuals, the gold standard of medical education was the university medical school. Only there, it was stated repeatedly, could a student receive his education (not simply training) from those who were actively engaged in research. Only through the university could doctors achieve the proper social status of liberally educated, true professionals. In universities, medical students could learn their science in laboratories, not in lecture halls. 'Knowledge lives in the laboratory', Charles Minot declared early in the twentieth century, and 'when it is dead, we bury it decently in a book'. In universities, men primarily engaged in the creation of new knowledge also taught clinical medicine and surgery. Universities had faculties, not simply collections of teachers. At mid-century, there were a number of university medical schools (and faculties) that had potential (or at least distinguished pasts): the University of Edinburgh, and University College and King's College, London, in Britain; the Universities of Pennsylvania and Harvard in the United States; Leiden and Groningen in the Netherlands. To turn university potential into modern educational reality required commitment and, above all, money. The university ideal for medical education was most evident in the German-speaking lands.

MEDICAL SCHOOLS: THE GERMAN LANDS

Modern-day Germany before the 1870s was a collection of independent states, kingdoms, and principalities. Although united by a common language, they were separated by religion (Catholic and Protestant areas), dialects, economic development, and local customs. The German language also extended to the Austro-Hungarian Empire, which included much of present-day Eastern Europe. Within this large but diverse area, a network of universities, some old, some new (e.g., the University of Berlin, founded in 1810) had developed during the eighteenth and early-nineteenth centuries. Within 'Germany', Prussia (whose capital was Berlin) was the largest, most powerful, and aggressive, and during the 1860s, diplomats throughout Europe concerned with the balance of power watched with fear and fascination to see how Prussia would consolidate its position within the German *Sprachgebiet*. It happened after Prussia's dramatic victory in 1870–1 over France, in the Franco-Prussian War. The 'Iron Chancellor', Bismarck, created a European 'Empire' by unifying the old German states and extending the German sphere of influence over much of Eastern Europe.

Bismarck inherited a vigorous network of universities, many of which had already developed distinguished medical faculties. German culture valued learning and systematic knowledge (for which the German word *Wissenschaft* loosely translates as 'science'). Already in the late 1840s, following the abortive revolutions of 1848, medical leaders such as Virchow had been calling for a single port of entry for doctors, through education in a university. With the abolition of the old 'practical' schools training *Wundaerzte*, the university ideal became dominant. At its best, the German system combined the virtues of *Lehrfreiheit* (freedom for professors to teach their own research) and *Lernfreiheit* (freedom for students to move from university to university, seeking the best from each).

The ideal was not always matched by reality. German universities (reflecting widespread values within German culture) were rigidly hierarchical, favouring professors at the expense of the lowlier *Privatdozenten*, young men who by their research had earned the right to teach within the universities. The routine tasks of teaching and examining often fell to those of this rank, and Jews, among others, might not aspire higher. As the German system developed, the grand lecture, delivered by the professor to hundreds of students, became too common, and clinical or scientific demonstrations were often remote from the view of the lowly student.

Despite the problems, the German universities were widely admired, and foreign medical students in their thousands spent periods ranging from a few weeks to two or three years, studying in the German-speaking lands. At mid-century, the migration was still a trickle, as many foreign students still opted for Paris. One doctor wrote in 1850 that there were only five Americans in Vienna, and between 300 and 400 in Paris. By the end of the century, the proportions had dramatically altered, and Berlin, Vienna, Leipzig, Munich, and the other major German universities enjoyed the patronage of hundreds of foreign students, in addition to servicing future doctors for greater Germany. For a half century, German was the principal common language of biomedical science, as Latin and French had been before, and English became afterwards.

Studies of the academic politics and budgets of several German universities – Berlin, Heidelberg, Leipzig, Vienna – have demonstrated how important powerful personalities were. A sympathetic minister of education could open up public coffers to build and equip new buildings, and hire new staff. Teaching hospitals and specialized clinics sprung up in German towns with small populations but big ambitions. Successful professors who published visible research, founded new journals, and attracted advanced students were in great demand. There was of course a general pecking order among the universities, and Berlin was always high on the list. But the fact that semiautonomous institutes represented academic disciplines within university structures meant that even smaller universities might hope to excel in one or two subjects. The *Lernfreiheit* enjoyed by students was duplicated in the professoriate by their career moves, almost always to universities offering purpose-built facilities, better income, more power. Late-nineteenth-century Germany was a good time to be 'Herr Professor'.

Heidelberg was particularly active in medicine and medical sciences at mid-century, recruiting Helmholtz in physiology, Jacob Henle in anatomy and microscopy, and Robert Bunsen (1811–99) – he of the burner – in chemistry. Liebig moved from Giessen to Munich when better laboratories were built for him; Virchow and Koch had special facilities offered them in Berlin. The emphasis on research encouraged specialization among the professors and this, in turn, attracted the foreign students, most of whom were already medical graduates. Budding pathologists went to work with Virchow or Cohnheim, hundreds of foreign students studied physiology in Ludwig's spacious laboratories in Leipzig, and Koch's group acted as a magnet for those interested in bacteriology. The clinical disciplines also began to become specialized: within medicine, Ferdinand von Hebra (1816–88) in Vienna attracted those interested in skin diseases, and Wilhelm Erb (1840–1921) and Carl Wernicke (1848–1904) developed famous neurological clinics in Heidelberg and Breslau, respectively. Surgery developed even more tightly knit specialties: ophthalmology and otolaryngology had important clinics in several German-speaking universities, as did orthopaedics, urology, and gynaecology. General abdominal surgery, now considered the province of the general surgeon, was then the object of the daring specialist surgeon. Theodor Billroth (1829–94) pioneered a number of new abdominal operations in his academic clinic, first in Zürich and then at the University of Vienna. All the surgical specialties benefited from the techniques of antiseptic and aseptic surgery pp. 157-59.

There were, of course, critics as well as admirers of the German system of medical education. Successful institutes or clinics sometimes became so large that students, even postgraduates, felt they were small cogs in a large wheel. The lecture-demonstration became too common for those wishing to learn by doing. German student culture, with its rigid codes of honour and love of duelling, did not appeal to many. After the Franco-Prussian War, French students preferred to stay at home. But the Americans, British, Spanish, Italians, Dutch, Russians, and Scandinavians came in droves. As Abraham Flexner, an enthusiastic but not uncritical student of the German university system, put it, 'With the outburst of creative energy characteristic of Germany from 1866 on, the German universities severally obtained scientific institutes and clinics equipped with the laboratories that became successively necessary and appropriate. The German conception of medicine as a university faculty, in a university equally bound to teach and to investigate, was thus admirably embodied in the equipment, spirit, and activity of the medical faculties' (Flexner, 1925, 33–4).

In 1872, the contrast between German and French values for medical education was starkly displayed. As a result of the Franco-Prussian War, Germany acquired the rich industrial lands of Alsace. They found in Strasbourg a large medical school, operating along French lines. Dismissing this as a 'trade school', a modern German university was established in its place. This new outpost of German imperialism was attractive to a number of distinguished German academics and the Kaiser oversaw the appointments: Friedrich von Recklinghausen (1833–1910) in pathology, Felix Hoppe-Seyler (1825–95) in physiology, and Oswald Schmiedeberg (1838–1921) in pharmacology. Most French staff of the older school declined to participate, leaving to join a new French school established in nearby Nancy. The student body, too, came for the most part from outside the area, as Alsatian students and doctors preferred to preserve the French way of doing things. Ironically, but more slowly, defeat in the Franco-Prussian War catalysed the modernization of the French university and medical education.

MEDICAL SCHOOLS: FRANCE

The power of institutional drag is prominently displayed in the later history of the French medical schools. Their basic form had been created in a time of revolutionary fervour, but the practical training that they offered from the very beginning had proved appropriate for the times. When the schools had been reorganized in 1794, the architects rejected medical theory as symptomatic of the corrupt medicine of the *ancien régime*. The integration of medicine and surgery was partly a response to the demands of the military, but also it was meant to abolish the older hierarchies within the medical orders. The unique educational experience that emerged – firmly based in the hospital and emphasizing the medical fundamentals of careful physical diagnosis and systematic postmortem examination – resonated throughout the Western world.

Ackerknecht's classic study of this period in French medicine ends in 1848, when, he argued, French medical education was being rendered old-fashioned by the newer German models. Many French observers recognized this, and the Societé de Biologie, established in that very year of revolution, 1848, by a group of reformist-minded young Turks, looked to the German integration of experimental science with medicine as the way of the future. Claude Bernard was an active founder and vice president of the informal society, whose membership included several well-placed clinicians and scientists including Pierre Rayer, later Dean of the Paris faculty of medicine; Paul Bert, Bernard's favourite pupil and his successor to the chair of physiology at the Sorbonne; Charles Robin, an energetic microscopist and influential professor in the faculty; and Charles Brown-Séquard (1817–94), Mauritian-born and American-educated, and a gifted experimental neurophysiologist with an eye for applying his laboratory findings in the neurological clinic.

Despite the society's collective admiration for developments in Germany, its members drew more immediate inspiration from a French philosopher, Auguste Comte (1798–1857), exponent of the doctrine of 'positivism'. Comte taught that the history of human thought revealed a progressive trend, from theological (supernatural) beginnings, through a second stage characterized as metaphysical, to its final glorious realization in the scientific work of the nineteenth century, the era of the positive. The Society of Biology was dedicated to bringing this positivistic spirit to the life sciences and to infusing medicine with these sciences.

Like several other informal scientific groups in the century, the influence of the society (which was relatively short-lived) can be found more in the subsequent activities of its individual members. They actively participated in what one historian has called 'the rise of the science empire in France', and another has described as the 'development of the modern university in France'. Despite the bitter pill that defeat in the Franco-Prussian War was for French pride, most historians see it as an important catalyst for social change. The Republican government that came to power afterwards recognized that a great deal of Prussian might was technological and scientific in origin. French universities retained many of their traditional structures and values, but science faculties were strengthened and scientific training more systematically merged into the educational experiences of French doctors.

After 1871, the French provincial universities developed quickly, even if Paris remained the central medical magnet. Its hospitals and scientific institutions continued to dominate French cultural and scientific life, and foreign students who went to France still gravitated to the capital. Late in the century, Jean-Martin Charcot's (1825–93) lectures and demonstrations still attracted a large following. His demonstrations were wonderfully theatrical and he was a clinician of international reputation, but he still operated largely within the framework of an earlier generation. The Institut Pasteur p. 163 was the principal French biomedical research institute and it remained an autonomous creation.

MEDICAL SCHOOLS: GREAT BRITAIN

What Flexner called the clinical, or hospital school, lasted longest in Britain. Even by the end of the century, most medical students would have been trained at a medical school attached to a general voluntary hospital. Despite moves earlier in the century to adopt a 'single portal' (which would probably have been a central examining body, rather than a university requirement for medical education), the older eclectic system of medical and surgical licensing survived. For the hospital medical students, this meant a split between teaching and the licensing examinations. The latter was in the hands of the Royal Colleges of Physicians and Surgeons in London, Edinburgh, Glasgow, and Dublin, and the Society of Apothecaries in London.

Standards of medical education had been placed in the hands of the General Medical Council, created by the Medical Act of 1858. During our period, membership on the council was dominated by medical and surgical élites drawn from the Royal Colleges and the universities. Many members of the council were sympathetic to the newer demands of a science-based education, but the council acted more in an advisory than an executive capacity. It inspected and commented on, rather than dictated what medical schools ought to teach.

Clinical teaching was practical and sound, if conservative, because clinical teaching staff were generally appointed from within the hospital and clinicians rarely moved from hospital to hospital. This meant that 'Old Boys', once in post, stayed until death or retirement. Clinical staff in the hospitals gave their time gratuitously, which required them also to maintain private practices. Many of those who taught the sciences – anatomy, microscopy, physiology, and pathology – were part-timers also in private practice, although this began slowly to change as the century wore on. Because students presenting themselves to the examining bodies had to offer evidence that they had taken science courses, the hospital medical schools were obliged to teach them. Histology gradually penetrated the syllabuses from the 1840s, anatomy and pathology were always seen as necessary, and in 1870 the Royal College of Surgeons passed a resolution requiring students to take a course in practical physiology.

This requirement, which was soon added to those of other examining bodies, was a turning point in British medical education. It obliged medical schools to teach experimental physiology and to create the space and resources to do so. It gave a few would-be biomedical scientists the possibility of carving out a career in science divorced from the everyday demands of practice. Michael Foster (1836–1907) was crucial in this professional development. After several years in general practice, he had become, in 1867, a professor of practical physiology at University College London, one of the most scientifically orientated medical schools in Britain p. 21. In 1870, he moved to Trinity College, Cambridge, as a fellow and praelector in physiology. Although without a proper university post in Cambridge until 1883, when a chair was created for him, he nevertheless managed to make physiology and the other medical sciences central to the university's medical curriculum. He created along the way a research school in physiology that produced a large number of outstanding experimentalists, such that by the turn of the century, Britain could rival Germany in the discipline. Although several German university towns no bigger than Cambridge developed clinical schools, Cambridge was felt to be too small to have a big enough hospital to provide adequate clinical facilities. Nevertheless, its medical school thrived, offering basic medical science training for a large number of students, who then went to the London hospitals (mostly University College Hospital or St. Bartholomew's Hospital) for clinical instruction, returning to Cambridge for final exams and the Cambridge M.B. degree. By the end of the century, Cambridge was as big as St. Bartholomew's in its medical student intake, a sign both of its local success, but also of the way in which medicine was projecting itself as a dignified liberal profession.

Cambridge remained unique in late Victorian England: Oxford modernized more slowly, and the University of London remained, despite moves to change it, solely an examining institution, not a teaching one. Some of its constituent institutions, including University College and King's College, possessed proper faculties, but degrees were granted through the parent university. Students from the London hospital medical schools – St. Bartholomew's, St. Mary's, Guy's Hospital, and the rest could, if they wished, take the university exams and receive the London medical degree. This became increasingly popular for the ambitious ones, but the thrust of medical education in Britain was to produce what was called the 'safe general practitioner', a student who on the day of his graduation had had training in basic medicine, simple surgery, and uncomplicated midwifery, and could be safely let loose on the public. For this purpose, in the 1880s, the Royal College of Physicians and the Royal College of Surgeons cooperated in producing what was called the 'conjoint exam', the Licentiateship of the Royal College of Physicians (LRCP) and Membership of the Royal College of Surgeons (MRCS), long the hallmark of the general practitioner. Those who aspired to consulting practices and hospital posts, took higher qualifications, the M.D., or the exams for Fellowship in the Royal College of Surgeons (FRCS) or Membership in the Royal College of Physicians (MRCP). The more prestigious fellowship in the College of Physicians (FRCP) was by election from among the membership.

The English system remained eclectic and piecemeal, and hardly satisfied Flexner's goal of all doctors being scientifically trained in a university setting. The Scottish medical schools were closer to Flexner's institutional ideal, but they failed to provide the resources to realize the research ethos that prevailed in the German universities. Medical schools in the English provinces – Manchester, Birmingham, Bristol, Newcastle, and Leeds – gradually developed a university setting, but they, too, continued to emphasize the practical at the expense of the scientific. Ambitious British medical graduates gravitated towards the German universities for postgraduate work, whether in the sciences or the medical and surgical specialities. Plans to introduce academic clinical units in medicine and surgery, on the German model, remained unrealized early in the twentieth century, and their birth had to wait until after World War I p. 303ff.

MEDICAL SCHOOLS: THE UNITED STATES

Ambitious American medical students transported the various British forms of medical education and licensing to colonial America and the early republic, and European styles were continuously brought back from Edinburgh, London, Paris, and other European centres. The political organization of the new republic handed the several states a good deal of power, which led to local variation in the regulation of medical men. In the early decades of the nineteenth century, *laissez faire* became increasingly the rule of thumb as market values ruled medical practice. Medical sectarianism reached its peak around mid-century. Although several older universities – the University of Pennsylvania, Harvard, and Yale – had medical faculties, they sometimes found it difficult to compete with the profusion of proprietary schools that offered medical training for a modest investment of time or money. Several of the various medical sects had their own medical schools.

Later in the century, women benefited from the casual nature of American medical education. Although the little medical school in Geneva, in upstate New York, closed its doors to women after Elizabeth Blackwell (1821–1910) exploited a loophole in their admission regulations to become the first modern woman medical graduate, several other small schools for women were opened in the later decades of the century, and by 1900 the United States had more women doctors than any other country.

It is symptomatic that an English woman had to go to a backwoods medical school in the United States to break down the barriers that had been built even higher in this age of professionalization. The less formal earlier centuries had allowed for a few enterprising women to practise medicine and surgery beyond the traditional confines of midwifery. The women from the mid-nineteenth century who wanted proper medical qualifications needed to be both ambitious and peripatetic. Marie Zakrzewska (1829–1902) trained in midwifery in Berlin before immigrating to the United States, where she obtained an M.D. from Western Reserve, in Cleveland Ohio. Mary Putnam Jacobi, née Mary Putnam, managed to get a medical degree from Paris. The first woman medical graduate from the University of Zurich, was a Russian, and Zurich proved to be a haven for many women. In the United States, as, eventually, in Britain, the easy, though not entirely satisfactory, solution was the foundation of medical schools for women. This solved the problem of exclusion from many medical schools and of segregated teaching in those schools that would admit them. These early pioneers argued not only their right to enter the profession, but the complementary right of women to have a female doctor should they desire it. Throughout the nineteenth century, women doctors mostly practised within those medical areas dealing with women and children: obstetrics, gynaecology, paediatrics, and school health. A number of them went into medicine from a religious calling, and trained in Europe or North America, but spent much of their lives in missionary work abroad.

The American Civil War (1861–5) undoubtedly helped medical orthodoxy because the dominant figures in both the Union and Confederate medical services were men who had been educated in the ordinary values and theories of traditional medicine. The Eastern states were most European in their medical (and cultural) outlook, and many of the young men who made European pilgrimages came from the eastern seaboard and its medical institutions. Recent scholarship has documented the extent to which Americans abroad were selective in the concepts and values they brought back. But the Parisian epoch in the first half of the century, and the German one in the second half, certainly left their marks on American medicine. A steady stream of American publications and translations from leading European authors testifies to a market for foreign books even among doctors who did not have the time or resources to spend time in Europe.

The traditional historical account of the reform of American medical education – and the triumph of the 'regulars' – credits Abraham Flexner's crusading zeal, from the very end of the nineteenth century and the early years of the twentieth. Certainly his surveys of medical schools in the United States and Canada (1910) and of Europe (1912) were highly influential. He preached above all the value of the German university system, and in the years after his reports, proprietary schools closed down with increasing speed. But to attribute so much to Flexner misses much that had gone on in the preceding decades. Not only had the older élite medical schools at Harvard, Pennsylvania, and Columbia (the College of Physicians and Surgeons) done much to adapt to the newer demands of scientific training, but several new schools, including the University of Michigan and, above all, Johns Hopkins, inculcated the values of scientific medicine from their very

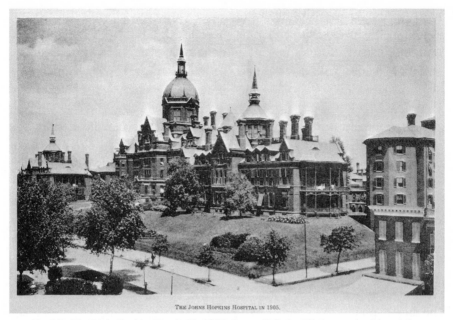

THE JOHNS HOPKINS HOSPITAL IN 1905.

Fig. 2.2. The Johns Hopkins Hospital in 1905. *Source: Bulletin of the International Association of Medical Museums* 9 (1926), facing p. 262. *Credit*: Wellcome Library, London (L0004916).

foundations. In different trajectories, each of them also admitted women medical students.

Flexner was, of course, aware that there were pockets of good in a sea of mediocrity. From the very beginning, Johns Hopkins was special and meant to be. Generously endowed by a Quaker railway magnate (whose first name *Johns* has created difficulties ever since), the university was opened to fanfare in 1876, with T. H. Huxley among other eminent participants. It was deliberately Germanic in its ethos, with a faculty that valued research. The medical school and purpose-built hospital were delayed for almost two decades (even at Hopkins the money was not inexhaustible), but when the hospital and medical school finally opened in the 1890s, its faculty knew they were part of a glorious experiment (Fig. 2.2). They also knew European medical training from the inside. William H. Welch in pathology, Franklin Paine Mall (1862–1917) in anatomy, John Jacob Abel (1857–1938) in pharmacology, William Henry Howell (1860–1945) in physiology, William Osler (1849–1919) in medicine, and William Stewart Halsted (1852–1922) in surgery had all done their European tour. From the very beginning, the medical school was not afraid to require an undergraduate degree from its students and its graduates began very quickly to people the posts of other progressive medical schools. On a smaller scale, the University of Michigan, Cornell, and other medical schools had bucked the trend and raised entry requirements, built laboratories and teaching hospitals, and hired faculty with a desire to contribute to medical knowledge.

HOSPITALS

As far as doctors were concerned, hospitals had been medicalized by the mid-nineteenth century. Hospitals were so closely identified with the education and activities of the medical professions that they seemed 'natural'. For doctors, at least, hospitals had lost much of the coercive, custodial capacity that Michel Foucault identified with the *hôpital general* and other institutions of the early modern state, where the sick poor were housed alongside beggars, prostitutes, orphans, fools, and madmen, in an amorphous gathering of deviants. During the eighteenth and early nineteenth centuries, such institutions had gradually become more highly differentiated: the mad were gradually separated from the bad, the sick poor were separated from the merely poor.

Many patients were undoubtedly less convinced that hospitals were simply about curing ills because there were still many hospitals associated with poor law and other regulative state functions, and the large psychiatric asylums that were beginning to spring up were rapidly becoming largely custodial rather than curative. Death rates in ordinary hospitals were still sufficiently high that they still carried the older popular image that they were 'gateways to death'. In Britain, Poor Law infirmaries and similar institutions were places where the infirm, demented, chronically ill, or simply old went when they had no other place to go. And at mid-century, hospitals remained primarily institutions for the care of the poor: the rich received their medical care elsewhere.

This class dimension gave hospitals their tone. Put simply, doctors in the middle of the nineteenth century cared for patients in hospital who came from a lower social order. Their patients were servants, unskilled labourers, porters, butchers, bakers, and candlestick makers. This simple fact helps explain power structures within the hospital, what Foucault called *pouvoir*. In a deferential society, of course, patients did as they were told or, frequently, did not do as they were told and were dismissed summarily.

There were, of course, other power relationships in the hospital, between the different orders of medical men, between senior and junior staff; teachers and students; and doctors and nurses, cooks, porters, cleaners, and other menial staff. In charitable hospitals, there were structures of control between those whose money supported the institution and all those who worked there. When the state, religious organization, or municipality paid for it, there were other pipers piping.

This latter format was more common on the Continent. Much of the hospital infrastructure was in the public domain, although in areas with strong Roman Catholic loyalty, many religious hospitals remained, and these were often used by wealthier individuals, whose bequests were important for the long-term continuity of the institution.

In Britain, the charitable hospital dominated. They were called 'voluntary hospitals' because benefactors volunteered their gifts and doctors volunteered their time. In the United States, hospitals were extremely scarce until the nineteenth century, although the two ones founded before the century's end (in Philadelphia and New York City) bore organizational resemblance to their English counterparts. The British voluntary hospitals survived, albeit under increasing financial pressures, until the nationalization of most hospitals under the National Health Service (NHS), after World War II p. 440. Parallel with the voluntary hospital system, another publicly funded system developed, mostly to take up the residuum, paupers, chronically ill, psychiatric patients, and those suffering from contagious diseases.

Hospitals in the mid-century West thus came in a variety of sizes, shapes, and financial circumstances. In virtually all of them, orthodox medicine prevailed. With the exception of the homeopaths, who founded a few hospitals, these institutions were a monopoly of the 'regulars', even in mid-nineteenth-century America. In Britain, the 1858 Medical Act denied doctors the more general monopoly many of them felt they deserved. It allowed for *laissez faire* to obtain in the wider medical marketplace. But only qualified doctors could hold posts in the voluntary hospitals as well as the medical institutions officially sanctioned by the state, Poor Law infirmaries, fever hospitals, and asylums for the insane. By mid-century, the hospital was a securely medical institution.

HOSPITALS: BUILT FORM

The institutional drag mentioned above is easily seen in hospital form. Unless one is prepared to tear down and start over from scratch, a building imposes some of its original functions on later generations. New hospitals continued to be built throughout the late Victorian period, but most of them at any one time were older structures, embodying different medical and social values. Notions of privacy, cleanliness, sanitary provision, surveillance, nursing, and medical functions, can all change faster than building structure. All medical hospitals always had a formal responsibility for patient care. In the eighteenth and early nineteenth centuries, hospitals had needed to accommodate increasing educational responsibilities. In our period, they assumed an increasing research function, but above all had to adapt to the newer demands of technology, nursing, medical, and, most important, surgical practice.

During the period, architects became more major players in hospital life. New hospitals were major projects, put out to tender, and their design was frequently discussed in architectural and medical journals. Many innovations were simply responses to technological improvements in general: central heating, electric lights, running water, and closed water closets. Other features of hospital building were more closely related to medical, surgical, and nursing demands. The British systematically noted, about 1860, that new hospitals tended to have lower death rates than old ones, and that death rates often increased as a new hospital aged. Florence Nightingale (1820–1910) trenchantly suggested that the solution was simple: tear them down and build them anew every decade or so.

This radical solution to hospitalism, as it was called, was never likely to be economically feasible, but Nightingale did get her way on a common ward design: the pavilion ward. Pavilion wards were not new, but they were not all that common in the mid-century. Nightingale returned from the Crimean War (1853–6) a national heroine, already depicted with her lamp, making her way among the beds of sick and wounded soldiers during the night. The American poet Henry Longfellow first dubbed her 'a Lady with a lamp'. She was a woman of definite ideas, with an indomitable desire to reform the world. Her twin passion, along with reform, was for statistics, and her writings are stuffed with facts and figures proving her points. Her leading ideas were developed in the 1830s and 1840s, reinforced by her Crimean experience, and more or less fixed thereafter. A mysterious illness confined her to her bed shortly after her return to England, but she spent the rest of her long life writing reports and letters, receiving visitors, and propagating her gospel.

The pavilion ward design was part of that vision, reinforced because it was the common makeshift design of the barracks and huts that she had experienced in the Crimea. It had important consequences for nursing, but, more generally, pavilion wards were healthier than the worst types they replaced. Working as she did within the context of miasmatic theories of disease spread, space between beds and a lot of free-flowing air were necessary

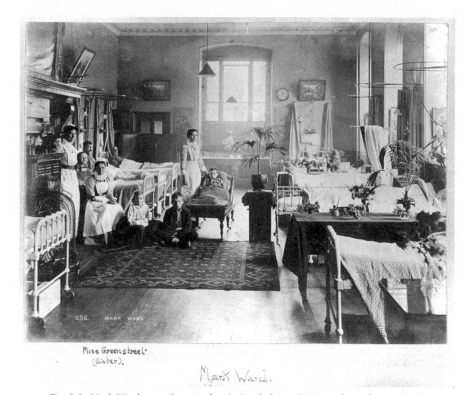

Miss Greenstreet
(Sister).

Mark Ward.

Fig. 2.3. Mark Ward, a pavilion ward at St. Bartholomew's Hospital, London, *c.* 1908.
Adult males and young boys are nursed together. *Source*: Photograph, Wellcome Library
Iconographic Collection. *Credit*: Wellcome Library, London (L0014166).

to keep the air pure, and so to prevent hospital infections, surgical gangrene, and the like. Miasmatists equated cleanliness with health and putrid
smell with disease, and the pavilion ward was easy to clean and ventilated
itself, if the large windows causing through-drafts were kept open. Later
observers noted winter temperatures of only a few degrees above freezing
in some of these wards (Fig. 2.3).

Pavilion hospitals were exceedingly land-hungry because the wards were
large, needed open space on each side for ventilation, and could not be more
than two stories high at the most. The ideal pavilion hospital consisted of a
central service block for cooking, laundry, and the like, with a series of wards
with about twenty-four beds each radiating out (Fig. 2.4). A number of
them were built in the middle decades of the century, but they were not very
adaptable to urban areas where hospitals were mostly needed. Advocates of
the pavilion design argued that doctors were the main beneficiaries of urban
hospitals because their location made it convenient to combine hospital and

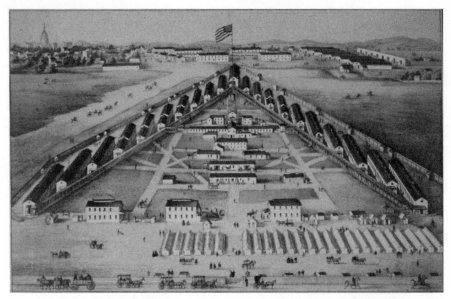

Fig. 2.4. Lincoln Hospital, Washington, DC. Archetypal pavilion hospital, having twenty-one ward blocks arranged in a 'V' with central administrative and service buildings. *Source*: Fry Print Collection. *Credit*: Yale University, Harvey Cushing/John Hay Whitney Medical Library.

private work. (They sometimes forgot that they were also more convenient for the urban poor who peopled them.)

The pros and cons of urban–rural, pavilion–conventional hospital design were played out on several occasions, rarely so publicly as when the medieval St. Thomas's Hospital was torn down in the 1860s to make way for a new railway station, a poignant instance of the new industrial order sweeping all before it. Nightingale was at the centre of the party insisting that it should be relocated in leafy suburban London, or even in rural Surrey. The medical staff, led by John Simon (1816–1904, p. 191), were almost entirely opposed, and the hospital governors recognized the impracticality of locating a hospital fifteen miles away from the patients it served. Several sites were considered, including some within the metropolis and some without. The site chosen, on the south bank of the Thames, opposite the Houses of Parliament, was practically the worst choice for a miasmatist, given the stench that often emanated from London's famous river, still a principal receptacle for sewerage. (The Embankment of the Thames had already been planned, and the hospital was eventually partially built on reclaimed land. The Embankment incorporated engineering works that took London's sewers out of central London to the east). Ward design was

154

primarily of the pavilion type, a minor victory for Nightingale and her supporters, and the wards were low-rise, although higher than she wanted.
She also got a nursing school in the new hospital, and the needs of modern
nursing guaranteed the longevity of the pavilion ward.

By the time the new St. Thomas's opened in 1871, the epidemiological
ideas that had made the pavilion so attractive were being undermined.
As hospital infections became identified with germs, not simply with bad
air, new methods of their control became possible. Even more significantly,
the demands of antiseptic and aseptic surgery, and the increasing use of
laboratories within hospitals for diagnostic and research purposes, brought
other issues to the fore within hospital design.

HOSPITALS: SURGERY

Surgery is now so intimately associated with hospitals that it is hard to
conceive that there was a time when the actual operation was a minor
part of the surgeon's hospital activity, and that even major surgery, such
as amputation of a leg, was more safely done elsewhere. When operations
in a hospital were performed, they were often carried out in the patient's
ward, sometimes in his or her own bed, or (especially if they were major)
in front of dozens or hundreds of students in the ordinary lecture theatre, turned into an operating theatre. Despite the serious limitations of
surgery, surgeons had gone a long way towards achieving parity with their
medical colleagues by mid-century. New operations had been pioneered,
for instance, tying arteries above and/or below a dangerous aneurysm, a
procedure based on physiological experimentation on the capacity of the
arteries to develop collateral circulation. Surgical debates about whether
it was better to amputate a leg with a compound fracture immediately or
reduce it and hope gangrene did not set in, filled the surgical literature in
the first half of the century. But all surgeons knew that surgical mortality for major operations was high, and they also knew that hospitals were
dangerous (if convenient) places in which to operate.

The control of pain during surgery had been possible since the public
introduction of anaesthetics at the Massachusetts General Hospital in October 1846. William T. G. Morton (1819–68) administered the anaesthetic
and John Collins Warren (1778–1850) performed the historic operation.
Anaesthesia was the first major medical advance to spread throughout
the West as fast as technology would allow (in this case, ships crossing
the Atlantic). Meticulous investigation has documented the early use of
anaesthesia in America, Britain, and Europe, and historians have correctly

pointed out that there was not a spontaneous uptake: wounded soldiers were often thought to do better with the stimulus of pain, anaesthesia during childbirth was (briefly) resisted, and the inevitable anaesthetic death came before coroner's courts and created medico-legal problems. On balance, the striking thing is how quickly the new procedure spread to out-of-the-way places. Ether was the first anaesthetic agent publicly used and chloroform was added by the Edinburgh obstetrician Sir James Young Simpson (1811–70) in 1847. These two chemicals provided the mainstay of anaesthesia until late in the century, when the local anaesthetics cocaine (its addictive qualities became only gradually realized) and procaine were added. Chemists and pharmacologists searched for other substances that might have anaesthetic properties without the problems associated with both ether and chloroform, but none of them replaced these two as general anaesthetics. Nitrous oxide, the 'laughing gas' of the early century, was also employed regularly in dentistry.

Hospital statistics suggest that anaesthesia probably had a detrimental effect on surgical mortality. Controlling pain gave surgeons longer to operate and, while they might be able to preserve delicate tissues more easily, it also meant that the open wounds were more exposed to the atmosphere and to unwashed instruments and hands. Like all important moments in medical history, Joseph Lister's (1827–1912) introduction of antiseptic surgery in 1867 has been scrutinized for precursors. There are some. In the 1840s and 1850s, the Hungarian obstetrician Ignaz Philipp Semmelweis (1818–65) was concerned with the high mortality among women whose babies were delivered in the teaching wards of the Allgemeinen Krankenhaus in Vienna. He also noticed that a friend of his had died of a dissecting wound, with symptoms very like those of the dying mothers. He further observed that mothers whose babies were delivered in the same hospital by midwives suffered a much lower mortality. He concluded, quite reasonably, that the medical students, who went from pathological dissection to delivery, might be introducing something into the birth canals of the unfortunate women.

By insisting that the medical students wash their hands in a lime solution between pathology and obstetrics, he managed to bring the mortality rates to a par. There were other interpretations to be put on his findings, however, and he remained an outsider and controversial figure. A retrospective hero, Semmelweis should be seen in his time as merely joining a list of obstetricians, dating back to the eighteenth century, who had made the unwelcome observation that puerperal fever seemed to be carried from patient to patient by the person delivering the baby. Since most of the observations (including Semmelweis's more systematic ones), had been made by males about males, the conclusion was not generally well received by the medical fraternity.

More generally, the mind-set that worried about hospitalism also saw virtue in cleanliness, and a number of surgeons routinely began to wash their hands and instruments before operating. In Britain, Robert Lawson Tait (1845–99) and Thomas Spencer Wells (1818–97) initially saw little new in Lister's antiseptic routine. Both Tait and Wells were beginning to perform ovariotomies, the surgical removal of one or both of the ovaries of a woman. Both men had good results of this major abdominal operation, with simple attention to cleanliness. Nevertheless, it was Lister who transformed surgical practice.

Lister was born into a prosperous Quaker family. His father, a wine merchant, was also an amateur scientist who invented an achromatic microscope, an essential tool in medical science in mid-century (and beyond). Lister attended University College and University College Hospital, where he proved himself an adept microscopist and published papers on fine structure and on inflammation. Deciding on a career in surgery, he went to Edinburgh for postgraduate work, becoming James Syme's (1799–1870) house surgeon (and son-in-law). In 1860, he obtained the chair in surgery at Glasgow, returning to Edinburgh as Professor of Clinical Surgery in 1869. He went back to London, this time to King's College, in 1877, where by the time of his death, he was the grand old man of British medicine, President of the Royal Society, and the first medical man to receive a peerage.

He spent his most productive, and happiest, years in Scotland. He developed what he called his antiseptic system of surgery in Glasgow. What this system actually entailed, and its theoretical basis changed over the years because Lister had the (common) tendency to project back into his earlier work changes and rationales that had taken place later. Consequently, his retrospective reconstructions do not always tally with his earlier published statements. His initial system had its roots in two sets of observations: the work of Pasteur on the common features of putrefaction, fermentation, and sepsis (putrefaction in living tissues), and the role of airborne substances in causing these vital processes; and the use of carbolic acid to disinfect, and thus render harmless, human faeces. Thus, carbolic acid as the disinfectant, and air as a source of surgical mischief, were his two main concerns. His antiseptic system, first published in 1867, used gauze soaked in carbolic acid solution to disinfect the surgical wound, and simultaneously protect it from the air. He also soaked his instruments in the solution and his reported results on joint surgery were impressive. He accepted that 'healing by first intention' (i.e., healing directly without pus and the formation of scar tissue) was very difficult to achieve after surgery, so contented himself with minimizing the dangers associated with 'second intention' healing. Indeed, he initially believed that a bit of suppuration, but not decomposition, was good for ultimate wound healing.

His early invocation of Pasteur's work has made it easy for later historians to assume that from the very beginning, he applied the germ theory of disease to surgery. Although he had used the word 'germ' liberally in the 1860s and early 1870s, it still had a more general medical usage, as any agent causing infection or sepsis. Only a decade or so later, when Pasteur's researches had matured, and Koch had come onto the scene, did Lister unequivocally equate the cause of surgical sepsis with bacteria. During that time, however, he continuously fiddled with his antiseptic system, experimenting with other antiseptic agents, using different concentrations of carbolic acid, and altering the timing of dressing change. He was utterly devoted to his patients, changing their dressings himself or entrusting it only to his closest disciples. He hated failure, but he declined to keep systematic statistics, so it was difficult for the world at large to know how revolutionary his surgical outcomes really were.

For all that, it was difficult to quarrel with an 'antiseptic' system because its opposite was a septic one. Resistance to Lister's work (soon called the 'Listerian system') came from surgeons who believed that exposing surgical wounds to air was better, and that simple cleanliness was all that was necessary to control surgical sepsis. His system had many problems, especially the irritating toxicity of carbolic acid. It often caused breakdown of the patient's wounds and irritated the skin and lungs of the surgeons. It required a supreme act of faith to adopt it, especially after he added to his repertoire a carbolic spray in the operating room. It is to Lister's credit that he inspired a group of young surgeons to take up his system. He also attracted a steady stream of foreign surgeons to come to Glasgow and Edinburgh, to observe the techniques and the results. His methods, or adaptations of them, were sufficiently well known among German surgeons that, when the medical statistics of the Franco-Prussian War were published, German soldiers fared much better at the hands of their surgeons than their French counterparts, who had been slower on the antiseptic uptake. Lister's most lasting contribution was to convince the world that the source of surgical infection came from without the body and, if it could be countered, or avoided, the wound would heal without major complications. As one surgeon put it, 'The best antiseptic is life' meaning that living, healthy tissues were naturally germ-free.

From the 1870s, antiseptic surgical techniques spread widely. Lister had a group of direct disciples, of whom the most distinguished was probably William Watson Cheyne (1852–1932), and the younger generation of surgeons had no difficulty accepting bacteriological explanations of wound sepsis and its prevention. Cheyne translated Koch's work into English and published the big book on antiseptic surgery that Lister never got around to publishing. More generally, where statistics were kept, antiseptic surgery could be shown to be safer. It also permitted a much wider range of operations to be performed, and gradually surgeons began to open the three body cavities (abdominal, thoracic, and cranial) that had been off-limits to traditional surgery. Especially in the academic surgical clinics in the German-speaking lands, organ after organ was exposed to the surgical knife. In Zürich and Vienna, Theodor Billroth (1829–94) and his students operated on the larynx, oesophagus, and intestinal tract. In Bern, Theodor Kocher (1841–1917) pioneered surgery of the thyroid (for which he won a Nobel Prize), but he also operated on bones, the spinal cord, and brain. In 1889, the Chicago surgeon John Murphy (1857–1916) removed an inflamed appendix. During the 1890s, William Macewen (1848–1924) in Glasgow and Victor Horsley (1857–1916) in London began to devote more time to the surgical removal of brain and spinal cord tumours.

As always, new surgical procedures were attended by higher risks, but as they became more routine, surgical mortality generally declined. Kocher's first thousand thyroid operations incurred a mortality of 14 percent; by the time he had done five thousand, it was under 1 percent. Both the statistics and the sheer volume of surgery are revealing. Mortality across the board was higher than would be acceptable today, but improvements were easy to demonstrate as the years passed. Surgery became safer as aseptic techniques replaced antiseptic ones. Aseptic surgery sought to prevent contamination of the surgical wound, rather than kill the germs with antiseptic substances. Aseptic techniques included careful sterilization of equipment (from the 1880s, generally by heat, in autoclaves that Koch made popular); the confinement of surgery to special areas of the hospital, where scrupulous cleanliness and disinfection could be observed; and the use of protective clothing – the gowns, masks, and gloves of modern surgery (Fig. 2.5). William Stewart Halsted introduced rubber gloves at Johns Hopkins in 1890, reputedly because his nurse (and fiancée) was allergic to antiseptics.

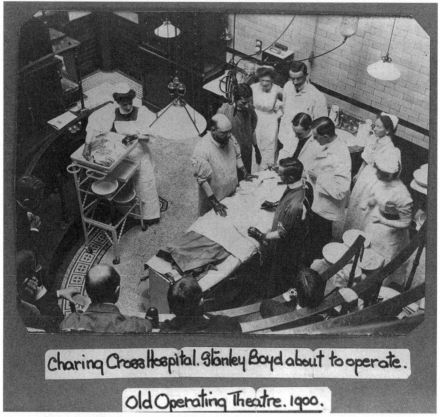

Charing Cross Hospital. Stanley Boyd about to operate.

Old Operating Theatre. 1900.

Fig. 2.5. Stanley Boyd, senior surgeon at Charing Cross Hospital, London, prepares to operate, 1900. Theatre staff wear rubber gloves and gowns over outdoor clothes, but no face masks or hats. *Source*: Photograph, Archives of Dr. Basil Hood (1876–1978). Wellcome Library Archives and Manuscripts. *Credit*: Wellcome Library, London (L0013050).

Because surgeons treated and sometimes definitively cured many conditions, such as cancer or gall stones, that physicians could only manage conservatively, the cult of the surgeon flourished. Hospitals had to provide the resources – theatres, recovery rooms, surgical nurses, and sterilizing equipment – for this modern miracle to enfold. Modern surgery was only one of many activities that pushed up hospital expenditure in the period. It had its upside, as well, because surgery greatly extended the social spectrum of hospital patients. Rich people, who a generation or two earlier would have been treated – even if they needed an operation – outside the hospital, now used these venerable institutions of medicine. Surgery made it easier for hospitals to develop private facilities that, in Britain and elsewhere, were run for the benefit of the more traditional service functions for the worthy poor.

160

HOSPITALS: NURSING

Like modern surgery, modern nursing is intimately associated with the nineteenth-century hospital. The word 'nurse' is replete with maternal and domestic associations, and hospitals always had individuals attached to them who looked after those who stayed there. Before the middle of the nineteenth century, hospital nurses were generally of either of two backgrounds. On the Continent, especially, nursing orders had long traditions and still carried on in our period. Those in these orders looked upon nursing as a calling, and their service to others was tied up with their vows. There were Protestant as well as Roman Catholic orders.

Secular nursing was of a different stripe. Charles Dickens (1812–70) created powerful, if affectionate, portraits of old style nurses in Sairey Gamp and Betsy Prig. This was part of a literary depiction of them as low-class women engaged in casual labour and with loose morals and a love of the bottle. Some of them undoubtedly fit the stereotype, and it was accurate at least as representing secular nursing as an informal occupation carried out by women who needed the work. Before the middle of the century, hospital nurses were routinely grouped with cleaners and other menials and, in fact, scrubbing the floors was one of their chores.

The transformation of nursing from a form of casual labour to a vocation, and a professional one at that, is associated (at least in the English-speaking world) with Florence Nightingale. More recent scholarship has widened our vision of nursing, and placed Nightingale within a movement that was gaining momentum independently of her. It is easier to show that her aims were not unique, and her methods were manipulative and often devious, than it is to reduce her to a historical footnote. Her ideas on nursing were formed on the Continent, before the Crimean War, and it was her observations of two nursing orders, one Protestant and one Catholic, that infused her later reformist ideals. She entered nursing (from a solid middle-class background) with a sense of religious calling. Her vision of nursing reform kept the vocational aspect, but was flexible and easily adopted within the increasingly secular hospital.

She achieved iconic status during the Crimean War, and a substantial fund was raised in her honour just after it. It provided the resources to found the Nightingale School at St. Thomas's Hospital in London, and to support 'Nightingale' activities in many other hospitals. She saw nursing reform as part of a more general plan to make hospitals safer and more effective. Her advocacy of the pavilion ward design has already been noted, and it had the double benefit of countering miasmatic-spread infections, achieved

161

through an emphasis on ventilation and generous spacing of beds, with that of nursing surveillance. By the end of the century, 'Nightingale' nurses dominated hospital nursing throughout the English-speaking world.

There were three main aspects of the Nightingale revolution. First, it made nursing a respectable occupation, even a calling, for women of genteel backgrounds. At a time when occupational opportunities for women were still relatively limited, nursing became a possibility, without the stigma of class and morals. 'Nursing' seemed a natural female occupation, so it reinforced gender stereotypes, even while offering respectable careers for middle-class girls. Second, nurses became a distinct order within the hospitals, divorced from the more menial tasks of cleaning, food preparation and distribution, and portering. Nightingales were of course concerned with tidiness, but they gradually acquired functions within the hospital that were instrumentally related to patient care, with 'nursing' in its modern sense. It is remarkable how many surveys, in the last century or so, have criticized facilities, plant, and even medical concern, and have remarked on the high standard of nursing care. Third, Nightingale nursing absorbed her vision of nursing discipline and calling, transformed in a secular context to ideals of professionalism. This meant that schools of nursing included formal education, not just training, so that nurses could play an active role in patient care. This professional ideal brought with it textbooks and journals, calls for formal regulation of qualification, and specialization, as nurses began to work exclusively in operating theatres, with children or the insane, and in the wider world. Doctors were concerned that all this activity was complementary, and subservient, to their own roles, and there were many clashes between medical and nursing staff over who would do what, who went on whose rounds, and who was responsible to whom. Nevertheless, the modern hospital is unthinkable without the modern nurse, and the increasing demands of postsurgical care, taking temperatures, dispensing medicines, and noting changes in a patient's status, increasingly devolved on nurses. The familiar modern experience, of remembering the nursing care more than the medical, has its origins in the nineteenth century.

RESEARCH INSTITUTES

Both medical schools and hospitals changed significantly during the second half of the century, but principally by adaptation of existing institutions with their own traditions and structures. The research institute, at least in the form it acquired late in the century, was new, a bricks and mortar legacy of the way in which medical science had sold itself.

As previously mentioned, the institute was the base unit of disciplinary organization in German universities. It enjoyed a different status from the ordinary divisions within universities in France, Britain, or the United States. The 'department' never had quite the cache or autonomy that a German institute enjoyed. These institutes were endowed by the state or other public authority, and were well equipped to carry out research in addition to teaching (advanced teaching was especially prized). Ludwig's physiological institute in Leipzig was a model. Built in the shape of an 'E', it had laboratories for elementary and advanced teaching and for research, as well as lecture rooms and a library. There was an animal room, stores for chemicals and other supplies, and offices for the professor and his staff. It was a little self-contained empire.

On an equal, or, mostly, smaller scale, this model was duplicated in many subjects (natural in addition to medical sciences and other disciplines) in the universities throughout greater Germany. It was these institutes, with their commitment to research and advanced training, which Flexner so much admired and thought embodied the highest ideals of the modern university. On a more modest scale, this model began to be emulated in Britain and the United States, as successful scientific entrepreneurs attracted notice and funds. From the late nineteenth century, medical research began to be deemed worthy of support, sometimes by the state, as in France and, reluctantly, in Britain, sometimes by wealthy individuals.

Within this general science movement, the Institut Pasteur stands out. Given Pasteur's shrewdness, its endowment can hardly be called fortuitous, but it was a spontaneous, international philanthropic response to his rabies vaccine. He seemed an international treasure and, once the appeal was launched, individuals from all over the world contributed to funds to build him an institute in which to pursue his researches without worry. The French state and municipality of Paris contributed the land on which to build his monument, but the endowment came from people who were moved by his work. He wanted it to be independent of the universities or other forms of control. Its opening in 1888 was widely reported at home and abroad, and rendered even more moving by the fact that Pasteur was so frail that his son-in-law had to read his speech for him. It emphasized the universal nature of scientific knowledge. The Pasteurs had an apartment on site, and although Pasteur did not do any significant research within his institute it became the centre of French biomedical work, the home to generations of 'Pastorians'. Pasteur died and was buried in that monument that bore his name. The institute enjoyed a generous endowment, but it was also expected to generate income through the ethical production of rabies, anthrax, and other vaccines and products of biomedical research.

Pasteur gave his name to other institutes founded in the next few decades, in France or areas of the French empire (Algeria, Vietnam). There was even a Pasteur Institute in British India, itself a tribute to the international reach of science and to Pasteur's revered name. The British succeeded in duplicating the Pasteur monument at home, though on a much smaller scale. Capitalizing on the importance of rabies vaccine for an island (which had greater control on the disease), Lister and other leading advocates of biomedical research were behind the plan to endow a private medical research institution in Britain. The appeal faltered until a rich brewer (of the Guinness family) gave a single large donation that allowed its trustees to find a site in London and build The British Institute for Preventive Medicine. It opened in 1891, changing its name to the Jenner Institute in 1898 and the Lister Institute in 1903. Its trustees avoided the word 'research' in its title because the antivivisection movement was strong in Britain, and chose for its successive eponymous honourees, two men noted for their practical contributions to human health. The Lister Institute was an important site of biomedical research in its early days (when funds were scarce in Britain), but it never had the endowment or international status to compete with the Institut Pasteur.

An American realization of the research institute ideal came shortly afterwards, through the largess of the Rockefeller Foundation, the creation of John D. Rockefeller (1839–1937) and his son John, Jr. (1874–1960). The Rockefellers made their vast fortune in oil, and their foundation became one of the most important sources of funding for health-related activities during the first half of the twentieth century. Before World War I, the foundation was concerned mostly with American philanthropy (the University of Chicago was an early beneficiary). Although Rockefeller had a personal homeopathic doctor, one of his key advisors, Frederick T. Gates (1853–1929), a Baptist clergyman, read William Osler's *Principles and Practice of Medicine* (first published, 1892). It contained elegant descriptions of disease, but little to encourage optimism about therapy. Gates convinced Rockefeller that biomedical research was a worthwhile humanitarian investment. The first major benefaction was the Rockefeller Institute (now Rockefeller University), opened in 1901, in New York City. Its staff were to devote themselves completely to research, and, to aid clinical research, Rockefeller built an adjacent hospital. Its medical staff could not engage in private practice, and the facilities were so lavish that it began to reverse the intellectual migration from America to Europe, attracting Jacques Loeb (1858–1924), who worked on biological tropism, Karl Landsteiner (of blood group fame), and Alexis Carrel (1873–1944), famous for tissue culture and surgical innovations, from Germany and France. The director of its laboratories, and effective director of the institute, was Simon Flexner (1863–1946), Abraham's younger brother and a creative investigator in serum therapy, virology, and epidemiology.

These highly visible institutes were manifestations of a wider public and private investment in medical research. They were complemented by laboratories in hospitals, medical schools, and universities throughout the Western world. They were at once part of the achievements of medical science, and witnesses to the faith that the public placed in it.

Disease and diseases

Nineteenth-century doctors had little trouble with disease. They were taught about it in medical schools and surrounded by it in their daily practices. Its existence provided them with their social *raison d'être* and bread and butter. The frequently repeated quip that the medical profession is the only one that seeks to render itself unnecessary (because everyone is healthy) is pious nonsense. Doctors need diseases, and if they did not exist, it would be necessary for them to create them. Preventive programmes for common diseases, such as smallpox in the nineteenth century or malaria in the early twentieth, were subtly resisted by rank-and-file practitioners because their disappearance would dent their livelihoods. In practice, doctors in all times can seek mightily to eradicate disease, knowing that there will always be work for them and their descendants.

We are now taught to appreciate that health and disease are not simply antithetic states, noninteracting Venn diagrams. Nineteenth-century doctors, too, appreciated that the boundaries between health and disease are rarely sharp. The lesion-orientated medicine of the French school had offered clearer guidelines for defining diseases, although often neglecting the subtlety of disease mechanisms. From mid-century, the physiology of disease (as opposed to its anatomy) acquired more prominence in medical thinking. Carl Wunderlich's (1815–77) work on medical thermometry was pursued within the context of what was called 'physiological medicine', a movement that emphasized the dynamics of disease, instead of its statics, and the subtle transitions from health to disease. Cellular pathology also encouraged physiological thinking within medicine, and Virchow

165

castigated what he called the older ontological conceptions of disease. These had underlay eighteenth-century disease classifications (nosologies). Virchow emphasized the primacy of basic cellular mechanisms, as revealed by the microscope.

In addition to the physiological–pathological dichotomy of disease, the functional–structural one was also important. There were many diseases for which there were no well-defined and consistent lesions. Melancholia and other mental disorders never quite conformed to the ideals of clinico-pathological correlation, and the brains of deceased lunatics often appeared normal at autopsy. Other diseases, notably hysteria, were quintessentially 'functional', and one psychiatric dictionary actually called 'hysteria' a synonym for functional disease. More generally, conditions, such as asthma, had symptoms without obvious lesions. A variety of psychosomatic explanations were posited. We look at the development of nineteenth-century psychiatry later p. 197ff. Curiously enough, hysterical symptoms more easily evoked psychosomatic aetiologies than did insanity, in which the functions of the mind (or soul) were disturbed. Throughout the century, doctors had reason to posit that mental disease was simply brain disease, the cause of which was yet undefined. Then, as now, it was possible to assume that functional or mental disease was caused by abnormalities at the chemical or molecular level: that these categories simply reflected current states of knowledge.

DIAGNOSING DISEASE

The four principal procedures of modern bedside physical diagnosis – inspection, palpation, percussion, and auscultation – were, as we have seen, routinized within the Paris hospitals in the first half of the nineteenth century. Only Laennec's invention of the stethoscope, which yielded *mediate* auscultation (*immediate* auscultation – placing the doctor's ear directly on the patient's body – was mentioned even by the Hippocratics), was new p. 42. Jean-Nicolas Corvisart extended Auenbrugger's earlier invention of percussion. The other two activities, looking and feeling, had always been a potential part of the doctor–patient encounter. Two points need to be remembered. First, they involved only the doctor's hands, eyes, and ears: touch, sight, and hearing. With a stethoscope in his pocket or bag, a doctor could perform the systematic examination advocated by Pierre Louis and the other high priests of French hospital medicine anywhere the patient was prepared to submit to the physical intimacy required. Second, this encounter involved only the brilliant, but simple, technology of

Laennec's invention, a tube of wood hollowed out and adapted for ease of carrying and for hearing high- and low-pitched sounds. Later nineteenth-century inventiveness improved the shape, convenience, and adaptability of the stethoscope, with binaural ear pieces and flexible rubber tubing connecting the shaft with what was called the 'bell' and the 'diaphragm', the parts placed onto the patient's body.

Manuals of physical diagnosis from the 1840s and 1850s indicate that medical students were being encouraged to learn these techniques, and those who went into general practice could have used them. Stethoscopes were commonplace by mid-century, even if patients' descriptions of their encounters with doctors suggest that auscultation was a rare event. (Even today, most family doctors, or general practitioners, use their stethoscope most commonly for measuring blood pressure, a twentieth-century procedure.) The discrepancy between systematic practice as taught within the hospital and the demands and possibilities of everyday practice persists.

That discrepancy widened in the second half of the nineteenth century. There were many new and important diagnostic aids introduced, but most of them were technologically sophisticated, labour intensive, and suitable only for the hospital or the specialist. They reflected the changes in disease concepts previously mentioned, and gave a higher degree of precision to many medical diagnoses. Their penetration into general medical practice was much slower.

The ophthalmoscope was one of the earliest of these instruments and typifies many of the features of diagnostic technology of the period. The British polymath Charles Babbage (1792–1871) – better known for his work on the computer, or analytical calculating machine – described a simple ophthalmoscope in 1847, but the modern instrument was introduced into medicine in 1851 by Hermann von Helmholtz. He developed it while working on the physiology of the eye (Fig. 2.6). It was one of several striking laboratory discoveries with an impact on medical diagnosis. The ophthalmoscope allowed doctors to examine the eye much more systematically. They could visualize directly the retina, optic nerve head, and the arteries that supplied the eye. The instrument also helped them evaluate the cause of defective vision. More than a half century ago, George Rosen chose ophthalmology as a fitting subject to examine the evolution of medical specialization. He noted the rise of societies and journals in the field, the development of special clinics, and the extension of eye surgery, all of which he argued were catalysed by Helmholtz's ophthalmoscope. Foremost among the medics stimulated by the new instrument was

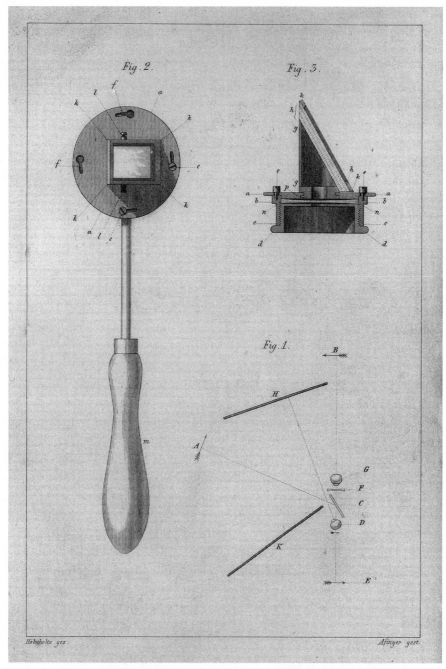

Fig. 2.6. Helmholtz's ophthalmoscope was devised to show that light entering the eye reflected back to its source and could form an optical (virtual) image of the retina. *Source*: H. Helmholtz, *Beschreibung eines Augen-Spiegels*, Berlin, 1851. Wellcome Library Early Printed Books. *Credit*: Wellcome Library, London (M0010474).

Albrecht von Graefe (1828–79), who before his early death from TB, established in Berlin a journal and a society in the subject, and pioneered a number of new operations for diseases of the eye.

The ophthalmoscope had value beyond the field of ophthalmic surgery, and the first two significant monographs on the instrument and its uses in Britain were by physicians. Clifford Allbutt's (1836–1925) 1871 treatise dealt with its use in diagnosing diseases of the kidneys and arteries and (Sir) William Gowers's (1845–1915) 1879 monograph showed how the ophthalmoscope was especially valuable as a diagnostic tool in neurology. Others in Britain and the United States, including the surgeon William Bowman (1816–92), had appreciated the value of Helmholtz's invention, but the expert use of the ophthalmoscope long remained just that: the tool of specialists, whether consultant physicians and neurologists, or those concerned with eye diseases, including their surgical treatments. Although Helmholtz's original paper was quickly translated into English, these two monographs did not appear until two decades later, a reminder of how long it could take for a complicated tool to make a more general impact within medicine.

Other mid-century diagnostic instruments also allowed doctors to see inside the body. The otoscope and the laryngoscope, for instance, made visualization of the inner ear, and the throat and larynx, respectively, much easier. They were simpler devises than the ophthalmoscope, easier to use even if the interpretation of what the doctor saw was always a learned skill. Their systematic use long remained in the hands of those who had a special interest in diseases of the ears, throat, and larynx.

More problematic was the vaginal speculum. It was an old instrument, dating back at least to Roman times. Its use became more common from the early decades of the nineteenth century and was associated both with the growth of gynaecological surgery and obstetrics, and the increasing identification of a variety of 'female complaints' with the uterus. Like most diagnostic procedures, it was first employed mostly in hospitals and on poor patients, only gradually diffusing out into the wider medical marketplace. The availability of submissive (and powerless) women in the Paris hospitals was one of the magnets of medical education there. Most women considered the speculum humiliating and painful, but it gradually became a mainstay in diagnosing disorders of the female reproductive tract, and with its use came complicated examination tables, with the familiar stirrups, to better enable the examining doctor to visualize the relevant organs.

Whether the medical gains were worth the moral costs was not obvious to all. In the 1830s and 1840s, the morality of speculum use was heatedly debated. A number of British doctors, including the physiologist and medical practitioner Marshall Hall (1790–1857), the obstetrician Robert Lee (1793–1877), and the ophthalmologist Robert Brudenell Carter (1828–1910), argued against its use except when absolutely necessary. Most doctors seemed more worried about the evil influence of vaginal examinations on women than any temptation that the situation might exert on the examiner. As Carter wrote in 1853, in an influential monograph on hysteria, 'I have, more than once, seen young women, of the middle classes of society, reduced, by the constant use of the speculum, to the mental and moral constitution of prostitutes; seeking to give themselves the same indulgence by the practice of the solitary vice; and asking every medical practitioner, under whose care they fell, to institute an examination of the sexual organs' (Moscucci, 1990, p. 116). Half a century later, Thomas Clifford Allbutt was still complaining of the too-easy resort to a vaginal examination for every woman's ills, and the male–female issue became part of the debate over female medical education and the right of the woman to have a female doctor, if she desired. Like other aspects of surgery, however, gynaecological surgery became much more common after the introduction of antiseptic and aseptic techniques. As the management of birth became an increasingly male-dominated specialism, the speculum and forceps were gradually accepted as part of mundane medical instrumentation.

These instruments were designed to allow the examining doctor to see inside the eye or body cavities. Other innovations approached diagnosis more indirectly. Trying to estimate the number of red blood cells provides a good example. We have already seen how the perception of the ratio of red and white blood cells led both Virchow and Bennett p. 121 to describe the disease leukaemia. Anaemia, literally, not enough blood, was an old medical term, especially associated with chlorosis, a disorder of young women who presented with extreme tiredness, loss of menses, and psychological problems. Chlorosis, like hysteria, was a diagnosis that virtually disappeared in the early years of the twentieth century and historians have sometimes linked the two. Physicians at the time also saw some parallels, especially in the age and gender of the patients and variable clinical course.

There were other kinds of anaemia, however, including a relatively rare form, called then (as now) 'pernicious', because it generally resulted in death. The blood was, as noted at the time, the only human tissue that it was easy to examine microscopically in living patients because a thin slide of it could be made at the bedside. The structure and colour of red blood cells were often reported in the clinical literature of the time, and a way of evaluating the number of red blood cells seemed desirable. Several attempts were made in the 1860s, and in 1877, William Gowers described his version of what was called a haemocytometer. It consisted of a graduated cover to a microscopic slide, to which a carefully diluted sample of blood was added. It gave an absolute number of red blood cells per cubic millilitre of blood, at a time when the concept of the 'normal' physiological value was being widely discussed. Gowers' haemocytometer attracted a good deal of attention, but it had problems. It took two hours or so to come to a conclusion, and it gave different values in the hands of other users, or even when a single patient was examined twice by the same person. It encouraged others to make improvements, and in the 1890s, the use of the centrifuge (an instrument designed for physics and chemistry) gave a reasonable value for the percentage of the total blood volume occupied by the red blood cells. The result of spinning the blood was called the haematocrit, and the value could be obtained quickly, assuming the equipment was available.

Other pathological conditions were looked for in the blood, as we shall see below. Another body fluid that attracted much attention was the urine. As early as the 1820s, the Guy's Hospital physician Richard Bright (1789–1858) had associated chronic disease of the kidney with protein (albumen) in the urine. The urine also offered clues to other diseases, such as diabetes, when it contained sugar, or bladder infections or kidney or bladder stones, when it revealed blood and pus cells. It became concentrated when there was fever and turned bright yellow when there was jaundice. Many of these observations were part of the received wisdom of clinical medicine, but systematically examining them became routine, at least in hospital patients. A number of chemical tests for components in the urine were introduced in the period, and learning how to examine the urine was the most common laboratory procedure that young house officers in teaching hospitals would have experienced. They would measure specific gravity, note the colour and clarity of urine samples, and look at it under the microscope searching for crystals, cells, and casts (collection of cells from the kidneys). By the century's end, there had been eight or ten chemical tests devised to measure urine sugar. Teaching wards frequently had primitive laboratories attached for this and a number of other visual, chemical, or microscopical examinations.

As pathophysiological mechanisms of disease were better elucidated, a number of clinical methods attempted to convert bedside findings to graphical form. The most basic was the fever chart, by the 1890s routinely hung at the end of the patient's bed. Traditionally, 'fever' had been considered as a disease in itself, diagnosed by the character and rate of the pulse, the flushed or pale skin, the patient's sweating or chills (or both), and other symptoms. Fever thermometers had been available since the seventeenth century, but they were large, cumbersome, and used only occasionally by enthusiasts. From the late 1850s, the German academic physician Carl Wunderlich turned medical thermometry into both an art and a science. A professor of medicine at Leipzig, Wunderlich used careful and systematic measurements of body temperature to distinguish between various forms of febrile illness, and to follow his patient's progress and response to treatment. Several of the fevers, notably typhus and typhoid, had been distinguished around mid-century on pathological grounds. Wunderlich's physiological approach further refined the important area of medical concern just before germ theory offered a new series of criteria to distinguish the fevers. His classic treatise of 1868, soon translated into the major European languages, established both the range of normal body temperature and its variation in many diseases. The Englishman, Thomas Clifford Allbutt, introduced a short-stemmed thermometer in 1870; it made taking a patient's temperature straightforward and gradually it became one of the nurse's tasks. While germ theory offered a new way of differentiating many fevers, it did not influence the routine taking of temperature in hospital patients.

The temperature chart offered a graphical record of the patient's course. Other graphical techniques, not so common, were also introduced into clinical medicine. The sphygmograph, invented by the German physiologist Karl Vierodt (1818–84) and perfected by the French physiologist Etienne-Jules Marey (1830–1904) in 1860, made it possible to have an objective record of the arterial pulse. It also provided a guide to irregularities of the heart beat that, later in the century, bore fruit in the treatment of heart disease and the development of the specialty of cardiology p. 283. Other instruments to record respiration, the strength of muscular contraction, and, eventually, blood pressure were all developed by physiologists or physiologically inclined physicians. The Italian Scipione Riva-Rocci (1863–1937), invented the modern blood pressure cuff in 1896, although its use did not become common until after World War I.

By the end of the century, the bacteriological laboratory was beginning to play a role in medical diagnosis. As germ theory became more widely accepted and specific organisms were associated with specific diseases, taking body fluids or tissues for culture became more commonplace. During the 1880s and early 1890s, this would more often than not have been for research purposes, or simply to confirm a diagnosis made by history and physical examination. As Western states became increasingly concerned with public health and the control of communicable diseases, public bacteriological laboratories were established to identify and monitor diseases such as diphtheria, scarlet fever, erysipelas, whooping cough (croup), and typhoid. These and several other diseases were part of the first group that, from 1889, were subject to compulsory notification in Britain, and other countries developed their own systems of disease notification and control. For the system to work, diagnostic standardization of the listed diseases was necessary.

In hospitals, bacteriological examinations would initially have been part of the pathology department's activities. The blood was also minutely examined in the whole range of infectious diseases. Richard Cabot's *Clinical Examination of the Blood* (3rd ed., 1900) devoted almost 100 pages to the blood variations in acute infectious diseases. These ranged from changes in the concentrations of the various kinds of white blood cells to the presence of bacteria in the blood.

The most dramatic change in diagnostic capability during the period came with the discovery of X-rays by Wilhelm Röntgen (1845–1923) in late 1895. Röntgen was a German physicist who was investigating the properties of cathode rays and stumbled on their remarkable ability to penetrate many substances, including human flesh. Probably no scientific discovery of the nineteenth century made such an immediate impact on the public's imagination. Röntgen made his initial discovery in early November. He X-rayed his wife's hand, complete with her opaque wedding ring, on December 22, in preparation for his lecture on this 'new kind of ray', to the Würzburg Physical-Medical Society on December 28, 1895. Her hand became one of the icons of the period and, despite the holiday production schedules of newspapers, by early January people from all over the world knew of this new scientific miracle.

The diagnostic implications of the X-ray were instantly realized, even if Röntgen was a shy physicist who was more interested in the experimental than the commercial potentials of his research. A clinical X-ray was taken as early as January 7, 1896, and reported in the February 22 issue of *Lancet*. Fractures could be more precisely diagnosed, foreign bodies located, gall stones and large renal calculi visualized, and the size of enlarged hearts estimated by the new procedure. X-rays were immediately applied to dentistry and, in 1898, Walter B. Cannon, still a medical student at Harvard, introduced bismuth compounds into the digestive tract to help visualize the outlines of the stomach and small and large intestines.

These important diagnostic modalities were in the short run overshadowed by the popular wonder of X-rays. 'X-ray proof' undergarments were quickly manufactured to protect modesty and a variety of skin conditions were subjected to the burning effects of X-rays. In 1896, Henri Becquerel (1852–1908) discovered the radiation associated with heavy metals such as uranium, and Pierre (1859–1906) and Marie Curie (1867–1934) added radium and polonium to the list of naturally radioactive elements. These were marshalled in the treatment of internal cancers, initially with great effect. What took longer was the realization that there were important safety factors to be considered as well. Acute radiation sickness limited the doses that could be given to many patients, and many of the early pioneers in the field, including Marie Curie, died of the long-term consequences of chronic radiation exposure. Safety procedures were only gradually put into place, and the modern perception of the dangers of radiation came into being only after the horrors of the atomic bombs were appreciated during World War II. Before the Great War, overexposure to radiation was experienced as a minor inconvenience for patients who were treated with it and for workers in the field. Risk-benefit analysis was not a visible part of the early world of X-rays.

All of these developments in disease diagnosis, and many more, changed the face of medicine during the second half of the nineteenth century. They made many diagnostic categories more secure and offered doctors better guidelines to treat the disease, or at least advise the patient what to expect. Two important points need to be remembered. First, most of these new diagnostic possibilities – the ophthalmoscope, Petri dish, sphygmograph, haemocytometer, and X-ray – came to clinical medicine through the combined result of biomedical research and technology. They were developed away from the bedside and applied there.

Second, they often required time and expertise to interpret their results. Unlike the important bedside tools of the French clinical school – inspection, palpation, percussion, and auscultation – they were not obvious bedside procedures. Medical students could be taught to appreciate and even rely on their findings. But no ordinary medical graduate would be expected to be expert in the taking and interpretation of bacteriological cultures, ophthalmologic findings, X-rays, and the esoteric curves of the sphygmograph. Inevitably, these developments encouraged specialization within medicine, and reliance of doctors on other doctors, and ultimately on non-medically qualified technical experts, in ways that were different, and more complex, than the traditional medical consultation. The doctor's simple use of his five senses at the bedside was being replaced by a much more collective enterprise.

THREE CHRONIC CONDITIONS

Most of the diagnostic innovations described above would have remained relatively esoteric parts of the medical world of both patients and their doctors. The 'germ' was fairly quickly assimilated into popular culture and X-rays made an immediate impact. The newer findings and reformulations of clinical signs and symptoms offered by other diagnostic procedures only gradually filtered into the medical textbooks, medical-school teaching and examinations, and practice. The interaction between diagnosis and disease can be best seen through specific examples. We take three here, TB, syphilis, and cancer, and will look at acute infectious diseases below.

'Tuberculosis' did not really come into being until 1882, when Robert Koch announced his identification of the tubercle bacillus. The word had been used before, but the chronic lung disease characterized by a productive cough, night sweats, loss of appetite, a peculiar kind of fever known as 'hectic', wasting, and general debility was known by other names, especially phthisis and consumption. Pulmonary phthisis was one of several diseases for which Laennec believed his new stethoscope could provide specific ('pathognomonic') criteria, listening to the upper regions of the chest, where the lesions of phthisis generally were situated p. 42. Many doctors came to rely on the stethoscope in diagnosing diseases of the lungs (and heart), but Laennec went one step further and united, on postmortem criteria, pulmonary phthisis with a number of other conditions in which the characteristic 'tubercles' associated with the lungs could be found in other organs. Patients dying with pulmonary tubercles often had similar lesions in their livers, intestines, brains, adrenal glands, spleens, kidneys, and skin. Laennec believed that these were manifestations of a single disease, the defining hallmark being the tubercle, wherever it was found.

Laennec's amalgamation of disorders that produced different symptoms and clinical courses was controversial, and many held that the tubercle resulted from more general pathological processes and needed to be considered as part of the diseases of the various organs where it occurred. Thus, pulmonary phthisis was generally regarded as a completely separate disease from intestinal TB, or TB of the glands, long called 'scrofula'. Laennec was closer to mainstream medical thinking when he assumed that the pulmonary affliction was a constitutional disorder.

Two major features of the disease seemed to bespeak its constitutional origins: its chronicity and its familial pattern. Along with gout, asthma, epilepsy, and scrofula, pulmonary phthisis helped define what doctors meant when they spoke of constitutional disorders. People were born with certain constitutions, whether delicate or robust; and from these innate features, either immunity from or susceptibility to these disorders flowed. Neither immunity nor susceptibility was absolute, just as the concept of constitutional does not naturally translate into the modern notion of genetic. Rather, people with certain constitutions tended towards certain diseases. Being born of consumptive parents labelled one as having a tuberculous (or phthisical, or consumptive) constitution. It did not mean the inevitability of TB, especially if those factors associated with its causation could be avoided. These factors included living in cold, damp climates and in dark and poorly ventilated houses. Stress and irregular hours were also detrimental. Certain kinds of work encouraged the disease to manifest itself. Sedentary occupations carried out in confined spaces, such as those that tailors and seamstresses endured, increase the risk; so did mining and other dusty occupations. Clerks were more likely to develop the affliction than farm labourers, urban dwellers more than rural ones, young adults more than the elderly.

These composite portraits of the 'typical' consumptive were frequently elaborated and discussed. After all, pulmonary phthisis was the leading killer of adults in the century. Its tendency to strike its victims in their early adulthood made it especially pernicious, taking away as it did the breadwinner with a young family or leaving children motherless. The reality of death from TB was a far cry from the romanticized version sometimes depicted in novels or paintings. Far from simply drifting away peacefully, the dying consumptive generally suffered agonies of breathlessness, sleepless nights, painful coughing, the regular salty taste of blood in the mouth and chronic diarrhoea. Maybe death from this disease was romanticized because it was too horrible to contemplate.

Despite its awfulness and its grim importance, TB also maintained a relatively optimistic presence in the massive medical literature on the subject. The disease was ever variable, even mercurial in its course. Young persons gravely pronounced consumptive sometimes completely recovered and lived to ripe old ages. Even spitting arterial blood, the sign that convinced the young poet (and medical student) John Keats (1795–1821) that he was doomed, was grim but not universally a harbinger of death. By the middle of the century, when reliable statistics began to be available, death rates from the disease were perceived to be dropping. Towards the end of the century, Arthur Ransome (1834–1922) noted with satisfaction that the disease was becoming less virulent, with a longer time between diagnosis and death (when that occurred). He calculated in 1896 that if the disease's incidence continued to decline at the same rate it had maintained since the 1830s, it would disappear completely within two decades.

Ransome was an experienced physician, critical of many of the claims made on behalf of medical treatments of TB over the years. Nevertheless, he saw ample reasons for optimism, and attributed the gains made on the disease to medical ministrations. Among nineteenth-century drugs, cod liver oil had the greatest staying power, but the antituberculous armamentarium was very large and ever changing. An ironic saying circulated among doctors that it was better to suffer from TB or cancer, where there were so many cures available, than the common cold, where there were none. The reverse of this was another common medical aphorism that one had to take a new remedy quickly because after a short time it lost its effectiveness.

In the 1880s, as we have seen, the chronic, constitutional disease, phthisis, changed into an infectious one, TB. Koch's tubercle bacillus gave the disease a new identity and aetiology. In the medium term, the infectious disease now finally called tuberculosis was the subject of extensive public health campaigns throughout the West. Ordinances against spitting in public were as much a part of these campaigns as the more visible and costly TB sanatoria. These latter became part of the folk memory of the disease around the turn of the century and were captured in a number of paintings and novels, most memorably in Thomas Mann's *The Magic Mountain*. Set just before the outbreak of World War I, Mann's novel ruthlessly captures the boredom, and alternating sense of hope and despair, of inmates caught in the throes of what later sociologists would call a 'Total Institution'. Such institutions – ships, prisons, boarding schools, insane asylums, leper colonies, and TB sanitaria – create their own repressive atmospheres, where the routine of daily life becomes the only physical reality, and the barriers between the institution and the outside world are impenetrable. The authority figures – officers, school masters, and doctors – take on a new significance for the inmates. Nineteenth-century states discovered the 'asylum', in the larger sense of the word, and used them to classify and segregate individuals believed to need treatment (or care, discipline, education, or some other prod). The tubercle bacillus made those suffering from TB into a group for whom segregation was in their, and society's, best interests.

There were continuities as well as breaks in the shift of tuberculosis from a constitutional to an infectious disease. The careful epidemiological work of earlier generations of doctors was not cast aside. The associations of the disease with class, occupation, economic status, and living conditions, were not abandoned. Nor, despite the bacillus, did the constitutional dimension disappear. Most people who came to autopsy showed signs of a primary tubercular infection and, if the bacillus was ubiquitous, idiosyncratic, innate factors must explain why some people remained well and others succumbed to the clinical disease. The sanatorium movement coincided in time with the rise of eugenics pp. 327–31 and these institutions discouraged the tuberculous from reproducing, as well as removing sources of infection from society at large.

The TB sanatorium was to have curative in addition to segregative functions. They were located primarily at high altitudes, where, as Ransome and others showed, cultures of TB bacilli did not thrive. Patients there spent long hours in the open air, consonant with the observation that living in close quarters encouraged the disease. They were fed rich diets to counter the emaciation that the disease caused and to try to create fat people, assumed to be less susceptible to the disease's ravages. They were eventually X-rayed regularly to follow the state of their lungs and treated with the latest medical or surgical innovation, including surgical collapse of the diseased lung or the artificial introduction of an inert gas into the lung space. And, as the records show, if they survived, many of them stayed behind to become nurses or gardeners or orderlies in the institution, as the outside world seemed too frightening, and doctors assumed (not without logic) that releasing patients to the same environmental conditions that had facilitated the disease in the first place, would merely result in a further breakdown and readmission.

Historical analysis of the decline of TB in the nineteenth century has tended to attribute it to a change in the virulence of the organism, and better social and nutritional conditions of Western populations. Doctors at the time were not blind to the latter factors, but they also believed passionately that their campaigns, public health measures, and sanatoria were important players in the process. There is probably truth in both interpretations, but what is certain is that TB stimulated a vast late-nineteenth-century movement, throughout most of Europe and North America, and that TB in 1914 was very different from the pulmonary phthisis that Laennec diagnosed with his stethoscope. He believed that its cause would never be elucidated, but Koch's bacillus provided a unifying agent for the tubercle in whatever human organ it was found and, in that sense, justified (but in ways he never dreamed of) Laennec's vision of a unified disease.

Syphilis, the second chronic disease, had its own crucial medical trajectory during our period. There were some striking medical parallels with TB. Both diseases were chronic ones, with long and variable natural histories. In both diseases, desperately ill patients sometimes completely recovered, which in turn encouraged doctors dealing with them. Both were disorders that could affect virtually every organ or system in the body and some of the chronic pathological changes in TB bore close microscopical resemblance to those of syphilis. Both had familial patterns and presented with formidable diagnostic challenges. If TB was for John Bunyan 'captain of all these men of death', William Osler summarized syphilis thus: 'Know syphilis in all its manifestations and relations, and all things clinical will be added to you'.

There were important differences, of course, in addition to the brute fact that they were recognized as two separate diseases. Syphilis throughout our period (and beyond) carried heavy moral overtones. The implicit stigmatization of the TB sanatorium was subtle compared to the moral baggage that syphilis bore. Much of the misogyny and many of the gender stereotypes that characterized social thinking of the period were starkly realized in the literature on venereal disease (VD). Prostitutes and loose women were commonly blamed for the high incidence of sexually transmitted diseases, as young men were excused from sowing wild oats and proper women were assumed to be naturally monogamous, with marriage and child bearing as their chief goals. When men spread syphilis, it was unfortunate, when women spread it, it was reprehensible.

Some of the moral overtones will be considered later, but the clinical and diagnostic issues were challenging enough. In the mid-nineteenth century, the relationship of syphilis with gonorrhoea was still sometimes in doubt. In the late eighteenth century, the surgeon John Hunter (1728–93) had inoculated a subject (maybe himself) with pus taken from the chancre of a syphilitic. The experiment resulted in signs of both gonorrhoea and syphilis, reinforcing the older view that gonorrhoea was merely an early stage of syphilis. The unity or distinctiveness of the two disorders continued to be debated for several decades, and inoculation experiments continued to be the principal means of investigating the natural history of venereal diseases.

The leading French venereologist, Philippe Ricord (1800–89), an inveterate inoculator, showed that the chancre of syphilis always bred true. He also divided syphilis into its three stages: primary, secondary, and tertiary.

The primary stage is the ulcer, or chancre, which other clinicians soon differentiated from a similar sore of another VD, chancroid, a less aggressive disorder. The secondary stage is characterized by a rash, fever, and more generalized sores, especially in the mucous membranes of the mouth and pharynx. Whether this stage was infectious or not was long debated. The third, chronic, stage was much more difficult to identify clinically. It manifests itself only years later, and was the basis of Osler's clinical pearl quoted above. Some of its microscopic manifestations were similar to those of systemic tuberculosis and, like TB, tertiary syphilis could appear in almost any organ of the body. In the arteries, it could lead to weakening of the vascular walls and aneurysms, especially in the aorta, the main artery leading from the left chamber of the heart. In the liver and other organs, a chronic inflammatory tumour, called a gumma, caused local destruction of normal function. In the nervous system, tertiary syphilis could produce damage that led to an unsteady gait and problems of balance. It was sufficiently distinctive to be described as a separate disease, variously called 'tabes dorsalis' or 'progressive locomotor ataxia'. Another form of chronic neurosyphilis revealed itself primarily through mental symptoms, including hallucinations and delusions of grandeur. Delineated early in the nineteenth century, general paralysis of the insane (GPI) became a common diagnosis in the ever larger psychiatric asylums that mushroomed from the 1830s pp. 198–9. All three major forms of tertiary syphilis were generally progressive and fatal, although other chronic changes to the joints, liver, or small arteries were also commonly found and were compatible with longer survival.

It was easy enough for careful clinicians to diagnose these conditions, with their striking physical findings, dramatic symptoms, and distinctive postmortem findings. Linking them to syphilis was a much more difficult affair. The chronic forms of syphilis occurred years after the initial infection, it affected only a portion of those who had had the disease, and syphilis was such a common affliction that many patients would have had it in their pasts (more than would have admitted to it). Ricord's post at the main French VD hospital, le Midi, allowed him to follow patients for years. Although doctors could readily produce chancres in human beings by inoculation (generally, but not always in patients who already had the disease), inoculation experiments in laboratory animals were singularly unsuccessful. From the 1870s, microscopists began to examine syphilitic discharges looking for some causative organism. They were met with regular findings but no consistency, as a couple of dozen bacteria were nominated as causes of syphilis during the last quarter of a century. Considering the complex natural history of syphilis, and in the absence of an agreed causative agent, it is remarkable that so much suggestive clinical, pathological, and epidemiological evidence had been assembled, linking together the disease in its multifarious forms.

Acute syphilis was most common among young adults, but syphilitic mothers often bore children with the disease as well. Victorians sometimes called this 'syphilis of the innocent', accurate enough in terms of the unfortunate newborn, though also implying that the parents were guilty. Syphilitic children began appearing almost as soon as syphilis (the 'Great Pox') was recognized in the late fifteenth century, and the relationship of congenital and neonatal syphilis to the health of both parents (and of wet nurses) was a topic of ongoing medical and domestic concern. Could a syphilitic father infect his child, or did syphilis in the newborn presuppose syphilis in the mother? Could wet nurses infect their sucklings, and/or vice versa? Congenital syphilis was not sexually acquired by the newborn. What nonsexual routes were possible in adults, especially supposedly chaste women? These questions, part medical, part moral, were still being discussed in the mid-nineteenth century.

The stigmata of congenital syphilis were there for all to see. Although many of the unfortunate children died, some survived and as they grew, they developed a variety of directly associated health problems. The English surgeon and shrewd medical observer Jonathan Hutchinson (1828–1913) grouped the triad of afflictions – notched teeth, inflammation of the cornea, and problems with inner ear function – that subsequently bore his eponym. The early cataracts were regularly noticed, and the problems of inherited syphilis worried many who were concerned with the future of the human race.

Most observers agreed that the real reservoir of the syphilitic virus (they used that word as simply meaning 'poison', without any biological connotation) resided with prostitutes. They reasoned that a promiscuous man would not infect many women, and these in any case would not routinely spread the disease further. A diseased prostitute could infect dozens, even hundreds of men, who (so the assumption went) would most likely infect only one further person: his wife. Get rid of prostitution and the syphilis problem would be more or less solved. Alternatively, syphilis would not be spread if prostitutes were disease free.

These were the two basic approaches. In France and some other places on the Continent, prostitution was accepted as a brutal fact of life. Brothels were licensed and the women who worked there regularly inspected. Many of the eminent French venereologists, including Ricord, were involved in examining and treating prostitutes in the specialist hospitals and clinics of Paris. They worked with the police in attempting to trace contacts and treat infected men as well. Much of the medical knowledge about the symptoms and natural history of the disease stemmed from this work. In Britain and in much of the United States, eradicating prostitution was the goal, and many reformers devoted time, energy, and money to reclaiming fallen women, offering them honest employment and, above all, instilling in them a sense of vital religion. Estimates of the number of prostitutes in London and other British cities sometimes put the number of prostitutes at 10 percent or more of the female population in the vulnerable age. Despite all the philanthropic activity, the problem seemed never to go away.

The one British experiment at controlling, rather than eradicating, prostitution, proved controversial. In the 1860s, the first of a series of Contagious Diseases Acts was passed. Although many of the Members of Parliament (MPs) who voted for the act assumed that it had to do with controlling cattle plague, then raging, the act passed. It was concerned only with the military and navy because the government was concerned with the morbidity that VD caused among troops. It allowed police to pick up suspicious women in areas around army and naval establishments and take them to medical clinics for compulsory examination and treatment, if disease was found. The act, and the publicity it aroused, catapulted the vaginal speculum into public view, even if British reserve guaranteed that euphemisms abounded. The word 'syphilis' was not uttered in Parliamentary debate for two decades after the first act was passed.

The act exposed flagrant double standards because nothing was done to the troops who used prostitutes, and it offended Victorian sentiment. The repeal campaign gathered momentum and took middle-class women who had spent their lives in domesticity to the platforms, turning them into public speakers and public figures. They argued that the act discriminated against women, that the diagnosis of VD was uncertain and its treatment equally so. They objected to the collusion between the police, state, and the medical profession. Above all, the Repealers argued that the act implicitly condoned prostitution, by trying to making it safe. Venereal disease was there to encourage chastity and punish immorality.

After two decades of heated agitation, Parliament rescinded the acts in Britain, although not from British India, to which they had been extended. The episode was one of several organized public protests against science and medicine during the period. Compulsory vaccination, animal experimentation, evolutionary biology: for many, these dimensions of modern thought, or of the alliance between the state and medicine, threatened traditional liberty and religious and moral values. Military efficiency, or public health, should not be purchased at too high a cost.

Ironically, the Contagious Diseases Acts were rescinded just before the diagnosis and treatment of syphilis were transformed by the laboratory. In 1903, Elie Metchnikoff and Emile Roux transmitted syphilis from a human being to a chimpanzee, making its experimental study easier. In March 1905, the German dermatologist Erich Hoffmann (1868–1959) prepared a slide from a small sore he had excised from the genitals of a young woman who had chosen an infected man with whom to celebrate the New Year. The pathologist Fritz Schaudinn (1871–1906) observed some thin, motile, and nearly transparent bacteria (a spirochete). Another smear from a second patient later that month produced the same organism. By the end of the year, other microscopists, having been shown what to look for, confirmed Schaudinn's observations. Barely a few months later, August von Wassermann (1866–1925) and his colleagues showed that the blood of syphilitic individuals produced antibodies that could be tested for serologically. This, the 'Wassermann test', was the first of several serological tests for the disease: during the interwar years, many countries made such tests mandatory for both partners before marriage. A positive result required treatment before the wedding day.

The treatment for syphilis had traditionally been mercury in one of several forms: hence the old bittersweet saying, 'Two minutes with Venus, two years with Mercury'. Mercury was difficult to administer and worse to take, either as a pill or rubbed into the skin. It was toxic and virtually impossible to disguise, an unfortunate consequence for a condition that was widely known as 'the secret disease'. The modern historical literature is generally cautious when judging whether mercury 'really worked', although three centuries and more of use reinforces the conclusion that both doctors and their patients believed that it did. It was finally rendered a second-line medicament through the chemotherapeutic work of Paul Ehrlich. Systematically examining a series of arsenicals, he and his Japanese colleague Sahachiro Hata (1873–1938) showed in 1909 that their 606th compound examined, named Salvarsan, was capable of killing the spirochete of syphilis without being too toxic for the patient. By 1910, when the drug was formally marketed, Ehrlich was a sick man, and the remaining five years of his life were spent modifying (Compound 914, Neosalvarsan had a better efficacy/toxicity ratio) and defending his new drug. Demand was high, but a few patient deaths, mostly from allergic reactions, clouded the picture. The fact that it was a treatment for a controversial disease, and that Ehrlich was a Jew in a time of rising anti-Semitism did not help.

In less than a decade, laboratory work had transformed doctors' diagnostic and therapeutic weapons. These developments made technological control possible. They did little to solve the continuing moral dilemmas surrounding sexually transmitted diseases (STDs), or to resolve issues of shame, guilt, and responsibility. They never disappeared, and indeed have been exacerbated in our age of acquired immune deficiency syndrome (AIDS).

It is a mistake to assume that cancer is only a modern anxiety, and that before the twentieth century, cancer was such a rare disease that it almost escaped lay notice, compared to TB and acute infectious diseases. Its pre-1914 incidence is generally difficult to ascertain because earlier diagnostic criteria are not easily translatable into modern equivalents, but its very real presence and its capacity to provoke dread, were solid enough. The early twentieth-century statistics of cancer mortality suggested that it had increased since the 1870s, in some countries by as much as 100 percent. Reported deaths from cancer certainly did increase during the period, but sober judges of the situation pointed out that a lot more cancer was being diagnosed, due both to increased medical awareness of the condition and, especially, to more patients suffering from malignancies coming to the surgeon's knife. In the mid-nineteenth century, a patient with abdominal pain and other chronic symptoms might never have come to autopsy, and his death diagnosis would have been that assigned by the doctor. Surgeons often diagnosed cancer – operable or inoperable – on the operating table.

The preceding paragraph was written as if 'cancer' were one disease. It is not, of course, and in ways radically different from tubercular infection, or syphilis, which could affect many different organs, cancer stands for many dread diseases. The language associated with these conditions – cancer, sarcoma, tumour, malignant, and metastasis – is mostly Hippocratic in origin, and had traditional and sustained uses within medicine. There was a special cancer hospital in early-nineteenth-century London and at the Middlesex Hospital there was a special ward by 1792. There was a French cancer hospital in the mid-eighteenth century. A diagnosis of 'cancer' was not uncommon in the nineteenth century, and it carried with it then much of the emotional baggage that it still retains. In 1885, the former president of the United States, Ulysses S. Grant (1822–85) was diagnosed with cancer of the throat. Reporters camped outside his house and spied and reported his last months in ways that make modern paparazzi seem almost tame.

The first American specialist cancer hospital was opened two years later, because a general hospital refused the offer of money to build a special cancer ward because the ward 'might seriously affect patients in other pavilions'.

Grant approached his end as dying patients often do, with dignity and stoicism, even though he was not a particularly religious man. We will examine the experience of another patient with cancer in more detail below, but the emphasis here will be on the ways in which pathologists and clinicians struggled to make sense of this cluster of diseases. From the mid-nineteenth century, they were concerned with a series of interlocking questions. Were cancers general or local diseases? Were they constitutional or environmental in origin? Did they spread by contiguity or through the blood stream or lymphatic system, or affect multiple sites because they were actually general diseases? Did they originate from the body fluids, tissues, or organs, or have their beginning in a single rebel cell? Were there important biological analogies between cancer growth and the growth of an organism during embryological development?

As in so much else in pathology, Rudolf Virchow was a major player, although even he found the answers difficult, and probably did not complete a major multivolume treatise on cancer, begun in the 1860s, because he was not satisfied with his own theoretical framework. His own speculations during the late 1840s had assumed that cancer cells somehow emerged out of an amorphous fluid, similar to the blastema that Theodor Schwann had postulated as the original origin of cells in early embryological development and in inflammation. Virchow's own elaboration of his 'cellular pathology' put paid to Schwann's theory of cellular genesis and pointed towards the renegade cell as the culprit in cancer. Other German pathologists were instrumental in the elaboration of the individual cell as the origin of the wildfire growth of cancer. Attention to the original embryological nature of cancer types had led to the broad division of cancers into carcinomas, derived from the cells of the outer, 'epithelial layer', and sarcomas, stemming from the middle, 'endothelial' layer. A classic paper by Wilhelm Waldeyer (1836–1921), in 1867, published in Virchow's own journal, outlined what a modern historian, L. J. Rather, described as an 'account of the genesis and mode of spread of carcinomas [that] is essentially the account that is found in all textbooks of oncology and pathology in use today' (Rather, 1978, p. 154). Waldeyer argued that carcinoma cells originate from normal epithelial cells, and that they transform (we would say 'mutate') directly, without any dissolution into some blastema-like fluid.

Further, he maintained, the carcinoma results from the multiplication of this original cell, spreading through local tissues by contiguity and to distant ones through the blood, lymph, or other body fluids. He stressed that cancerous epithelial cells (carcinomas) never transform into cancerous connective tissue cells, but that they stimulate the proliferation of these connective tissue cells that give carcinomas their gross and microscopical forms.

Like most classic papers in science and medicine, Waldeyer's achieved its status only gradually. Its propositions were not accepted by all pathologists and clinicians, but it was well-known and provided a framework for cancer research. It remained essentially a descriptive account of the behaviour of cancer cells, without venturing into the murky waters of *why* these biological events occur. It left others to investigate why cancer happens in the first place.

There were almost as many explanations as there were investigators, but four main types of aetiological theories dominated late-nineteenth-century medical thinking. Virchow's student Julius Cohnheim (1839–84) postulated that cancer was caused by remnants of embryological cells – 'rests' – that were sequestered in normal adult tissue and, for unknown reasons, these cells could begin later in life the process of differentiation that was normal in the fetus, but abnormal in the later organism. It had the virtue of drawing on the fact that rapid cellular reproduction is characteristic of early embryological development, as it is of cancer. Cohnheim was a pathologist of international repute who had first observed diapedesis, the migration of white blood cells through the capillaries in inflammation, and whose textbook of pathology was widely translated and used. His 'rest' theory explained much, but had little direct evidence to support it.

A number of clinically minded commentators noticed that their patients were unusually anxious, and attributed the origin of cancer to the demands of modern living. 'Stress' could cause cancer just as it could cause neurasthenia and other disorders of Western civilization. They believed that cancer (at least most forms of it) was relatively rare in nonwhite races, and that it was just one more burden of modern technological life. By the end of the century, more systematic surveys of cancer throughout the world suggested, however tentatively, that cancer was widespread, even though it took different forms in different cultures. From this mass of clinical and epidemiological date came the perception that breast cancer is more common in women who have not borne children and that uterine cancer is more common in women who have had many offspring. Surveys were also done relating cancer incidence to occupation, socioeconomic status, and gender. Although environmental or economic causes did not seem precise, the very ubiquity of cancer suggested to many doctors that no simple cause was likely to be forthcoming.

A third cogent theory related carcinomas to chronic irritation. Chronic irritation, whether mechanical or chemical, was known to cause cell proliferation, and sometimes these cells showed some of the abnormal forms of cancer cells. The chronic inflammation theory drew on the well-known phenomenon of the precancerous lesion, such as a mole, ulcer, or lump in the breast. It was most easily related to the parts of the body that could be seen or felt, such as the skin, mouth, or breasts, but alcohol was presumed to be a chemical irritant, and stomach cancer seemed more common in heavy drinkers. The relationship between 'benign' and 'malignant' tumours was all important, and the chronic irritation placed cancer within a natural historical continuum, whereby the development of malignancy was a gradual process. It encouraged the investigation of environmental factors, such as badly fitting dentures or dietary substances.

From the 1880s, a fourth theory of cancer was elaborated: that it was contagious and caused by germs of one kind or another. There were many striking similarities in the minute pathology and clinical presentation of various cancers and chronic bacteriological diseases, such as leprosy and, above all, TB. Like cancer, TB seemed to 'metastasize', and the small tubercles found throughout the body had microscopic features that were similar to the cellular appearance of some cancers. The analogy between TB and cancer was noted long before Koch's discovery of the bacillus, and once tuberculosis was accepted as an infectious disease, the model stimulated the search for the parasitical causes of cancer. Syphilis, too, offered pregnant analogical speculations, and the American surgeon William Bainbridge (1870–1947) reported in 1914 coming back from a trip to discover a thirty-one-year-old patient of his anaesthetized on the operating table, about to have his tongue excised for what Bainbridge recognized as a chronic syphilitic lesion.

Worry about 'cancer houses' – dwellings where several members of the same family came down with cancer – and the possibility that cancer patients ought to be isolated in the way that TB victims were, was widespread. Like syphilis before the spirochete was discovered, cancer suffered not from too few, but too many, putative causative agents. Both clinical and laboratory evidence was rich and never conclusive, but the parasite paradigm was so powerful that it stimulated the foundation of German

(1900) and American (1899) cancer foundations, in addition to an abortive International Association for Cancer Research (1906). The historical volume of Jacob Wolff's *Science of Cancerous Disease* (1907) is more than 700 pages long and almost half of it was devoted to parasitical theories. In Britain, the main players in the Imperial Cancer Research Fund (1902) were more devoted to the chronic irritation theory.

It is significant that the major goal of these initiatives was research. Cancer was an enigma and many thoughtful doctors would have agreed with Bainbridge, when he concluded that 'The true, or even a satisfactory working explanation of the nature of cancer has not yet been discovered' (Bainbridge, 1914, p. 121). It was a subject that, from the late nineteenth century, has always attracted research funds. It was a disease to be dreaded, but one that, from the 1880s, was also full of hope. Much late-nineteenth-century surgery was cancer surgery, as a radical excision seemed the best prospect of a cure. The breasts and uterus seemed especially prone to cancer, one reason why women came under the surgeon's knife more than men. With the coming of X-rays and radiation, other therapeutic modalities offered hope. A subsequent century of biomedical research has made significant gains in understanding cancer's aetiologies and offering new therapies. The diseases that go under the name of 'The Big C' still occupy the same grim place in public perception.

PREVENTING DISEASE

As we have seen, there were preventive programmes mounted against TB, VD, and, to a lesser extent, cancer during the late nineteenth century, but what was generally called 'public health' had its modern origins earlier in the century, and shared more with other reform movements of the early industrial period than it did with the public health services in place in the age of the science and technology of bacteriology. The ideological roots of nineteenth-century public health are most clearly seen in Britain, the first industrial nation. The early public health movement there drew its membership from a wide swathe of professional and other middle-class groups: lawyers, clergymen, teachers, wealthy landowners, and business entrepreneurs, in addition to doctors. By the end of the century, most of this voluntary contribution had dropped away, and the actual work of public health was more firmly in the control of trained professionals: doctors, public analysts, inspectors, engineers, and laboratory technicians.

As mentioned earlier, the key figure in this early public health movement was Edwin Chadwick, a lawyer who had been Jeremy Bentham's last secretary and imbibed Bentham's commitment to reform society along the principles of utilitarianism, whose philosophical principles Bentham elaborated p. 86. Bentham died in the year that cholera became epidemic in Britain for the first time. The year 1832 also witnessed the passage of the First Reform Act, which extended the vote and redistributed Parliamentary representation better to reflect the population shifts that the urbanization of the Industrial Revolution had brought about. Traditional historical consensus has accorded the cholera the status of catalyst of the public health movement. Certainly the epidemics, especially the first two (1832 and 1848), occurred in years of political and social turmoil, and they heightened consciousness of the threat that epidemic diseases posed. Like most epidemics, cholera was prevalent among the poor, but it took its toll in all ranks of society. It also killed quickly and nastily, generally in a day or two after the victim became ill. People could be well in the morning and dead by nightfall, following violent diarrhoea, cramps, and, towards the end, bloody stools that contained pieces of the bowels. The badly dehydrated bodies took on an eerie bluish tint and were perceived to decompose especially rapidly (Fig. 2.7).

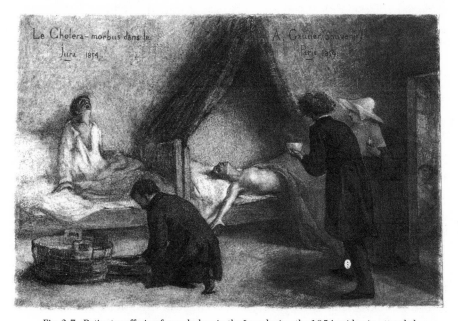

Fig. 2.7. Patients suffering from cholera in the Jura during the 1854 epidemic, attended by Dr. Paul-Ferdinand Gachet (1828–1909). *Source*: Pencil and charcoal drawing by Amand-Désiré Gautier, Paris, 1859. Wellcome Library Iconographic Collection. *Credit*: Wellcome Library, London (L0012076).

Although 1832 and 1848 were two important years in Chadwick's career, coinciding with his appointment as secretary of the New Poor Law Commission, and as a member of the General Board of Health, respectively, cholera did not occupy a unique place in his social philosophy. It was, after all, simply one of a cluster of epidemic diseases, called by him 'filth diseases', all of which emanated from the same basic cause. Chadwick was an ardent miasmatist – 'All smell is, if it be intense, immediate acute disease', he wrote – who attributed epidemic filth diseases to the overcrowded and insanitary conditions in which the poor lived and worked. His solutions were direct and simple: clean water piped into houses and excrement removed, suspended in water, in glazed pipes that would not allow any seepage into the soil. In a fit of bureaucratic tidiness, he suggested that the guano-rich faeces could be pumped into the country for treatment, and the fertilizer sold to farmers at a profit, the latter helping to pay for the system of sanitary improvements. With the modest addition of running water and privies to the dwellings of the labouring poor, Chadwick believed that the incidence of epidemic filth diseases could be more than halved, with commensurate increases in productivity and diminution in the poor rates. Rich and poor alike would benefit.

Social unrest and bad harvest characterized the 1840s – they were known grimly as the 'hungry forties'– and a pressure group that called itself the Health of Towns Association advocated reform on the back of a continuing barrage of sombre social statistics. That association, and Chadwick's Board of Health represent the culmination of the older combination of lay-dominated public health agitation in Britain. The initial 1848 board consisted of three laymen, and it was given only advisory powers unless death rates in an area were usually high or 10 percent of the rate payers (i.e., property owners) petitioned for the board to intervene. The beginnings of medical domination of the public health movement were embodied in one of the consequences of the act that created the board: the obligatory appointment of a Medical Officer of Health for all districts with an annual death rate over 23 per 1,000, and the permissive power for local health boards to appoint one should they see fit.

The board under Chadwick's guidance was nothing if not energetic. He was a man obsessed with efficiency and fully convinced that ill health (from preventable disease) was one root cause of high taxes and low levels of production and wealth. He believed that centralization of power and decision making was the only way forward and in the *laissez faire* political and economic atmosphere of mid-century Britain, he inevitably made many enemies. His fall from power was sudden and unexpected, coming as it did in the very year of the third British cholera epidemic, 1854. He was pensioned off to a long and frustrating retirement and replaced in a reconstituted board by John Simon (1816–1904; his family was originally French and his last name has the accent on the second syllable), who since 1848 had been the successful Medical Officer of Health for the City of London. By an anomaly of British politics, the City of London had fallen outside the remit of the 1848 Board of Health, so Simon had been able to work outside the sphere of Chadwick's influence.

Simon had achieved much in London through his personal magnetism and a liberal conviction that men of goodwill could be educated to act in the public interest. He was certainly shrewder politically than Chadwick, and during his two decades in central government (1854–76), Simon masterminded the development of what by the 1870s was the most comprehensive system of public health administration in the world. A surgeon and pathologist by training, Simon appreciated the complexity of disease within individuals as well as populations. Whereas Chadwick remained a miasmatist until his death in 1890, Simon adjusted to the newer teachings of germ theory. Simon's impassioned writing contrasted with Chadwick's heavy bureaucratic style. At the same time, Simon came to believe that compulsory legislation was necessary for effective sanitary change. A good example is provided by the gradual development of the system of compulsory public vaccination for smallpox. Simon examined the European dimensions of smallpox in the 1850s and showed through comparative analysis of statistics that the only way to protect against the disease was through a universal policy of mandatory infant vaccination. Accordingly, the British vaccination laws were gradually broadened, vaccination becoming in succession free, nonpauperizing, universal, and, eventually, compulsory. By 1871, the system was in place. It necessitated establishing sources of safe vaccine, appointing public vaccinators, creating a bureaucracy to oversee the service and legislating mechanisms to pay for it. It has been called a Victorian National Health Service. Parents who failed to comply could be prosecuted. Simon defended compulsion on pragmatic grounds: it was the only way to protect the whole community, but it went against the traditional tenets of liberalism and *laissez-faire* and provoked an organized antivaccination movement, reminiscent of the campaign to repeal the Contagious Diseases Acts. The vaccination laws were eventually relaxed in 1907 (by which time smallpox was no longer perceived as a serious threat) with the introduction of a conscientious objection clause, and subsequent immunization policy in Britain has followed suit.

Although the vaccination scenario provides the clearest instance of the tensions between individual freedom of choice and the collective good, it is by no means the only one, and by the end of Simon's regime, a whole range of social legislation had been effected, touching such issues as child labour, dangerous trades, sewage disposal, water supply, nuisance removal, food adulteration, and housing. The Public Health Act of 1875 consolidated existing legislation and provided the framework for British public health administration until after World War I. Simon had effected a shift from Chadwick's environmental, engineering approach to a more medical one, and germ theory further medicalized public health, just as public health further medicalized ordinary life. John Snow's brilliant epidemiological investigations during the 1848 and 1854 cholera epidemics had shown that cholera was not simply one of an undifferentiated class of filth diseases, but specific and spread through faeces-contaminated water. His mapping of cholera cases around a single contaminated well in Broad (now Broadwick) Street in Soho, in central London, implicated this source for a local outbreak that caused isolated cases further afield from individuals who had drunk its waters. He further investigated the relative cholera incidences in houses supplied with water from two separate London water companies, one which took its water from downstream the Thames, after the sewers of London had been emptied into it, and the other, which both filtered its water and took it upstream. The statistics were impressive: almost thirteen times the likelihood of contracting the disease from the contaminated water, and in houses that were often in the same street and shared similar social and environmental conditions. Snow's work convinced a lot of people that clean water was a desirable commodity, but, then, that had hardly been in contention, and his work was recognized for its power only during the decades to come.

Further public involvement in the control of epidemic diseases followed in Britain. A network of publicly funded infectious diseases hospitals was initiated from 1867, adding control of disease (through isolation) to the curative functions of the hospital (Fig. 2.8). Compulsory medical notification of key infectious diseases was enshrined in legislation in 1889. By the century's close, under the banner of 'Notification, Isolation, and Disinfection', a comprehensive system of infectious disease control was in place, by this time, with the benefit of germ theory.

The British experience highlights a number of issues that can be seen, *mutatis mutandis*, throughout Western societies. In France, the public

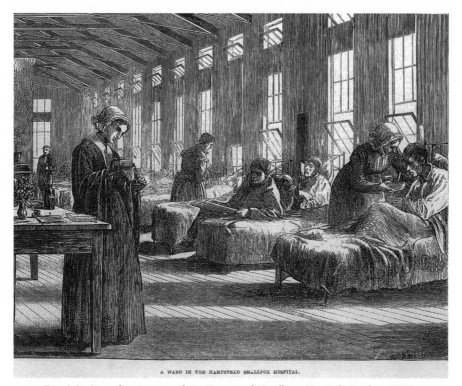

A WARD IN THE HAMPSTEAD SMALLPOX HOSPITAL.

Fig. 2.8. A pavilion-type ward in Hampstead Smallpox Hospital, London, 1871.
Source: *Illustrated London News*, 59 (1871), p. 335. *Credit*: Wellcome Library, London
(L0006796).

health movement of the early nineteenth century was closely identified with a small group within the medical profession. Hygiene as a subject was legitimized with chairs in the reorganized medical schools of the 1790s and Napoleon was an enthusiastic advocate of vaccination, even if it remained voluntary in civilian populations. Even before cholera hit, yellow fever in Cadiz and Barcelona led to a strengthening of national boundary protection through quarantine and inspection. As we have seen, Louis René Villermé's investigations from the late 1810s of the relationships between poverty, overcrowding, and disease, quantified social inequality p. 92. His massive study of health conditions among textile workers was a classic, appearing two years before Chadwick's chief work. Villermé's social diagnoses were stark, his solutions less so, as he argued the liberal case for education and enlightened employers to provide workers with decent wages and working conditions. In return, workers should exercise sobriety, honesty, and frugality. He excepted children as being helpless and in need of state protection, although the child employment regulations of 1840 were bland and policed only by unpaid volunteers. A succession of central and municipal boards, including an active Conseil de salubrité de Paris (1802) and the Central Sanitary Commission of 1820, provided administration, especially in times of epidemic crises, although political instability and wide shifts in state ideology hindered sustained continuity. *Médecins de quartier* provided medical care for the poor in addition to public health services.

Whereas Chadwick had looked for inspiration to a centralist French model of social administration, by the time of the Third Republic (1870), Britain was clearly more advanced in the field than France. Nevertheless, the prestige of Pasteur and Pastorianism benefited French public health efforts, and the Consultative Committee on Public Hygiene was revitalized in the 1870s. Henri Monod (1843–1911), a career administrator, became Director of Assistance and Public Health, and along with several Pastorians, such as Charles Chamberland (1851–1908), provided effective representation in government circles. Professional public health associations and private pressure groups advocated a variety of reforms, especially in pronatalism and child welfare. Compulsory smallpox vaccination was belatedly introduced into the French armed forces in 1876 (there had been devastating epidemics during the Franco-Prussian War), and from 1887 children were required to possess vaccination certificates before they could enter public school. A number of public health issues, including notification of some infectious diseases, were consolidated by the law of 1902.

In the German-speaking lands, the Enlightenment concept of Medical Police had received its fullest expression in Johann Peter Frank's (1745– 1821) massive *System einer vollständigen medicinischen Polizey* (9 vols., 1779–1827), which discussed virtually every aspect of human life from the womb to the tomb. Frank's was more a vision of what might be than a description of any society that has ever existed, but the close association between the medical profession and the state in the early-nineteenth-century German lands guaranteed an audience for the teaching of public medicine. Despite this long tradition of public service among doctors, and the flurry of legislation during the cholera epidemic of the 1830s, most historians date the modern German public health movement to a slightly later period. In 1847, Max von Pettenkofer (1818–1901), a young doctor turned chemist, received a post in chemistry at the University of Munich. His lectures and experimental work gradually turned to disease causation and prevention, and his chair was translated into one in hygiene in 1865, the first in the subject in the German lands. An institute was subsequently created for him, partly to stave off attractive academic offers elsewhere. Pettenkofer was by nature an experimentalist, devoting much ingenuity to determining a variety of conditions that facilitated or prevented the spread of contagious diseases. Late in his career, he argued, against Koch, that the cholera bacillus was not the simple 'cause' of cholera, famously swallowing a flask containing the bacilli without serious consequences. His approach to prevention was always broadly environmental, though none the less effective for that. He was the key player in the dramatic improvements in public health in Munich.

Except for a short period in Würzburg, Virchow's career was centred on Berlin. His analysis of the causes of the 1848 typhus outbreak in Upper Silesia (p. 92) had argued radically (though still within the liberal mould) that only a more fundamental social reorientation could prevent such epidemics: education, universal democracy, workers' cooperatives, and progressive taxation. Although some of his youthful radicalism softened with age, he never lost his liberalism or his commitment to sanitary reform. Both as a member of the Berlin City Council and of the Reichstag, he put into practice his beliefs about the political dimensions of health (and of medicine). The Berlin sewage and water systems were overhauled under his watchful eye. In Hamburg, the 1892 cholera epidemic catalysed similar reforms. German unification helped centralize public health activity: a Reich Health Office was established in 1873, although it took some years before it functioned efficiently. Compulsory vaccination was introduced to the civilian population in 1874, a legacy of the freedom from smallpox enjoyed by the vaccinated Prussian army in 1870–1.

In the United States, with its expanding frontier and division of political powers between central, state, and local governments, public health activity was more piecemeal. Among the more active states were Massachusetts and New York, and New York City has its own unique history of health administration. Lemuel Shattuck's (1793–1859) classic Massachusetts *Report* of 1850 was in the older statistical, sanitarian mould, though more wide-ranging than Chadwick's 1842 volume. Like Chadwick, Shattuck came to public health from outside of medicine, motivated as he was by his religious convictions. Shattuck called for the establishment of a Board of Health with wide-ranging powers relating to hospitals, factories, vaccination, water supply, and burial practices. It took almost two decades of agitation before such a board was established in Massachusetts, and then with fewer powers than he had envisioned.

The American Civil War (1861–5) dramatically demonstrated the role of social disruption and deprivation in the spread of epidemic diseases, and most states began to establish health boards in its aftermath, by which time industrialization was in full swing. Central government activity had largely been directed at quarantine, to which both the fear and the reality of yellow fever and cholera contributed. State and local resistance to central interference finally crumbled in the 1870s, when a yellow fever epidemic swept from the port city of New Orleans up the Mississippi valley. Although the resulting National Board of Health had a short and unsuccessful life, an older institution, the Marine Hospital Service, took over its quarantine brief, and just before the outbreak of World War I, it was transformed into the United States Public Health Service. Bacteriology stimulated the field dramatically, as is evidenced by the career of Charles Chapin (1856–1941), active in Providence, Rhode Island, and subsequently as a lecturer in public health at the Harvard School of Public Health. Although Chapin's *Municipal Sanitation in the United States* (1901) dominated the field for more than a decade, he cautioned public health officers against the trap of using bacteriological concepts too loosely.

The great wave of immigration, especially from Eastern Europe and Asia, in the decades before World War I, heightened concern about the spread of 'imported' diseases and led to increased surveillance and physical examination of immigrants. The demonstration that TB could be spread through milk obtained from tuberculous cows encouraged inspection of herds and pasteurization of milk. We have already mentioned 'Typhoid Mary' (p. 131) the asymptomatic Irish kitchen worker named Mary Mallon who infected a number of people with the bacillus and exposed (as had compulsory vaccination) the stark dilemma of balancing individual freedom and community health. That Mallon was poor, Irish, and a lone woman, undoubtedly made it easier for public health authorities to incarcerate her, but hardly solved the ethical issues. Compulsory disease notification exposed the potential tension between the doctor's divided responsibility to the patient and the community as a whole.

Karl Marx once defined the 'best' country as the one with fewest diseases, laws, and crime. The development of modern public health suggests that, at least within societies as we know them, diseases and laws can be inversely related. Time and again, diseases were identified within the context of unregulated human relationships. Permissive legislation proved inadequate to address the issues of housing, water, sewage, food adulteration, pollution, employment, education, and a host of other factors that nineteenth-century sanitarians correlated statistically with disease and premature death. The mere availability of a vaccine did not eradicate small-pox. Showing that cholera was spread by contaminated water did not produce clean water. Demonstrating that overcrowded, substandard housing could kill did not convince many landlords to repair their tenements, or employers to raise their workers' wages. Only when laws began to acquire what John Simon called 'the novel virtue of the imperative mood' could more systematic change occur. Even then, change was evolutionary, not revolutionary. Death rates were beginning to drift down by the century's end, and the real contribution of public health services should not be doubted. On the other hand, the most consistent positive correlation with disease and death uncovered by nineteenth-century investigators was that of poverty, and medicine as a social institution has never effectively challenged the fundamental issue of economic inequality.

MENTAL DISEASE

For many individuals in the nineteenth century, the phrase 'mental disease', if examined closely, would have seemed at odds with traditional theological beliefs. Christianity tended to equate the 'mind' with the immortal 'soul', our soul/mind being what survives after death. (The French use the same word, *âme*, for both soul and mind.) Consequently, a diseased mind (soul) was a matter for the clergyman, the result of sin, possession, witchcraft, or some other affliction of the spirit.

In practice, disturbances of mental functions and behaviour were common and routinely included in disease classifications. Psychiatry was in fact one of the earliest specializations within medicine, 'mad-doctors' being a visible component of the early modern medical landscape. Shakespeare's audiences would have responded to the sight of Edgar, in *King Lear*, taking on the form of 'Poor Tom-o-Bedlam'. The incidence of mental disorders is such that psychiatry today is sometimes said to occupy half of medicine, and the situation was probably not very different a century or two ago. Private madhouses, catering for paying patients, developed long before middle-class people suffering from ordinary diseases of the body would have paid for hospital care.

That the middle or upper classes would pay to have a troublesome relative looked after in a madhouse reflects the stigma always attached to 'mental' disease. Even today, our language perpetuates the difference between mental and physical disease. We *are* mad, insane, schizophrenic, hysteric, or alcoholic. We *have* TB, cancer, or heart disease. These diseases happen to us. Conditions that were formerly grouped within the 'mental' category, such as epilepsy, still grammatically share in both camps: one *is* an epileptic, but also can *have* epilepsy.

Historians traditionally have dated the birth of 'modern' psychiatry to the elaboration of 'moral' (i.e., psychological) therapy by several individuals in the closing years of the eighteenth century. Philippe Pinel in France, the Tuke family in Britain, and Vincenzo Chiarugi (1759–1820) in Italy, all 'discovered' independently, and at about the same time, that mentally disturbed individuals responded better to subtle psychological ('moral') measures than they did to restraint, bloodletting, and the other physical remedies generally prescribed for the mad. Moral therapy created a model that continued to infuse psychiatric writings and practice throughout the nineteenth century. It was not self-evidently a medical innovation. William Tuke (1732–1822) and his grandson Samuel Tuke (1784–1857), the leading players in creating the York Retreat as a psychiatric hospital, were Quakers and laymen. Pinel was of course a doctor, but he ran his asylums, the Salpêtrière (for women) and the Bicêtre (for men), along lines that deemphasized the medical in favour of systematic nursing, common sense, and kind firmness.

By the 1830s, doctors had assimilated moral theory within their therapies, and asserted their control over the insane. Doctors in France, Germany, Britain, and the United States established psychiatric societies during the 1840s, and these, along with specialist journals and hospitals (generally called 'asylums') ensured a distinct identity for those doctors concentrating on diseases of the mind. Psychiatrists (they were generally known by such terms as 'alienist', 'mad-doctor', 'nerve specialist', or 'asylum doctor') retained a buoyant optimism during the middle decades of the century. Psychiatric categories were extended to encompass a number of conditions or behaviours that would earlier have been deemed sinful or criminal. Thus, kleptomania, alcoholism, monomania, and nymphomania came under the ken of the psychiatrist, varieties of what James Cowles Prichard (1786–1848) in 1835 dubbed 'moral insanity', that is disturbances of the emotion, affect, or behaviour. In earlier times, 'madness' was deemed to include a clouding of the rational faculties, reason being the distinctive characteristic of human beings. An increasing social acceptance of psychiatric expertise in the early decades of the century, along with the promise of early diagnosis and treatment within the asylums, brought with it the belief (among the psychiatrists) that the number of individuals suffering from mental disorders would soon diminish.

The reverse happened. By the century's end, asylum populations throughout Western Europe and North America had increased far more rapidly than the population at large. There were many more asylums and their average size was larger. The situation in England and Wales was typical: in 1850, there were twenty-four publicly funded asylums, each with an average population of about 300 inmates. By 1890, there were sixty-six asylums, and each held an average of 800 patients. Psychiatric opinion was divided about whether this was a triumph or a failure: the result merely of better diagnostic methods, appropriately expanded diagnostic categories, and the transferral of insane paupers from the work houses to the asylums, where more humane care was available; or whether psychiatric disease was actually on the increase. By the end of the century, most psychiatrists shared the widespread perception of an increasing psychiatric burden. Three major factors reinforced this conclusion. First, the asylum had demonstrably failed as an institution of active psychiatric cure. Despite an extensive literature debating the merits of 'nonrestraint', a therapeutic programme championed in the 1830s by John Conolly (1794–1866), by the end of the century, nonrestraint had lost its novelty. Many asylum superintendents tried Conolly's programme, but most of them concluded that his powerful description of an asylum with a level of nursing care and administrative control that made physical restraint of violent patients unnecessary, was idealistic and impractical. There were simply too many suicides and acts of violence to permit his utopian vision to dominate. At the same time, the asylums gradually filled up with chronically ill, long-term patients, and asylum psychiatry became too much of an administrative specialty, as superintendents struggled to meet budgets, ensure that sanitation and basic necessities were in place, and deal with the daily grind of keeping a large 'total institution' running. Having been established with great optimism early in the century, by its end, asylums had become drab, highly regimented institutions whose primary function was to keep dangerous or awkward people off the streets.

A second factor made the failure of the asylums more easily explained: the increasing hereditary cast of social thought from mid-century. Early-nineteenth-century reform movements had often assumed that human nature was pliable (the French evolutionist Jean Baptiste Lamarck had argued that organisms are also very plastic and liable to change dramatically over time). These earlier, essentially optimistic philosophies were gradually replaced by the much more hard-nosed notions of hereditarianism. Francis Galton (1822–1911) was a leading figure in this shift. He devised a number of techniques for measuring the relationship between parents and offspring, and concluded that heredity (rather than environment) plays a large part in such characteristics as height, hair colour, physical vigour, and 'intelligence'. His family pedigree studies emphasized the extent to which various diseases, in addition to longevity, run in families. In 1883, he coined the word 'eugenics' to describe his science of good breeding, and he believed that social policy ought to encourage individuals with desirable characteristics to have more children. The negative part of eugenics programmes discouraged the undesirable from reproducing, through segregation in asylums, prisons, or hospitals for the mentally defective, or, in the twentieth century, through sterilization of individuals thought to be mentally, physically, or morally defective (p. 329).

As psychiatrists began to enquire more closely into the pedigrees of their patients within the asylums, they found what they were looking for: stigmata in the ancestries. Many patients reported (or asylum staff could determine in other ways) that parents, grandparents, uncles, or other relatives had drunk too much, had a brush with the law, been addicted to opium, were epileptic or suicidal, had produced an illegitimate child, or possessed some other socially undesirable attribute. These findings fit powerfully into the paradigm that the French asylum psychiatrist Benedict Augustin Morel (1809–73) had elaborated in his *Traité des Dégénérescences* (1857). Morel believed that 'poisons', in which he included alcohol, opium, miasms, the poison of cretinism, and other substances, could stimulate a downward spiral within a family. Their effects were cumulative over the generations, leading from excesses or simple nervousness in one generation, to frank addictions or criminality, to epilepsy, madness, and idiocy, as the generations unfolded. Several later social investigators ratified Morel's model, after the eugenics movement gathered pace, and degenerationism was given powerful literary expression in the series of novels by Émile Zola (1840–1902), scandalous for their frank depiction of French lowlife, sexuality, and criminality. The contemporaneous medicalization of homosexuality and other sexual proclivities occurred within this context of degeneration and late-century anxiety.

There was a third area of psychiatric unease, and this was largely outside the asylum walls. Even as asylums filled up as fast as they were built, increasing numbers of individuals were being diagnosed as suffering from a variety of incapacitating 'functional' disorders. Two were especially prominent, neurasthenia and hysteria. Neurasthenia was the diagnostic brainchild of the fashionable New York neurologist George Beard (1838–83). Its name harked back to the eighteenth-century system of John Brown (1735–88), who had grouped all diseases into two grand clusters, those with too much 'excitability', sthenic ones, and those with too little, the asthenias. Beard combined the latter term with the prefix for 'nerve' to describe a disease he attributed literally to nerve weakness, or exhaustion. Neurasthenia was largely a middle-class disorder, the result of the increasing pace of life of people who had burned the candle at both ends and suffered from what we still call 'burnout'. What is a metaphor for us was a stark physiological truth for Beard. Neurasthenia was essentially a disease of civilization, which is why Beard thought the disease was largely confined to advanced, Protestant countries. Although the disease affected both sexes, Beard believed that high-flying businessmen and professionals were particularly prone. Sufferers eventually reached a state of collapse and exhibited the cluster of symptoms that are still all about: tiredness, disturbances of sleep, palpitations, dizziness, headache, disorders of the bowels (diarrhoea in some, constipation in others), loss of appetite, various aches and pains, dyspepsia, and a general feeling of malaise. Although neurasthenia was not a form of insanity, it could easily lead in that direction if allowed to go unchecked (and untreated).

Three kinds of therapies were commonly advocated: rest, graded exercise, and electricity. Exercise was frequently prescribed for men, rest for women, including the 'rest cure' advocated by the Philadelphia physician and novelist, Silas Weir Mitchell (1829–1914). Under Mitchell's direction, a patient would be put completely to rest, denied all forms of stimulation (such as books or writing paper), and looked after hand and foot. Some women undoubtedly liked the attention and release from responsibilities, but others, such as the novelist Virginia Woolf (1882–1941), found it excruciating and demeaning. The rest cure and related therapies were institutionalized in spas, hydropathic establishments, health resorts, and nursing homes throughout the West. The one most common characteristic of their clients was that they could afford to pay.

If men and women were both susceptible to neurasthenia, in women the same cluster of symptoms was often diagnosed as hysteria. By the nineteenth century, this old diagnosis had been shorn of its traditional explanation as the consequence of a wandering uterus, but it was still commonly diagnosed. Hysteria carried more moral censure than neurasthenia. If neurasthenia was a disease of men who had worked too hard, hysteria was the disease of a women with too little to do. It was commonly perceived as a disease of idleness, of impure thoughts, and too much reading of French novels. No other nineteenth-century diagnoses reveals so much about the social and biological status of women. Doctors generally agreed that males could sometimes suffer from hysteria, but it affected only effeminate males who, like hysterical women, also betrayed the same self-centredness, emotional instability, and moral deviousness.

Jean-Martin Charcot did more than anyone to establish hysteria as a viable diagnosis in males. He also made its more common female manifestations a major medical spectacle. Charcot's weekly demonstrations of hysterical women before hundreds of medical students and foreign visitors in the amphitheatre of the Salpêtrière, put hysteria even more firmly on the map. He was, he thought, the master, producing hysterical symptoms at will on his patients, through hypnotism, pressure on sensitive points (especially just above the ovaries), and medical dominance. The photographic record produced some of the most famous images within nineteenth-century medicine. We now know that Charcot was as much manipulated by his patients as were they by him. They enjoyed the attention (and payments) and were consummate actresses, able to swoon or adopt contorted poses on command. Nevertheless, Charcot's fascination with hysteria produced at least two lasting results. First, it finally established hysteria as a psychological disorder. Neurasthenia had always been a convenient physical model for disease, nerve weakness having some physical cause. Charcot made hysteria into a psychiatric disorder, what he called a disease of 'ideas'. He made explicit the notion that the mind can be diseased.

His second psychiatric legacy was his influence on Sigmund Freud (1856–1939). Freud studied for several months in Paris, and these months were crucial for his own psychological development. They encouraged him to take the therapeutic potentials of hypnosis seriously, and when the economic demands of marriage meant life as a medical practitioner rather than a medical academic, both hysteria and hypnosis were waiting for him. The underlying principles and practices of what he came to call 'psychoanalysis' were laid down in the 1890s. Freud then collaborated with another Viennese medical practitioner, Josef Breuer (1842–1925), using hypnosis to treat hysterics. He also undertook a kind of self-analysis, through an intense correspondence, including analysis of his own dreams, with a Berlin ear, nose, and throat surgeon, Wilhelm Fliess (1858–1924). His notions of psychosexual development, the role of sex in the causation of hysteria and other neuroses, the interpretation of dreams, and the psychopathology of everyday life, have become part of modern culture. As a Jew at a time of rising anti-Semitism, Freud was always something of an outsider, and most doctors thought he was far too obsessed with sex. Nevertheless, he found a number of disciples, many of whom immigrated to the United States during the Nazi era. Although Freud came to psychoanalysis through neurology and psychiatry, many of his disciples were not medically qualified, with the subsequent blurring of the distinction between psychiatry as a medical specialty, and psychoanalysis and other forms of psychotherapy. That the public still confuse psychiatry and psychology reminds us that these issues have not been resolved, and mental illness has a different status to physical disease.

Whereas Freud took psychoanalysis into nonmedical directions, his contemporary Emil Kraepelin (1856–1926) attempted to establish a scientific psychiatry within the framework of medicine. Kraepelin spent his life within the German university system, at Leipzig, Dorpat, and Munich, where he headed a psychiatric institute. His textbooks, translated into most European languages, provided the basic classification of psychiatric diseases that still resonates. In particular, he differentiated between the 'minor' disorders, the neuroses, and the major ones, the psychoses. He pulled together various earlier descriptions of severe mental disturbance, which he grouped under the name of 'dementia praecox'. This was renamed 'schizophrenia' in 1911 by the Swiss psychiatrist Eugen Bleuler (1857–1939), and more than any other psychiatric disease, has become what most lay people mean when they speak of 'madness'.

Medicine and society

DOCTORS AND PATIENTS

The scientific and clinical transformations of medical practice during the nineteenth century worked their way into the relationship that patients experienced with their doctors. The physical intimacy of certain diagnostic and therapeutic procedures, the unfamiliarity of some diagnostic equipment, or the more ready suggestion of an operation, all were new to a patient from the 1850s or 1860s. Even the setting of the doctor's office and examination room gradually changed.

Historical convention assigns the dramatic shift in doctor–patient relationship, and power, to the nineteenth century. This typology, most strikingly enunciated almost three decades ago by Jewson, places the hospital at the centre of medical practice, and generalizes from the power structures that gradually obtained there. As we have seen, Jewson argued that relationships before the nineteenth century favoured patients and those after the nineteenth century favoured doctors (p. 56ff). The evidence is much more subtle. Hospitals always favoured doctors, not so much because of the care that was taking place there, but because of the nature of the hospital population. The poor were often in hospital because they had no choice, and did what they were told, or rebelled in their own ways and risked dismissal from the hospital, in the eighteenth and nineteenth centuries. That more medical care took place in hospitals in the latter century made the power that hospitals bestowed on doctors more commonplace, but did not necessarily signify the wholesale transformation postulated by Jewson.

Outside the hospital, and for middle-class patients, the changes were much more gradual and individualized. The health histories of many middle-class patients in the nineteenth century are known. Charles Darwin (1809–82), for instance, spent his adult life as a kind of valetudinarian. He consulted lots of doctors, went to health spas, and recorded his daily symptoms in a notebook. He was not alone, but was probably typical in taking the medical advice that suited him, or that produced visible results, quietly neglecting advice that interfered with the daily life he wished to live. Despite advice by doctors, he always held that a couple of slices of bacon at breakfast would do him no harm.

The surgeon's knife, which Darwin never experienced, was the single most important change in medical therapeutics during the century. The therapeutic modalities of physicians altered only gradually and, even if their advice carried more weight, it was easy to set aside, or follow only haltingly. As more conditions came under the realm of surgery, doctor–patient relations shifted, for surgery was often a matter of life or death, and was attended with pain and uncertainty. The medical history of Emily Gosse is a case in point.

In 1857, Emily Gosse, wife of the naturalist Philip Henry Gosse FRS (1810–88) and mother of literary critic and poet (Sir) Edmund Gosse (1849–1928), died of breast cancer. She was fifty-one years old and Edmund wrote movingly about his mother's illness and death in *Father and Son* and his *Life of Philip Henry Gosse*. It was often the child Edmund, aged six, who provided company for his sick mother. Ironically, Philip was enjoying some scientific success, was about to be elected a fellow of the Royal Society and had obligations to fulfil that forced the otherwise devoted couple to be apart. Like her husband, Emily was deeply religious (they were members of the radical protestant sect the Plymouth Brethren) and prayer, sometimes shared with Philip and Edmund, was an important way of coping with her painful and fatal illness. Despite their faith, the Gosses did not rely on prayer alone and sought medical help from a range of orthodox and irregular practitioners as her condition worsened.

In April 1856, Emily was troubled by discomfort in her left breast and possibly a lump, which she interpreted as some kind of bruising. A female friend urged her to see her doctor, Edward Laseron, a former missionary and a Brother. When she came home from seeing Laseron, she told her husband (as recounted by Edmund): '"He says it is – "and she mentioned one of the most cruel maladies by which our poor mortal nature can be tormented. Then I saw them fold one another in a long silent embrace, and presently sink together out of sight on their knees, at the farther side of the bed, whereupon my Father lifted up his voice in prayer.' Edmund was no more able to use the word 'cancer' when he continued his narrative and reported asking his parents at breakfast the next morning 'What is –?' . . . Receiving no reply, I looked up to discover why my question was not answered, and I saw my parents gazing at each other with lamentable eyes.' Edmund's retrospective fear was nothing compared with the dread felt by his parents despite their resolution to accept God's divine will.

Emily and Philip visited Dr. Henry Hyde Salter (1823–71), a distant relative of Philip. Salter recommended surgery and suggested they consult London's leading surgeon, James Paget (1814–99). Paget wished to operate immediately to try to remove the tumour. Emily was afraid of the pain and attendant risks associated with surgery and they opted instead to follow up Salter's other suggestion, an American, Dr. Jesse Weldon Fell (1819–89) who offered a new, nonoperative means of curing cancer for which he claimed an 80 percent success rate. On the Gosses's behalf, Salter attended one of Fell's open days designed to demonstrate the efficacy of his treatment to London's medical élite, a circle he was anxious to join. Salter was aware of Emily's dread of surgery and apparently sufficiently impressed with Fell's show. His treatment for cancer of the breast consisted of the application of ointments of zinc chloride or lead iodide to which he added the root of *Sanguinaria canadensis*, a plant reputedly used by the Cherokee Indians. Emily may have dreaded the surgeon's knife but Fell's treatment was not without considerable pain 'at times . . . scarcely supportable', despite his firm assurances to the contrary.

Fell had left New York two years before (1855) after a long-running dispute with the New York Academy of Medicine of which he was a founder member, and some disparagement of his cancer treatment. He had set himself up in London in unfashionable Pimlico and like a true quack begun to offer his 'secret medicament' to a fearful cohort of mostly poor cancer sufferers, although in December 1856 he moved to Warwick Square and began an attachment to the Middlesex Hospital. Here a trial of his remedy was undertaken, he having decided to shake off the trappings of quackery and reveal its constituents. The results of the Middlesex trial were mixed, the treatment (which was not particularly original) was about as successful as operative surgery, but attended with considerable pain. By this time however, Emily was dead and Fell had what he wanted, a lucrative specialist private practice among the higher echelons of society.

When the Gosses visited him in his rooms in Pimlico he offered a photographic record of previous cases to explain what he did and how it worked. While they were there, he was conveniently able to demonstrate the condition of a tumour from a middle-aged patient: 'We saw the large tumour, dark, hard, and apparently dead, deeply scored across, and divided by a distinct line of demarcation from the white living flesh around.' The patient apparently declared 'that the pain of the process was not worth speaking of'. In Emily's case, he opined that application of the ointment would be sufficient and if after a few months the tumour had not faded away, as he predicted there was no cause for concern, there would be no deterioration in her condition and tumour removal could be undertaken. All this was exactly what Emily hoped to hear. The Gosses returned home, prayed, and decided to put Emily in the hands of Fell.

From May 12th until the end of August, Emily travelled across London from their home in Islington to Pimlico three times a week. Fell applied his ointment and Emily learned all too quickly that far from being pain free, she suffered from a 'gnawing or aching in the breast'. In consolation for this distress she was able to use the hours spent travelling to distribute the religious tracts she wrote and engage fellow passengers in conversations designed to bring them to God. At the end of August, Fell gave Emily a supply of ointment so she could continue to treat herself and she left London with her family for South Wales.

When the Gosses returned to London in early October Emily was much worse, greatly fatigued by the return journey, a marker if one were needed, for her rapid decline. Fell decided that the second phase of the treatment was necessary and the tumour should be removed. Emily (with Edmund) moved to lodgings in Pimlico for easier access to Fell and he began applying nitric acid with a sponge to the skin of the left breast, followed by a series of small incisions approximately a centimetre apart into which a plaster of a 'purple mucilaginous substance' was introduced. Each day the incisions were deepened and dressed with this plaster until they were sufficiently large to allow strips of fabric coated in the same stuff to be inserted. Emily was in great distress and failing visibly. She could not sleep without opiates and would 'wander up and down her chamber, resting her head, from time to time, upon the mantelpiece or against the wall'.

After four weeks the cuts had reached two-and-a-half centimetres in depth and Fell changed the nature of the dressings and after two further weeks the tumour 'dropped like a stone out of a basin . . . . There it lay on the table, a hard and solid block of black substance resembling in size and shape a penny bun; deeply scored on one surface and on the other nearly smooth. And then on the breast, was the corresponding cavity, raw and lined with pus, but presenting an apparently healthy appearance'. It was only an appearance. Fell reported another smaller tumour within the cavity. The whole, tortuous process had to be repeated he said and the patient submitted. After a further four weeks, the second tumour came away. This time examination revealed two more. A weak but querulous Emily asked Fell for an explanation: 'But how do you account for this spreading of the disease'? He responded 'Oh, 'tis in your blood'. Emily could not countenance further treatment in Fell's hands and she returned home to Islington a few days before Christmas 1856. Gosse too was puzzled and disappointed; the idea of a constitutional disease was 'contrary to the statements we had all along relied on'. 'What is the use of a merely local treatment of a disease which is seated in the blood?' he asked. By this point, it was merely a rhetorical question.

After he brought his wife home, Philip engaged Dr. John Epps (1805–69) to be her final physician. Like Fell, Epps had trained in orthodox medicine before turning to an alternative system, in his case homeopathy. Indeed, by the 1850s, he had become the leading practitioner of homeopathy in London. Epps could do little except try to control Emily's pain while she concentrated on ensuring her husband would take proper spiritual care of himself and their son. She asked for her photograph to be taken so that Edmund would have a tangible reminder of her (Fig. 2.9).

Late on Monday, February 9, 1857, a little over ten months since she began her treatment under Fell, Emily Gosse faintly told her husband 'I'm going home – I must go home!' A little later she asked 'I shall walk with Him in white; won't you take your lamb, and walk with me?' repeating the last sentence, which Philip assumed applied to Edmund. He held his wife in his arms as Monday night slipped into Tuesday morning and apparently

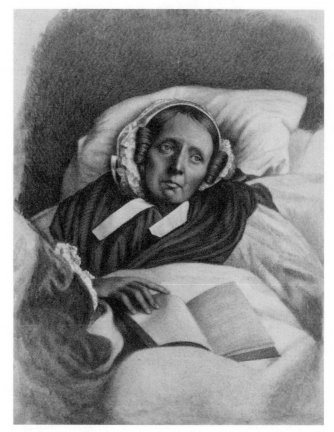

Fig. 2.9. Emily Gosse on her deathbed, 1857. *Source*: *The life of Philip Henry Gosse, F.R.S.*, by his son Edmund Gosse. London, 1890. Shelfmark Adv.c.82.5. Interleaved illustration no. 50. *Credit*: By permission of the syndics of Cambridge University Library.

ready for death she whispered 'Open the gates! Open the gates, and let me in!' He closed her eyes, knelt by her bed, and prayed.

Gosse retained his dignity after Emily's death and restricted his comments on Fell to suggesting that his ointments had been 'much overrated'.

Emily Gosse's last illness contains both individual and universal elements. It reminds us that a diagnosis of cancer was dreaded long ago, and that it, and other grave diagnoses, created shock waves, even in the deeply religious. Individuals who could afford it generally sought a second medical opinion if the first one was alarming or unsatisfactory. Pain and suffering were not routinely embraced, even among those who might nevertheless strive to find meaning in them. Our forebears were no different from people today in wanting to live until death seemed inevitable or the pain became unbearable. Unorthodox treatments are still embraced, if they seem more effective or less painful. Hope has always been an important element of medical care. Fell was not alone among doctors in promising a great deal, and in having a ready explanation when his treatment failed.

Emily Gosse suffered from a disease that killed her within a year. Rothman's sensitive study of tuberculous patients in nineteenth-century America recounts longer-term interactions between patients and their supporting networks, including families, neighbours, and doctors. The twin stories of Deborah Fiske and her daughter would have been played out in thousands of nineteenth-century families, and few doctors would not have had the management of consumption as a common part of their practice. In Rothman's account, doctors and their patients shared similar visions of how consumption expressed itself and the general parameters of how best to deal with it. Even after Koch's bacillus entered the equation, climate remained important, the sea voyage, immigration to the hot dry regions of the American Southwest, or sanatorium treatment in the cooler mountains, all expressing shifting versions of an underlying theme.

Childbirth offers another window on medical care during the century. Jalland has used the letters, diaries, and other personal papers of a group of wives, daughters, and sisters in British political families. Dying in childbirth remained a highly visible possibility throughout the century, and it coloured young women's attitudes towards marriage. Her work reveals how doctors had variable reputations among the powerful families of Britain. Their pros and cons were discussed, and recommendation obviously helped build and sustain an active practice. Male attendance at birth was the norm, not the exception, although the doctors were supposed to supervise only the actual birth and, not infrequently, they arrived just too late. Midwives or, more commonly, the 'monthly nurse', hired to stay the first month after a child's birth, were booked beforehand and often supervised the early stages of labour. Husbands, at least in Jalland's sample, were with their wives during the labour and birth, a convention that had to be rediscovered more recently after childbirth moved into hospital delivery rooms. Prince Albert had been with Queen Victoria during the births of their children, although it caused comment in the *Lancet* when he first did it in 1841. Perhaps, as in the use of chloroform as an obstetric anaesthetic, commoners followed where royalty led. The middle-class families in Jalland's study uniformly considered pregnancy and birth as normal, physiological events. The pathologization of childbirth, commonly enunciated in the United States, was associated with the concerted campaign, led by obstetricians, to move delivery into the hospital.

Jalland's women chose their doctors carefully and were not afraid to seek second opinions, or even change medical attendants, if they thought it desirable. However, they seemed in general to have been satisfied with the care they received, although mothers or sisters of young wives pregnant for the first time were more regular sources of practical knowledge. And when they complained of their doctors, sometimes it was for the vagueness of what their doctors told them. As one of them wrote, after a Dr. Hayes had examined her with a speculum and told her that her pregnancy was going normally, '[Dr Hayes] has been most aggravating – in the way of never letting me know what he really wants me to do, and even when he gives me a direction he only gives it vaguely. "You must lead a very careful life for the next few days." And then when I try to ask him what he means, I have the greatest difficulty in discovering whether stairs matter, or drives or walks or indeed anything' (Jalland, 1986, pp. 141–2). Edith Lyttleton clearly wanted more, not less, medicalization of her pregnancy.

One cannot, of course, generalize about doctor–patient relationships on the basis of a few examples, but it seems likely that the most important determinants were the class and social status of the patient, and the personality of the practitioner. If a disease or condition was not amenable to surgical correction, it was almost inevitably managed rather than cured. But the management of disease certainly improved during the century. Doctors had few powerful drugs, but their judicious use could do much to help the patient. Besides, doctors were well aware of the self-limiting nature of most illness. The Boston physician Jacob Bigelow (1786–1879) elaborated on the self-limited nature of much disease in a famous address in 1835, although most doctors were reluctant to espouse the doctrine publicly. It would have been bad for business. Among the drugs mentioned by Jalland's women were boric acid, brandy, bromide, castor oil, champagne, ergot, laudanum, morphia, opium, port wine, and quinine. Three opiates and three alcoholic beverages: not exactly high tech, but likely to have produced a certain amount of patient satisfaction.

Fee-paying patients could pick and choose their doctors; the evolving professional ethics of the day gave doctors less choice. The rhetoric of medicine, evoked on speech days and graduation ceremonies, in admission ceremonies and eponymous lectures at medical gatherings, proclaimed that medicine was a thoroughly altruistic profession. Young doctors were reminded that they were obliged to treat anyone who sought their help. Formal and informal codes of ethics provided guidelines on the duties (and rights) of the profession, generally within a contractual framework that had

characterized the classic late-eighteenth-century writings of Thomas Per-
cival (1740–1804) and Thomas Gisborne (d. 1806). A formal code of ethics
was central to the formation of the American Medical Association in 1847,
and the General Medical Council, created in Britain under the terms of the
1858 Medical Act, devised a set of acceptable and unacceptable behaviour
in doctors. As the century wore on, issues like advertising and touting secret
remedies were deemed outside the bounds of professional activity. At the
same time, many doctors were incensed at the large range of proprietary
remedies available for over-the-counter purchase. These were investigated
in both Britain and the United States early in the twentieth century, and
roundly condemned by doctors, who also knew well that many of the tonics
they dispensed or prescribed were similar in ingredients and physiological
effects to the quack remedies they were denouncing. The regulation of sexuality was always contentious: procuring abortions was relatively easy to
condemn (except when the life of the mother was threatened), but offering
contraceptive advice was also deemed unethical.

Throughout the nineteenth century, the marketplace was crowded, especially in major cities. This continued to give patients more choice and made
it harder for the profession to unite against the experiments in national
insurance that were introduced in Germany, Britain, and elsewhere from
the 1880s (p. 345ff).

MONOPOLY AND THE LIBERAL MEDICAL PROFESSION

As liberalism developed during the nineteenth century, it furthered the
comfortable assumption that professional groups possess two principal
characteristics: esoteric knowledge and altruistic codes of behaviour. The
knowledge gave them the right to autonomy and internal regulation
because 'lay' people are not competent to judge them, lacking the knowledge base. The disinterested behaviour guaranteed that society received
value from the profession's activities. Doctors have their patients' best interests at heart, and thus deserve society's trust. 'The profession of medicine
is distinguished from all others by its *singular beneficence*', remarked Sir
William Osler. This is one version of the historical scenario. An alternative
account takes its cue from George Bernard Shaw's quip that 'All professions
are conspiracies against the laity' and argues that professions are really
concerned with power. Professional rhetoric of disinterested service is in
reality empty, and professions have primarily their own members' power
and incomes in view. From either perspective, a profession may hold that it
deserves an occupational monopoly, either policed by the state or, 'natural',

211

as a rational public recognizes the greater claims of the properly qualified professional. Many doctors argued as forcefully as they could that it was irrational and dangerous for anyone to trust his or her health to the ministrations of a herbalist, wise woman, itinerant drug peddler, or homoeopath.

Strict occupational control ran counter to the tenor of nineteenth-century liberalism, which valued freedom and individualism over regulation and centralization. As Ramsey has summarized it: 'Briefly, where laissez-faire liberalism flourished, de jure monopoly was generally weak or non-existent; where mainstream liberalism was strongly committed to reform from the center, monopoly was only weakly challenged; and where liberalism failed, professional monopolies were at their tightest' (Ramsey, 1984, p. 229).

The medical profession in nineteenth-century Europe and North America offers an instructive instance of Ramsey's generalization. Traditionally, the regulation of medical personnel and the control of standards had been in the jurisdiction of the relevant college, academy, or collegium. In many Old Regime German states, the healing 'professions', including midwifery and pharmacy, were tightly regulated alongside other occupations. In Britain, where Adam Smith's *Wealth of Nations* (1776) had elaborated the classic statement of economic *laissez-faire*, the guilds had lost much power and occupational freedom was the norm. The Royal Colleges of Physicians and Surgeons controlled the practice of physic and surgery in London, as did similar institutions in Edinburgh, Glasgow, and Dublin. Outside the major cities, an open medical marketplace more or less reigned, and even within areas of collegiate jurisdiction, the prosecution of irregular practitioners and quacks was expensive and seldom resorted to. The colleges were obliged to pay for their own legal costs to police their monopolies. A weak medical licensing system gradually evolved in the United States in the decades after the American War of Independence at a state or local level.

It was in France where the medical profession enjoyed most protection during the nineteenth century. The law of Ventôse (March 10, 1803) created two orders of medical men, those with a doctorate of medicine or surgery from a medical school, and the more practically trained *officiers de santé*, meant for rural areas and more routine medical work (p. 138). Only holders of one of these qualifications could practise medicine and charlatans could be prosecuted. The higher grade of student trained in Paris, Montpellier, or Strasbourg at one of the three degree-granting schools to survive the revolution. The more haphazard way in which *officiers de santé* obtained diplomas from departmental medical boards was never popular

212

with élite doctors or state officials, although both the grade and the law of Ventôse remained in force until 1892. This was despite repeated liberal criticism that the monopoly was virtually impossible to enforce adequately, and the law hindered freedom, both of enquiry and choice.

Napoleon exported both the law of Ventôse and a hostility to guilds wherever French conquests were successful. In the annexed German states of the Rhineland, the medical profession had long been protected by the state, and many physicians were actually civil servants. Despite some economic advantages to this arrangement, there could be drawbacks, such as the duty to practise wherever the state dictated, and the *Kurierzwang*, the obligation to treat any person in urgent need. Liberal German voices, such as those of Alexander von Humboldt (1769–1859) and, from 1848, Rudolf Virchow began to challenge the restrictive shackles of the old order, arguing that social reform and universal education would produce a populace that would chose their doctors wisely and, in any case, the freedom to choose (*Kurierfreiheit*) was fundamental, both for doctors and their patients. The Prussian *Gewerbeordnung* (trades ordinance) of 1869 finally opened the medical marketplace, and it was extended throughout the Reich in 1871. It permitted a rapid increase in all kinds of irregular healers, who often formed their own occupational associations. In Berlin, there were thirty-four regular doctors for every full-time empiric in 1879; by 1903, the number had dropped to just over three.

Most observers interpreted the *Gewerbeordnung* as a blow against medieval protectionism, while at the same time recognizing that in public health and medical care, a complete *laissez-faire* could be detrimental to the public's welfare. In practice, the state continued to protect the regular professional by limiting the sphere of irregulars, who could not treat VD or cancer, administer injections, or use narcotics. The liberal German system was finally ended by the Nazis, not from any particular regard for scientific medicine, but because the preservation of collective health was decreed as more important than individual freedom (p. 373ff).

The German system of the 1870s bore striking similarities to that that had been obtained in Britain after the Medical Act of 1858, although the British approached the issue of monopoly from a different perspective. The 1858 act, finally passed after more than two decades of discussion and several abortive bills in Parliament, was another triumph of liberalism. It perpetuated the eclectic system of education and licensing that had gradually grown up between the universities, hospital medical schools, and medical corporations, but failed to outlaw irregular practice. Irregulars could not misrepresent themselves, while the annual Medical Register of legally qualified doctors in theory gave the public access to the information necessary to make sensible medical choices. The act also granted the profession a good deal of autonomy by establishing the General Medical Council (GMC), with jurisdiction over malpractice and 'infamous conduct' (e.g., advertising, molesting patients, or collaborating with irregulars), along with an advisory role in medical schools' curriculum and examination standards. The GMC was also responsible for compiling and ensuring the accuracy of the Medical Register. Only doctors on the register could hold various public posts, such as public vaccinators, Medical Officers of Health, Superintendents of Lunatic Asylums, Poor Law Medical Officers, and consultants in the voluntary hospitals. State patronage of medicine is considered further below.

In the United States, the early licensing laws proved ineffective and, by mid-century, alternative medical groups, such as homeopaths, eclectics, and Thomsonians (who emphasized the curative powers of the plant *Lobelia inflata*), vied with the regulars for professional hegemony. Proprietary schools of all stripes were founded in great numbers, with the consequence that the 'doctorate' was devalued. Joseph Rhodes Buchanan (1814–99), sometime dean of the Eclectic Medical Institute of Cincinnati, sold hundreds of diplomas by mail order. After the American Civil War (1861–5), new licensing regulations began to be passed in most states, and although some of these laws recognized unorthodox practitioners, the regulars were the greatest beneficiaries. We have seen how the foundation of Johns Hopkins University in 1876 introduced a deliberate Germanic research ethos into American higher education (p. 148ff). Ironically, even as the internal reforms gathered apace during the last decades of the century, homeopathy and eclecticism continued to enjoy popular support. Of equal or greater long-term import, osteopathy and chiropractic began their own successful careers. Andrew Taylor Still (1828–1917) established osteopathy in the 1870s and Daniel David Palmer (1845–1913) set up as a magnetic healer in the 1880s and developed his techniques of spinal manipulation over the following years. He established his school of chiropractic in 1898. In Abraham Flexner's famous survey in 1910 of medical education in the United States and Canada, he looked at orthodox as well as alternative schools. The majority of schools of both kinds failed his 'gold standard' test, the model provided by the best University Medical Faculties in Germany. Many small American schools closed in the wake of post-Flexnerian reforms.

Although France stands out as a notable exception of continued state protection of the medical profession (along with the regulation of many other occupations), a general convergence can be seen in many European countries and the United States. Liberal ideals prevented medical monopolies from being enshrined in law, even if the state officially entrusted regular doctors with overseeing public health provision; treating dangerous conditions, military personnel, and VDs; and manning government health departments and hospitals. There were several factors at work. In the middle decades of the century, medical associations were established in many localities: the Provincial Medical and Surgical Association (forerunner of the British Medical Association) in 1832; the American Medical Association (AMA) in 1847; and the *Berliner medicinische Gesellschaft* in 1860. Many of these served a mixture of educational, professional, and political ends, and helped provide a collective voice for the profession. The growth of science and technology within medicine changed medical education, diagnosis, and therapy (especially surgical); yoked medicine to ideologies of progress; and distanced 'regular' practitioners from what we now call 'alternative medicine'. In Britain, the rise of antivivisection groups undoubtedly drew doctors closer together. Government health insurance schemes gave the palm to regulars, as did public investment in disease surveillance and prevention. Thus, although consumer choice prevailed in most localities, the orthodox profession was stronger, more coherent, and more powerful than it had been at the beginning of the century.

PAYING THE DOCTOR

'Medical instruction does not exist to provide individuals with an opportunity of learning how to make a living, but in order to make possible the protection of the health of the public.' So Virchow told his students, though most of them would not have listened. Throughout history, most doctors have assumed that a patient satisfactorily helped within the context of a fee-for-service transaction represented the acme of their aspirations. There could be sufficient room for idealism in the helping, but the practice of medicine was the way the doctor actually made his living. For every doctor who threw himself into public health, medical research, or full-time academic work, dozens tested the waters of the world outside. During the nineteenth century, that outside world changed, as new forms of paying for health care emerged or older forms changed their character.

There are four principal kinds of economic relationship between doctor and patient: (1) fee-for-service; (2) charity; (3) prepayment through mutual aid associations, or private insurance; and (4) payment regulated by local or central government, through taxes, social security contributions, or a combination of the two.

Traditionally, either fee-for-service or charity accounted for most medical encounters, and throughout the nineteenth century, most individuals who were comfortably off simply paid for medical care as and when they needed it. Doctors who practised successfully among the rich often became rich. At the same time, most doctors devoted some time to charity, either seeing poor patients *gratis*, charging only what the patient could afford, or working within a charity hospital, dispensary, or infirmary. In Britain, the voluntary hospital system, which developed from the early eighteenth century, provided hospital treatment for the worthy poor. These hospitals were financed by charitable giving from the well-to-do, who enjoyed the benefit of recommending suitable patients and governing the institution. Medical and surgical élites eagerly sought honorary posts in the voluntary hospitals, even though the direct financial rewards were minimal because such posts brought prestige, offered teaching and clinical research opportunities, and were good for their private consulting practices. Until the end of the nineteenth century, when pay beds for rich patients began to be introduced, these hospitals were exclusively for the indigent, and the well-to-do were treated primarily at home, although doctors sometimes took patients into their homes or used private nursing establishments. Operations were sometimes performed in hotels.

As we have noted, aseptic surgery, trained nurses, and other aspects of modern care eventually brought all classes into British hospitals. On the Continent, the class distinction was never so clear-cut, as many hospitals admitted patients from a variety of economic circumstances. In the United States, too, most hospitals, even those founded on the British voluntary model, incorporated pay beds, even if these were few until the end of the century. In all countries, however, charitable giving was encouraged, through organized religion, individual conscience, or direct solicitation from the charitable institution. And in all countries, most hospital patients were poor.

Charity, however, was never enough. For one thing, it was often targeted at selected groups: orphans rather than beggars, injured workers than raving lunatics, church-goers than strangers, the worthy rather than dirty poor. It was also dispensed with a price: recipients were supposed to be deferential to their economic and social betters, even while being preached the virtues of self-reliance. Many families that could cope economically in good times could not stand the trials of illness, injury, or death of the breadwinner. For these, mutual aid associations could provide a measure of economic and social continuity. Medieval guilds developed extensive networks of mutual assistance to provide support for a variety of domestic crises. In the seventeenth and eighteenth centuries, a number of more general schemes were proposed and insurance companies were prepared to insure human life in addition to property or ships.

The nineteenth century witnessed a dramatic increase of mutual aid associations, often within the context of the workplace. Some employers contributed to them: Josiah Wedgwood, for instance, had helped support a model scheme of social insurance among the workmen in his highly successful pottery factory. The Société philanthropique de Paris encouraged workers to establish aid societies. One of the major functions of the nascent trade union movement was to provide help in times of hardship. In Britain, the harshness of the New Poor Law of 1834 further stimulated the self-help movement. This was an intended consequence and between 1835 and 1845, new friendly society chapters were established at the rate of three a week. In the second half of the century, medical clubs were formed with the sole purpose of employing a doctor to provide medical services for their members.

Many medical practitioners resented these developments. The salaries on offer were perceived as modest and being the employee of a working-class group hardly appealed to professional self-esteem. On the other hand, the overcrowded profession guaranteed competition for patients and meant that medical clubs were able to find willing doctors, even if only at the beginnings of their careers and with eyes to private practice in the long term. Importantly, mutual-aid groups weaned participating doctors off the fee-for-service model and on to one of capitation, by which the doctor was paid for the number of patients for which he was responsible, not the number of consultations he had with any particular patient. Because medical clubs and other forms of mutual-aid society were varied in their constitutions and autonomous in their contractual arrangements, it is difficult to estimate national figures of how many people paid for their health care in this way. Nor is it easy to evaluate the quality of service provided by club doctors. Claims that it was poor were generally made by nonparticipating doctors who distrusted the whole structural base. What is clear is that contract practice expanded substantially in Britain, France, Germany, and elsewhere within Europe, during the second half of the century, and was beginning to make a more modest impact in the United States.

These contractual practices also provided continuities with the fourth type of economic relationship between patient and doctor, through the medium of social security. It has already been noted that the state had long provided a variety of medical and other welfare services for the really destitute through the Poor Laws or *assistance publique*. Michel Foucault has stressed that such state activity was more concerned with public order than the humanitarian relief of distress, and many historians have examined the processes whereby the undifferentiated category of social dependence – beggars, vagabonds, orphans, widows, the elderly, and the mad – was gradually untangled, with a variety of more specialized institutions replacing the *hôpitaux généraux* and their equivalents after the process Foucault called the 'Great Confinement'.

Superficially, early social security systems might seem to be merely a further extension of state activity in the area of medicine and welfare. The more striking continuities, however, are with the mutual-aid associations described, though with the difference that the state as a player made. The prototype national sickness insurance scheme was that that Bismarck got through the Reichstag in 1883. There had been earlier industries, mining, for instance, which had been required by Prussian law to institute compulsory sickness, accident, and burial insurance for workers. The 1883 sickness insurance bill, combined with ones for accidents (1884) and old age pensions (1889), were designed by Bismarck to secure the loyalty (he had no great desire for their love) of workers who were being increasingly exposed to socialist ideas. The Social Democratic Workers' Party was equally distasteful to the Iron Chancellor, although antisocialist legislation of the same period had been unsuccessful in keeping Social Democrats out of the Reichstag.

The Sickness Insurance Bill made mandatory insurance in a number of industrial occupations and was extended in subsequent years to many other occupational groups. Hospital and doctors' services were both included, along with income compensation for lengthy illness. Whenever possible, the administrative facilities of existing mutual-aid societies were used, and detailed arrangements varied, depending on the size and wealth of the schemes. Most used capitation payments, although in some instances a fee for service structure prevailed. Initially, only workers were covered, but as the scheme began to be expanded, dependants were sometimes included. Although the state had legislated for it, it made no direct contributions, with payments coming from employees and employers.

Bismarck pushed through the legislation without consulting the medical profession. Initially there was little protest, partly because the profession had no powerful central organization, partly because the legislation for the most part covered industries with strong traditions of mutual assistance. As the schemes began to be extended, however, insurance practice became increasingly important for practitioners and dissatisfaction with capitation arrangements, levels of remuneration, and terms of service surfaced. The Association of German Doctors for the Protection of Their Economic Interests, known as the *Leipziger Verband*, was established in 1900 through the activities of Gustav Hartmann to argue the doctors' case. It has been estimated that in 1900, 80 percent of medical practice was still private, fee-for-service, but the trend was downwards.

In France, *mutualité* in the nineteenth century had a chequered history. The legal status of mutual-aid societies was affected by the Napoleonic Criminal Code forbidding associations of more than twenty persons. This tended to drive them underground, although it is estimated that there were no fewer than 262 in Paris alone in 1846. Some liberalization occurred during the Second Empire, though political activities of the mutual societies were outlawed. There was further expansion in the Third Republic, by which time the legalization of strikes and the rise of syndicalism had largely separated political radicalism from mutualism. In the two decades before World War I, the friendly societies experienced rapid growth at a time when the concept of national pensions, accident provision, and health care for the indigent was being widely debated, though within a context of widespread suspicion of anything German, including Bismarck's programme. More general social security schemes were not instituted until after the Great War.

The British looked on the German schemes with more interest, although the growing resistance of German doctors was widely reported in the British medical press. A Royal Commission sat between 1905 and 1909 to examine the operation of the Poor Laws, and while the majority of the commissioners recommended their continuation, a famous minority report, written by Beatrice Webb (1858–1943) and other dissenting commissioners, argued for more universal, nonpauperizing systems of social relief. Beatrice and her husband Sidney Webb (1859–1947) campaigned for a state service of medical care. In the event, the social legislation passed by the Liberal Government between 1905 and 1911, was influenced by the German model. Unemployment and old-age pension were covered in separate acts. The National Health Insurance Act of 1911 built on the existing mutual-aid societies, using their collecting facilities and membership lists, but extending compulsory insurance to almost all workers whose wages fell within the specified bands. The existence of the voluntary hospitals seemed to justify the decision to provide only general practice services under the act. Unlike the German scheme, however, the state contributed to health insurance, along with workers and their employers. Dependants were not initially covered, but the capitation system of payment was taken over from the mutual-aid societies.

We have already seen that contract practice was never popular with medical élites, and the British Medical Association was initially hostile to the 1911 act. It was unable to marshal widespread resistance, however, and doctors actually benefited from the new arrangements because the availability of state funding meant that capitation fees were double the pre-1911 average. An almost incidental clause in the act specified that a penny in each pound should be spent on medical research, whence derived the systematic state support of medical research in Britain, through what became the Medical Research Council (MRC). As in Germany, the scheme was gradually extended to more groups, such as agricultural workers, and remained in force until superseded by the National Health Service Act of 1946.

In the United States, contract practice and insurance schemes developed gradually in the second half of the nineteenth century, and the German experiment was watched with interest by some, and alarm by others. The AMA flirted with such ideas briefly, and national health insurance schemes were debated extensively in the years surrounding World War I. By then, however, the AMA was firmly against any form of legislated health insurance, and the war made it easy to dismiss it as un-American, Germany being the enemy. American social security and her embryonic 'welfare state' were largely products of the world economic crisis of the 1930s.

These varying national experiences point to some general themes. First, health care cannot be separated from other aspects of social life, such as unemployment, industrial accidents, and the dependence of old age. Second, systems of social security were linked historically with industrial life and strife, including trades unionism and other forms of mutualism, to which governments felt ambivalence to the degree to which mutualism had political dimensions. Initially, social security was concerned primarily with industrial workers and only gradually extended to other groups. The extent to which social security has been universalized happened later. Finally, despite notable individual exceptions, the medical profession has collectively resisted rather than led in the field. Doctors' assumption that private fee-for-service practice produces the best care persisted throughout the nineteenth century, and is still powerful today even if higher costs and a more general philosophy of risk spread through private insurance mean that third-party payments are the norm.

THE NATIONAL AND THE INTERNATIONAL

Despite differences in timing, intensity, and response, Western nation-states faced similar fundamental changes during the nineteenth century. The processes of urbanization and industrialization transformed the ways in which people lived and worked. Both industry and commerce became more international, a process given concrete embodiment in the regular series of Great Exhibitions, Expositions Universelles, International Expositions, or World's Fairs, as they were variously called. These monumental international occasions, initiated by the Great Exhibition in London in 1851, were held regularly in major Western cities throughout the century and beyond. They attracted tourists and official delegates in their hundreds of thousands, and, like the modern Olympic Games, inevitably left behind tangible legacies in the host cities. For the Great Exhibition in London, (Sir) Joseph Paxton (1801–65) constructed his daring (and beautiful) Crystal Palace, an enormous edifice of steel and glass, housed in Hyde Park, in the centre of London. There were displays from thirty-four countries of 'arts and manufactures' in the older sense of the phrase, divided into four categories: manufactures, machinery, raw materials, and fine arts. The underlying theme of the Great Exhibition and the subsequent celebrations was material culture, in which science, technology, and invention played prominent roles. The Great Exhibitions were so stunningly successful and profitable that there was keen competition to host them. World's Fairs provided occasions for peoples from many nations to celebrate the marvels of the age, not least the way in which modern transportation made travel by land and by sea so much easier than it had ever been. In the face of regular wars involving Western powers throughout the century, these moments of international cooperation (or friendly competition) were tangible monuments to social and material progress.

That same year, 1851, also witnessed two other international gatherings, these within medicine and its underlying sciences. Between them, they expose both the power and the tensions of the transnational within medicine. The international currency of nineteenth-century medicine was science. As already noted, this notion of science was not confined to the laboratory, but could encompass bedside practice or the statistical investigation of social conditions. It was above all to be based on carefully acquired, public, and objective knowledge. It brought foreign students in their numbers to the Paris Medical School in the first half of the century, and to the German universities in the second half, a process facilitated by those very improvements in travel and communication that made the World's Fairs so successful.

The first of these meetings, held in Paris, was called an International Sanitary Conference, and it was concerned with cholera. If quicker travel made the world seem smaller, the cholera pandemics reminded people that epidemics do not respect national boundaries. Despite historical experiences with bubonic plague, repeated eighteenth-century outbreaks of smallpox, or the New World's encounters with yellow fever, the impact of cholera on nineteenth-century perceptions should not be underestimated. For one thing, the pandemic of the 1820s and early 1830s was anxiously watched as it moved inexorably across Asia and the Middle East into Europe and North America. Cholera was the first disease to force doctors to think globally, and it is no accident that the first world maps depicting disease were produced in the 1830s, and they had cholera as their focus. Its European appearance coincided with the heyday of British anticontagionism, when commercial ideologies of free trade and medical and social evidence favouring miasmatic patterns of epidemic spread pointed in the same direction. Within this framework, quarantine was an outmoded, medieval practice with no real place in the modern world. As the leading international maritime carrier of goods and people, Britain and her merchant navy had the most to lose from the costs and disruption of quarantine. As a relatively small island, she had potentially the most to gain in terms of disease control because foreign imports of disease spread by people or fomites could in theory be controlled at port. Mediterranean ports, including the French and Italian, were long familiar with quarantine regulations and, throughout the century, travellers in the Middle East risked spending time in a lazaretto, should they have been in an area of dangerous epidemics. Lazarettos were looked upon as necessary inconveniences of travel there.

If epidemic disease was spread through the medium of the air, as miasmatists held, quarantine was useless or worse, creating the potential for further disease spread through crowded quarantine conditions. It is a measure of the anxiety that cholera generated, combined with the observed role of port cities in its slow spread from India to Europe, that the British adopted quarantine in the 1830s, despite the general dominance of anticontagionist sentiment. Although cholera first entered the country through a port, Sunderland, on the northeast coast, the later consensus was that quarantine

Table 2.1. *International Sanitary Conferences, 1851–1938*

Number	Venue	Dates	Principal Focus
1	Paris	July 27, 1851–Jan. 19, 1852	Cholera
2	Paris	April 9–Aug. 30, 1859	Cholera
3	Constantinople	Feb. 13–Sept. 26, 1866	Cholera
4	Vienna	July 1–Aug. 1, 1874	Cholera
5	Washington	Jan. 5–Mar. 1, 1881	Cholera, yellow fever
6	Rome	May 20–June 13, 1885	Cholera
7	Venice	5–Jan. 31, 1892	Cholera, plague, yellow fever
8	Dresden	Mar. 11–Apr. 15, 1893	Cholera
9	Paris	Feb. 7–Apr. 3, 1894	Plague
10	Venice	Feb. 16–Mar. 19, 1897	Plague
11	Paris	Oct. 10–Dec. 3, 1903	Plague, cholera, yellow fever, malaria
12	Paris	Nov. 7, 1911–Jan. 17, 1912	Plague, cholera, yellow fever
13	Paris	May 10–June 21, 1926	Plague, cholera, yellow fever
14	Paris	Oct. 28–31, 1938	Plague, cholera, yellow fever, smallpox, typhus

Source: Bynum, W. F. 'Policing Hearts of Darkness: Aspects of the International Sanitary Conferences', *History and Philosophy of the Life Sciences*, 15 (1993), 421–34.

had not been effective during the first cholera epidemic, and Britain slowly developed a marine sanitary procedure for its ports that emphasized inspection and occasional isolation, but not wholesale and routine quarantine.

In this strategy, Britain tended to be at odds with the international community. Systematic modern attempts at international disease control began with that first International Sanitary Congress of 1851. It was the first of fourteen such congresses, ending with another one in Paris, in 1938 (Table 2.1). Initially, despite the 'international' title, these conferences were largely European affairs. At the first conference, only Turkey (actually straddling the Eurasian border) represented the non-European parts of the world, and of the ten other countries that sent delegates, four were independent Italian states (this being before Italian unification). No German state was represented. The United States did not participate until the fifth conference was convened in Washington and a not entirely successful attempt was made to place yellow fever on an equal footing with cholera as a disease requiring international action. Several New World governments sent representatives to the Washington meeting, but the earlier conferences remained fundamentally European in their composition and concern, with the regular addition of delegates from Turkey, Egypt, and British India, and, eventually, the United States and Japan.

In the 1870s, the opening of the Suez Canal introduced another variable in the equation because British India was generally reckoned (although not by the British) to be the universal source of epidemic cholera. Many ships passing through the Canal were *en route* to or from there, and the British and French were the two dominant European influences in Egypt, with the French government holding a much more positive attitude to the sanitary value of quarantine than the British. Even Koch's discovery of the cholera bacillus in 1884 did not resolve the scientific questions for more than a decade; the political ones took even longer. These conferences were after all not simply medical, they were medico-political. In the early meetings a medical man from each country was paired with a diplomat. For our generation, confronted with AIDS and bovine spongiform encephalopathy (BSE), the mix of the medico-scientific and the political is still familiar (Ch. 4).

The sanitary congresses represented the cutting edge of official medical internationalism because the exchange of sanitary conventions by participating countries was the theoretical outcome. Over the years, many of the international superstars of scientific medicine represented their countries: Robert Koch, Max von Pettenkofer, and August Hirsch (1817–94) for Germany; Emile Roux, Leon Calmette (1863–1933), and Adrian Proust (1834–1903) for France; and William Gorgas (1854–1920) for the United States. The British India representative for the 1885 Rome conference, Joseph Fayrer (1824–1907) left an amusing account of the mix of medicine and politics in his autobiography. Fayrer had been asked to act as technical and diplomatic representative, which posed a slight problem as the technical delegates were intended to work apart from their diplomatic colleagues. That his name was omitted from the opening ceremony when attendees' names were read out in alphabetical order of their countries further added to his problems, protocol and etiquette being important elements in offsetting the heat of ensuing disputes. Much of his time was spent discussing cholera: 'The chief subject discussed both morning and afternoon was land quarantine. The English delegates opposed it, and the proposal that it should be abolished was passed unanimously, with the exception of the Turkish delegate . . . . On the 25th [May 1885] the discussion commenced by a proposition . . . that arbitrary time in quarantine of ships is unreliable and useless, and that it does harm by preventing the adoption of more rational measures. The Turks, French, Danes and others opposed it . . . . On the

26th sea quarantine was discussed, and M. Broudardel proposed that sanitary measures were most important in prevention of cholera at ports, and I supported him. On the whole, though vigorous opposition was made to the abolition of quarantine, many, French included, appeared desirous of conciliating and conceding.' At times his exasperation and experience got the better of him. He described the suggestion that the presence of cholera in a port ought to lead to the disinfection before embarkation of 'all the luggage of every passenger who leaves Calcutta, Madras, or Bombay' as 'impracticable'. As for improving conditions on the Red Sea pilgrimages, after some apparently sensible dialogue he described discussion of the idea of onboard baths – 'fancy douching 1000 men in a troopship!' – as 'twaddle' and 'unworthy of the assembly'. With that established, the session was thankfully brought to a close (Fayrer, 1900, pp. 452–6). It wasn't all work however; most evenings he went out seeing the sights with colleagues or attending official receptions and dinners.

The 1885 conference was notable as the first after Koch's announcement of his discovery of the cholera bacillus. Koch was there in an official capacity, but his work did not provide a ground for international agreement. Indeed, it was not even mentioned in the published proceedings of the meeting.

The gradual extension of disease under discussion can be seen from Table 2.1, but no international disease, except plague, generated quite the heated debate that cholera had done in the second half of the century. By the time plague broke out in Mongolia in the 1890s, and spread from India and Hong Kong to many Western countries, including Australia, South Africa, and the United States, cholera was largely confined to its older Asian habitats. Plague's outbreak coincided with the discovery of its mode of transmission, through the rat-flea, and the identification of the causative organism. It led in ways that cholera never had, to a new appreciation of the value (at least psychological) of quarantine: when plague broke out in San Francisco in 1900, Texas instituted quarantine measures against goods and people from California. As Major Greenwood remarked in the 1930s: 'We are all the dupes of words or of their emotional colour. One may easily demonstrate that in India in 1918 influenza destroyed in a few weeks far more lives than plague consumed in as many years, but the word 'influenza' is emotionally colourless, while to all of us the mere name of that sickness which, scorning any adjectival qualification, is so emphatically *the* plague, brings a faint thrill' (Greenwood, 1935, p. 289).

Towards the end of the century, after ten sanitary congresses (one of them, the third, lasting more than seven months), modest progress was made. Even the British began reluctantly to sign international sanitary conventions. On other fronts, international humanitarianism was established. Henri Dunant (1828–1910) founded the International Red Cross in 1863, after observing atrocities at the Battle of Solferino, and the first Geneva Convention, dealing with the neutrality of those caring for the wounded in war, was signed by twelve nations in the following year. At the same time, developments in weaponry could make modern warfare even more brutal. These official and humanitarian manifestations of internationalism were paralleled by the social and intellectual fare offered by the second series of international clinical and scientific congresses that were held with increasing regularity from the 1850s (Table 2.2). This international movement began gingerly, with an international statistical congress, also in 1851, more about demography and reporting disease than mathematical statistics. Some of the early congresses were small affairs, with only a few delegates from outside the host country. Paris and Brussels vied with each other for the honour of hosting the greater number of the inaugural meetings, in which French was still the official language, and in many instances a first gathering led to a cycle, with a four-year interval as the norm. The general medical congresses that began in Paris in 1867 became particularly grand occasions, the seventh, held in London in 1881, attracted more than 3,000 participants from seventy countries ('every land in which scientific medicine is practised'). Most of the international giants of medicine and medical science were there: Virchow, Pasteur, Koch, Kölliker, Charcot, in addition to Lister, Simon, and the other British luminaries. At every congress, even ones in clinical subjects, 'science' was top of the agenda, and the increasing specialization within both clinical and scientific disciplines can be seen from the growing list of topics covered, including: hygiene (from 1852), ophthalmology (1857), otology (1876), TB (1888), dermatology (1889), physiology (1889), psychology (1890), gynaecology and obstetrics (1892), cancer (1906), and tropical medicine (1910).

Sharing knowledge was furthered by frequent translations of books and papers into other languages, a process catalysed by expanding markets for medical books and journals, and rendered more useful by the disappearance of Latin as the *lingua franca* of scholarship. Medical dictionaries helped to standardize word meanings; significantly, the great *National Medical Dictionary* (1890), edited by John Shaw Billings (1838–1913) in the United States, included French, German, Italian, and Latin terms alongside English ones. The *Index Medicus* (1879) was also Billings's brainchild. Attempts were made to agree on international disease classifications and

Table 2.2. *International Medical Congresses, 1851–1912*

Subject	Year of First Meeting	Host City
Sanitation	1851	Paris
Statistics	1851	Brussels
Hygiene and demography	1852	Brussels
Ophthalmology	1857	Brussels
Veterinary medicine	1863	Hamburg
Anthropology	1865	Spezia
Pharmacy	1865	Brunswick
Medicine	1867	Paris
Otology	1876	New York
Laryngology	1880	Milan
Criminal anthropology	1885	Rome
Tuberculosis	1888	Paris
Dermatology	1889	Paris
Physiology	1889	Basel
Psychology	1890	Paris
Gynaecology and obstetrics	1892	Brussels
Alcoholism	1894	Brussels
Leprosy	1897	Berlin
Dentistry	1900	Paris
Surgery	1902	Brussels
Care of the insane	1902	Antwerp
Unification of heroic remedies	1902	Brussels
Milk	1903	Brussels
Habitations	1904	Paris
School hygiene	1904	Nuremberg
Physiotherapy	1905	Liège
Cancer	1906	Hiedelberg
Pellagra	1906	Turin
Occupational diseases	1906	Milan
Sleeping sickness	1907	London
Epilepsy	1909	Budapest
Tropical medicine	1910	Manila
Comparative pathology	1912	Paris
Eugenics	1912	London

Source: Garrison, F. H. An Introduction to the History of Medicine, 4th ed., Philadelphia: Saunders, 1929, p. 789.

the growth of biologicals – vaccines and antisera – created urgent issues of standardization. Microbiological and entomological taxonomy acquired new significance as germ theory developed and new disease vectors were discovered with regularity.

Competing with the scientific spirit of internationalism was the competitiveness engendered by flagrant nationalism in this period of imperial expansion. As Germany and the United States began to overtake the British in industrial output, and the scramble for Africa gathered momentum, national pride or anxiety could heighten both personal and collective tensions. The well-known antipathy between Pasteur and Koch was not simply the idiosyncratic manifestation of two strong personalities creating a new and powerful discipline, but also the mutual distrust of a Frenchman and a German. The impressive achievements of what came to be called 'tropical medicine' (see below) offered new possibilities to nations seeking to make tropical countries safe for the white races. The implication of the mosquito in the transmission of both malaria and yellow fever, just at the century's close, was especially exciting, but pitted Ronald Ross (1857–1932) from England and India against Giovanni Grassi (1854–1925) from Italy, in their battle for malarial kudos. The Spanish liked to remind the Americans that Carlos Finlay had argued for the mosquito transmission of yellow fever before Walter Reed and his compatriots went to Havana. The Nobel Prizes, instituted in 1901, were cosmopolitan in their recipients, but sometimes exacerbated personal and nationalistic rumblings among those not chosen. Before the awards were suspended during World War I, sixteen individuals were awarded Nobel Prizes in medicine or physiology. Not surprisingly, five were German, three were French, and two were Russian, with a single individual each from Britain, Italy, Spain, Sweden, and the Faeroe Islands. The recipients, clinicians and scientists, can be roughly divided in half (the proportion of scientists today would be much higher). Pointing towards the movement we associate with biomedical scientists today, one of the Frenchmen (Alexis Carrel) worked in the United States and one of the Russians (Elie Metchnikoff) in France.

Few of these discontents seriously disturbed the widespread perception that science was both progressive and international, and it was in the assimilation of its methods and results that the practice of medicine would become so. The speed with which news of Pasteur's rabies vaccine, Koch's tuberculin, von Behring's antidiphtheria toxoid, and Röntgen's X-rays spread to both profession and public, testified to the achievements of the age, in science, medicine, and communication.

Doctors and the state

By the end of the nineteenth century, the institutions and practitioners of medicine were much more closely intertwined with nation-states than they had been a half century previously. We have already seen several examples: in the provision of medical services for the poor, in contractual forms of payment, in the regulation of medical licensing and qualifications, the surveillance of medical schools, compulsory smallpox vaccination, the notification of infectious diseases, and the policing of international diseases, especially cholera. A large number of doctors received part or all of their incomes from public funds, including practitioners participating in national health insurance schemes, Medical Officers of Health, public analysts, and, on the Continent, many medical academics. At one level, these changes can be grouped as part of the growth of modern bureaucracy, of which individuals today regularly complain. They also enjoy many of its benefits. None of these incursions of the state into the medical marketplace happened accidentally. Someone or some group had to identify a problem, campaign for its solution, and ensure that the necessary legislation was enacted. Then, as now, no legislation was universally acclaimed. Proprietors of medical schools that folded in the wake of American reforms as advocated by Flexner lost their livelihoods. The provision of clean water had to be paid for. Many doctors opposed any form of contractual medical care, or its regulation by statute. Further, despite all these changes, fee-for-service medical provision still governed the lives of most doctors and their patients.

There were three other major areas of interaction between doctors and the state that need brief mention. All of them were in place before the Great War, and their effects continued long afterwards. The first was the medical policing of national borders. While this was the more local dimension of some of the issues that had been thrashed out in the International Sanitary Conferences, it went further. It was most obvious in countries with well-defined barriers, especially the sea. In Britain, it involved the development of a Port Health Authority medical service, with routine inspection of goods and people coming from infected or simply 'dangerous' areas. The fact that Britain escaped the later cholera pandemics was cited as evidence that the British system of vigilant inspection worked, and that wholesale quarantine was unnecessary, but the British officials were also on the lookout for smallpox, typhus, and other communicable human diseases, in addition to contagious diseases of farm animals. In the wake of Pasteur's rabies vaccine, that disease was also scrutinized, and isolation of dogs and other carriers

229

of the virus became the preferred method of prevention. Rabies was more difficult to control in countries with land borders, but systematic maritime inspection developed in other major European ports, including Hamburg, Antwerp, and Marseilles.

It was in the United States that this move had the most visible impact. The late nineteenth-century pogroms in Eastern Europe, continuing deprivation in Ireland and mass immigration from Italy encouraged millions of the tired and the poor to try their fortunes in the New World. These immigrants went to the East Coast of the United States, hoping that the pious words on the Statue of Liberty were literal. On the West Coast, similar waves from Asia, especially China, hoped to build better lives in America. In the middle decades of the century, American immigration policy had been fairly lax. After all, it was a country of immigrants (even then Native Americans did not count for much). With the rise of hard-line racial thinking from the 1840s, the development of a culture of 'native' (European-origin) Americans, and the growth of American cities, with ghettoes and the health problems of urban life, attitudes changed. One way of policing the border was through medical inspection, and millions of immigrants, many of them speaking no English, were subjected to medical inspection on Ellis Island in New York, and other major ports. Tuberculosis, VD, and typhus were the principal diseases looked for, but other conditions could also result in quarantine or a refusal of admission. A more stringent quota system was eventually put into place, whereby the immigrant influx was not supposed to alter the existing racial balance of the United States, but before the Great War, doctors were the chief gatekeepers. From this service, much of the modern public health infrastructure developed in the decades leading up to the Great War.

A second area in which doctors interacted with the state was that of employment and workmen's compensation. With the development of heavy industry – ship building, iron and steel manufacturing, mining, and railways – and the concomitant trades unions movement, the question of who was responsible for industrial accidents and diseases loomed large. If a man and his family were pauperized because he had an accident through no fault of his own, or had pulmonary disease after long hours in mining or other dusty trades, it seemed irrational to support him out of general taxes, especially if the employer had been lax in effecting safety regulations. These were delicate matters, of course, especially in an atmosphere of *laissez faire*, and the negotiation of workplace safety standards and compensation was a long and protracted affair, differing widely in different industries and different countries. Inevitably, doctors were involved in assessing the extent of the injury or disease, judging its likely cause, and in providing (in many industries) basic medical care for employees. Protecting children in the workplace had been one of the earliest issues of British social concern, and factory surgeons among the earliest to quantify the extent of injury, disease, and death acquired in the line of work. Railway accidents were an early cause of especial concern, and compensation for both injured workers and passengers was championed by Thomas Wakley (1795–1862), the crusading founder of the influential weekly medical journal, the *Lancet* (1823; Ch. 1). That he was also a coroner gave him ample experience in adjudicating in industrial fatalities.

The laws and social conventions developed only gradually, but by the 1880s, workmen's compensation legislation began to be passed, and the British model was eventually adopted in the United States. In these and other European countries, the examining doctor was juxtaposed between the victim, employer and the state. As in many instances of nineteenth-century medical and social legislation, the structures and procedures seem naïve by contemporary standards, but they do represent another area in which medical knowledge was pressed into the service of the state.

A third major arena in which the state was vitally concerned was in the twin structures of the armed forces and tropical medicine. These were related not simply because many nineteenth-century wars were fought in tropical areas of the world, but also because military and civilian practice in these areas was closely intertwined. The relationship between tropical medicine and the military was most striking in the British case, but as European imperialism gathered momentum from the middle decades of the century, German, French, Belgian, and Portuguese governments established permanent colonies in Africa and Asia. The Dutch had long had interests in Southeast Asia, and Spanish involvement in South America continued even after many South American nations achieved independence. The Americans arrived on the imperial scene slightly later, wresting territory from Spain in Cuba, Puerto Rico, and the Philippines after the Spanish-American War (1898).

Careers in military medicine never had much prestige after the Napoleonic Wars, but many doctors on the Continent had routine military experience early in their careers. In Germany, the Friedrich-Wilhelms Institut in Berlin offered free medical education to young boys, in return for military service afterwards. Virchow and Helmholtz were among its many outstanding products. In Paris, the Val-de-Grâce, France's premiere military medical school, enjoyed resources and good students throughout the century. Osborne's work has been instrumental in analysing the careers and achievements of French military doctors (Osborne, 1994). In Britain, doctors had enjoyed lower status than ordinary officers, and while many Scottish and Irish graduates of Edinburgh saw the military as an opportunity for experience and employment early in their careers, the Army Medical Department suffered from chronic underfunding and low morale. The medical services during the Crimean War (1854–6) came under heavy criticism, both in the wake of Florence Nightingale's exploits and the serious logistical difficulties that had been encountered. Getting medical supplies and personnel to where they were needed had proved almost impossible to achieve. Britain had traditionally relied on a volunteer army, and many of the medical officers who went to the Crimea had volunteered out of patriotism, a sense of adventure, or because they had nothing better to do. Typhus and cholera proved to be the most serious medical problems, and the French army also suffered from scurvy. Deaths from disease were about five times those from enemy fire, a reasonable improvement over the figures from the Napoleonic period, but unacceptable for a public that, for the first time, could read about the campaigns in the newspapers the day after they happened, thanks to the telegraph and the presence of journalists.

Following Parliamentary enquiries, the old Army Medical Department was given a formal military status (it had been a civilian department of government), under the War Office, and an Army Medical School was opened at Chatham. It subsequently (1863) moved to larger quarters at Netley, where recruits for the Army Medical Corps (it received a Royal charter in 1898, becoming the Royal Army Medical Corps, RAMC) went for special training before being posted to their stations. Independent from the RAMC, and more prestigious than it, the Indian Medical Service (IMS) was the medical department of the Indian Army, in addition to being responsible for providing doctors for the large European population in India. IMS officers also treated wealthy Indians, a pattern common in imperial domains throughout the world. IMS recruits also underwent training at Netley, where Edmund Parkes (1819–76) and (Sir) William Aitken (1825–92) were prominent among a largely distinguished faculty. Parkes' *Manual of Practical Hygiene* (1864) drew on his experience in India and the Crimea; it was adapted to the needs of army medical personnel and went through multiple editions and translations. Aitkens' *Science and the Practice of Medicine* (1857) remained in print as a popular textbook until the 1890s. It too, had extensive coverage of the exotic diseases encountered in tropical climates, in addition to sensitive speculations about the geography of human diseases and the role of the environment in their causation.

The environment had traditionally played a central role in explaining the differing disease pools in temperate and tropical climates. Individuals bound for India, Southeast Asia, Africa, or the West Indies would have known that they faced the risk of serious illness or death. Central Africa had been particularly difficult for Europeans to operate in, one reason why in the 1870s, so much of it (and its vast natural resources) remained up for grabs. Curtin has found that, from the 1840s, some diminution of mortality among British troops can be found (less among the French). He attributes this to the increasing use of prophylactic quinine, and better discipline and camp hygiene. Even so, mortality rates remained staggeringly high; coming down with malaria (see below) was distressingly routine, and yellow fever, amoebic dysentery, and a variety of other fevers, made survival there for more than a year or two a less than fifty-fifty proposition. The environment, with its lush vegetation, high temperatures, aggressive vermin, swamps, oppressive humidity, and rotting organic matter, was sufficiently uncomfortable that it seemed rational to attribute disease and death to the cumulative effects of the environment. That those who survived often gradually became more resistant to the spectrum of disease was explained by 'seasoning': acclimatization of the same kind that plants and other animals could achieve. A number of societies from the 1830s more systematically sought to investigate the mechanisms, causes, and limits of acclimatization, a topic with vast economic implications, to say nothing of vital importance, for the future of permanent European conquest of the darkest parts of the Dark Continent.

Tropical medicine was thus of vital importance to imperial or would-be imperial governments. Quinine has been named by one historian as a 'tool of empire', along with the telegraph, breech loading rifles, and (especially in India) the railroad. Both the explorer and missionary David Livingstone (1813–73) and the Welsh-born American explorer and adventurer, (Sir) Henry Morton Stanley (1841–1904) who 'found' Livingstone in Africa ('Dr. Livingstone, I presume?'), placed great store in quinine (Fig. 2.10). Monographs on the 'diseases of hot climates' never fail to recommend it, though there was much debate on dosage, frequency, length of the course, and on whether it could be reserved as a curative, rather than taken regularly as a prophylactic. It had originally come from the cinchona tree, native to Peru and other parts of South America (hence, one of its early names, Peruvian Bark). South America was still the major source until the

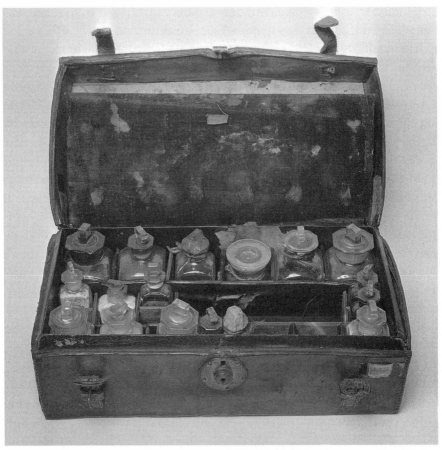

Fig. 2.10. David Livingstone's medicine chest. After losing a similar chest on his last expedition, he wrote: 'I had a fit of insensibility, which shows the power of fever without medicine.' *Source*: Wellcome Historical Medical Museum. *Credit*: Wellcome Library, London (L0007376).

middle of the nineteenth century, when the Dutch managed to establish plantations in Java. The British planted some cinchona trees in India, as well, but Indian production never was adequate even for Indian needs.

The transition from 'diseases of hot climates' to *Tropical Medicine*, (the title of Sir Patrick Manson's [1844–1922] classic 1898 textbook), took place through the 1890s, and involved two principal conceptual shifts. First, not the inorganic features of an oppressive climate, but living organisms, were implicated in the causation of many tropical diseases: malaria, schistosomiasis, filariasis, sleeping sickness (trypanosomiasis), amoebiasis, and many others, were shown to be parasitical disorders, caused not by bacteria but by other kinds or organisms, especially protozoa and worms. In the preface to

234

Tropical Diseases, Manson distinguished what he called the traditional 'cosmopolitan' diseases caused by bacteria, such as the bacilli of TB, typhoid, or cholera, and the parasitical diseases of the tropics. Bacterial diseases were ubiquitous in their potential: cholera, plague, or leprosy, another bacterial disorder with a strong tropical presence, could occur anywhere, but had largely disappeared, in the wake of 'civilization' and 'the improved hygiene that has followed in its train'. In contrast, many of tropical diseases had strict geographical distributions. That they were also caused by different classes of organisms was no accident.

The second feature that set off many tropical diseases from the 'cosmopolitan' infectious diseases was their more complicated chains of spread. In particular, they often had complicated life cycles requiring an intermediate host. Manson had done pioneering work in China in 1877 on the role of the mosquito in the spread of filariasis, known familiarly as elephantiasis, from patients' vastly swollen legs due to lymphatic obstruction. He showed that the causative parasite (a nematode) could be transmitted from a patient to a mosquito, through its bite. Believing that female mosquitoes bite only once before they lay their eggs and die, he postulated that the mosquito's eggs become infected with the parasite, which is then transmitted back into human beings who drink the water.

A fuller account of the relationship of the mosquito to the worm's life cycle was not worked out until the 1890s, by which time various other insect vectors – ticks, flies, and fleas – were being implicated in the spread of a variety of diseases. Both the complex life cycles and the insect vectors helped demarcate tropical medicine from old world bacteriology, and medical entomology and parasitology became important fields in their own right. At this highpoint of imperial competition, Manson, an intense British patriot, believed that the discipline had much to offer Queen Victoria's government. His hand was strengthened by the work of his protégé, Ronald Ross, in India.

Ross was Anglo-Indian, that is, born in India to British parents and raised there until his school days. His father was an officer in the Indian Army, and although the younger Ross was always interested in literature, art, and mathematics, his career in medicine was decided by his father. An undistinguished medical student, he failed his examinations the first time around, but finally managed to qualify in medicine and to get an ordinary posting in the IMS to the Madras Presidency (those to Bengal were the most prestigious). He spent a dozen desultory years in India, mostly doing what colonials of all occupations did: amusing himself with the local offerings, in the case of southern India, shooting, fishing, golf, and tennis. He also learned mathematics, which was useful in some of his later epidemiological work. His real inspiration came during his second furlough to London, when he met Manson, who showed him how to observe the malaria parasite in blood smears, first identified in 1880 by the French colonial army doctor, Charles Laveran (1845–1922). Manson was convinced that malaria was spread by mosquitoes, although he still held that females bite only once. Ross returned to India, with a pocket microscope he had designed, determined to prove Manson's 'grand induction'. It took him almost three years of dogged and frustrating work, as the IMS had little appreciation of his researches, and the biological and clinical problems that confronted him were formidable. The breakthrough came on August 20, 1897, when he observed some dark pigment in the stomach of a mosquito he had just dissected (he had dissected hundreds before). He recognized it as the elusive malaria parasite, and between then and late 1898, he worked out a life cycle of the parasite in mosquitoes, using birds as his animal model. By the time he left India in February 1899, Europe knew of his work, through Manson's careful publicity. Within two years, the mosquito had been implicated in the spread of yellow fever, by Walter Reed (1851–1902), an American army medical officer, and his colleagues in Havana.

The impact of these two discoveries on the visibility and funding of tropical medicine was huge. *Mosquito or Man?* was the title of a survey of progress in tropical medicine published by Sir Rubert Boyce in 1909. The book's subtitle is significant: *The Conquest of the Tropical World*. Malaria and yellow fever were the two very diseases prevalent in hot climates that affected Europeans the most, and they could be controlled, so it seemed, by simply getting rid of the appropriate mosquitoes, relevant species of Anopheles for malaria, *Aedes* ae*gypti* for yellow fever. The tropics could be made safe for Europeans, literally conquered through tropical medicine and its attendant sciences.

There were some early successes in controlling each of these diseases. William Gorgas made Havana much healthier, and local antimalarial campaigns in Egypt and Malaysia were encouraging. Ross spent the rest of his life arguing that, with adequate resources, the problem could be solved everywhere. The successful building of the Panama Canal beginning in 1904, after a disastrous French attempt two decades previously, was further vindication (Fig. 2.11). The French had been defeated by the very two diseases, malaria and yellow fever, that now seemed tamed or, at least, tameable.

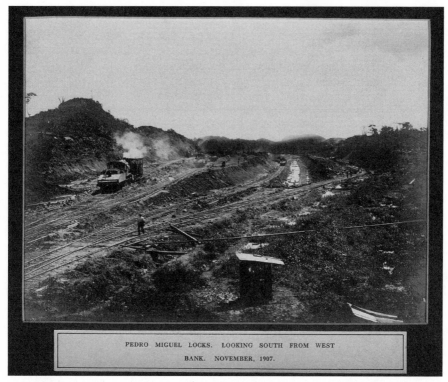

PEDRO MIGUEL LOCKS. LOOKING SOUTH FROM WEST BANK. NOVEMBER, 1907.

Fig. 2.11. Constructing the Pedro Miguel locks, Panama Canal, 1907. Mosquito control and the use of nets and screens helped keep workers nearly free from malaria and yellow fever. *Source*: Photograph, Wellcome Library Iconographic Collection. *Credit*: Wellcome Library, London (V0030214).

Despite the early optimism, the diseases proved more formidable than the isolated successes suggested. Resources were always in short supply, and the mosquito proved remarkably resilient to human effort, even with cheap coolie labour available. An early systematic experiment at a military cantonment at Mian Mir, in India (now in Pakistan) carried out between 1901 and 1904 yielded important results, but all of them depressing. The malaria campaign there was sponsored by the Royal Society and had been sanctioned by Ross, although it was later bitterly attacked by him as being badly planned, shoddily executed, and stopped too soon. In fact, it was planned in addition to contemporary knowledge allowed, and failed for reasons that are easy to understand in hindsight. It showed that mosquitoes have longer flight paths than had been assumed (so larger areas must be cleared for control to be achieved), that monsoon rains quickly renewed mosquito breeding sites, that crop irrigation, necessary for economic prosperity, was

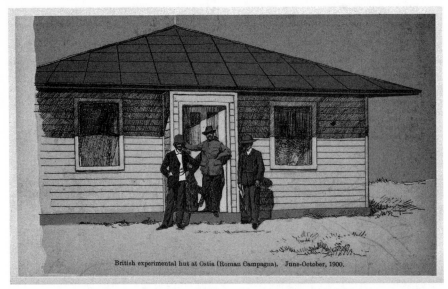

British experimental hut at Ostia (Roman Campagna). June-October, 1900.

Fig. 2.12. Researchers outside the British experimental hut near Ostia, Italy, to verify the mosquito-malaria theory, June–October 1900. *Source*: Photoprint with watercolour by Amedeo John Engel Terzi. Wellcome Library Iconographic Collection. *Credit*: Wellcome Library, London (V0022613).

a constant source of breeding sites, and that one could not protect the military without also paying attention to the large number of camp followers as well (wives and children of the Indian soldiers).

Mian Mir and other early experiences with mosquito control in India convinced the medical officers in the IMS that the older tried and trusted remedy of prophylactic quinine represented the most effective use of scarce resources. In Italy, also with malarious areas, free quinine, combined with what the Italians called 'bonification', that is, drainage and reclamation of swampy land, worked, but Italy had financial resources that were not readily available in British India (Fig. 2.12). These and related issues continued to permeate debates about malaria eradication throughout the early decades of the twentieth century. The only thing that all parties agreed on was that it was a difficult disease to eradicate, or even control, in many parts of the world.

Malaria continues to be a major scourge in the modern world. In the short term, however, it encouraged Western governments to invest in tropical medicine. Manson convinced the Colonial Secretary, Joseph Chamberlain (1836–1914) to release government funds to help establish the London School of Tropical Medicine (1899), just after Liverpool had stolen the march on London and established a school of tropical medicine of its own. Before the outbreak of World War I, there were schools of tropical medicine in Germany, France, Belgium, the Netherlands, and the United States, in addition to research stations in India, Indochina (now Viet Nam), the Sudan, and Malaysia. They represented tangible monuments to the power of medicine and medical research, in the scramble for imperial power and wealth. Knowledge of the aetiologies and pathology of many of the exotic tropical diseases was dramatically increased before the outbreak of the Great War. It was mostly fought on familiar terrain, the mud of Flanders and elsewhere, but when the combatants ventured further afield, as in the Dardanelles or Mesopotamia, the continuing power of the diseases of hot climates still prevailed.

Chronological table for chapter 3: 1914–1945

Year	Medical and scientific events	Contemporary events	Nobel prize in physiology or medicine
1914	Alexis Carrel performs first successful heart surgery on a dog; Henry Dale describes neurotransmitter acetylcholine in ergot	Outbreak of First World War; Opening of Panama Canal	Robert Bárány 'for his work on the physiology and pathology of the vestibular apparatus'
1915	Alexis Carrel and Henry Dakin describe irrigation treatment of gunshot wounds	Gallipoli Landings	Money allocated to the Special Fund
1916	Walter Gaskell names the involuntary nervous system; Margaret Sanger founds the first American birth-control clinic in Brooklyn; Marie Stopes's *Married Love*	Battle of the Somme; Einstein's *General Theory of Relativity*	Money allocated to the Special Fund
1917	Carl Jung's *Psychology of the Unconscious*	Russian Revolution; United States enters War	Money allocated to the Special Fund
1918	Start of influenza Pandemic	End of World War I	Money allocated to the Special Fund
1919	British Ministry of Health established	Treaty of Versailles signed; Ernest Rutherford splits the atom	Jules Bordet 'for his discoveries relating to immunity'
1920	Establishment of Tavistock Clinic, first U.K. centre for teaching and deployment of Freud's psychoanalytical ideas	League of Nations founded; regular American radio broadcasting established	August Krogh 'for his discovery of the capillary motor regulating mechanism'

Year	Medical and scientific events	Contemporary events	Nobel prize in physiology or medicine
1921	E. G. Banting and C. H. Best isolate insulin; Marie Stopes opens first birth-control clinic in the United Kingdom	Treaty agreed for formation of Irish Free State	Money allocated to the Special Fund
1922	State Institute for Racial Biology founded at Uppsala	USSR established; Benito Mussolini takes power in Italy; T. S. Eliot's *The Waste Land*	Archibald V. Hill 'for his discovery relating to the production of heat in the muscle'; Otto Meyerhof 'for his discovery of the fixed relationship between the consumption of oxygen and the metabolism of lactic acid in the muscle'
1923	Albert Calmette and Camille Guerin develop the Bacille Calmette Guérin (BCG) vaccine for tuberculosis	Turkish republic formed—end of Ottoman Empire	Frederick G. Banting, John Macleod 'for the discovery of insulin'
1924	International Society of Medical Officers of Health organized in Geneva.	Hitler's *Mein Kampf*	Willem Einthoven 'for his discovery of the mechanism of the electrocardiogram'
1925	Sir Ronald Ross opens British Mosquito Control Institute at Hayling Island	Term *Art Deco* derived from International Art Exhibition, Paris	Money allocated to the Special Fund
1926	First enzyme (urease) crystallized by American biochemist James B. Sumner; G. Richards, and W. P. Murphy use liver in the diet to treat anaemia	General Strike in Great Britain	Johannes Fibiger 'for his discovery of the Spiroptera carcinoma'
1927	Philip Drinker and Louis Shaw develop the 'iron lung'	Charles Lindbergh pilots *The Spirit of St. Louis* solo across the Atlantic	Julius Wagner-Jauregg 'for his discovery of the therapeutic value of malaria inoculation in the treatment of dementia paralytica'

Year	Medical and scientific events	Contemporary events	Nobel prize in physiology or medicine
1928	Alexander Fleming discovers penicillin in a mould; Albert Szent-Gyorgyi isolates vitamin C; G. Papanicolau develops Pap test to diagnose uterine cancers	Stalin's first Five Year Plan	Charles Nicolle 'for his work on typhus'
1929	Henry Dale and H. W. Dudley demonstrate chemical transmission of nerve impulses; Werner Forssmann develops cardiac catheter; M. J. Sakel introduces insulin shock to treat schizophrenia; Hans Berger develops the electroencephalogram	Wall Street Crash; start of Great Slump	Christiaan Eijkman 'for his discovery of the antineuritic vitamin'; Sir Frederick Hopkins 'for his discovery of the growth-stimulating vitamins'
1930	Hans Zinsser develops immunisation against typhus	The planet Pluto discovered	Karl Landsteiner 'for his description of human blood groups'
1931	Androsterone isolated in crystalline form in Germany (synthesized three years late)	Japanese invade Manchuria; Oswald Mosley founds 'New Party' in Britain	Otto Warburg 'for his discovery of the nature and mode of action of the respiratory enzyme'
1932	Armand Quick introduces a test to measure the clotting ability of blood; Gerhard Domagk describes the first sulpha drug, Prontosil	F. D. Roosevelt promises 'New Deal' in United States	Sir Charles Sherrington, Edgar Adrian 'for their discoveries regarding the functions of neurons'
1933	W. S. Feldberg and J. H. Gaddum demonstrate acetylcholine is so-called vagus stuff	Adolf Hitler appointed Chancellor of Germany	Thomas H. Morgan 'for his discoveries concerning the role played by the chromosome in heredity'
1934	Chemical structure of vitamin B1 (isolated from yeast in 1932) worked out; ascorbic acid synthesized	Beginning of Long March under Mao Zedong in China	George H. Whipple, George R. Minot, William P. Murphy 'for their discoveries concerning liver therapy in cases of anaemia'

Year	Medical and scientific events	Contemporary events	Nobel prize in physiology or medicine
1935	Development of prefrontal lobotomy to treat mental illness; first blood bank set up in the United States at the Mayo Clinic, Rochester	Italy invades Ethiopia	Hans Spemann 'for his discovery of the organizer effect in embryonic development'
1936	Ugo Cerletti describes electro-convulsive therapy	Beginning of Spanish Civil War	Sir Henry Dale, Otto Loewi 'for their discoveries relating to chemical transmission of nerve impulses'
1937	Development of vaccine against yellow fever by Max Theiler and of first antihistamine by Daniel Bovet; Charles Dodds describes a synthetic oestrogen (stilboestrol)	Sino-Japanese War begins	Albert Szent-Györgyi 'for his discoveries in connection with the biological combustion processes, with special reference to vitamin C and the catalysis of fumaric acid'
1938	New Zealand Social Security Act provides pioneering state medical service; John Wiles develops the first total artificial hip replacement, using stainless steel	Austria incorporated into Reich	Corneille Heymans 'for the discovery of the role played by the sinus and aortic mechanisms in the regulation of respiration'
1939	Vitamin K isolated and synthesized	Outbreak of World War II; end of Spanish Civil War; release of *Gone with the Wind* and *The Wizard of Oz*	Gerhard Domagk 'for the discovery of the antibacterial effects of prontosil'
1940	Howard Florey and Ernst Chain develop penicillin as an antibiotic; Karl Landsteiner describes the Rhesus factor in blood	Scandinavian and Netherlandish countries fall to Nazis; The Blitz	Money allocated to the Main Fund and Special Fund
1941	Norman Gregg links rubella in pregnancy with cataract and other abnormalities in children; Selman Waksman coins the term 'antibiotic'	Hitler attacks Soviet Union; Japanese attack on Pearl Harbor	Money allocated to the Main Fund and Special Fund

Year	Medical and scientific events	Contemporary events	Nobel prize in physiology or medicine
1942	World Health Organization (WHO) set up as an agency of the United Nations; Report by William Beveridge paves the way for the establishment of a National Health Service in Britain	Nazi death camps erected in occupied territories	Money allocated to the Main Fund and Special Fund
1943	Willem Kolff develops first kidney dialysis machine; Selman Waksman describes the antibiotic streptomycin	Soviets retake Stalingrad and defeat Nazis at Battle of Kursk	Henrik Dam 'for his discovery of vitamin K'; Edward A Doisy 'for his discovery of the chemical nature of vitamin K'
1944	Alfred Blalock performs first blue-baby operation	D-Day June 6	Joseph Erlanger, Herbert S. Gasser 'for their discoveries relating to the highly differentiated functions of single nerve fibres'
1945	Liverpool School of Tropical Medicine conducts first clinical tests of Paludrine against malaria	End of World War II; United States drops atomic bombs on Hiroshima and Nagasaki	Alexander Fleming, Ernst Chain, and Howard Florey 'for the discovery of penicillin'

3　Continuity in crisis: medicine, 1914–1945

CHRISTOPHER LAWRENCE

Overview

At the turn of the eighteenth and nineteenth centuries (see Ch. 1), a medical revolution took place during two cataclysmic social upheavals: the Industrial Revolution, and the French Revolution and its aftermath. By contrast, for medicine in the West, the period beginning in 1914 and ending in 1945 might be summarized as one of stability, consolidation, and growth. There is an apparent paradox in this. The fifty years prior to the Great War (see Ch. 2) saw what many considered a second medical revolution (mainly based on the growth of basic science) accompanying monumental and rapid change in many other areas of life. Yet this revolution occurred during a period of relative social stability, certainly in Europe and to a lesser extent, America. The period 1914–45 on the other hand saw violence and social unrest more profound than anything since the early modern period. It saw two world wars and two interwar decades unanimously, then as now, designated as years of crisis. Medicine participated in the crises of these years, indeed in some areas, for better or for worse, it shaped them and was at the forefront of addressing them. Nonetheless, the medical institutions created and the ideas and assumptions established before 1914, largely remained intact in this period and were built on rather than being jettisoned or radically modified.

In the interwar years, orthodox medicine consolidated its authority in all areas: the home, the hospital, local and central government, the community, and industry. Universities and their associated hospitals were increasingly made into the seats of medical education and the sites where standards of care were set. Hospitals grew in size and number and their business-like management increased. Specialization continued apace. Technologies used in diagnosis and treatment grew in variety and size, and abounded. Surgery flourished although it saw no radical innovations of the sort that characterized the periods before and after the two wars when brain and heart surgery, respectively, were introduced. Laboratories became increasingly important as centres for diagnosis and seats of research. Funding for clinical medicine and for research increased markedly. Money came from industry, government, and philanthropic agencies (especially the latter). In 1913, the Rockefeller Foundation was established. The foundation had a huge effect on medicine in this period. Medical manufacturing industries, especially the pharmaceutical industry, expanded rapidly. Drug companies became larger and introduced new forms of organization, management, and marketing. All these various sorts of change were often seen as evidence of 'modernization' or 'modernism' and their vital force, whether deemed spiritual or commercial, was usually found to lie in America. These changes were approved of by many. Some regarded them with dismay. In this respect, medicine was no different from any other cultural phenomenon of the time.

In the industrial nations, the health and efficiency of workmen and the armed forces remained priorities. On the public health front, provision for welfare was expanded and established in new areas. How much all this did for the sick and the well in industrial societies is hard to judge. People in many places were living lengthier and healthier lives for sure, but how much this owed to medicine as opposed to diet, better living conditions, and shorter working hours is a subject of much debate. For the sick too, except in a few clear-cut cases (notably the insulin treatment of diabetes), it is hard to judge how much better treatment was in, say, 1930 than 1910. Also during these years, the goal of international cooperation was lauded if not always attained.

This monochrome picture of sustained growth fails to capture the upheavals in medicine that were part of broader social cataclysms, of which war, the establishment of the Soviet State and the rise of fascism are the most obvious examples. For convenience, these will be dealt with separately although not necessarily because they did not partake of a common thread. For the most part, a single story can be told about this period, but one that had huge national variants. For simplicity, too, a separate section on internationalism will include accounts of colonies and also independent countries into which Western medicine was imported, but that had autonomous non-Western cultures. China is the obvious example. Again, however, the connections with the main theme will be made.

HEALTH AND DISEASE

One thing that did change in the interwar years and that affected the nature of medical practice in much of the Western world was the pattern of disease, particularly epidemic disease. The picture was, however, largely one of a continuation of trends that had been established before 1914. Practitioners of Western medicine in many parts of the world between 1914–45 expected to encounter exotic infectious killers such as plague, yellow fever, and malaria. In much of Europe and North America, however, the incidence of many acute infectious diseases caused by microorganisms was declining. The death rates in nearly all the common ones fell strikingly. Around 1900 a doctor in a Western city might well see cases of tetanus, typhoid, and rabies even. In some places, notably Russia, typhus or cholera still occurred. Physicians in the United States might discover smallpox among unvaccinated immigrants. Those in the southern states might see cases of hookworm and malaria. But between the wars a doctor practising in London, Vienna, Sydney, or New York would be extremely unlikely to see anything so exotic. A practitioner would see a large number of patients with infectious disease, especially children – notably cases of diphtheria, whooping cough, measles, rheumatic fever, and scarlet fever – but would be most struck (unless he or she was particularly incompetent or unlucky) by the decreasing number of deaths in these cases. The prewar fall in mortality in these conditions continued uninterrupted (including during the wars). Morbidity fell too, particularly after the 1930s. Historians, epidemiologists, and clinicians debate how far this decline was owing to changes in virulence, improved nutrition, or medical measures. Many chronic infectious diseases also continued to show a decline in incidence and mortality. This was true of tuberculosis (TB) although it remained frighteningly common among the poor and malnourished, and in immigrant populations. In many communities, however, bovine TB disappeared. Between the wars venereal disease (VD) seems to have persisted with little change in incidence. Around 1930, sexually transmitted disease (STD) clinics in England and Wales recorded nearly 10,000 cases of gonorrhoea and a similar number for syphilis (obviously many cases were in both categories). Those doctors who were seeing fewer infectious diseases and their patients living longer were watching the modern Western morbidity and mortality pattern taking shape. The diseases of maturity and old age (e.g., cancers and cardiovascular conditions) began to compete for prominence with those attributed to microorganisms.

The decline in the familiar infections was, in a puzzling manner, accompanied by the appearance of new epidemics or, perhaps, the resurgence of very old ones. 1918–19 saw a worldwide outbreak of influenza of frightening virulence. A known disease, it was formerly regarded as benign and physicians once joked 'Quite a godsend! Everybody ill, nobody dying'. The postwar pandemic killed those in the prime of life and the global death toll has been estimated at anything between 30–100 million. Poliomyelitis, which had been recognised before the war, devastated America, which suffered a severe epidemic in 1916. In New York over 9,000 cases were reported. Occurring as it did in middle-class homes in addition to the slums, health workers held the fly to be the agent accountable for transmission. Polio continued to break out sporadically in the 1920s and 1930s although worse was to come in the 1950s. To doctors at the time, the most enigmatic of the epidemics was the global outbreak of encephalitis lethargica that appeared in Europe at the end of World War I and that swamped the world in waves over the next ten tears. Producing myriad neurological symptoms, lethargy, and frequently resulting in death (one third of acute cases died) or chronic disability (notably Parkinson's disease), its cause was an acknowledged mystery. Most authorities now deem it a sequel of influenza.

World War I, 1914–18

THE MODERN WAR MACHINE

For medicine two wars started in 1914: one on the battlefield and one on the home front. They were not, however, separate wars. Historians are far from united on the role of or effect on medicine in either case. There are two related issues to consider when writing the history of the Great War and medicine: one general and one particular. This observation applies to both wartime fronts. At the general level there is a problem of the relation between the war, medicine, and modernization. The question is this: in what way were recognizably modern forms of organization brought into play in the war and how far did medicine utilize and promote them? Further, to what extent did any military-induced medical modernization spill over into peacetime? This latter question applies especially to Europe, for in America the war had less effect on social change, and much more powerful forces, such as industrial and commercial reorganization and philanthropy, were effecting modernization. At the particular level it is important to explore how various wartime problems were seen to be medical issues, and how far solutions to such problems were temporary and how far they too were carried over into peacetime. In doing so, it is necessary to recall the first question and explore how far the problems of wartime were addressed with solutions that incorporated and brought about modern ways of doing things.

Modernity has been described as including among other things 'the growth, differentiation and integration of bureaucracy and other organizational and managerial systems; the standardization and routinization of administrative action; and the employment of experts to define and order such systems' (Cooter and Sturdy, 1998, p. 1). This modern or technical rationality, the rationality of unification and uniformity, depended heavily on science to transform older, traditional ways of doing things so as to bring about socioeconomic efficiency. Such ideas, applied to business, industry, education, government, and so on, were also embodied in modern armies that, ideally, were constructed as efficiently organized killing machines. Civilian and military societies in the modern era were becoming increasingly similar. It might be argued in more than jest that, in the first half of the twentieth century, a nation's belligerence (or at least preparedness for war) could be measured by the extent and efficiency of its welfare system: making men and women fit for war was making them fit for work. World War I, it has been argued: 'vastly extended the forms and processes of modernity: the size of bureaucracies, the numbers of managers, the extent of the integration of civilian and military spheres, in addition to the scale and sophistication of the mass manufacture of armaments and the routinized treatment of their effects on human bodies. The waging of war was thoroughly industrialized . . .' (Cooter and Sturdy, 1998, p. 4). What part did medicine play in this 'rationalization'? One historian argues that 'it enhanced military efficiency by reducing wastage from disease and by improving the return of casualties to active service' (Harrison, 1999, p. 3). Medicine also contributed to the 'standardization of men' by physical and mental examination of recruits and by the calculation of dietary requirements. Perhaps more important, doctors, nurses, medical technicians, ambulance drivers, cooks, and cleaners thought of themselves (if they bothered to think about it) as being in some sort of massive hierarchical team. This was new. Before the war such people had perhaps been conscious of working on their own or with a small number of other individuals. Now they constituted a huge machine. Except in isolated places this mentality was one of the war's greatest legacies.

These sweeping generalizations should not, of course, obscure the fact that the details of wartime organization by no means always conformed to modern rationality. The hopeless inefficiency of so many wartime arrangements and the traditional methods by which so many haphazardly planned goals were brought about are easily catalogued. Rehabilitation, for example, was one area where truly modern approaches were worked out, but one in which economic constraints restricted ideal solutions. Modernity was resisted in addition to promoted. In some quarters, even by World War II (1939–45), older martial values deemed sickness to be weakness and unworthy of serious attention. Nonetheless, generalizations about modernization serve to indicate a changing sense of how many professionals and legislators considered that war and peacetime life should be managed. Most of the examples that follow are from British history, but where possible German, French, Russian, and American case studies will be used.

THE BATTLEFRONT

The war broke out in the summer of 1914 with Germany prepared and Britain and France partly prepared for battle. It was the first major war for a century and had been long expected in a Europe pervaded by the ethos of martial culture. Many had hoped for it; others saw it as the end of civilization. It involved all the major powers and nearly every European country. Asians, Australasians, and Americans were drawn in. Soon after war began, the stagnant western front, 'a machine for massacre', was established (Hobsbawm, 1996, p. 25). Guns, gas, rain, rats, lice, and microbiological pathogens ensured there would be ample work for medical personnel. The numbers of dead were terrifying. Estimates vary but at least 1.5 million French and somewhat more Germans died in battle or from its effects. Many of these victims, of course, received medical attention (if only briefly in some cases) before they died. Such fatalities add to the massive numbers of nonfatally wounded and sick recorded as receiving medical care.

Medicine played a greater part in World War I than in any other previous encounter. As one author has observed of the British army: 'To a greater extent than in any previous war, medicine was involved in selecting, preparing and maintaining Britain's war machine. Men were vetted for military fitness, immunized against infections and trained in camp sanitation; sick and wounded were tended; disease incidence was monitored; and research into old and new military medical problems was actively conducted' (Hardy, 2001, p. 59).

Famously, it was the first major war ever, in which more combatants died of wounds than disease. Preventative medicine worked. Sanitary measures and vaccination against cholera, typhoid, paratyphoid, and smallpox conspired to keep these diseases from the western front. Typhus too was absent where elaborate delousing was enforced. Dysentery took its toll, however, particularly in the Near East, and especially Mesopotamia where the British surgeon Sir Victor Horsley (1857–1916), who met his death there, described the conditions as 'grossly insanitary and inhuman'. Malaria took large numbers out of action in Macedonia. Venereal disease wreaked havoc everywhere. According to rumours at the time, the Austrian army had 1.5 million men rendered noncombatant by VD. The German army in the field had, in fact, comparatively low rates (most VD it turned out was contracted in the homeland if not the home). One of the highest incidences was in the Canadian Expeditionary Force, which had 28.7 percent of its troops with VD in 1915. Taking the efficiency view, military commanders had to decide whether allowing their troops access to prostitutes was better for morale than VD was worse for it. No coherent answer appeared among any of the combatant powers. Some officers pondered whether prohibiting prostitution encouraged masturbation (an 'enslaving habit') and homosexuality: vices seen as far worse for morale than adulterous, but heterosexual, intercourse. Various approaches to the containment of VD were adopted. All soldiers were repeatedly told of the terrible symptoms. British soldiers were not paid during treatment. The Americans and Dominions either issued or told soldiers about prophylactic packs, sometimes containing condoms, usually chemicals to be applied during washing after intercourse. The French relied on medically inspected, regulated prostitutes (they were supposed to be inspected twice weekly by physicians); an option that the British public (and thus the army) could not stomach (p. 182). The Germans did not condone this, but never quite condemned it either, with their army running brothels in occupied territory.

Mortality and morbidity statistics for the United States army were particularly impressive. In the American Civil War, sixty-one in a thousand deaths were from disease; in the Great War it was seventeen per thousand. American troops from country areas, however, suffered severe epidemics of measles, mumps, and meningitis. Matching the 1.5 million Germans who were killed (nearly a million more were reported missing) was an almost similar number who died of disease. Clinical medicine claimed its successes. Among British soldiers 82 percent of the surviving 'wounded' and 93 percent of the 'sick and injured' were returned to some form of military duty. The death rate from wounds among American troops was half that of Civil War levels.

The war saw a vast increase in, and reorganization of, the British military medical services, overseen and orchestrated by the surgeon Sir Alfred Keogh (1857–1936), Director-general at the War Office, and Sir Arthur Sloggett (1857–1929) who carried out the Director-general's duties in

France. Given the duration and unanticipated nature of the war, the reorganization was a qualified success; the qualification being that civilian medical services suffered. Enormous numbers of medical workers were mobilized. At the outbreak of war the Royal Army Medical Corps (RAMC) numbered less than 20,000 of all ranks. At the end of the war there were 13,000 officers and 154,000 other ranks. In Germany, links between military and civilian medicine had long been strong. Conscription existed before the war and all medical graduates had encountered, and many had internalized, military values and discipline.

In Britain, volunteer nurses were hastily recruited and equally hastily trained to work at home and abroad. These members of Voluntary Aid Detachments (VADs, usually unpaid) included many daughters of the gentry and aristocracy. Indeed, women in all countries were, as one nurse testified 'as eager to get to the front as any boy' (Mary Borden in Higonnet, 2001, p. vii). Thousands of American women volunteered even when their country was neutral. In Britain, the British Medical Association (BMA) was put in charge of recruiting doctors. Those working in hospitals that cared for the armed forces were given ranks that reproduced the civilian social order: general practitioners (GPs) became lieutenants, consultants became colonels. Likewise, chief administrators of voluntary hospitals were given commissioned ranks and chief administrators of Poor Law institutions became quartermasters.

The British War Office, at first, would not allow women doctors to serve abroad so they formed their own voluntary organizations to do just that. Impressed by the work of the Woman's Hospital Corps (WHC) in Paris, the War Office invited the WHC to set up a hospital at Wimereaux in France. The Scottish Women's Hospitals organization established a hospital at Abbaye de Royaument where, at one time, three operating theatres were working all day and two of them at night. The hospital's reputation was sufficiently high for wounded men to ask to be sent there. The War Office, however, continued to discriminate against women in terms of, among other things, status and pay. Similar discrimination occurred in the U.S. army where women were not granted commissions even though women in many states had obtained the right to vote by 1917. One way or another, however, many American women doctors involved themselves in the war.

Certainly for the British, and presumably other armies of the time, the success of medical arrangements at the front ultimately depended on good relations between medical and combatant officers. At Gallipoli and in Mesopotamia, medical officers were excluded from meetings with

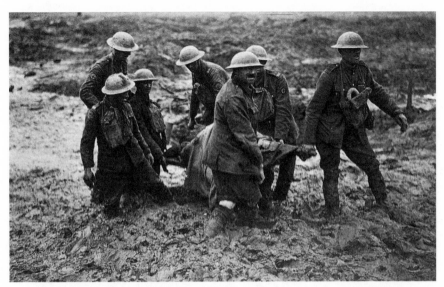

Fig. 3.1. British army stretcher bearers, World War I. *Source:* Photograph, Wellcome Library Iconographic Collection. *Credit:* Wellcome Library, London (L0006421).

headquarters staff and consequently the sick and wounded received treatment slowly 'because the General Staff had not made adequate arrangements for medical transport and hospital facilities' (Harrison, 1999, p. 2) On the western front, treatment of the wounded in the British army began with stretcher bearers who were trained in first aid, particularly the arrest of haemorrhage (Fig. 3.1). They carried the injured to a Regimental Aid Post (RAP) where the Regimental Medical Officer (RMO) would clean the wound, perform emergency amputations, and splint fractures. Basically, he was making the severely wounded fit to travel. This job was no sinecure. By 1917 'the death rate among RMOs and regimental orderlies was reportedly as high as 40 per month' (Whitehead, 1999, p. 184). Many of the RMOs advanced to the trenches to take part in the action. Next up the line from the RAP was a Field Ambulance (FA) which relieved the RAP of sick and wounded and treated men so they could be sent down the line for more extensive management. The FA was divided and subdivided into various sections and had at its disposal motor-driven and horse-drawn ambulances. From here the wounded were transported to Casualty Clearing Stations (CCS). These clearing stations, originally designed as sorting stations, later 'expanded into the forward areas to take, in some cases, up to 1,000 patients, provided with nursing sisters and all specialist facilities' (Laffin, 1970, p. 215). The CCS was basically involved in the business of saving life or getting soldiers back to the front. From the CCS the wounded were evacuated to base hospitals. Significant in these arrangements is the institutionalization of triage, teamwork, specialization, hierarchy, and large-scale communication. This experience encouraged some medical workers to attempt to promote these innovations in peacetime. To a great extent, however, they were unsuccessful. The institutionalized interests of older modes of management remained resistant to change.

Wound management was obviously central to medical work of war. As is well known, surgeons at the front encountered injuries of a sort they had never seen before. Unlike the Boer War in which wounds on the sunny dry veldt healed easily and where expectant treatment succeeded, the Flanders's mud, full of gas gangrene bacilli and tetanus spores, did not collude with the healing power of nature. Henry Souttar (1875–1964), a young British surgeon, later famed for trying mitral valvotomy for heart disease thirty years before it became accepted practice, noted in 1914 that, 'the ordinary rules of surgery did not apply' (Whitehead, 1999, p. 206). Surgeons soon cottoned on to the fact that immediate treatment was better than waiting. Routine use of antitetanic serum after wounding solved the tetanus problem, but the civilian procedures of antiseptic and aseptic surgery seemed almost useless in the face of gas gangrene. Geoffrey Jefferson (1886–1961), a surgeon of the time and later one of the distinguished neurosurgeons of World War II, called the degree of failure of aseptic surgery 'staggering'. It was soon recognized, indeed predicted by some like Almroth Wright (1861–1932), that antiseptics could not sterilize the deep, muddy, macerated wounds of Flanders. Early, complete excision, rather than pouring antiseptics into the wound, was soon adopted. Later, the method of treating wounds developed by Alexis Carrel (1873–1944) and Henry Dakin (1880–1952) was employed. Tubes were installed in the wound and sodium hypochlorite continuously administered. Although the method had its opponents, the incidence of gas gangrene definitely fell with its use (surgeons from the United States were particularly impressed with the method and imported it into civilian practice).

Integral to the use of new techniques were new social orderings. Protected operating units close to the battle lines were established. Nonetheless, recovery from gunshot wounds could be long. Head wounds had a dreadful mortality (Jefferson had comparatively excellent figures of 36.7 percent). Chronic infection led to sinuses and sequestration of bone and a life of invalidism. It was, said Jefferson, a 'bitter tale', for surgeons were aware at the time that the problems, despite relatively quick recovery after surgery, lay in chronic infection, not with their lack of skills at the operating table.

Jefferson estimated that only four in a series of twenty-eight deaths were due to the brain injury. It was held at the time that war-wound cases needed a systemic bactericide. However, there was no agreement that an effective drug existed. Some thought highly of *therapeutic* vaccines – antisera raised against septic agents (on the model of diphtheria antiserum, (p. 134)).

Other measures had an important place in obviating a fatal result after injury, notably blood transfusion and the use of gas and oxygen anaesthesia rather than the employment of ether or chloroform. The war provided opportunities for surgical experts to promote their subject. In 1915, the Boston surgeon Harvey Cushing (1869–1939) who was at the forefront of the creation of neurosurgery as a specialty, joined the 'Ambulance Américaine' (American military hospital) in Paris (America had not officially entered the war at this point). Cushing visited several hospitals and was shocked by the way the wounded were moved and how 'things were badly disorganized' (Fulton, 1946, p. 395). He also operated, war providing him with opportunities to try out new techniques, such as the use of a nail and a magnet to remove shell fragments from the brain (it worked). Cushing's work on the classification and treatment of head injuries was widely admired. Wartime concentration on neurosurgery did not, at first, impact substantially on civilian medicine. For all his prominence, Cushing was unable to get the Rockefeller Foundation to fund a neurological institute. Such was the postwar consciousness of American surgeons, however, that in 1919 William J. Mayo (1861–1939) could announce to the American College of Surgeons that 'a new surgical specialty of neurological surgery had now been founded.'

By previous standards the management of wartime, crippling limb injuries was a spectacular success. In Britain, by 1918, 20,000 beds in twenty Military Orthopaedic Centres under the direction of Robert Jones (1858–1933) had been created. An 800-bed hospital at Shepherd's Bush, London, was the hub of this 'empire'. At the front, at Jones's instigation, the various splints that he had devised with Hugh Owen Thomas (1834–91) were brought into use. Thomas's splint for fractured femurs was seen 'by officers and men alike as virtually a sacred object ('St. Thomas's splints')' (Cooter, 1993, pp. 106–7). From being a marginal medical discipline, orthopaedics became a premier specialty. Similar changes in status occurred in the United States, Italy, and Germany. This specialty formation involved far more than the training of skilled experts in the management of war wounds. War provided the opportunity for experts to modernize their discipline's organization and integration into the war machine.

Besides evacuating the wounded, the fundamental job of doctors at the front was to prevent disease. The British army was highly efficient in this respect and had personnel especially delegated for sanitary duties: purifying water, filling in latrines, and disinfecting clothing, for example. The French, according to British accounts, were much less well organized in these matters and after departing a trench, left filth and stench behind them. Indeed, it was not until November 1916 that the French army established sanitary squads. Lapses of sanitary attention among British troops resulted in dysentery and typhoid. Neglect of delousing procedures was followed by trench fever, a highly contagious rickettsial disease. Rats were a problem, carrying various diseases, notably infective jaundice. The RAMC appointed Rat Officers. In spite of medical and sanitary attention, cold and rain led to frostbite and trench foot, a painful condition marked by blackening and death of surface tissue. The issuing of orders in 1915 regarding basic foot hygiene reduced the incidence of the disorder in the British army.

In their management of disease all the major armies set great store by science, particularly laboratory science that, when the war was over, was given great credit for the solution or management of various pathological problems. Bacteriologists and physiologists were prominent in the British and American forces; pathologists were prominent among the Germans. The British had a Mobile Bacteriology Laboratory on the western front in 1914, and laboratories were soon a part of the management of any outbreak of infectious disease. Men who had been in contact with cerebrospinal fever spent three weeks in isolation where nasal swabs were taken to check for meningococcal bacteria. After an outbreak of epidemic jaundice in the Second Army, Captain Adrian Stokes (1887–1927) identified a spirochete carried by rats as the responsible agent. In 1918, a British Committee chaired by Major General Sir David Bruce (1855–1931) reported that the rickettsia associated with trench fever were carried by lice. The work of an American Commission under R. P. Strong was taken to have proven this.

If bacteriologists were prominent in the British army, pathologists were at the forefront of German researches. Unlike their British and American counterparts, German pathologists were specialists, separated from clinical medicine. Following Rudolph Virchow (1821–1902), they were strong advocates of a morphological approach, 'the post-mortem analysis of static pictures of organs, tissues and cells' (Prüll, 1999, p. 132). Around 1900, in response to the rise of bacteriology, German pathologists began to emphasize the significance of the human constitution. At the outbreak of the war, the head of the pathological institute at the University of

Freiburg, Ludwig Aschoff (1860–1936), organized a programme to pursue *Kriegspathologie* (war pathology). Aschoff advocated immediate routine autopsy on all dead soldiers to ascertain the cause of death and to create mortality statistics. The war, he said, offered the chance to carry out extensive postmortem research on material rarely encountered in peacetime: bodies of once fit young men. The effects of vaccination and injuries, for example, could be comprehensively studied. Besides this, said Aschoff, war pathologists could study constitutional pathology. By weighing, measuring, and examining bodies and organs, the normal constitution and the effects of war could be reconstructed. Aschoff's aims were shared by most German pathologists.

The programme was implemented and Aschoff was put in charge. German institutes of pathology were the institutional seats of the operation. Pathologists and dissectors were organized and dispatched to the field and military hospitals at home. Specimens were sent to Berlin, Munich, and Vienna to be sorted, registered, and exhibited. In 1921 there was a register of 70,000 postmortem reports and 6,000 specimens in Berlin. On the basis of such work, one German pathology professor contrasted the healthy young men who had been strengthened by the catharsis of war with the 'urban, degenerate human material' usually encountered in civilian life.

In Britain, scientists, notably engineers, physicists, and chemists, had made themselves important to government from the early days of the war. Physiologists, too, were seeking to expand their role, but up until then their researches were not seen to have any significant part to play in the activities of the state. The Medical Research Committee, later Council (MRC), was founded to research into TB; soon funds were diverted to physiology. Physiology was valued by a small sector of the pharmaceutical industry and by doctors in so far as it constituted a part of the preclinical curriculum. The first large-scale German gas attack at Ypres in April 1915 was to change this. Two days after this attack the respiratory physiologist John Scott Haldane (1860–1936) was summoned to the War Office where he was asked to visit France and investigate. After examining soldiers and attending a postmortem he identified the gas as chlorine and its clinical effects as being produced by inflammation of the lungs.

Haldane's work was the first step in the recognition of the physiologist as a valuable expert within the machinery of government. At the War Office, Alfred Keogh established an Anti-Gas Department over which, slightly later, the physiologist Ernest Henry Starling (1866–1927) took charge.

This department looked into the design of respirators and, despite its name, the potential of various chemicals for offensive use. Liasing with the Royal Engineers in France, the department drafted in the physiologist C. G. Douglas (1882–1963). Keogh also turned to the Royal Society, which formed a Sectional Committee on Physiology. In June, the government set up a Ministry of Munitions with a Scientific Advisory Group that included the physiologist William Bate Hardy (1864–1934) who undertook to collect physiological data 'on the suitability of a wide range of chemicals for use as weapons.' In June 1916 the new ministry established an Experimental Station at Porton Down and nine months later a physiology department was included there under Joseph Barcroft (1872–1947). Many of these disparate initiatives were rationalized in 1917 under the Chemical Warfare Department of the ministry in which physiologists played a major role.

As the war entered its third year and there was a pressing need to return men to the trenches (and to reduce military pensions), physiologists began to investigate the therapeutics of gas injuries and they became convinced of the value of oxygen. As a result of this, 4,000 cylinders of the gas were to be made available in France. The Director of Gas Services in France noted that 'A great saving of manpower was effected in this way.' Physiologists made themselves invaluable to government in other areas: in researches on efficiency in industry and as expert advisors on food policy. The British government certainly took more note of its food scientists than did the German authorities; the latter perhaps to the detriment of the German people (some German physiologists at this time showed little interest in vitamins, a largely British discovery). The moral that the British government and the military drew from all this was that scientific research had a vital part to play during war and not just in periods of peace in preparation for war. For physiologists there were permanent gains, notably, 'the rise in status and authority of the MRC' over whose policy in the postwar years they had considerable influence (Sturdy, 1998, pp. 68, 73, 78).

Shock was another condition that attracted the attention of physiologists. In 1916 the National Research Council in America asked the Harvard physiologist Walter Bradford Cannon (1871–1945) to establish a physiology committee to develop research programmes into the health and safety of the forces (for his early work, see (pp. 117, 173–4)). Cannon made shock a priority. At first he worked in his department, but after the United States entered the war in April 1917 he joined the Harvard Base Hospital No. 5 unit. Cannon's physiological work with patients and in the lab did not result in acceptance of the therapies he advocated, but his presence in Europe contributed to a strong sense among physiologists of their being an international community. Cannon collaborated extensively with British workers. Internationalism in medicine and science was a prewar invention but the interwar years saw it being strenuously promoted.

Research into heart disease by British physiologists and clinicians also proved valuable to the military and the government. 'Soldier's heart', a not very clearly defined syndrome, of which breathlessness was the most important symptom, had been known long before the war began. Many accounts of its cause had been given and these usually tied it down to an anatomical abnormality. Many recruits were rejected as unfit for service because they had a heart murmur, which was always considered a sign of valve damage. At the beginning of the century, drawing on the work of experimental physiologists, clinicians interested in heart disease began to stress the importance of understanding functional rather than morphological disturbance. To investigate cardiac disorders they used the polygraph and the newly invented electrocardiograph (ECG). At the end of 1914, a considerable number of soldiers were being sent back from France with symptoms of heart disease. The British authority on heart disease at this time, and who had been at the forefront of the new approaches, was a former GP, James Mackenzie (1853–1925). In 1915 in a memorandum distributed by the War Office, Mackenzie stated his views on soldier's heart. In line with modern opinion, he regarded it as functional and insisted that cardiac murmurs might not signal anything seriously amiss. A murmur did not prohibit recruitment of a man who could exert himself without distress.

At Mackenzie's suggestion, at the end of 1915, the War Office established a hospital for the treatment and study of soldiers deemed as having heart disease. Originally at Mount Vernon hospital, Hampstead, London, it was later moved to Colchester in Essex. On the staff was Mackenzie's protégé and wizard of the ECG, Thomas Lewis (1881–1945), who from 1916 was also on the permanent scientific staff of the MRC. On the basis of a study of about 1,000 soldiers, Lewis distinguished a functional disorder of the heart called 'effort syndrome', the symptoms of which were 'exaggerated manifestations of healthy response to . . . effort' (Howell, 1998, p. 92). All that was needed to ensure a return to duty, Lewis said, were graded exercises. At first hand, American physicians studying the British work found similar symptoms in their troops that they christened 'neurocirculatory asthenia' and for which they recommended rest and discharge to civilian life.

The creation of effort syndrome had got men back to the front and saved the government money. It would do the latter again in peacetime. The

British Ministry of Pensions was formed in 1916 and was put in charge of the administration of disability pensions in the following year. At the end of the war Lewis was appointed to the ministry as an honorary consulting physician in cardiovascular disease. He set up courses and trained deputy commissioners. An outpatient clinic was established at University College Hospital, London, for reports on, and treatment of, heart cases. Response to effort, which had been the criterion for fitness to fight, was now made the criterion for entitlement to a pension. In brief, the new method of assessment cut down numbers of recipients considerably. There was a further consequence of this postwar development. A number of the physicians involved in the assessment formed a Cardiac Club, which was to form the nidus for the formation of the specialty of cardiology in Britain (p. 283). The lessons of the war and soldier's heart are that, once again, the proponents of a modern scientific medicine were perceived as valuable experts by government and were incorporated into its machinery. In turn, institutions associated with this sort of medicine, the universities and the MRC, were favoured. Further, specialty formation was promoted.

Another disorder that was created in the war, or an old one that was re-created, went under the name of 'war neurosis' and, in some places, 'shell shock'. Soldiers showed similar symptoms in all armies although the disturbance of behaviour had various explanations and some denied that it was a medical condition at all. 'Shell shock' was the name given by the Cambridge psychologist Charles Samuel Myers (1873–1946) to men under shell fire who were left 'blinded, deaf, dumb, semi-paralyzed, in a state of stupor and very often suffering amnesia' (Shephard, 2000, p. 1). Shell shock provides a window into the state of psychiatry, neurology, and specialist advice at the time. Essentially, experts could not agree. Some proposed somatic explanations: that a shell bursting a few yards away did serious physical damage to the nervous system. Others, of a psychoanalytic persuasion, found continuities with prewar hysteria; a position that could stigmatize sufferers as effeminate. Yet other psychiatrists saw only cowardice or malingering. Among the European powers, the British seem to have been most sympathetic to sufferers. In Germany, fear of malingering was widespread and the German Association of Psychiatry 'overwhelmingly refused to recognize war neurosis as an independent mental illness' (Eghigian, 2001, p. 107). The French openly regarded it as hysteria and saw it, says one historian, as 'artificial and perverse' (Roudebush, 2001, p. 253). Therapy mirrored theory. In Britain, everything from electric shocks to psychoanalysis was tried. The latter, famously and successfully, in the case of the poet

Siegfried Sassoon (1886–1967). But, like soldier's heart, two things were driving management: returning men to the front and pensions. The German military authorities briefly flirted with Freudianism because it seemed to be the approach most likely to get men back into action. Consistent with their contempt, the French paid no pensions; the Germans paid pensions only until 1926 when Weimar finances could no longer bear the burden. The British and the Americans paid in full, although often grudgingly, avoiding payment when possible.

THE HOME FRONT

There is debate as to the effect of the war on the health of citizens in the various nations. In Britain and Germany (after a rise in 1914), the infant death rate continued to fall. In France, there was a steady rise. The birth rate fell everywhere in Europe; in France it fell alarmingly. The Red Cross sent 400 infant welfare units to France. Overall, the war drove every nation to ponder its infant welfare services. Germany's worry about the declining birth rate resulted in the illegitimate children of soldiers killed in service receiving pensions. In Britain, female mortality fell (except during the influenza of 1918), but in Germany it rose, particularly in 1917. Death rates among people over sixty years old in London, Paris, and Berlin rose sufficiently for it to be called a 'demographic crisis' (Hardy, 2001, p. 54). It is known that grief has an effect on the survival rate of the elderly. Civilian health probably improved in Britain; rigorous antidrink laws (passed in the interests of efficiency in the munitions industry) reduced alcohol consumption. Everywhere cigarette smoking increased enormously. Factory work, everywhere, particularly in the munitions industry (where toxic chemicals were employed), was desperately demanding and often dangerous, no doubt with detrimental effects on health. Illegitimacy rates rose. Communities policed potentially unfaithful women. In Britain, the statutory separation allowance that a soldier's wife might expect could be withdrawn were she to be adulterous. In Germany, the Prussian war ministry issued leaflets cautioning soldiers wives to be faithful to their husbands. By the time of the German collapse, starvation took its toll on the nation and rickets reappeared. Babies called *Kreigsneugeborene* (war infants) were underdeveloped, with symptoms of restlessness and automatic grasping movements. During the war and just after, the Russian people suffered more from starvation and from physical and mental disorder than the citizens of all the other nations combined. Typhus, cholera, and malaria attended famine in that country.

The Rockefeller Foundation, newly established in 1913, sent aid to the tune of $22,000,000 to Europe during the war years. Food was sent to Belgium on chartered ships when that country faced famine after the German invasion. Supplies were also sent to Poland, Serbia, Armenia, Syria, Montenegro, and Albania. The foundation supported the Red Cross and was interested in prisoners of war.

It was anticipated even before the war that many casualties would be treated back in the homeland, a situation bound to affect civilian medical services. In Britain, at the outbreak of war there were 9,000 beds in military hospitals, but as early as 1907, in preparation for war, the RAMC 'made arrangements to set up 23 Territorial hospitals with a minimum of 500 beds each in existing public buildings throughout the country' (Richardson, 1998, p. 98). Together, this meant that in August 1914 there were about 20,000 beds ready for the use of the armed forces. The War Office issued appeals for further accommodation and many private buildings including Lambeth Palace, the London residence of the Archbishop of Canterbury, offered space. The Canadian Red Cross hospital was based in the grounds of Cliveden, a stately home in Buckinghamshire. The Red Cross was one of many voluntary organizations (e.g., The Order of St John and the Soldiers and Sailors Help Society) involved in the medical war effort. Rivalry between these bodies ensured 'unco-ordinated activity' that produced 'a chaotic dispersal and waste of scarce resources' (Abel-Smith, 1964, p. 254). Only intervention from the War Office saved the situation.

By the end of 1914, 73,000 wounded officers and men had arrived in England. The War Office had got its bed estimate quite wrong. Huts were erected and workhouses taken over (their inadequate facilities shocked voluntary hospital consultants who had never before been in such places). Evicted paupers, by and large, were given a bad time. Sick civilians were neglected. Military service was made compulsory in 1916 and doctors were called up whether they liked it or not. Apart from a lull in early 1916 the demand for more beds did not abate. In 1917, 700,000 wounded officers and men were transported home. In August of that year there were over 300,000 beds for servicemen and by the end of the war over 350,000. Voluntary hospitals were not keen to admit patients with VD, and by November 1918 the army had opened twenty VD hospitals with accommodation for 11,000 sufferers. In the United States, so-called progressives saw the war as a moral crusade that offered the opportunity to instil the values of hard work and respectability into the American male. President Woodrow Wilson had linked sexual purity and masculinity by urging soldiers to keep themselves 'fit and straight in everything and pure and clean through and through'. The focus of progressive reforming zeal was military training camps at home. These were notorious, however, during the Mexican conflict of 1916, for rampant alcohol abuse and VD. A special Commission on Training Camp Activities (CTCA) was set up. The CTCA developed a sex education programme that urged self-control. The commission also initiated a chemical-prophylaxis scheme, and failure to report for chemical prophylaxis within three hours of sexual contact was made a court-martial offence.

Doctors and nurses in Britain were in very short supply at home. In 1915, Charing Cross Hospital admitted women medical students for the first time. By 1917, more than half the medical profession had been called up. Scarcity meant that women doctors began to get jobs in voluntary hospitals for the first time. The entry of the United States into the war brought some relief in the form of extra doctors and nurses.

Standards of care and accommodation in hospitals in Britain varied widely. Conditions in hutted camps, which had 47,500 beds by the end of the war, could be dreadful. The influenza epidemic of 1918 tested civilian services to the limit. In December 1918, 10,000 died in London of the disease. Disabled servicemen were being discharged at the rate of one thousand a month; 'incapacitated and thrown aside with a trifling pension', as a contemporary journal observed. The organization of a rehabilitation service did not begin until 1917. 'In no respect', says one historian, 'had the burdens of war [in Britain] been fairly shared' (Abel-Smith, 1964, p. 281). Officers got priority over other ranks; young active males came before the elderly, women, and children. Minor conditions in soldiers took precedence over TB in civilians. Young doctors served abroad and lost their practices; many consultants kept their private patients and in addition were paid generous salaries for nominal military duties.

The war saw the beginning of the transformation of the French hospital system. On the eve of the war, hospitals in that country were institutions for the very poor and had none of the signs of middle-class admission that were already visible in American and Britain. A great deal of the care of the poor in hospitals was for 'social' rather than for 'medical' reasons. More than in other countries, French hospitals preserved social distinctions. The financial stresses of caring for civilian and military victims put the hospitals to the test. Masses of temporary hospitals were set up by the state-run Service de la Santé Militaire, the Red Cross, municipal councils, and private charities. Costs soared. The total budget of the Assistance Publique in Paris increased from 51.5 million francs in 1914 to 166.2 million in 1919. Provincial cities were forced to take out huge loans to pay for their hospitals. The Hospices Civils de Lyon was bankrupted. These pressures were to have profound postwar consequences.

A central concern among all the belligerent powers was, at least during the war, rehabilitation. Underlying all rehabilitation strategies was the assumption that work (for men) was the most fulfilling of human activities. Sometimes, thinking explicitly in terms of the conservation of energy (and thus of humans as machines), those involved in rehabilitation sought to find what an American philosopher called the 'moral equivalent of war' that was, he said, 'analogous . . . to the mechanical equivalent of heat.' In other words, the question was: how were the manly energies once devoted to killing to be converted into the energies of self-fulfilling citizenship? As one American rehabilitator put it: 'The end and purpose of the new conception of the Nation's duty is complete restoration of the disabled and their re-establishment in civil life as self respecting, useful independent citizens' (Price, 1998, pp. 6, 10). The first concerted attempts to reintegrate the permanently disabled soldier into civil life began in the Great War. Hundreds of new prosthetic devices were designed all over Europe and America. These devices were not designed, as had previously been the case, to resemble the limb visually, but to mimic it functionally: to enable what Americans called 'veterans' to work. In Germany, attempts were made to standardize prosthetic devices so that parts were interchangeable, just as were the parts of weapons produced by the modern munitions industry. It was envisaged that a variety of end devices, such as hammers or files, would be made so that the workman could switch tasks. The collapse of Germany that followed the war's end laid these plans, at least temporarily, to waste. What is important here is to take note of the modern technocratic mentality underlying them.

Between the wars

INTRODUCTION

For the most part, the massive organizational changes visible in the medicine of war were not carried over to peacetime. Obviously some were strictly wartime contingencies. Others, however, simply could not be rooted in civilian life. Most of the doctors who had spent their wartime years in the forces and thus employed by the state, showed no inclination for anything other than private practice back home. In most countries, the idea of state service in peacetime conflicted with long-standing conservative medical traditions. Medical specialties, such as orthopaedics that had become highly organized in wartime, generally failed to hold on to the full extent of those gains. As indicated, however, changed attitudes were carried over in some quarters, notably in the approval of governments of the role of medical laboratory sciences in diagnosis and treatment, and of the value of basic scientific research. Such approval did not always translate into substantial funding.

This section deals with the nexus of relations constituted by the hospital, university, and industry. Following is a section on medicine in the community and those issues broadly covered by the terms 'public health' and 'welfare'. Hospitals and related institutions are dealt with first, not because these were the places where most sickness was treated, but because these were the seats, and the increasingly important seats, of medical power. These were the sites at which the majority of the medical labour force was trained, where medical technologies where created, and where medical and scientific knowledge was made and reproduced. They were the places from which medical policy and action in the community stemmed. They were thus the most important seats of modernization in medicine.

Modernization was by no means everywhere warmly embraced in medicine any more than it was elsewhere. Many observers both inside and outside occupations that were built around health and disease deplored, or in some cases found mildly uncomfortable, the sorts of changes that modernization was effecting in medicine. Modernization in medicine was largely recognized in two related phenomena: first, changes of scale and organization, and second, reductionist approaches to knowledge and the technologies seen to be associated with such approaches. Some of the responses to these things are dealt with in the following text, but here it is useful to note that a great deal of interwar critical thinking about medicine and, indeed, about society at large was structured by holist perspectives. Significantly, the word 'holism' was coined in the 1920s and came to mean a variety of things. The term was not used frequently at the time (the word 'organic' usually serving in its stead), but the concepts it seemed to refer to were prominent in cultural debate at all levels. Broadly speaking, the word and its congeners were applied as a contrast to reductionist views; the notion that all phenomena whether in the scientific or social realm could be understood by reference to one or more fundamental constituents. The idea that a person's illness, for example, could be more or less fully explained by reference to a bacterium seemed hopelessly myopic to some. Holist concepts referred to the seeming fact that things were greater than the sum of their parts. Modernization was frequently the butt of holistic criticism and modern society was often condemned as atomistic. But modernizers could turn holist ideas to their own ends. In all domains holistic concepts were used normatively; as prescriptions for goal-directed action. Among the sciences, embryology was particularly informed by this mode of enquiry, but it can be found in all the interwar disciplines, including physics. It was very much a relative concept; one group's holistic approach could be seen by another as reductionist. Thus Walter Bradford Cannon, the American physiologist who in the 1920s coined the term 'homeostasis' to describe the organism's internal environment and the integrative activity maintaining its constancy was, as he recognized, guided in his work (and social thought) by holist ideas. Yet Cannon was committed to animal experiment, a mode of investigation regarded by some (also guided by holist ideas) as reductionist, immoral, and fruitless. As a source of political analysis and action, holistic concepts were employed to argue that the ideal community was an organic whole; as such, these concepts were appropriated by the political left and right who variously found utopian societies in the past or the future. Nazi thought was awash with holistic concepts, but the Nazis by no means had a monopoly on them.

Without doubt, the holistic ideas that permeated these years, and that evaporated with incredible rapidity after World War II, were responses to the crises of the time. They were means of understanding them, ways of making sense of a world splintered by the Great War, before which some sort of harmony had seemed to reign. They were ways of galvanizing responses (even if only nostalgic retreat) to these crises. In medicine, holist ideas were used by modernizers, but were more obvious among conservatives and critics of change. Many clinicians used holist ideas to lament what they saw as the disappearance of the caring face-to-face bedside encounter. In doing so, they invoked the healing power of nature as being as important as drug therapy or surgery. They stressed how disease should not be seen only in terms of laboratory categories and how knowledge of the whole patient was important. Holism in medicine had a powerful historical dimension. In Britain, America, and France, a strong neo-Hippocratic movement developed in which that ancient Greek physician was held to have embodied all that was best in medicine: bedside observation, expectant therapy, and the management of individuals not disembodied diseases. Sometimes, the seventeenth-century English doctor Thomas Sydenham (1624–89) was enrolled in this movement. Similar developments occurred in Germany where Paracelsus (*c.* 1493–1541) was added to the list of worthies. Holistic reconstructions of the medical past often situated the doctor as priest and sought to restore him (medical holism was a very gendered ideology) to that role both as a healer of the sick and as a saviour of modern society. This was particularly true in Germany. The historical dimension of holism was less the creation of a new tradition that, for example, English surgeons had done in the nineteenth century and was described in Chapter 1, but rather the vigorous reassertion and refashioning of an older one (for doctors had long traced their art back to Hippocrates).

Medical institutions

THE HOSPITAL – CATHEDRALS OF MEDICINE

Between the wars, the position of the hospital as the cathedral of medicine was consolidated. More and more people who would once have been treated at home were being treated in hospital. The university hospital became increasingly prominent in medical education and the seat, in theory at least, of medical excellence. Simple factors, such as the high price of some therapies, often contributed to the concentration of resources in a single hospital or specialized centre that often combined research and therapy. Radium, for example, was expensive and cancer treatment with radium was often concentrated in one place, sometimes supported by charities, such as the American Society for the Control of Cancer (1913) or the Franco-Anglo-American Anti-Cancer League of 1918. In France, a network of specialized cancer centres was set up. Therapeutic efficacy thus began to be identified with high technology and multidisciplinary centres.

In the move to hospital medicine, as in almost everything else in clinical medicine at this time, America took the lead. In 1909 there were nearly 4,500 thousand hospitals in the United States containing over 400,000 beds. By 1923 there were nearly 7,000 hospitals with over 750,000 beds. Thereafter, a new trend set in; hospitals decreased in number but increased in size. In 1932, in the United States there were over 1 million hospital beds. The patient composition of hospitals changed in both Europe and America. Middle- and even upper-class folk who once would never have dreamed of entering a hospital began to be treated there in large numbers. Doctors, especially in America, increasingly practised some or all of the time in hospitals. In the United States in 1929, of the 140,000 or so practising doctors nearly 100,000 were attached in some way to a hospital.

This story of hospital expansion was repeated everywhere. There were over 100,000 beds in voluntary hospitals in England, Scotland, and Wales in 1938. Beds per thousand of population in these institutions increased from 1.49 in 1921 to 2.12 in 1938. Length of stay in the same period fell by a quarter to eighteen days. Teaching hospitals averaged over 500 beds. Hospitals with less than 100 beds were very common. In the public sector, in-patient provision increased, and by 1938 public hospitals contained 176,000 beds. Local authority involvement in hospital development continued. In Bradford, Yorkshire, a 600-bed municipal hospital was opened in 1922. In Germany, most hospitals were supported out of public (insurance) funds. In 1885 in that country there were 1,706 public hospitals with 75,000 beds; by 1927 there were 2,964 hospitals with a massive 314,019 beds. Around 1930, Germany had 833 private hospitals with 44,310 beds. Establishing a private hospital required state authority. France probably saw the most profound change because none of the modernizing trends visible in the hospitals of many countries before the war had been apparent in France. Here, massive reform and growth occurred simultaneously. Between the wars, dozens of modern hospitals were built.

If science, for present purposes, can be identified with laboratories, technology, and systems of management, it can be safely said that it moved into major hospitals in a big way between the wars. Once again, it was in America that change was most pronounced. American hospitals fell victim to the efficiency movement that was based, said its protagonists, on the scientific study of production and management. The hospital was described at the time as a 'health factory' and as a 'health manufacturing plant' that 'specializes in the conversion of the non-producing and wealth absorbing sick men and women into wealth producing citizens' (Berliner, 1985, p. 136). Trends that had begun before the war intensified. Showpiece hospitals everywhere began to use sophisticated accounting systems and management methods borrowed from business. Patient records increased in length and became standardized. Graphic information, such as ECG printouts and glucose tolerance curves, hand-drawn in diabetic cases, proliferated. Between 1900 and 1925 the number of graphs per patient, per day, increased tenfold at the Pennsylvania Hospital (Howell, 1995, p. 52).

Hospitals were increasingly fractionated into departments, again notably in the United States. Old departments were dismembered: a once single surgery department might have satellites of, for example, neurosurgery; ear, nose and throat surgery; accident surgery; and gynaecology; and medical departments might have cardiology and gastroenterology units. New departments might be formed out of new technologies or scientific disciplines. X-rays, which had proved their worth in the war, formed the nucleus of radiology departments. Medical biochemistry took off in the 1920s and was the core discipline behind biochemical laboratories that joined pathology and bacteriology laboratories in providing diagnostic services for clinicians on the ward. Diabetic clinics were formed after the introduction of insulin. Departments often not directly run by doctors, such as those of dietetics and physiotherapy, were also established. Paramedical workers – physiotherapists, X-ray technicians, laboratory assistants, and medical social workers – outnumbered the medically qualified. In the United States in 1929, about 1.5 million people were engaged in health work, of whom only 143,000 were doctors.

SPECIALIZATION

The predominance of the hospital was intimately related to the growth of medical specialization. Experience gained in the European base hospitals of wartime furthered this development, which had quite different forms in different places. In America, GPs began to disappear as doctors of all sorts began to specialize. In the United States as early as 1915, only 23 percent of graduates stayed in wholly general medicine. In the United States, specialist practitioners treated their patients both in and out of hospital. In Britain and some other parts of Europe, specialization widened the divide between GPs practising in the community and consultants working in hospitals. The interwar years saw the proliferation of specialist regulation in Europe. In 1930 the Dutch Medical Association created a committee to register specialists and to specify training requirements. By the early 1930s, Italy, Hungary, Germany, Sweden, Turkey, and Belgium were considering or had passed specialist-regulating powers. The Danish Medical Association kept a list of all recognized specialists. In France, however, specialists proliferated without check until after World War II.

In America, the family doctor was disappearing. It is not hard to see why. A report of 1932 showed that full-time specialists had an average annual income of $10,000 and GPs one of $3,900. The comfortably off went directly to consult a specialist rather than call a GP. Among the poor, dispensaries and clinics offered specialist advice in return for teaching and research opportunities for junior staff. It was the mass of wage earners in the United States that made most use of the GP. One of the reasons for the differences with Europe, where GPs remained, was that in many European countries welfare schemes tied patients to practitioners. In the United States, welfare schemes scarcely got off the ground. Fundamentally,

271

however, the move to specialize in America must have been driven by the modernizing impulse that affected all areas of life.

By the 1920s, American specialties displayed gross diversity in their educational routes and certification methods (where they existed). Much of the initiative for regulation came from professionals, perhaps from concerns about standards, and also fear of competition. Formal specialization in the United States began with the formation of the American College of Surgeons in 1913 that conferred fellowships on 1,059 surgeons in that year. Founding members discussed various ways of certifying competence at large. Surgeons who were experienced and capable saw this as a good thing; those who dabbled in surgery saw a threat of professional control. In Europe, a higher qualification in surgery acquired from a professional body that limited practice, either legally or by consent, was common. To many American doctors the formation of the college was undemocratic, smacked of monopoly, and, it was said, demonstrated 'medical snobbery' (Stevens, 1998, p. 92). The college's examination, while defining competence, was not binding on anyone; patients and hospitals were free to employ any surgeon they cared to. The college, however, in addition to its examining activities, developed, with monetary help from the Carnegie Foundation, a hospital standardization programme.

Following the surgeons, internists (practitioners of internal medicine) strove to distinguish themselves by an educational qualification above that required for general practice. The American College of Physicians was set up in 1915. The college only had a small number of fellows. The contrast with Britain is striking. Membership of the Royal Colleges of Physicians in Britain was a mandatory rite of passage for anyone wanting to achieve success in *any* medical (as opposed to surgical) area. There was no such thing as specialty of *internal* medicine in Britain. *General* medicine in Britain comprehended a variety of areas that in America were distinct specialties. In the United States, practitioners in say, psychiatry, paediatrics, pathology, or neurology had a strong sense of specialist identity distinct from internal medicine. The American College never played anything like the part that the British colleges did in setting educational standards and in certification.

In 1916 the American Board for Ophthalmic Examinations was created. This was America's first 'specialty board'. It examined and certified ophthalmologists but made no attempt to control practice by licence. By the end of 1925, the board had certified 501 physicians, while about 1,300 doctors were practising ophthalmology on a full- or part-time basis. In 1924 the otolaryngologists formed an examining board – the only one formed in the

1920s. Standards in the subject gave rise to concern. The popularity of tonsillectomy and the high incidence of ear defects (many men rejected for the draft had ear problems) made otolaryngology a popular choice as a specialist sideline for GPs. More speciality boards were formed in the 1930s. A year after the establishment of the British (now Royal) College of Obstetricians and Gynaecologists in 1929, American specialists in these subjects formed a single board to certify practitioners. Operative intervention of some sort at childbirth (including caesarian section) was becoming common and there was real concern that the unskilled, notably in general practice, were causing deaths. The paediatricians followed the obstetricians in the same year. Other specialties followed suit.

To some doctors in Britain, specialism was a term of opprobrium when applied to anything other than surgery or general medicine. Others saw division of medical labour as necessary, desirable, and inevitable. These two views were embodied in the struggles between the Royal Colleges that wanted to keep medicine unified and the emerging specialist groups that favoured some division. Allegiances to the colleges remained, however, and the Membership of the Royal College of Physicians (MRCP) or the Fellowship of the Royal College of Surgeons (FRCP) remained the gateway to consultant practice even if that was as a specialist. An equivalent movement to the American creation of specialty boards never really got off the ground in Britain. Although some medical consultants specialized in areas such as cardiology, neurology, and neurosurgery, they were an élite few, confined to the major hospitals and had no special degree or diploma in their subject. Psychiatry in Britain, says one historian, 'was still regarded as more a public service than a respectable clinical subject' (Stevens, 1966, p. 42). There were moves to upgrade the status of psychiatry in these years. The Conjoint Board set up a Diploma in Psychological Medicine in 1920. In 1923 the Maudsley Hospital, an independent school of London University, was opened to provide early psychiatric treatment and research and teaching in psychiatry. In America, psychiatrists (formerly alienists) developed a strong sense of identity in these years, albeit with ambivalent feelings about neurology and psychoanalysis. The American Psychiatric Association was formed from an older organization in 1923. The subject's status increased within the profession as a whole (as measured by its incorporation in the curriculum), and in the public eye. The psychiatrists were united with neurologists in a board formed in 1934.

Confirming earlier trends, specialism in France grew much as it did in America rather than Britain. It flourished both inside hospitals and outside them. By 1935, 52 percent of doctors in Paris – nearly 4,000 practitioners – were specialists. Surgeons and gynaecologists at 15 and 16 percent respectively, topped the list. Paediatricians were a close third at 13 percent. Women made up 7 percent of specialist practitioners. Over 95 percent of élite Paris doctors were specialists; a situation English doctors would have regarded with contempt. What began as a metropolitan phenomenon in Paris moved to the French provinces where, by 1935, similar figures can be found. In 1930, fourteen professorial chairs in clinical specialty fields were in existence at the Paris Faculty of Medicine.

Little needs to be said about specialization in Germany. It had been accepted as a good thing before the war and all universities had separate clinics in medicine, surgery, paediatrics, obstetrics and gynaecolgy, psychiatry (sometimes also neurology), dermatology, otology, and ophthalmology. A similar organization existed in universities in Sweden, Denmark, Holland, and Switzerland. One new feature of the German scene, no doubt arising from economic circumstances, was the tendency for university professors (who were of course specialists) to establish private clinics, for example, the Charité in Berlin, a university hospital, opened private wards.

HOSPITAL PRACTICE

Perhaps one of the most striking features for anyone entering a major hospital in, say, 1925 and who had not visited one for thirty years would be the presence of new, often large technologies. The X-ray machine is the obvious example, but an Electrotherapeutic Department might well be visible, presided over by a radiologist or a medical electrician. Here, there would be installed such things as sun lamps (Finsen lamps) for delivering ultraviolet (UV) light to patients with, for example, skin diseases or to children with rickets (Fig. 3.2). Victims of cancer in the 1920s might be treated by deep X-ray machines, 'radium collars', and 'radium bombs'. In the 1930s, those with gynaecological or head and neck tumours might meet another radium-based device, the 'external beam machine'. In the late 1930s, polio sufferers might be found in iron lungs. A large ECG machine might be installed in a basement although, later, smaller more portable versions that could be brought to the patient's bed would be in evidence (Fig. 3.3). Any hospital that aspired to be modern would have a special room with apparatus for eye testing. Patients with suspected thyroid disorders might be taken to a biochemical laboratory where they would breathe air into a 'Douglas bag'. From this, a technician or perhaps a physiologist would take samples and measure the oxygen and carbon dioxide content with a van

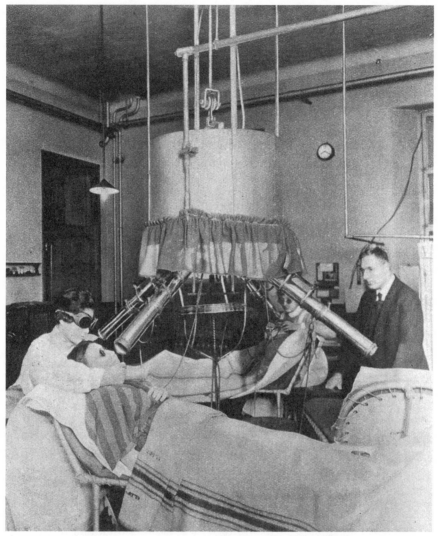

Fig. 3.2. Finsen lamp treatment, Guy's Hospital, London, 1925. In order for the UV rays sufficiently to penetrate the skin, a section of rock crystal was held in place by a nurse and water circulated to prevent burns. *Source: Illustrated London News*, 166 (1925), 16. *Credit:* Wellcome Library, London (L0016005).

Slyke apparatus (p. 307). The Basal Metabolic Rate could then be calculated and thus a laboratory measurement could be added to a clinical judgement.

On a smaller scale, patients would encounter many technologies at the bedside. A good number of these had been invented before the war, but their wholesale importation into medicine was an interwar phenomenon. Besides the familiar stethoscope and one or two other scopes and speculae,

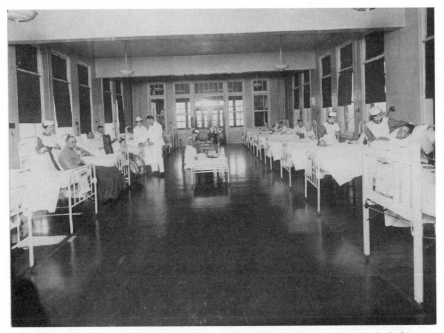

Fig. 3.3. Nurses and medical staff carry out tests and attend patients at the bedside in a ward at Long Hospital, Indianapolis, Indiana, *c.* 1920–5. *Source and credit:* Photograph, Indiana University, Purdue University Indianapolis, University Library Special Collections and Archives.

patients might now have their blood pressure taken with a sphygmo-manometer. By the outbreak of World War II, this might have become a routine investigation. Many patients with suspected neurological disorders would have a lumbar puncture. The cerebrospinal fluid might be examined microscopically by a junior doctor in a ward side room. Pus cells would provide evidence of meningitis. He or she might also estimate the protein present with an Esbach's tube (another test for meningitis). But the fluid might also be sent to a bacteriology lab for culture and a Wassermann reaction (for syphilis) and to a biochemical lab for variety of tests (in the 1920s raised chloride levels were recognized as being a strong indication of tuberculous meningitis). Patients with suspected gastrointestinal disorders might be required to swallow a 'Sahli's' tube so that their gastric hydrochloric acid could be measured before and after a 'test meal'. Although taking blood with a syringe for haemoglobin estimations and cell counts had been instituted before the war, the practice became much more common after it. By this time, too, blood would also be sent to a biochemistry department where, by 1930, a technician could perform at least thirty tests. The introduction of insulin in 1923 was accompanied by a large demand for blood sugars. At the Edinburgh Royal Infirmary, blood glucose tests performed per annum jumped from twenty-one in 1921 to 682 in 1923. By 1930, they had reached 1,197. The routine use of blood tests or X-rays on nearly every patient was a late-twentieth-century phenomenon, however, and many patients might enter and leave hospital without any investigation beyond physical examination at the bedside.

One set of tests already routinized before 1914 and that retained a routine presence and increased in importance after that date was done on the urine. The vast majority of these tests gave normal results. The post–World War I period, however, revealed a trend to multiple analyses. At the Pennsylvania hospital in 1909, 73 percent of patients who had a urine test had it done once only. By 1930, 70 percent had more than one test. Multiple examinations were, of course, common in diabetics even before the introduction of insulin. What was happening here, and it can also be witnessed in blood testing, is that the criteria used in monitoring a patient were being subtly altered. Laboratory data were displacing the patient's own assessment or unassisted clinical judgement as measures of the career of an illness. In the process, definitions of disease were being changed.

Before the Great War, the use of X-ray, except in special instances (war, legal cases, and sometimes fractures), seems, rather like urine examination, to have had as much symbolic value as it had a practical one. It signalled that medicine was scientific. Only in the interwar years was it made a regular part of patient management. In 1900 at the Pennsylvania and the New York hospitals, scarcely anyone had an X-ray. A decade later it remained an unusual event. Fewer than one in ten admissions were X-rayed and some of those images were made, says one historian, 'out of medical curiosity' (Howell, 1995, p. 112). By 1925 at the Pennsylvania Hospital, the number had risen to one in three (a figure excluding patients admitted for relatively simple, 'routine' procedures, notably tonsillectomy). The management of suspected fractures constituted a large part of this leap in numbers. At the same hospital in 1910, a quarter of suspected fractures were X-rayed and by 1925, with a couple of explicable exceptions, every single suspected fracture was X-rayed. Such routine became part of a new concept of what constituted proper care. For a hospital this meant employing a specialist radiographer perhaps to replace an enthusiastic resident who took X-rays when there was time. The move to routine X-ray use was not easily achieved, however, and was not seen as an obvious and necessary transition at the time. For reasons discussed in the following text many physicians viewed the growth of routine, specialism, the laboratory, and technology with apprehension.

HOSPITAL NURSING

Many of the contradictions and struggles that characterized pre–World War I nursing (p. 161–2) were featured in the postwar years. Nurses, their employers, doctors, and the public continued, often with little resolution, to engage in contests that had been part of nursing since the late nineteenth century. The image of the nurse as self-denying angel (and occasionally as sinister creature) was still used to anchor nurses in nineteenth-century ideals of womanhood (and keep down their wages). Conflicts still gravitated around the poles of occupation and profession, qualified and unqualified, hospital and community, and apprentice-trained and formally educated. Further unresolved issues involved unionization, general versus specialist nurses, and male and female questions. Two powerful, usually related assumptions, sometimes questioned and tested, sometimes taken as self-evident, were still important in this period as they were before and after. One was that that the general nurse should be the first goal of any training (and that the product of any other sort of training was second-rate); the other was that the hospital was the appropriate site for such training. These assumptions have been, until recently, uppermost in the historiography of nursing, hiding from view the labour of such workers as domiciliary nurses, public health nurses, mental nurses, and so on.

The need for nursing labour and the demands for better education for nurses were central to many conflicts in this period. For the most part, nurses were trained as residents in hospitals. In most places, this meant that nurses were poorly paid and received very little in the way of formal education. Training, practical experience, and cheap labour amounted to the same thing. In America, this way of doing things began to be challenged and the suggestion that nurses should have a formal education like doctors was seriously considered, and in a few places put into practice. Comparatively speaking, American nursing in one or two areas saw quite marked transformation in these years. The leaders of American nursing entered the Great War already strongly identifying themselves with their occupation and espousing professional autonomy and broader cultural values, such as efficiency, the desirability of a college (university under-graduate) education, and its socially elevating power. They marshalled support from doctors and other professional groups, gradually shedding the aid once offered by wealthy, philanthropic women. Nurses involved in wartime organization began to promote nursing as a career for college women (partly to ensure a postwar nursing élite). The independence and power of nurses can be measured by their success in persuading officials to establish an Army School of Nursing. A campaign for military rank gave them ambiguous status. They had the title of officers and the authority to command in matters pertaining to their professional responsibility, but without the pay or benefits of other officers. In America, struggles for registration occurred within individual states. By 1923, state nurses' societies had secured some type of regulation in all forty-eight states. The attitude of the medical profession towards nurses varied enormously. Some doctors were immensely supportive of educational reform and professionalization, others drew on older perceptions. In 1923 the liberal, reforming, academic Boston doctor Richard Cabot (1868–1939) observed, approvingly, how in 'the motive for nursing there is contained the deep desire that no one else shall have a harder time than we do' (Woods, 1987, p. 157). This sentiment, when internalized by nurses, was eminently exploitable. American nurses were much more vocal than their British counterparts in denouncing poor schools and inadequate training. The greater flexibility of, and competition within, the American educational system led to developments unthinkable in other places. Universities in the United States began to offer degrees in nursing or college degrees in other subjects and a nursing diploma. Not surprisingly, the Rockefeller Foundation took an interest in nursing. A report published under its auspices in 1923 recommended broad reform in nursing education, recognizing that in hospital schools 'the health and strength of students are frequently sacrificed to practical hospital exigencies.' Consistent with its philosophy of supporting education and science-based professionalism, Rockefeller conceived of nurses being trained 'to conform to standards accepted in other educational fields.' In 1923, the foundation directors resolved to commit $175,000 to establish a university school of nursing at Yale. Developments endorsed by the American medical profession and by American society at large made specialization in nursing unremarkable in ways it would not have been in, say Britain. Nurse anesthetists, for example, were acceptable. America, between the wars, had a surplus of nurses but there were shortages in rural areas. Overall, the conditions of work and training for most American nurses showed little change from prewar days. Nurses with higher educational backgrounds did well, however. They worked in the private sphere or gained appointments at high prestige hospitals where advanced skills were in short supply.

To confine a discussion of British nursing to the interwar years is some-what unsatisfactory. It marks no period for the working nurse remarkably different from the pre-1914 years and the early post-1939 ones. Long-term continuities are much more striking than change. Indeed, in some respects, for all that World War I did for women and, at first sight, for nurses, it might just as well not have happened. British nursing, like its counterpart in America, took its colour from society at large. The war cer-tainly changed many women's perceptions of their place in society. Women workers had become more assertive during the war. In Britain, after the armistice, many nurses who perhaps had little in common with their sis-ters in the great voluntary hospitals, joined unions such as the National Asylum Workers Union and the Poor Law Workers' Trade Union. The war had an important consequence on paper for British nurses. In 1919 the General Nursing Council was set up by statute (in the face of opposition) to maintain a register of all trained nurses. This measure in part resulted from occupational pressure in response to the flooding of the market by VADs and worries about competition. It was also an administrative accompani-ment to the formation of the Ministry of Health and the centralization of health policy. Hailed by some as a coming of age of British nursing, from another perspective the register looks as conservative and class-ridden as the society that gave rise to it. It came as near to creating a closed shop as any profession would dare that did not wish to be stigmatized as a covert trade union. It contained a general register and supplementary ones for men, and nurses caring for the mentally ill, sick children, fever patients, and the mentally deficient. Education of nurses was not a priority of the council. In this area it was virtually powerless anyhow, except for devis-ing an examination and admitting those who passed it to the register. It did not prevent practice among unregistered nurses. Control over nursing education remained firmly in the hands of hospital schools. As in America, the life of the ordinary working nurse changed little although she would have had around her more younger women and fewer widows and married women. For a variety of reasons in the interwar years, not least because medical practice became more technologically complex, large acute care hospitals experienced a nursing shortage even though numbers of nurses increased. There were over 111,000 female nurses in Britain in 1921 and over 138,000 in 1931. Male nurse numbers in these years jumped from 11,000 to 15,000. Probationers were an essential source of cheap labour, but hospitals found it difficult to attract them in the face of financial diffi-culty and the increasing opportunities for women elsewhere. The nursing life for many remained restrictive and severely disciplined. No movement for university undergraduate education appeared (let alone postgraduate as in the United States). In line with the views of the élite of the medical profession, specialization was not set as the highest goal to which a nurse could aspire unless it was in an area such as dietetics. This latter, perhaps, was seen as a woman's natural sphere.

NEW DISEASES

Doctors in hospital in the interwar years continued to use most of the diagnostic categories of the prewar period and a good many of the same treatments. There were important innovations though, and many subtle conceptual shifts in thinking about disease and therapy. Physiological or functional thinking about disease, especially when this could be quantified by technology or be based on the experimental laboratory sciences, became more prominent. An older use of the term 'functional', applied to any condition that could not be identified as organic, was gradually marginalized. Diseases such as neurasthenia and 'weak heart' were no longer seen in any hospital that thought itself modern, although these conditions remained a handsome source of income when diagnosed by private practitioners in wealthy private patients.

Medical specialization is sometimes seen as 'natural', as though it was the forced consequence of new and more knowledge. The reverse is more the case. Specialization is often a goal sought after by practitioners within general medicine or surgery who seek to change knowledge often by employing new resources, such as the X-ray or the laboratory. In the mid-twentieth century such developments were overwhelmingly associated with élite hospital doctors. An extremely good example of the various new forces at work within and outside medicine is seen in the refashioning of pernicious anaemia. Described by many observers in various ways in the late nineteenth and early twentieth centuries, pernicious anaemia was a name given to a disorder said to have protean manifestations. It was agreed, however, that all cases showed a diminution of red blood cells and the appearance of blood cells of unusual form (megaloblasts). For many among the older generation of élite clinicians around the time of the Great War, the disease was seen as the product of various social and personal factors, such as overwork, the stresses of modern life, and excessive drinking. Thus, concerned as they were with the disease's haematological dimensions, which could be investigated in the laboratory, they also saw the disorder as part of the 'moral matrix' of patient's lives (Wailoo, 1997, p. 117). That is, the disease provided the physician with the opportunity to fulfil the older role as counsellor in addition to that of healer. This view of pernicious anaemia was challenged by the rise of specialism. Specialists of various sorts claimed that their expert knowledge of an organ, system, or technique gave them privileged insight into the disease. All agreed that there were blood changes in the disease, but many saw them as epiphenomena. The real cause lay elsewhere. Surgeons claimed splenectomy (removal of the spleen) cured the disease. Gastroenterologists said the problems lay in the gastric mucosa and that hydrochloric acid was a beneficial remedy. The disease (if there was a single entity) also manifested neurological symptoms and, unsurprisingly, neurologists discovered the cause in disintegration of the nervous tissue. In other words, doctors who were active in marking out special areas of expertise, found the essential fault of many general diseases to lie in the physiology of a particular tissue, organ, or system.

By the 1920s, Harvard University and the Boston hospitals constituted a major centre for the most up-to-date medical research offering opportunities for combined ward and laboratory studies. Here, two clinical researchers, George Minot (1885–1950) and William Murphy (1892–1987) obtained a great deal of time, space, and resources to study their chosen field: pernicious anaemia. In 1926, in *The Journal of the American Medical Association* (JAMA) they announced that they had fed a large number of pernicious anaemia sufferers liver and had restored them to health. The therapeutic focus of their study was diet and the measure of its efficacy was symptomatic and haematological improvement. What ensured the success of their claim was the involvement of the Eli Lilly pharmaceutical firm. This involvement resulted in an unappreciated transformation in the understanding of pernicious anaemia. The interwar years saw new relations develop between drug companies and academic medicine. Close bonds were forged with the result that firms marketed tests and therapies devised in academic environments. By 1928, Eli Lilly was marketing 'Liver Extract No. 343' with the approval of the 'Harvard Pernicious Anemia Commission'. What was marketed, however, was not just a drug but a definition of what pernicious anaemia was. Physicians trying the extract reported satisfactory results in many cases although not in all. A study from Michigan reported a 20 percent failure rate. What happened, however, is that so dramatic were the results of therapy in many cases that physicians began to describe patients who did not respond to liver extract as 'atypical' or not even suffering from pernicious anaemia at all. The therapy was being turned into a diagnostic test. Some physicians found this objectionable. It smacked of empiricism rather than scientific understanding. The problem of how to account for unsuccessful treatments was dealt with in various ways. One worker classified unrelieved neurological cases as 'combined system disease' (Wailoo, 1997, p. 127). What is important here is that the reconstruction of a disease was intimately related to the rise of physicians having a laboratory interest in haematology, the expanding power of drug companies, and the large-scale transformation of academically generated and approved therapies into commercial commodities.

Cardiology provides another example of the creation of a disease entity. This specialty, as noted previously, was developed in prewar days as clinicians brought ideas from the physiology lab to bear on cardiac function, often by using the ECG. 'Heart attack' was a disease first defined in the interwar years as part of the formation of the specialty. A large number of figures were involved in the framing of the disease, but all were prominent practitioners, often with academic posts at large hospitals: notably James Herrick (1861–1954), professor of medicine at Rush Medical College, Chicago; Evan Bedford (1898–1978), a research scholar at the London Hospital; John Parkinson (1885–1976), a consultant at the same institution; and Harold Pardee (1886–1972) of the Medical Clinic of the New York Hospital. Chest pain of cardiac origin, infarction of heart muscle, and thrombosis in the coronary artery were well-known clinical and pathological phenomena before the Great War. Only in the interwar years, however, were they assembled into one disease, today's 'heart attack'. Characteristic ECG findings were slowly associated with the disorder, and by the end of the 1920s doctors in hospital who had never seen the disease were diagnosing it everywhere. Such diagnostic innovations often took a long time to reach GPs, especially those trained in older ways of viewing disease. When knowledge of this and other conditions did arrive at the periphery, it further encouraged the predominance of the hospital and specialization, as patients with a tentative diagnosis of heart attack were referred to hospitals for further investigation. Ironically, some of the figures involved in defining 'heart attack' were opposed to specialization.

The move to use modern laboratory-based physiological thinking at the bedside can be exemplified in many areas. Renal disease was reconceptualized clinically in this period, showing once again the shift from morphological to functional approaches. Bright's disease, for example, began to be edged out by talk of 'renal insufficiency'. Tests of dye excretion and urea concentration began to complement microscopic examination of the urine. Thomas Addis (1881–1949), a Scottish physician appointed to the staff of the new Stanford University medical school in 1911, became a world authority on the condition. His book, *The Renal Lesion in Bright's Disease* of 1931, used the word 'lesion' to mean disordered structure *and* the amount of lost function. Nephrology was not recognised as a specialty in America until well after World War II, but in the 1930s many individuals (clinicians and scientists) devoted their research time to renal problems.

As in cardiology, new conceptions of disease in nephrology and other areas were largely brought about by joint laboratory and clinical work. Laboratory studies will be dealt with in more detail in the following text, but it is important to note how many long-standing clinical and pathological-anatomical entities were now being envisaged physiologically and biochemically. Biochemistry began to displace physiology in some areas as a premier resource for thinking about disease. This was particularly true in the constitution of a whole new category of disorders: the diseases of metabolism. Medical textbooks began to use the latter as an organizing category comprehending conditions such as diabetes and obesity. The study of the body's acid base balance was made central to human biochemistry. At the bedside, diabetes, diabetic coma, and clinical signs, such as Cheyne-Stokes respiration, were increasingly conceived and managed in the light of the blood's actual or potential acid base imbalance (during the Great War it was in these terms that Walter Bradford Cannon attempted to understand shock). Directors of up-to-date clinical biochemistry laboratories in hospitals offered bicarbonate reserve measurements as a service to clinicians who wanted a guide to the acid base of their patients' blood.

In one area, the study of internal secretions, physiology continued to have a prominent profile in clinical work. This study was firmly established by the beginning of the period covered by this chapter. Nonetheless, biochemistry was made into an increasingly important tool for investigating the endocrine glands. Chemical synthesis in particular was profitably applied to the subject. Examples of some of the work done in this area brings out the dominance and cooperation of university departments and hospitals developing in this period. In 1922, on the basis of animal experiments and chemical techniques, Frederick Banting (1891–1941) and Charles Best (1899–1978) isolated an internal secretion from the pancreas, insulin, that was involved in the control of blood sugar levels. Banting was a clinician and his laboratory work was done in the physiology department of John J. R. Macleod (1866–1935) of the University of Toronto. Macleod took no great part in the work, but crucial to it was the skill of the biochemist James B. Collip (1892–1965). In 1925, Collip isolated an active parathyroid extract. Insulin was synthesized in 1926 by J. J. Abel (1857–1972), professor of pharmacology at Johns Hopkins University. Likewise, the active principle in the thyroid gland, named thyroxine, was isolated in 1914 (on Christmas day) by Edward Calvin Kendall (1886–1972), biochemist at St. Luke's Hospital in New York City. It was synthesized in 1927 by the biochemist Charles Harington (1897–1972) of University College London, and the experimental pharmacologist George Barger (1878–1939) of the University of Edinburgh. In the 1930s, Kendall and his colleagues isolated a number of steroids from the adrenal cortex. Deoxycorticosterone acetate was synthesized in America in 1937 and in 1939 it was used to treat Addison's disease by implanting pellets of it in the abdominal wall.

Most of the 'classic' diseases associated with hormonal deficiency or excess had been described before the period covered by this chapter, but in 1932 the American surgeon Harvey Cushing described his eponymous syndrome. Cushing's disease, a pituitary-based affliction, was defined in the context of Cushing's neurosurgical work. Endocrinology hardly existed as a specialty in this period. The conditions that textbooks of endocrinology described had been mainly appropriated by other specialists, for example, growth disorders by paediatricians, diabetes by internists or general physicians, thyrotoxicosis by neurologists, and problems of sexual behaviour by psychiatrists. Specialist gland doctors flourished on the lucrative margins of medicine.

Psychiatrists, if not describing new diseases, certainly revisited old ones. Using ideas derived from experimental psychology and physiology, notably Pavlov's work on reflexes, models of the mind were produced that rooted it in both the biological and social worlds. In America, one of the architects of psychiatry's increase in status was Adolf Meyer (1866–1950) who viewed mental disorders with a wide-angle lens, seeing them as maladjustments rather than diseases. In 1926, Meyer wrote 'The wider field of psychiatry now includes mental and behaviour problems outside as well as inside hospital walls.' Meyer's concept of maladjustment was, says one historian, the 'master paradigm' of the 'American School' of psychiatry of the 1930s (Pressman, 1998, p. 21). Within it patients were to be *restored* as functioning citizens. For proponents of this model, the shell-shocked soldiers of the war provided ample evidence of its truth. Psychiatry in America was setting itself up as the healer of a deeply troubled world. By the 1930s, psychiatry to some still appeared to lack the sound scientific basis that seemed to be rewarded by therapeutic success elsewhere in medicine. This truth was confirmed for many by the massive dichotomy between the extremes of psychiatric therapy. On the one hand, some psychiatrists, using the new synthesis that gave mind a material base, created aggressive physical therapy. On the other, some adherents of psychoanalysis favoured 'the talking cure' even in conditions such as schizophrenia.

Disciplines devoted to the study of the mind including psychology, psychotherapy, and psychoanalysis, flourished in these years. Most of them had techniques and technologies, often used by doctors or in settings with medical connections, for dealing with deviance and maladjustment. Child guidance clinics, for example, largely deriving their legitimacy from psychology and psychiatry, were founded in these years. There were 233 of them in America by 1935. Psychiatric clinics devoted to psychotherapy were opened, such as London's Tavistock Square Clinic in 1920. Psychoanalysis was riven by conflict over practice and theory. Splinter groups repeatedly formed new orthodoxies, and from outside, critics ridiculed its claims to scientific status. In the United States, psychoanalysis was developed almost exclusively within medical circles. Freud tried unsuccessfully to persuade Americans that the discipline was not medical (pp. 202–3), and after trying to have a 'detailed discussion with New Yorkers' on the matter, discovered that they 'betray just as low a level in this question as in other matters' (Schwartz, 1999, p. 175). Nonetheless, ego, superego, and so on became household words among educated Americans in the 1930s. In Washington, Harry Stack Sullivan (1892–1949) developed psychoanalysis as a tool (based on 'interpersonal theory') for treating severe psychosis. In Europe, psychoanalysis was much more widely diffused as a therapy and had many lay practitioners. Institutions for training psychoanalysts were widely established (e.g., the Berlin Institute founded in 1920). In Budapest and Berlin, Melanie Klein (1882–1960), a Viennese woman and not a doctor, developed the theory and practice of child psychoanalysis.

THERAPEUTICS

Although there were therapeutic innovations between the wars, to a great extent doctors still drew on the therapeutic arsenal that was available to them before 1914. Leeches, for example, continued to be used. Doctors continued to rely on aspirin, quinine, mercury, potassium iodide, iron, and potassium bromide. Salvarsan, arsphenamine, and neoarsphenamine remained popular in the treatment of syphilis. Within the new cardiology, digitalis was reassessed. Vaccines and sera stayed popular and diphtheria antitoxin remained the flagship of this sort of treatment. Various sera for the treatment of pneumococcal pneumonia were produced in the 1920s after the introduction of the prototype by the Rockefeller Institute's Rufus Cole (1872–1966) in 1913. These agents were produced commercially and also in European research institutes and United States public health departments. Only after World War II was there a massive jettisoning of old drugs from the pharmacopoeia. Although commercially produced, standardized preparations were increasingly available, hospital pharmacies continued to compound many of their own drugs. The market and the laboratory, however, did begin to have an effect on drug production. Combined clinical and experimental work led to the introduction of new agents. Insulin has already been noticed. After trials it was fairly widely available by late 1923. Problems of cost, however, meant that many patients received less insulin than they might be expected to handle. It was usually given in conjunction with a strict diet, and a good number of patients left the hospital with their symptoms controlled but their weights (often very low) no greater than when they were admitted. Like liver extract, insulin was soon marketed commercially, a variety of drug companies competing for sales. Vitamins, a number of which were discovered just before the Great War, were brought into use. Antihistamines were developed in the 1930s.

Optimism, following Ehrlich's work that many more specifics against infectious agents would be discovered (p. 183) was scarcely fulfilled, but a large number of synthetics, some of them effective, were introduced by drug companies. A drug that combated sleeping sickness (trypanosomiasis) was produced in Germany in 1916, and agents effective against malaria were synthesized in the 1920s. Not until the 1930s were any drugs introduced that were generally regarded as a significant innovation in the management of common bacterial diseases. These were the sulphonamides, the first drugs universally agreed to work in bacterial infections, notably pneumonia and meningitis. Attempts to treat cancers as analogous to parasites and to develop chemicals to target malignant cells were agreed to be relatively unsuccessful. Radium and surgery remained the treatments of choice. Penicillin was developed during the 1939–45 war and is dealt with there.

The persistence of the chemical tradition in German therapeutics alerts us to differences in national medical 'styles' during a period in which moves to homogeneity might seem predominant. Nowhere is this better illustrated between the wars than in French hydrological medicine, or thermalism, as it dignified itself. The French had always been a nation of spa visitors, drinking and bathing in the waters for medicinal (and other) reasons. The French medical establishment had, for the most part, long endorsed the virtues of its national waters. What is striking about the interwar years is

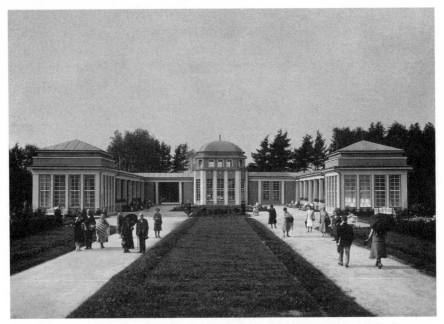

Fig. 3.4. Franzenbad Spa, Czecho-Slovakia. Visitors promenade the two paths leading to a C-shaped building that houses the Natalie Spring, 1930s. *Source:* Silver gelatin photograph, Wellcome Library Iconographic Collection. *Credit:* Wellcome Library, London (V0029817).

how intensely medicalized hydrotherapy became (Fig. 3.4). A vast industry was created with government, commercial, medical, and scientific backing. National pride, a long-standing tradition of spa visiting, and competition with Germany all played their part in this glorification of a national product. In 1913, an Institute d'Hydrologie with six laboratories was opened in Paris. By the 1930s, every medical faculty in France had professorial chairs in hydrology. The values of French waters were pretty well taken for granted and professors of hydrology devoted much of their time to collecting increasingly refined clinical evidence of their virtues. Chemists brought their latest tests to bear to discover, for instance, the presence of radioactive elements, rare gases, and the catalytic properties of colloids in the waters. Physiologists investigated spa products by injecting them into animals. It was estimated that there were 500,000 visitors to French spas in 1938. Hydrology also demonstrates how comfortable the French medical profession was with specialization. Different waters were said to have particular uses in particular diseases, for example, Vichy water in digestive ailments. Many doctors welcomed this opinion and turned themselves into experts on the diseases benefited by particular waters. Although spa visiting was popular in Italy and Germany, it was nowhere as near as medicalized as in France. In Germany, hydrology, where it existed, was a branch of physiotherapy. In America and Great Britain, spa visiting scarcely existed other than recreationally and there was no comparable science of therapeutic waters.

Psychiatry saw some of the most startling therapeutic innovations in these years. In 1917, for example, an Austrian doctor, Julius von Wagner-Jauregg (1857–1940) described his malarial treatment for general paresis (the final neurological stage of syphilis). The high fever of malaria was held to weaken the syphilitic spirochete. Results seemed impressive and Wagner-Jauregg received the Nobel Prize in Medicine in 1927. Pyretic therapy became something of a fashion in a variety of conditions. In the 1920s, an optimistic psychiatric profession in America that was endeavouring to synthesize mentalist and physicalist approaches to mental disorder, 'embraced a disparate array of therapeutic interventions that ranged from psychotherapy and occupational instruction to glandular therapy and colon surgery' (Pressman, 1998, p. 39). This variety, of course, reflected the fact that factions – sociological, psychoanalytical, and neurophysiological to name but three – within the profession pushed different approaches.

The origins of psychosurgery lay in research carried out in the lab of the Yale physiologist John F. Fulton (1900–60) in the 1930s. Fulton had described how a brain operation had altered the behaviour of two chimpanzees. In 1935, a Portuguese neurologist, Egas Moniz (1874–1955), practising in Lisbon organized a young surgeon, Almeida Lima, to carry out leucotomy (severing pathways between the brain's frontal lobes) on psychiatric patients. Moniz reported some success and the procedure was taken up by a partnership of a neurologist Walter Freeman (1895–1972) and a surgeon James Watts (1904–94) in Washington, DC. After several years they had performed thousands of such operations. Between 1936 and 1951, close to 20,000 patients had some form of psychosurgery in America (most of them after the war). In 1949, Moniz received a Nobel Prize for his work. For various communities, the apparent success of psychosurgery had many uses. For physiologists such as Fulton it could be used to show how medical advance was based on laboratory investigation (notably Pavlov's work). For psychiatrists who favoured organic explanations of mental illness, it was a vindication of their view.

Enthusiasm for psychosurgery soon led to the extension of its use for the treatment of everything from melancholias to severe, long-standing schizophrenias – a condition said to be characteristic of the so-called forgotten patients on the back wards. In Europe, Moniz tried his procedure in the national psychiatric hospital. In America, it was moved from private practice to the state system (the usual direction of the spread of innovation in that country – most physicians *au fait* with medical advance worked in private practice). Results were admittedly mixed and large sections of the medical profession in America and elsewhere were hostile. Psychosurgery was not the sole somatic therapy introduced during these years. Others included the 'shock' therapies that produced fits by injecting a convulsant or insulin, or by applying electric voltages to the head (electro-convulsive therapy, ECT). Between 1935 and 1942, 75,000 patients in the United States had received some form of shock. Overinflated records of cure using these therapies were caused by and contributed to psychiatric optimism in these years.

The controversy over psychosurgery and other treatments was the public dimension of an important contest that had gone on within the medical profession for some years and that embodied so many of the changes that medicine had undergone by this period. The issue had been set up in the prewar years and involved two questions: how were therapeutic claims associated with new drugs to be tested, and how were standards, such as constancy of composition of drugs, to be maintained? In fact, the latter question was addressed at first rather more earnestly than the former. From at least 1900, there had been concern in many quarters that drugs did in fact contain what they were claimed to contain. This issue will be dealt with later under the pharmaceutical industry (pp. 318–23). Here, we look at the clinical problems surrounding assessment of claims to efficacy. Traditionally, new drugs had been introduced by individual physicians who had relied on their clinical skills to evaluate them. From about 1900 on, and ever more noisily in the 1920s, academic physicians at university medical schools, sometimes in association with government research-funding agencies (e.g., the MRC in Britain), claimed that individual reports of efficacy were not a satisfactory mechanism for assessment. A drug's evaluation, it was said, should be based on experimental knowledge of its action and clinical investigation by a team of laboratory scientists and experts in therapeutics. Such proposals were not easily implemented. For a start, many university clinicians remained wedded to the ethos of clinical individualism and did not find collaboration and having to *share* responsibility an easy thing. Nor were there, in the 1920s and 1930s, clear protocols for carrying out tests (e.g., using controls) such as those developed in the 1940s. In an era far less regulated than our own, agreeing on uniform methods of assessment, let alone imposing them, was almost impossible. Many clinicians saw any such move as a further attempt to increase the dominance of the medical school and the laboratory in medical life: a move that was resented and resisted.

In Britain, the control exerted by the MRC enabled it to demonstrate, by example, how it considered a new agent should be assessed, even if its preferences could not legally be enforced. Soon after insulin was isolated, the MRC sent Henry Dale (1875–1968), the director of the biochemical department of the National Institute for Medical Research (NIMR), to Toronto to investigate. The MRC was granted the British patent to oversee insulin production, so it effectively had control of assessment and of quality. Several drug companies including Burroughs Wellcome, Allen & Hanbury, and British Drug Houses produced the hormone in Britain. Control of insulin supply enabled the MRC to demonstrate to doctors how it considered drugs should be tested. In 1923, seven university hospitals were chosen to carry out trials. In Edinburgh, insulin was put in the hands of Jonathan Meakins (1882–1959), the full-time professor of therapeutics. Meakins had hospital beds at the Royal Infirmary of Edinburgh under his control in addition to a biochemical laboratory. On his team he had another clinician, a physiologist, and a biochemist. They reported their very favourable verdict on the drug's efficacy in spring 1923. Their report documented animal experiments to standardize dosage, and clinical trials on large numbers of patients, monitored by biochemical tests. Remarkable though the efficacy of the drug was, what is also noteworthy is that the MRC was making a statement about how drug trials should be carried out and who should do them.

The words 'trials' and 'controls', in use at this time, did not have the same meaning as they did in the randomized controlled trials conducted after 1945 (p. 414). The word 'control', when used at all, had a rather different meaning, as the following example brings out. The growth of knowledge of internal secretions had produced a sizeable industry devoted to so-called organ therapy: the marketing of organ extracts usually for oral consumption and said to contain active hormones. Such products were advertized in the popular and medical press alike and were regarded with disdain not to say revulsion by academic clinicians. In Britain, in the mid-1920s, perhaps in response to insulin's cost, various independent doctors, usually in general practice, began to claim that the feeding of raw pancreas was just as effective as insulin therapy. This conclusion, they said, was upheld by their patient's well-being. The academic medical establishment reacted in horror. Such observations, it said, were made by individuals without access to laboratory tests and were thus not to be credited. What was at issue here were two ideologies. First, an older one, that valued individual clinical experience gained in the community and that took great account of the patient's subjective reporting. Second, a modern one, that valued hospital-based observation on a large number of patients by a team of clinicians and basic scientists, and that used laboratory tests to monitor a patient's progress and animal experiments to determine a drug's action and efficacy. Only in these circumstances, said proponents of the latter view, were trials properly 'controlled', that is managed. As in the case of pernicious anaemia described in the preceding text, ideas of what a disease was, how to identify it, and how to monitor its career were all undergoing change.

In 1931 the MRC attempted to increase its control over the introduction of new drugs with the decision to establish a Therapeutic Trials Committee. This body was charged with the operation of a scheme under which academic or commercial laboratories could submit new remedies for clinical trial. The composition had to be stated. Drugs accepted were sent to one or more clinicians for testing and successful results published in the medical press. An unsatisfactory report was communicated privately to the manufacturer. Although not legally constituted, the committee acted as a gatekeeper. Many drugs never got past the stage of first acceptance. In the period 1933–9, the committee oversaw the introduction of calciferol for rickets, digoxin for atrial fibrillation, and stilboestrol for menstrual disorders.

In America, there were, perhaps, greater numbers of academic doctors keen to control therapeutics, but also a mentality more resistant to legislative interference. In 1906, the American Medical Association (AMA) had created the Council on Pharmacy and Chemistry to judge the claims of drug manufacturers. The council took a jaundiced view of a commercial world that bombarded the market with drugs, good and bad, but found equally shocking the inability of ordinary practitioners to discriminate among preparations; a prescribing freedom over which it had no control. Attempts by American physicians to produce gold standards in treatment only revealed the depth of the problem. A Cooperative Clinical Group formed in 1928 by a number of academic physicians to study the problem of treating syphilis, ran into insurmountable difficulties. It endeavoured to overcome the problems associated with observations by lone individuals by pooling of data, but it discovered that even reports of practice from university professors revealed 'Astonishing variations' (Marks, 1997, p. 55).

Before 1938, control of drugs in America was regulated by the Food and Drug Act of 1906. This gave the federal government very limited powers. The Food and Drug Administration (FDA) sought greater powers to address the truth of therapeutic claims, but ran into a morass of objections and difficulties in framing administrative arrangements. A scandal catalysed action. By 1937, the side effects of the new sulphanilamide drugs were causing concern. One drug company, S. E. Massengill began to market a sulphanilamide as an elixir with ethyl diglycerol, a known toxic antifreeze. One hundred and six deaths followed its use and in 1938, the Federal Food, Drug and Cosmetic Act was passed. The act required firms to demonstrate drugs were 'safe for use' with respect to the labelling (Marks, 1997, p. 71).

SURGERY

Surgery had developed the profile of a powerful therapy by the turn of the nineteenth and twentieth centuries. By this time abdominal and cranial surgery had been created. The interwar years did not see any transformations of such profundity. Nonetheless, surgeons extended their grip on the body's interior (Fig. 3.5). Blood transfusion and better anaesthesthetic and aseptic techniques made operations safer as did specialization and the weeding out of less competent practitioners. Blood transfusion was usually by the direct method (donor to patient) until the 1930s. The first blood bank was established in 1937 at Cook County Hospital in Chicago. Local and regional anaesthesia were widely practised. The first academic chair of anaesthesiology was created at Harvard in 1928, and Henry K. Beecher (1904–76) was appointed its first professor. For surgeons, the white gown and rubber gloves became *de rigeur*. The use of blood chemistry, for instance to measure urea before prostate operations, improved patient selection. Surgeons also retained their place as muscular heroes in the public imagination. Through Hollywood they were to gain additional romantic gloss.

German surgical preeminence declined and more and more European surgeons took time to study in America. The first meeting of the International Society of Surgeons after the war was held in Paris in 1920. It excluded members of the former central powers and eliminated German as an official language. Members from excluded counties were invited back to Madrid in 1932. The society met every three years until 1938 when the venue was changed at the last minute from Vienna to Brussels because of the German occupation of Austria.

Surgeons created increasingly sophisticated versions of old operations and devised new ones for what were once purely medical conditions. Gastric

293

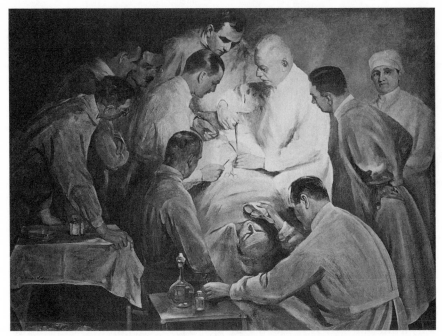

Fig. 3.5. Ernst Bumm (1858–1925), Professor of Gynaecology at the Charité Hospital, Berlin, operating on a patient while an anaesthetist administers ether dropped onto a gauze mask from a bottle, 1920. *Source:* Photogravure, Wellcome Library Iconographic Collection. *Credit:* Wellcome Library, London (L0002549).

resection for peptic ulcer became popular. The Dutch surgeon, Jan Schoemaker (1871–1940), was the acknowledged master of gastric surgery, and surgeons from all over Europe and even America came to The Hague to see him operate. His mortality rate of 5.5 percent for resection of benign ulcers was considered exceptional (some clinics had a 25 percent mortality). Appendectomy became common, almost fashionable. Artificial pneumothorax for pulmonary TB was virtually routine in sanatoria. Removal of lobes of the lung for chronic bronchial disease was occasionally practised. Lumbar sympathectomy for arterial insufficiency of the lower limbs came into common use until new drugs replaced the technique after World War II. Frontal lobe operations, as noted, seemed a good way to treat madness. Operations were created for conditions that are no longer deemed to exist. The London surgeon, Sir Arbuthnot Lane (1856–1943), advocated removal of the colon to rid the body of the focal sepsis that caused rheumatism, enfeeblement, and all other manner of complaints. The heart remained a no-go area except in wounding. One or two bold operators, such as the London surgeon, Henry Souttar in 1926, attempted to correct mitral stenosis by widening the valve opening with their finger, but they rarely tried more than once. Not everything changed: many anaesthetics were still administered by medical students and ether or chloroform (rarely used in America) were often given by simply tipping the fluid onto cotton wool and allowing the patient to inhale. In America, a unique occupation was created, the nurse anesthetist.

Surgery continued to change its institutional location to the hospital. The size and availability of the facilities (e.g., a large, well-lit operating space and autoclaves), administrative efficiency, and access to other services, such as radiology and biochemistry, made surgery in the patient's home look primitive. It was not only the variety of operations and the place of surgery that changed, there were changes in scale. A study of a Pennsylvania hospital has shown that in 1900 the total number of operations performed was 870 and in 1925 it was 4,180. The author of this study notes that in 1895 'the most frequently performed operation was excision of cervical adenitis [inflammed neck glands], usually tuberculous, which was done only 25 times. Three decades later in 1925, surgeons performed 1,356 tonsillectomies and/or adenoidectomies, 234 appendectomies, 98 inguinal hernia repairs, and 39 thyroidectomies' (Howell, 1995, p. 59). A 1932 national study found tonsillectomy to account for about a third of all operations. Tonsils, like the colon, were held to harbour foci of sepsis. Everything from insanity to arthritis was ascribed to these pockets of filth. Tonsillectomy was an important source of income for many practitioners. In spite of all these gestures to modernity no one had much idea of the long-term outcome of these operations; surgical record keeping was in a sorry state. In America, the College of Surgeons soon got on the case and embarked on a mission to upgrade and standardize clinical records.

THE UNIVERSITY MEDICAL SCHOOL

As noted, the university medical school and an associated hospital became more prominent in this period. Obviously much more so in Britain and the United States where they once represented but one possible place to receive a medical education. With varying success in these countries, attempts were made to establish full-time professorial chairs in clinical subjects. In France, too, educational reformers increasingly came to the view that teaching and research should be integrally related in universities, a position long established in Germany. By now, nearly all teaching in the basic medical sciences, such as in physiology, was done by full-time researchers. Many medical schools added lectureships and sometimes chairs in new subjects recently added to the preclinical curriculum, such as biochemistry or physiological chemistry, as it was also known. Philanthropic money played a huge part in the reorganization of medical schools in some countries.

In Britain, the Haldane Report (1913) on University Education in London had been shelved during the war. The report was in favour of the full-time model of medical professorships and the proscription of private practice. Its implementation began in 1919 when full-time directors of medical and surgical units started work. At St. Thomas's Hospital a part-time director of a surgical unit also started in 1919. Whole-time directors of medical and surgical units started at the London Hospital in 1920. The cost of these units was borne in part by the University Grants Committee (UGC). These grants were conditional on various other changes being made at the schools. At St. Bartholomew's, for example, there were to be improvements made to clinical teaching, and laboratories to be established in relation to the wards. St. Bartholomew's solved the first problem internally and the second through a grant of £10,000 from the Trustees of the Sir William Dunn Fund (which also funded a school of pathology at Oxford). Other schools soon followed suit. T. R. Elliott (1877–1961) was appointed professor and Director of the Medical Unit at University College Hospital in late 1920. Louise McIlroy (1878–1968) was appointed to a chair in obstetrics and gynaecology at the Royal Free Hospital in 1921. The Royal Free admitted only women medical students until 1947. McIlroy had a distinguished career behind her before the appointment, but getting on in London medicine was far from easy for either men or women. The unit system may have appeared meritocratic, but promotion could still depend on connections and educational background as it had in the Victorian world and still did in the voluntary sector. The few women who were successful in London medicine often had to rely on their upbringing and string pulling in addition to their talents and hard work.

Outside London, universities instituted full-time professorships on their own initiative. As noted, Jonathan Meakins was appointed Professor of Therapeutics at Edinburgh in 1919. By 1944, there were seven medical units in England and Wales. For the most part, the men and women who held these chairs had distinguished research records. For instance, Hugh MacLean (1879–1957), medical professor at St. Thomas's, was an authority on the hot subject of the day, acid base balance. Those who approved of the unit system regarded the hospital world outside of it as consisting of antique survivals. The American educationalist, Abraham Flexner (1866–1959), whose famous *Report* and 'crusading zeal' for reform was dealt with in the last chapter, noted disapprovingly in 1925 that in British hospitals, 'promotions are usually made on the basis of seniority [i.e., not a research record], inbreeding is common' (Flexner, 1925, p. 28). The unit system was not greeted with universal approbation. Some consultants approved of promotion by the seniority system as due reward for loyal service. Such doctors gave their time voluntarily to teach and practise in the hospitals and regarded the full-time professors with a degree of disdain. This discomfort was part of a more general uneasiness with modernization.

Academic medicine in Britain seemed just about capable of taking off but it was philanthropic money, noticeably Rockefeller money that kept it airborne. In 1919 the foundation created a division of medical education. This was presided over by Richard M. Pearce (1874–1930) until 1930, and then by Alan Gregg (1890–1957). Both men were shrewd operators. Both were proponents of academic medicine and both acted by singling out like-minded powerful allies at home and abroad. They commissioned many surveys, carefully choosing sympathetic observers. In Britain, Pearce relied heavily on Sir Walter Morley Fletcher (1873–1933), Secretary of the MRC. Pearce earmarked the London University College complex (university, hospital, and hospital medical school) to be the flagship of modern medicine in Britain. Between 1920–3 it received a massive £1,205,000 from the foundation. Among other things, Rockefeller aided the unit system by raising the number of beds. It endowed an institute of zoology and comparative anatomy. It funded laboratories at St. Thomas's, the London Hospital, and the Royal Infirmary of Edinburgh. At Cambridge, it funded pathology and biochemistry. There were always strings, of course. Pearce would never advise his trustees to cough up unless the end was to be what he called a 'true university clinic'. Such a programme was far from parochial. Pearce had, he said, worked out a programme that he 'considered wise for the Empire, the Dominions and the Colonies' (Fisher, 1978, p. 36).

Medical schools of the university type had developed in Germany, Scandinavia, Holland, and German-speaking Switzerland, well before the war. In structure, German medicine remained unchanged. Flexner surveyed European medical education and in 1925 considered that, by 1910, German medicine had reached its zenith and he saw signs of decline. He still thought that the German universities stood 'as a group the best organized, the best equipped, and the most soundly conceived that exist.' However, he observed that the war 'administered a serious check to university medicine in Germany.' It was being said, he reported, that 'Personal, sectarian, and reactionary machinations have . . . become more mischievous; anti-Semitism is no longer disguised; the authority of the state has declined, that of cliques has become more powerful.' In addition, he added that money was lacking and 'apparatus, supplies, animals, books, periodicals are well nigh unobtainable.' The financial reverberations of German inflation, he noted, had made 'serious difficulties' for countries such as Switzerland, Denmark, Holland, and Sweden (Flexner, 1925, p. 38). Medical schools in Europe received Rockefeller money. Belgium got 4.5 million dollars. Significant amounts also went to Brazil, Lebanon, Australia, and other areas of the Pacific.

Flexner saw very little change in the French system after the war. The French professoriate he viewed as orientated totally to practical teaching and without scientific interests as he conceived them (i.e., laboratory work). He thought the whole system 'hostile to youth, originality, abundance or surprise.' With the exception of twenty-one 'scattered services' at the disposal of the Paris faculty, hospitals and universities had no official ties. The French system did not make for the 'team work' he found supported by the German and American university systems (Flexner, 1925, p. 22–3). 'Nowhere in Europe', he concluded, 'has ambitious youth a harder road to travel.' Although the French received half a million dollars from Rockefeller, they turned down $12 million so as not to accept full-time restrictions.

In 1925 Flexner observed that the medical schools of America, 'now fewer in number . . . are almost all in form, and sometimes in fact, university departments' (Flexner, 1925, p. 44). In America, in these years, proprietary medical schools gradually disappeared. In 1920 there was one women's school, three black schools, five homeopathic schools, and one eclectic school. There had been fifty-five such schools in 1900. The universities drove change in America where there was no equivalent of European educational ministries to initiate and orchestrate reform. University presidents and medical faculty deans, in pursuit of the survival and honour of their institutions or personal glory or the improvement of health care, or whatever, saw in the sorts of changes made at Johns Hopkins and Harvard, models for elevating the profile and standards of their schools.

Modelling nonclinical subjects on the continental university pattern was one thing, creating full-time clinical appointments in hospitals that were local philanthropies was quite another. As in Great Britain, hospitals had to be approached diplomatically by universities for the right to attach a hospital post to a university appointment. Hospitals, of course, might have much to gain in the way of prestige (and therefore voluntary donations) from such an arrangement. But they also might impose conditions that those seeking laboratory and clinical facilities might find irksome. Hospitals might, for instance, ban animal experiments on their property for fear of offending subscribers. The full-time professorial system did make headway in America, but not without resistance, notably from clinicians who in many places stuck out for the right to do private practice for personal gain. All full-time professors in America could see private patients, but fees went to the medical school. A full-time group was established in medicine, surgery, and paediatrics at Johns Hopkins in 1913. Other chairs followed and by 1924 there were, for example, full-time posts in psychiatry and obstetrics at Hopkins; medicine, surgery, paediatrics, and obstetrics at Yale and at Washington University in St. Louis; and medicine at McGill University in Montreal.

There was, of course, no central government support for university clinics in America. Universities, unless they were state schools, had to rely on their own funds and philanthropy. The Rockefeller philanthropies, ever the supporters of science and modernization, found masses of money to promote change. Between 1919 and 1921 Rockefeller Senior (1839–1937) gave the General Education Board $45 million for medical education. The board funded most of the first full-time chairs. To the dismay of the Reverend Frederick T. Gates (1853–1929), Rockefeller's advisor in business and philanthropy, the board aided state universities; psychiatry and paediatrics were established at Iowa State University. Canada received $10 million for remodelling. The AMA opposed the full-time plan. In 1914, the chairman of its Council on Medical Education called it 'grotesque'. The objection that the 'best brains' in medicine would not work under such a system was an objection to any sort of restriction on clinical freedom.

MEDICAL EDUCATION – QUALIFICATION AND LICENSING

Although the basic structure of undergraduate (or in the U.S., the M.D.) medical education was pretty well settled in many places by 1918, the consequences of war wrought economic havoc with the details. This latter was particularly true of Germany and Austria. Writing of scientific institutes in these countries in 1925, Flexner recorded that while the price, for example, of chemicals had risen by 50 percent, the budget of some scientific institutes had decreased by a third. He observed that 'the former full-time worker and teacher now supplements his income by any form of drudgery obtainable ... apparatus, and supplies, whether for teaching, care of the sick, or research are inadequately obtained.' He further noted that the 'throng of young enthusiastic workers, willing on hard terms to take the risks involved in an academic career . . . has been gravely injured.' Nonetheless, student

299

numbers climbed. Although costs had increased in the smaller European countries, Flexner was impressed in general and thought it 'an astonishing fact that small countries like Switzerland and Holland . . . continue to support medical faculties worthy of comparison with the corresponding institutions in Germany at their prime.'

France, he thought, 'can hardly be said to have held its own.' However, he considered the French type of organization and instruction more able to weather economic hardship than the highly developed and expensive forms of education and research of the northern universities. In Britain, costs had risen, but again, partly because of the more relaxed educational arrangements, it was easier to return to prewar ways of doing things. Indeed, no doubt because of his approval of government funding of professorial units and research, Flexner thought 'some headway' had been made in that country. When speaking of America, his customary and apparently detached tone turned into a hymn of praise. In 1910, he said, 'the country was, like England, far behind the times.' However, by the 1920s he could record that in spite of rising costs 'the leaders in medical education undertook far more than was anywhere else undertaken.' If things improved at all, they certainly got worse again in the Depression. A League of Nations report on medical education in 1933 was not surprised 'to find a crisis when a crisis exists in all spheres of human activity' (Bonner, 1995, p. 337). During the interwar years, Western medical education became more uniform largely owing to the increasing adoption of the German model. An American report of 1932 evidenced the business-like attitude informing medical reform in that country in its welcoming of efforts to 'standardize medical education'. Americans, indeed, took medical education worldwide very seriously, producing numerous reports, many backed by Carnegie or Rockefeller money. These reports are extremely revealing of American attitudes. Before the Great War, Americans found many virtues to exist in European education, after it they found most of these virtues at home.

In general, in this period, older forms of nonuniversity education were slowly killed off. There was, however, by no means close agreement everywhere on detailed course content (in the United States there was not even agreement on whether medicine should be an undergraduate or postgraduate course – which it was). Debate, argument even, persisted over the amount and nature of the basic science material and laboratory work that should be included in the medical curriculum. Just about everywhere it was assumed that a medical education should qualify a student to be a safe GP and that further education was required for specialists. The idea of general practice requiring special training was one that was largely discussed after World War II. Women made little progress, indeed, in some places there were marked reverses. Saving their places for young men returning from the front, London hospital medical schools that had admitted women in wartime closed their doors in the 1920s. The proportion of women in German medical schools dropped by 17 percent between 1923 and 1928. In America in 1910, 4 percent of medical students were women. By 1930 the figure had crept up to 4.4 percent. In the 1930s things began to pick up for women in parts of Europe, but looked no brighter in America.

In the United States, a minimum of two years' college work was required for admission to medical school. By the 1930s, of the seventy-five approved institutions in the United States and Canada where a full medical education could be obtained, only a tiny handful were not university schools. To practise in the United States required education at an approved school and a state license; many, but not all, of these latter were recognized all over the country. There were six medical schools in America (in Illinois, Massachusetts, and Missouri) not recognized by any other state than their own. Medical courses lasted a minimum of four years. Black students made little progress under the new regime. In 1938, 1.6 percent of all U.S. medical students were African American. Nine-tenths of these were enrolled at the two accredited black schools of Meharry in Nashville, Tennessee, and Howard in Washington, D.C. Opportunities for internship and residency for them were almost nonexistent. In general, young men from poor backgrounds found it harder to enter medicine as costs rose, the curriculum lengthened, and night schools disappeared.

In Britain, medical education was based on a group of resolutions adopted by the General Medical Council in 1922. This stipulated a fairly basic premedical education often far below that required by universities. The result was that, in London for example, there was a heterogeneous student population. A London hospital might have on its wards: students from Oxford with the B.A. degree that they needed to graduate in medicine at their own university; London University students intending to take a degree; and students with the minimal General Medical Council (GMC) requirements – insufficient alone for London University matriculation, but enough to proceed to the conjoint diploma of Membership of the Royal College of Surgeons (MRCS) and Licentiateship of the Royal College of Physicians (LRCP). By the interwar years new, 'red brick' universities in big provincial towns such as Birmingham and Sheffield were turning out large numbers of medical graduates. British medical education lasted five years, but matriculating British students were usually required to have more in the way of knowledge of the basic sciences than their German and transatlantic counterparts. Registration with the GMC was usually by degree, but the vestiges of apprenticeship persisted in the various qualifications that could be obtained from the Royal Colleges in England, Scotland, and Ireland (a separate country after 1921), and also at the apothecaries' institutions in England and Ireland. Observers from the Rockefeller Foundation who scrutinized British medical education in the 1920s found it sadly neglectful of the laboratory sciences and, in general, hopelessly backward compared to an American one. As in America, standardization reduced opportunities for the poor, and entry to the profession became overwhelmingly middle class.

In Germany, where all medical education was at a university, matriculation required graduation from one of the *Höhere Schulen* or secondary schools attended by about 15 percent of the population. In an attempt to expand educational opportunity in Germany, a law was passed shortly after the war to suspend, by 1930, the special preparatory schools used by the well born and well to do. Some Germans thought this had led to a lowering of standards with the result, as recorded in an American report, 'that the student body in medicine is less well educated than formerly and that many students are entering medicine now for vocational, financial, and social rather than professional opportunities.' In Sweden, where secondary school fees were small and universities free, peasants and artisans had the opportunity of studying medicine. In Germany, medical education lasted six years with a further compulsory year of practical experience. Because universities were state institutions, graduation was equivalent to a license to practice.

In France, university admission was secured by passing the baccalaureate examination after completing courses at a secondary school. Unlike anywhere else in the world a student might matriculate with an intention to study medicine after an almost entirely classical education. This was because all students were required to spend one year in the science faculty studying physics, chemistry, and natural history before proceeding to a nationally decreed five-year medical course.

Senior American doctors were generally pleased with the clinical education offered in their schools, but criticized the teaching of therapeutics and preventive medicine. They also criticized overspecialization. Their criticisms have a current ring about them. Therapeutics' teaching was denounced because it failed to impart knowledge of the treatment of common disorders. Mirroring this, American graduates complained about the large amount of time spent in the study of rare diseases. They felt the psychological aspects of disease were neglected and, as summarized in a 1932 report, they thought that in hospitals there was 'an impersonal attitude toward most of the patients.' American medical students were possibly the most closely supervised in the world. By 1923 there were sufficient positions for every graduate to serve an internship although this was not obligatory.

Americans condemned a feature of medical education in Britain that the British took pride in; its primarily practical character. British students spent lots of time with patients on a one-to-one basis. This, Americans considered, was the product of the desire to produce safe GPs and the medical needs of the colonies. The new professorial units described in the preceding text played little part in teaching because of their relatively small size and sparse distribution. Americans also thought British students had insufficient supervision. German students had the greatest freedom to choose their degree of supervision and the shape of their courses before proceeding to qualification, as long as various requirements were satisfied. This was a consequence of the persistence of the *Lehrfreiheit, Lernfreiheit* principle (p. 140), which could result in courses such as hygiene and pathology not having requirements for attendance but having an obligatory examination. Clinical teaching was largely by lecture demonstration conducted by a professor with a patient in an amphitheatre full of students. Anglo-American observers described German medical education as 'highly theoretical'. In 1919 the writer Karl Kautsky (1854–1938) echoed what Americans approved of in medicine, but turned it into a criticism condemning German medical education for having become a 'mass industry'. Universities, he said, were mere 'educational factories' (Bonner, 1995, p. 334). Training in Austria, Switzerland, the Netherlands, and Scandinavia was similar to that in Germany. In France, clinical education remained with the structure it had been given shortly after the revolution, and its teaching commenced simultaneously with instruction in the medical sciences. As in Britain, first-hand contact with patients was regarded as paramount. The Americans thought the result of such a system was 'obvious' and deeply unsatisfactory: teaching of the medical sciences was 'slighted'.

FURTHER EDUCATION

On both sides of the Atlantic in these years, the main assumption underlying educational reform was that a first medical qualification was for general practice and that any further instruction should be directed at potential specialists. There was, however, a growing sense that the knowledge and

303

skills of GPs might require updating. Medical postgraduate qualifications and institutions, mostly in the university sector, expanded considerably in this period, and institutions, such as professional colleges, fostered this growth. American philanthropic money was once again much in evidence in the promotion of advanced study.

Although in America by 1914, there was a handful of university medical postgraduate schools and a number of proprietary schools (several of poor quality), many American would-be specialists went to Europe to train. This was to change. Specialty practice in America was fostered by the growth of residency. Residency, established in few prestigious university hospitals before the war, was based on the German hospital 'assistantship'. It was a sustained period of specialty training following internship (this latter was not at this time an obligatory part of medical training). America began to get its specialist training in some sort of order in the later 1920s. The Council on Medical Education of the AMA published a list of approved residencies in 1927 (1,699 in 270 hospitals). Nonuniversity hospitals predominated over university graduate schools (Stevens, 1998, p. 156). In 1915, a year after its foundation, the Mayo clinic at Rochester, Minnesota, established a three-year training plan for postgraduates. This soon became a three-year degree programme of the University of Minnesota. By the 1930s, several universities had residency programmes that provided advanced training in clinical subjects leading to higher degrees, such as Master of Surgery, which was offered at the University of Toronto. Universities also set up advanced courses in public health work, the medical sciences, and hospital administration; this latter was surely a measure of hospital commercialization. At a less academic level, short extension courses were devised by various alliances of universities, state medical societies, and State Boards of Health (that in some instances bore the costs) to update specialists and refresh GPs.

Similarly in Britain, where there was central government involvement from the new Ministry of Health, attempts were made to create programmes in local hospitals to provide continuing medical education for 'panel' doctors. Also in Britain, as in America, new higher degrees were established, supplementing older ones. An increasing number of graduates strove to obtain one or the other of them. The new universities adopted traditional models, installing the M.D. or M.S. (Master of Surgery, sometimes ChM) and such like degrees. Licensing bodies in special subjects gave diplomas in radiology, ophthalmology, and tropical hygiene, among others. Two new institutions merit special attention. During the 1920s, there were repeated recommendations that a postgraduate school of medicine be set up. This was achieved in 1935 when such a school was opened at the Hammersmith Hospital in West London. It had whole-time professorships in medicine, surgery, pathology, and obstetrics. Most interesting about this development is that the Hammersmith was not one of the élite teaching hospitals but a municipal (public) hospital, the new school being partly funded by the go-ahead London County Council. The Hammersmith teachers put on courses that large numbers of students from the colonies attended, many in search of the higher qualifications of MRCP or Fellow of the Royal College of Surgeons (FRCS). Oddly for a country with an immense empire, British funding of research and teaching in tropical medicine looks comparatively small. By contrast, for a country without one, American funding in the guise of Rockefeller money was enormous. It appears ironical then that it was Rockefeller money that established the London School of Hygiene and Tropical Medicine, a postgraduate school, which opened in 1929.

In Germany, there had been an unofficial plan of continuing education since the beginning of the century. This was revived in the interwar years and training was given in hospitals and supplemented by radio talks and a special journal. For those intending to proceed to a higher degree in Germany, this remained the university M.D. The examination was something of a formality requiring a thesis and an oral examination. In France, there was no organized effort to keep the main body of the profession informed of current methods of diagnosis or treatment, but most clinics and lectures at hospitals were open to all practitioners. In continental Europe, there seems to have been nothing like the proliferation of the named specialist diplomas that graced Britain and America. In general, to attain specialist status, clinical attendance or residence in relevant, usually university-based, departments was required followed by committee approval.

Medical research

CLINICAL RESEARCH: NONINFECTIOUS DISEASES

As in so many other areas of medicine, these years saw philanthropic money pour into research. Although the name 'Rockefeller' immediately comes to mind, by 1930 there were forty major foundations worldwide funding various medical fields. Myriad charity-based research enterprises flourished, especially those devoted to cancer and TB. The British Empire Cancer Campaign, for example, was established in 1923. In all fields, workers put short research or travel programmes together from a variety of sources, such as equipment grants from their universities and bursaries established by local people. The extent of clinical research, however, was tiny compared to post–World War II developments. In Germany, as noted, economic and other factors began to cramp the research tradition. In Britain and America, it continued to grow, but not always easily. In many places, clinical researchers still felt themselves to be beleaguered minorities. Although a full-time clinical professor in a venerable old hospital might find some support among the staff, often there was indifference and occasionally hostility. More than once, modern ideas of how to carry out investigations rubbed up against older ones. The idea of teamwork that had been heavily promoted before the war began to be realized in many places although the lone clinical researcher using modern laboratory methods persisted. Indeed, by post–World War II standards, the isolation of insulin looks like 'string and sealing wax' science. Compared to postwar years, the U.S. government stood aloof from the funding of medical research although the National Institutes of Health (NIH) was established in 1930. In spite of claims by scientists, governments largely paid little more than lip service to medical research as the means to national health and greatness. In Britain, where governments did commit money to medical investigation throughout this period, investment was insignificant compared to the funds poured into armed forces research. The latter has been estimated at £2.8 million in 1932. In 1932–3 the grant-in-aid for the MRC was a twentieth of this at £139,000.

As before the Great War, the principal laboratory sciences drawn on by clinical workers were experimental physiology and bacteriology. However, prior to 1914, the physiology used by researchers to create new models of disease was, broadly speaking, one of pressures, rhythms, and electrical activity. Hence the introduction of, for example, the sphygmomanometer and the ECG into clinical medicine. After the war, as physiology became more orientated to chemical activity, so too did clinical research develop a strongly biochemical (including endocrinological) dimension. The home of this new direction of physiological research was the United States, notably New York and Boston. Thus it was that ambitious young researchers who had once made the trip to Germany now found a new site of pilgrimage. In North America, a number of schools, including Chicago, Cornell, Yale, Harvard, Johns Hopkins, Rochester, Minnesota, and Western Reserve, were acknowledged as preeminent. The Rockefeller Foundation facilitated domestic and transatlantic traffic to these centres by providing one-year scholarships for young, but proven, workers. The principle goal of any student's voyage was the hospital of the Rockefeller Institute in New York. Here, under Rufus Cole and the second director Thomas Rivers (1888–1962), appointed in 1937, researchers were expected to investigate specific diseases on the ward and in the laboratory. Rivers's own work was widely acknowledged as having contributed to the understanding of viral disease. In the laboratories, visiting scholars might collaborate with Donald Dexter van Slyke (1883–1971), a physiologist who was studying blood gases and acid-base balance, and reconceptualizing older clinical entities in metabolic terms (not with the approval of all clinicians). Such work had its technological payoff in biochemical tests that could be done in a lab using blood collected at the bedside. Similar lessons might be learned at Harvard with Otto Folin (1867–1934) who was devising comparatively simple methods for estimating substances, such as sugar, in the blood. While in Boston, of course, an ambitious young surgeon might visit Harvey Cushing to learn how to operate on the pituitary. From such centres, the newly initiated would travel home in the hope of converting colleagues and hospital managers to the modern, American, way of doing things.

At Vanderbilt University in Nashville, Tennessee, one of Cole's resident physicians, George Canby Robinson (1878–1960), became dean in 1920. With Rockefeller and Carnegie money, Robinson designed a new hospital and medical school complex built so that laboratories, wards, and university departments were all within short walking distance. The first building opened in 1925. At Vanderbilt, the surgeon Alfred Blalock (1899–1964) used the new facilities to produce widely cited studies of shock that combined observations on patients on the ward and in the operating theatre with experimental work on dogs carried out in the laboratories. A significant dimension of the Vanderbilt story is that Robinson, a scientifically educated clinical researcher, was also major subscriber to the view of the 'patient as person' and the 'individual as a whole'. This philosophy challenged what it saw as the depersonalizing elements of academic medicine. Robinson intended the holistic approach to be realized in the architecture of Vanderbilt where all aspects of care would be integrated under a single roof.

Nothing on this scale occurred in Britain, but attempts were made in various quarters to introduce American ways of doing things. Little in the establishment of the transatlantic medical style would have taken root at this time without the MRC and not, perhaps, even then without Walter Morley Fletcher, the council's dynamic and diplomatic secretary. Fletcher was a product of the élite, Trinity College, Cambridge, school of physiology. An extremely gifted organizer and shrewd medical politician, Fletcher's administration at the MRC was permeated by an ethos he had grown to savour at Cambridge. This identified disinterested research in pure science as the surest path to knowledge from which, it was said, tangible progress would follow. Biochemistry, the science of his close Cambridge friend, Frederick Gowland Hopkins (1861–1947), was earmarked by Fletcher as most deserving of support. To some, Fletcher's view had a morally superior, ivory-tower tone and smacked of a superciliousness still associated with the ancient universities. Certainly, to many clinicians at the Royal Colleges who approved of a 'try-it-and-see' style of research based on individual experience at the bedside, Fletcher's attitude seemed to amount to frank contempt for rather more traditional approaches. Fletcher once recollected that, in 1914, he met a government minister who observed, 'Well doctor I don't hold with research. If we want to stop disease we must give the people better grub and less dirt.' Fletcher said he agreed but wished the minister 'could tell me what better grub was and what less dirt was – for I knew no way of finding out those two things except by persistent scientific work.'

By mobilizing people in high places and maginalizing the unsympathetic, Fletcher managed to either directly control or give advice on the use of an incalculable, but very large, amount of the money spent on medical research in Britain. By his death in 1933, he had established an administration that he hoped would run on rails that ran forever. In fact, his successor, Edward Mellanby (1884–1955), was not particularly sympathetic to Cambridge nor indeed basic research. Beside the MRC's own money, no Rockefeller penny missed Fletcher's eye. Dunn money was turned to medicine by him, and medical charities looked to him for advice. Not surprisingly, the research, individuals, and institutions funded by the MRC had a distinct profile. For example, freed for administrative reasons in 1919 from its original obligation to fund research into TB, the MRC took little further interest in this leading killer. Where possible, Fletcher ensured money only went to workers (even when their studies were clinical), with impeccable basic science backgrounds. The MRC's own National Institute of Medical Research (NIMR), established at Hampstead in 1920, initially had departments of bacteriology, applied physiology, medical statistics, biochemistry, and pharmacology. Under the directorship, from 1928, of Sir Henry Dale it attained the same world status as the Rockefeller Institute. With Otto Loewi (1873–1961) of Graz, Dale gained a Nobel Prize in 1936 for work on the chemical transmission of the nervous impulse carried out at the NIMR. Unlike the Rockefeller Institute, the NIMR had no hospital. There is no known reason for this. Perhaps Fletcher did not care to see money going to clinical medicine that might have gone to laboratory research.

Between the wars, attitudes to issues, such as patient consent, seem grossly negligent by today's standards. Consent was routine in most places for most surgical operations, but not for clinical research. The use of patients in hospital to try out new procedures and drugs without asking permission, unless anything obviously dangerous was being attempted, was common-place, even the norm in these years. There were no formal guidelines in America, for instance, until the 1940s. Before rushing to judgement, how-ever, at least two things need to be borne in mind. First, most innovations would have been seen at the time by researchers as interventions in the patient's interest. Distinctions between experiment and a useful new treat-ment or test are by no means always clear today, and they certainly were not in a period when clinical research was being defined. For the most part, the employment of new remedies and their assessment, without consent, by blood test, X-rays, and more dangerous procedures, such as lumbar punc-ture, would have been regarded as good clinical management even though the results might appear in a learned journal as a research paper. Sec-ond, even though patients in public (including voluntary) hospitals were increasingly seeing themselves as having the treatment they were entitled to by right, the ethos of charity still reigned. In many places, the most senior doctors still gave their hospital services voluntarily and in turn deference was expected of the poor. It was not only deference that was expected, but, by a sort of reciprocity principle, compliance in the promotion of medical progress. How far the poor knew of, or agreed to, this principle is impossible to know fully. Many of them may have done so.

Nonetheless, beyond these grey areas, surgical operations without con-sent and human experimentation beyond the (then) normal bounds did go on at this time and not just among the Nazis. Although some episodes have only come to light recently, the charge of 'human vivisection' and the use of 'human guinea pigs' applied to the interwar years are not ret-rospective accusations, but contemporary ones. Between the wars, a great deal of anxiety was expressed that doctors might operate on people for non-therapeutic reasons. To a great extent these concerns were related to the antivivisection movement. In his Pulitzer Prize–winning novel of 1925, *Martin Arrowsmith*, Sinclair Lewis (1885–1951) described the work of a medical researcher sent from a fictional research institute in New York to test a serum on a plague-ridden Caribbean island. Planning to use the serum on only half the population to determine its efficacy, in contrast to an untreated half, he is told by the governor that 'as far as possible I shall certainly prevent you Yankee vivisectionists coming in and using us as a lot of sanguinary [i.e., bloody, he was being polite] . . . corpses.'

Many of the scandals surrounding human experimentation in these years concerned the use of prisoners, soldiers, and children, notably orphans, often with respect to vaccine testing. The following examples are from America, not because physicians there were particularly culpable in this matter, rather it is because historians have studied the subject in that country. In 1921, a New York journalist published an account of researchers using 'orphans as guinea pigs'. According to this report, a paediatrician and two colleagues withheld orange juice from babies at an orphanage to study scurvy. The children developed symptoms of the disease. This was not a clandestine study but published in a medical journal. Although something of a fuss was made, the authors were exonerated, the journal *American Medicine*, using the reciprocity principle, commented that the orphans had made a 'large return to the community for the care devoted to them'. In the 1930s, controversy raged around several trials of various polio vaccines during which children died. The most notorious human experiments conducted in these years, and continuing long after, were in the Tuskegee Syphilis Study begun in 1932. Rewarded in kind and money, black males in Alabama had the career of their disease studied until 1972 when public outcry brought the investigation to a halt. The men had been kept in ignorance of the purpose of the study, and penicillin, introduced in the course of the research, was withheld so as not to interfere with the disorder's supposed natural course.

As noted, holistic concerns were prominent among those who expressed concerns about the apparent trajectory of interwar medicine. Critics, however, did not have a monopoly on the perspective. Holistic interests drove the research of many modern-minded, academic clinicians. Like conservatives, they showed great interest in the bodily constitution of the sick and well, but they chose to study it in the laboratory as well as on the ward and to quantify their knowledge of it where possible. Paradoxically, it was the success of bacteriology that heightened this awareness. Bacteriological data alone, it was acknowledged, could not explain unequal disease distribution among people of different age, sex, social status, ethnic group,and so forth. Doubts about bacteriology's capacity to explain all aspects of a disease were often expressed in terms of a soil (*terrain* in France) and seed metaphor. Knowledge of the soil (i.e., the body or constitution), it was said, was as important as knowledge of the seed (the invading microbe). Work in

310

the basic sciences both drew on and fuelled holistic approaches. Cannon's work on homeostasis and studies of the integrating activities of the nervous and endocrine systems, seemed to bear out the importance of the study of the whole in addition to the parts. Although scientifically pursued, many of these studies were loaded with the cultural freight of the interwar years; concerns with race and national efficiency became increasingly prominent in them.

Between 1920 and 1950, over 400 articles were published by students of the human constitution in the United States. Like so many other holist-inspired investigations, constitutional inquiries evaporated after World War II. One of the most prominent of the many students of the constitution between the wars was the American George Draper (1880–1959). A man with impeccable training in physiology, pathology and clinical research, Draper spent most of his working life in the Constitution Clinic at Columbia University that he founded with private financial support during the Great War. Draper developed a taxonomy of constitutional types based on anatomy, immunity, physiology, and psychology. By the late 1930s and 1940s, constitutional studies in America were focusing on mental and nervous disorders and on the physique of persons working in different occupations. Later still, race and gender difference attracted attention and was notably present in the widely read studies of William Sheldon (1899–1977) who held posts at a number of American universities until he replaced Draper on his retirement in 1946.

Such approaches were not the prerogative of Americans. In Germany, the field of constitutional pathology that had been established by Ludwig Aschoff during the Great War (p. 259), was pursued by him and his pupils. Students of the subject made links to anthropology and statistics, and turned their focus from the soldier to the worker. Walter Koch (1880–1962), a student of Aschoff's, observed: 'Occupational pathology is actually the war pathology of peace.' Such studies took on an overt racial dimension, and warriors and labourers were increasingly contrasted with enfeebled civilians.

The interest of constitutionalists in mental disease overlapped with that of psychiatrists. In America, clinical research in psychiatry became as prominent and, perhaps, almost as respectable and exclusive as research into physical medicine at an élite institution. Rockefeller money and scientific approaches, infused with holistic ideas and ideals, transformed American psychiatry in this period, at least in its higher reaches. The reason for this lay in the wider programme of the Rockefeller Foundation. In academic medicine, physicians aimed to arrive at new understandings of disease through laboratory studies. But the vision of the foundation was to integrate the researches of the laboratory with the behavioural, psychological, and social sciences to achieve understanding (and hence management) of society and its problems at the broadest level. Underlying these goals was the belief expressed by Raymond Fosdick (1883–1972) in 1936, the year he became president of the foundation, that 'Body and mind . . . are one and indivisible.' Given the esteem in which the foundation held medicine generally, psychiatry, the avenue to mental health, was the obvious target through which to realize its wider ambitions. The foundation's programme in psychiatry began in 1932 and lasted twenty years. Approximately $16 million were spent on it, mainly in establishing departments. Money supported research into such fields as epilepsy, delinquency, conditioned reflexes, schizophrenia, industrial psychology, neuroanatomy, genetics, and sex. The programme certainly produced detailed research findings and was a massive help in raising the status of psychiatry, but, as to the achievement of its broader goals, its proponents had to admit at the end, there was nothing to show.

CLINICAL RESEARCH: INFECTIOUS DISEASES

Just as biochemical analysis can be seen as tying together research into noninfectious disease, in these years, so was bacterial typing the thread that united work on the infectious distempers. It was acknowledged by this time that the great age of bacterial discovery was well past and microbiological research was, broadly speaking, orientated to the goal of breaking down the great bacterial groups, streptococci, staphylococci, and so forth, into their various types. This was carried out using culture, chemical, agglutination, and serological techniques. Biochemical analysis was used to identify the substances that made bacteria type-specific. This was a project that fed into both the basic sciences and clinical practice. It can be traced in the study of the mechanisms of bacterial action and immunity, in the creation of new diagnostic tests, and in epidemiology and therapeutics. What is significant here was the successful use of technologies to stabilize laboratory phenomenon, say, the culture of the haemolytic streptococcus from cases of scarlet fever. When such activities could be consistently reproduced (and thus exported to other laboratories) they could, in turn, be used as the basis for more refined and coordinated inquiry.

Research into pneumonia and scarlet fever provide good examples of the interactions of lab and clinic in these years, but an analysis of work on typhoid and TB would have been similarly illuminating. As indicated, at the Rockefeller Institute and Hospital in New York, Rufus Cole and his co-workers began a project in 1912 that classified the pneumococcus (one of the agents causing pneumonia) into three serotypes. This work also associated pneumococcus types and their pathogenic activity with specific substances in their capsules later identified as complex polysaccharides. These findings fed into basic and applied biological research on bacteria. Rockefeller workers also developed type-specific antisera for pneumococcal pneumonia and for which they claimed good therapeutic results. Doubts were cast on these, however. The trial methods were open to criticism and the pneumococcus was known to be associated with highly variable mortality and morbidity. In spite of doubts, pneumococcal antisera continued to be tested on both sides of the Atlantic, and in some places throughout the 1920s and early 1930s, they were enthusiastically endorsed.

Typing research had other ramifications, notably in the study of scarlet fever (scarlatina), a disease in which the streptococcus had a highly contested role. It was known by this period that some streptococci had haemolytic activity – the power to break down or *lyse* red blood cells – when cultured in the laboratory. Cultures of haemolytic streptococcus proved an invaluable basis for further research. In the early 1920s a series of papers, notably those produced by George (1881–1967) and Gladys Dick (1881–1963), from the University of Chicago, claimed that there was an association (although some critics said not a fully proven one) between scarlet fever and the presence in the throat of haemolytic streptococci. The Dicks used a bacterium from a nurse suffering from scarlet fever and (by a circuitous route) were able to induce the disease in two out of ten volunteers. Using a toxin obtained from haemolytic streptococci, the Dicks found that a red reaction developed at the site of its injection in those who had never had scarlet fever. Although known to be occasionally unreliable, the 'Dick test' for susceptibility to scarlet fever was turned into a valuable public health and epidemiological research tool.

In reality, in this period it was recognized that a detailed classification of streptococci had not yet been agreed on. Resolution of this taxonomic muddle had potentially practical consequences, some clinical. Questions asked included: was puerperal sepsis (childbed fever), caused by a specific strain of streptococcus? If so, was a specific cure possible? Many attempts were made to develop antitoxins to scarlet fever, puerperal sepsis, and rheumatic fever, another disorder largely agreed in the late 1930s to be caused by the haemolytic streptococcus. These antitoxins were passive sera, raised in horses, analogous to the diphtheria antitoxin and used for immediate treatment. Some (particularly those for scarlet fever) were held to be successful and marketed by drug companies. Around this time, Rebecca C. Lancefield (1895–1981) addressed the problem of streptococcal typing by employing immune sera. Using this method she identified five groups, of which most strains of haemolytic streptococcus causing human disease (including scarlet fever) belonged to group A. This proved an invaluable classification for further research and the group was quickly divided into many serotypes by Frederick Griffith (1881–1941). However, no specific type was consistently associated with scarlatina.

The foregoing outlines the style in which bacteriological research was still largely pursued on lines laid down before the Great War. Such an account is only partial for it fails to take notice of the ways in which laboratory work and epidemiology were also informed by holist ideas in these years. A couple of examples will suffice. The first explores a follower of Eli Metchnikoff (1845–1916), the Russian immunologist at the Institut Pasteur in Paris (pp. 132–3). Metchnikoff was one of the few prewar bacteriologists who laid as much stress on the *terrain* as the seed. Metchnikoff had endeavoured to describe the *terrain* in concrete immunological terms that could be used to create therapeutic technologies. He died in 1916, and in the interwar years his ideas were pursued by his friend (and after 1918, head of his laboratory), Alexandre Besredka (1870–1940), also a Russian. On the basis of laboratory and clinical work, Basredka developed a view opposed to the prevailing antibody theory of immunity, which he regarded as an account based only on the body's fluids and which he called the 'test tube' model. Besredka described infectious disease as a complex interaction between bacteria and the body's cells, tissues, and organs. On the basis of this, he developed various bacterial products for vaccination. These he named *antivirus* which, he said, stimulated the natural (nonantibody) immunity present in the normal body. His views were not well received among immunologists. Nonetheless, Basredka's antivirus was used by doctors to treat boils, cutaneous anthrax, infected burns, impetigo, and so on. Pharmaceutical companies took up its production. Basredka's ideas did not survive World War II. His approach shows, however, that alternative immunological models were available for research and technological exploitation. His work should not be regarded as an oddity, not least because of its stress on the *terrain* not the germ, had strong affinities with the holist ideas used by French clinicians.

Another attempt to counter bacteriological reductionism was the programme of constitutional serology advocated by Ludwik Hirzsfeld

(1884–1954), director of the State Hygiene Institute in Poland. Hirzsfeld, whose theories are too complex to describe in detail here, attempted to use natural blood group antibodies (isoagglutinins) as a measure of constitution. He endeavoured to correlate them with disease (notably diphtheria, which he studied in Vienna and Berlin) and also susceptibility to disease using the Schick (a skin test for immunity to diphtheria) and Dick tests. His studies also included an ethnic dimension, drawing on, for instance, the work of research expeditions, notably to Greenland and Manchuria. Hirzsfield's approach was a mélange of reductionist and constitutional studies. After all, the idea that serology could be used to discover biological types was itself reductionist, and indeed, Hirzsfeld considered such types were genetically determined. Serology was just a feasible way of discovering them. Two general points stand out, however, that are not peculiar to Hirzsfeld. First, his work indicates the international interests of these years because he was able to draw on huge numbers of studies on race, blood type, constitution, and disease (the German Society for Blood Group Research, founded by Otto Reche [1879–1966] in 1926, was established mainly to distinguish race in the test tube). Second, although his conceptions of constitutional pathology were rejected after World War II, Hirzfeld's studies show how deeply such concerns had penetrated laboratory enquiry in addition to clinical medicine.

Hirzsfeld's work drew on epidemiological research. This discipline was transformed in these years and an 'ecological point of view', as it was called at the time, became predominant. Epidemiologists broke with pre-war understandings of epidemic diseases (and their control) based solely on bacterial properties. The exception was France where Pastorian approaches had consistently admitted of environmental inducements to bacterial virulence, and in that country, therefore, the transition to the new epidemiology was relatively seamless. Elsewhere, the lab as the epidemiological court of appeal lost favour as the conditions created there were seen as artificial. A new experimental epidemiology was established in which large populations of laboratory animals were exposed to infection under 'natural' conditions. Part of the explanation for this move lay in new disease patterns. Influenza and encephalitis lethargica were clearly not distributed like the old waterborne diseases, such as typhoid, in which 'bacteria tracking' had proved its worth. But again, wider holist concerns were at work shaping the discipline. Britain and America were the principle homes of the new epidemiology that was increasingly dominated by mathematical approaches. The British drew on the statistical approach (biometrics) to inheritance developed by

Karl Pearson (1857–1936) at University College London. Major (his given name) Greenwood (1880–1949), of the MRC's statistical unit, was the foremost proponent of the new methods and, interestingly, he admitted that he had searched for inspiration by 'looking into' Thomas Sydenham. This was a typical neo-Hippocratic move in these years, usually associated with reactionaries. Greenwood, however, was no reactionary; most doctors were pretty ignorant of arithmetic, never mind the new statistics. The new epidemiology started to add all sorts of elements into the explanation of epidemics: host factors, the environment, and the time and space between outbreaks. Microbial agents were seen as components of a 'state of equilibrium' rather than intruders. 'Complexity' was the word associated by Simon Flexner (1863–1946, brother of Abraham) in 1922 with epidemics. Although epidemiologists of this generation did not name their approach 'holistic', it was called that in the 1950s by a member of the community.

BASIC SCIENCE RESEARCH

Scientific work carried out far from the bedside was seen by many in these years as vital to future prevention and treatment of disease. Those working in laboratory sciences often based their claims for support on the position that research not immediately practically applicable, would one day yield clinically fruitful results. This position was developed in the late nineteenth century, and by the interwar years had become more widely, if far from universally, accepted. It is impossible to survey the whole of interwar basic science research here. However, cancer research provides a very good example, both of the organization of research and its rhetorical and technical impact in the public sphere.

The importance of basic research was a message extensively employed by those concerned with cancer from the 1920s onwards. Experts claimed that new understandings of the biology, biochemistry, and genetics of cells would soon be transferred to an understanding of 'deviant cells'. Various assumptions, the origins of which lay in the nineteenth century, underlay such claims. These were that cancer was a disease originating in cells, perhaps even one cell; that these cells could migrate; that therapy necessitated the elimination of every single cell; and that cancer was a unitary phenomenon. That is, whatever the cause, morphology or clinical course of a cancer, all were manifestations of one fundamental pathological process. Cure for cancer in these years was thus publicly associated with research in cell biology and high-technology therapy.

In the 1920s, researchers abandoned prewar theories of innate 'resistance' to tumours (based on rejection studies) when it was accepted that rejected cancer transplants were simply rejections of foreign tissue. Genetically uniform animals (i.e., those that did not reject transplants) became a major research tool. Importantly, the tool obviated variability, making it possible to exchange tumours and mice between labs that were working on different agendas. Thus, networks of researchers were built up. Studies of malignant growth were coupled with researches into artificial carcinogenesis using such things as hydrocarbons and radiation to induce tumours in the laboratory. As biochemistry began to become a visible science in clinical medicine during the interwar years, cancer workers turned to it in the hope that studies would reveal different metabolic pathways in normal and malignant cells. By the mid-1930s biochemists had elucidated 'intermediary metabolism' or enzymatic pathways of key life processes. By the late 1930s, experts were admitting that they could find no differences in the metabolic pathways of normal and malignant cells; differences seemed to lie only in proliferation rate. Between the wars, the pursuit of cell biology as the route to understanding cancer had done more for the understanding of the biology of the cell than it had for comprehending or curing malignancy.

Basic science, like clinical research, had its critics. From within the profession there were those who, although wholly in favour of laboratory investigations in principle, felt that, in what were times of economic stringency, money might be better devoted to more immediate patient-orientated projects. Many clinicians felt the basic sciences, especially physiology, occupied far too much time in a medical curriculum better devoted to practical work. Some within the profession felt that scientists occasionally tackled problems that were best addressed by common sense or at least straightforward economics. As noted, Walter Morley Fletcher thought the problems of nutritional deficiency were only soluble through scientific research. In contrast to this view, Thomas, Lord Horder (1871–1955), a St. Bartholomew's Hospital physician and perhaps the greatest English diagnostician of the day, believed, as he said in 1936, that you should, 'Look after the accessibility of food and nutrition will look after itself' (Horder, 1937, p. 152). These various doubts about basic sciences research were as nothing compared to the campaigns of the antivivisectionists. These continued unabated everywhere between the wars. Their public impact was perhaps less than before the Great War, however, because it was widely perceived that animal experiments had been vital to the production of vaccines, which were seen to have saved the lives of thousands of fighting men. Nonetheless, British experimental physiologists whose disciplinary history was very short, felt much threatened by antivivisectionist campaigns in the 1920s. Like so many embattled medical workers and scientists in this period they cele-brated the imagined longevity of their 'tradition' and its supposed 'found-ing' by William Harvey (whose work on the circulation of the blood was published in 1628), and they 're-created' his experiments and recorded them on silent film.

The pharmaceutical industry

The history of the pharmaceutical industry in the years covered by this chapter repeats many of the themes that have been identified in medicine at large. By 1914 the industry's modern structure, its ways of operating, and the ideas and assumptions informing research, production, and mar-keting were in place. The interwar years saw consolidation and growth in all of these areas. Quantitatively, changes were mainly confined to the wax-ing and waning of companies, to mergers and takeovers, and to changes in national fortunes. Qualitatively, synthetic chemicals, such as Salvarsan and the sulphonamides, began to become as important as the 'biologicals' – vaccines and antisera – on which the creation of the modern industry had largely been based. Vitamin preparations were an important source of income for pharmaceutical companies everywhere. In the United States, the wholesale vitamin market grew from less than $5 million in 1925 to nearly $100 million at the start of World War II. Hormones were econom-ically important too. New commercial relations were established, notably between companies and farmers and slaughterhouses supplying raw mate-rial to industry. In sum, during these years drug production became 'big business'. More and more were people exposed to mass-produced prepa-rations. Less and less did doctors, the local pharmacists, and hospitals compound their own prescriptions. Modernism transformed everything it touched. As in other areas, many welcomed it and some were suspicious.

On the eve of the Great War, modern, large-scale machine production was being used by some companies as were modern managerial techniques. The biggest companies, especially in Germany, were funding research and long-term development. They had also formed the beginnings of a network of relations with the medical profession, academic scientists, and government officials. For drug companies, as for the medical profession, science was presented as evidence of trustworthiness. Drug companies even produced journals that followed academic models. In 1914, the German industry was the powerhouse of innovation and production, supplying both Europe and America. The United States was becoming a large producer, but did little in the way of the development of new products. For a small country, the Swiss industry was comparatively large. British and French companies lived in the shadow of Germany.

The war years deprived Germany of its markets and the patents which gave it monopolies, even in the United States. This opportunity was grasped by American companies who began to fund research into new drugs in a systematic way. Formerly, American firms lay far behind those of Germany in terms of innovation. The strength of the American industry lay in its scale of production, quality control, and its exploitation of new markets. The infringement of the Salvarsan patent opened the floodgates. America (which did not enter the war until 1917) relied entirely on German suppliers for Salvarsan. The British blockade severely curtailed supplies of a drug that American physicians had come to take for granted. The drug was synthesized and then manufactured in the United States in 1915. England, France, Japan, and Canada followed suit. Dermatological Research Laboratories (DRL) that produced Salvarsan, or Arsenobenzol as the new product was known in the United States, won the contract to supply the U.S. armed forces. It built a huge production facility and eventually a profit to match. Salvarsan production infringed the German patent and legal squalls followed. The net result, however, after the United States entered the war, was a government bill effectively allowing firms to infringe any German patent they cared to.

The American move into new product development saw a massive expansion of a class of relationships that had been established in that country before the war but at that time had no great public impact; that is, between the drug companies and the universities. This, of course, was not a move confined to the pharmaceutical industry. In 1927, industrial laboratories of all sorts in America employed 19,000 researchers; by 1940 the figure was 58,000 (Swann, 1988, p. 15). In the 1920s and 1930s, firms such as Eli Lilly, Merck and Company, Abbott Laboratories, and ER Squibb began to employ university-trained researchers and to contract with university departments for specific services. Companies also founded research institutes, such as the Merck Research Laboratory. These were halfway houses between pure research establishments and product development laboratories. The Merck research team (largely composed of organic chemists) was one of the most powerful in America. Among its successes was Lewis Sarett's synthesis of cortisone in the 1940s.

By the end of World War II, nearly fifty companies in America were subsidizing biomedical research projects at universities. For the universities, collaborative effort brought money to their coffers, support for academic departments, and younger scholars by way of fellowships and so forth. In 1931 Merck spent $146,000 on research and in 1940 it spent $906,000. For the industry, research collaboration brought profit and a degree of respectability. For the doctor and the public, these interactions resulted in numerous new therapeutic agents in large, standardized quantities. These included hormones, vitamins, anticonvulsants, anaesthetics, sedatives, and chemotherapeutic agents. All was not sweetness and light, of course; university workers in particular worried about the shady reputation of some companies, and also about commercial remuneration and secrecy where disinterestedness and freedom of knowledge exchange were meant to be the norms. In *Arrowsmith*, Sinclair Lewis fictionalized how scientists expressed alarm and dismay when one of their number joined a drug company. Described as a 'damned pill-pedlar', the firm made 'excellent antitoxins' and also a new cancer remedy 'possessing all the virtues of mud',

Despite the war, the German pharmaceutical industry continued to flourish. It was based largely on chemical synthesis which had its origins in Germany's industrial supremacy in synthetic dye production. In 1916, in the therapeutic laboratory of the former dyestuffs company Friedrich Bayer and Co. at Elberfeld, William Roehl (1821–1929), a former pupil of Ehrlich, synthesized an agent, suramin (marketed as 'Germanin'), from the dye trypan red that was active against the trypanosomes of sleeping sickness. In the 1920s, Bayer developed the antimalarials plasmoquine and mepacrine. Further success followed when, in the late 1920s, Heinrich Hörlein became director of a huge pharmaceutical research operation based in several laboratories that combined the established method of chemical synthesis with physiological investigation and animal testing. In 1932, Gerhard Domagk (1895–1964) and Fritz Mietzsch (1896–1958), synthesizing variants of red azo dyes, discovered that those containing a sulphonamide group had a systemic effect on streptococci. One of the compounds was patented by Bayer as 'Prontosil' in 1935. From this, the soluble agent sulphanilamide was soon produced by two French scientists, and Bayer's patent was effectively undermined because many variants of sulphanilamide were synthesized and patented throughout the world: in the United States by Merck, Sharp & Dohme, Squibb, and Lederle; in Switzerland by Ciba; in England by Burroughs Wellcome and also May and Baker whose variant named

693 is discussed in the following text. In 1939, Domagk was awarded the Nobel prize for his work but Hitler had forbidden Germans to accept this reward and Domagk was arrested. He received it in 1947. The most interesting thing about the award, however, was the acrimony it caused. The synthesis of Prontosil was an industrialized invention, a modern collaborative exercise, to which the older system of individual recognition seemed inappropriate to other workers involved.

Compared to the size of the country's population, the Swiss pharmaceutical industry's world prominence between the wars was remarkable. True to their prewar history, the Swiss continued to rely on chemical agents rather than 'biologicals'. High-powered chemical research and synthesis were central to the strategy of the major firms. Hoffmann-La Roche suffered a setback during the Great War when its main manufacturing plant in Grenzach, just over the border, was closed down by the German authorities. The collapse of the lucrative Russian market threatened extinction and the firm was only saved by conversion to a public limited stock company in 1919. After this, the firm flourished by concentrating on vitamins, hypnotics, and analgesics. At the end of World War I, a dyestuffs company, Sandoz, switched its attention to pharmaceuticals. An academic biochemist, Arthur Stoll (1887–1971), built up a research department. In 1918 he produced ergotamine, which was marketed as 'Gynergen' for controlling postpartum haemorrhage. Modelling themselves on the six German dyestuffs and drugs manufacturers (including Bayer) that had merged in 1925 to form the powerful IG Farben conglomerate, the Basel firms Ciba, Sandoz, and Geigy united to form a combine that divided activities and pooled profits.

Britain, and to a greater extent France, were minor players in the drugs' league between the wars. In 1914, the British drug companies, often family-based and concerned with protecting their markets, relied heavily on continental suppliers. Indeed, during the war, many major contracts to supply the armed forces had to be given to U.S. companies, although Burroughs Wellcome was making its own brand of Salvarsan ('Kharvisan') soon after the American synthesis. Reputable drug companies in Britain also faced fierce competition from unscrupulous manufacturers because Britain's regulatory laws were notoriously lax or nonexistent. The Therapeutic Substances Act of 1925, based on German and American models, helped rectify this. In brief, the British drug industry, for economic reasons and deep-seated managerial traditions, saw nothing like the expansion seen in America. Its most remembered moment, M&B 693, underlines this. M&B 693 was a sulphonamide that was very effective against a variety of cocci.

It was developed in May and Baker's laboratories in Britain over two years beginning in 1936. But it hinged on a German development and a recent French takeover of the British company. In 1932, some years after the introduction of the German antimalarial, plasmoquine, the British drug journal *The Extra Pharmacopoeia* noted: 'England should have done it!' The French pharmaceutical industry was generally based on small companies and relied more heavily than it cared to admit on German suppliers at the start of the Great War. Things did not change much after that with French companies continuing to rely on importing finished or semifinished drugs. The country saw nothing like the change in scale seen in America.

For a number of doctors and other observers, the pharmaceutical industry represented one of the unacceptable faces of modernization. There was scarcely anyone, of course, who did not welcome the easy availability of preparations whose content, strength, and probable action could be relied on. These were a blessed relief from the multitude of drugs of unknown composition (especially the agents of so-called organotherapy) marketed with exaggerated claims of efficacy. Nonetheless, aspects of the drug industry were unsettling. Some saw in commercial research the potential corruption of what was held to be disinterested scientific enquiry. Others saw in the industry the (by now familiar) evils of mass production and mass marketing with a consequent degradation of the worker and consumer, that is, the further erosion of creative labour and informed choice. Significant here, however, is that some clinicians regarded these things as damaging the best management of their patients. It was yet another force perceived as corroding good medical practice. One of the responses to modernization at the bedside was the defence of the view that people needed to be treated as individuals; that their complaints were unique and should be managed accordingly. Standardized remedies, some argued, obliged doctors to treat all their patients in the same way rather than their being able to tailor their prescriptions and doses to the needs of individual sufferers. Such an argument was not usually solely about therapy. It was part of a wider view that condemned standardization in general and saw it as the road to the regimentation that would destroy individualism on the small scale and produce the worst political consequences on the large one. In 1936, the English physician Lord Horder, said that recently medicine had seen an 'invasion' (a word with chilling overtones) of 'mass methods', the results of which were 'very disappointing'. In consequence, he added, 'We had to start all over again, working out the particular case'. Fascism and communism were also mass movements and therefore not solutions to social malaise for they did not attend to the individual. Horder noted: 'It is for this reason that I have dealt [critically] with mass movements as efforts towards restoring that sense of security which is essential to national and to international well being. The analogy from Medicine is all against treating the crowd, and all in favour of treating the individual.'

Welfare

CRISIS YEARS

By 1939, even allowing for the Depression, a great many people in industrialized nations had better incomes, housing, education, and welfare provision than they would have had in 1914. The term 'welfare state' was probably made common currency in the English language during the 1930s. Material gains were continuations of trends that had begun long before World War I. These developments occurred at an international level, for the similarities between nations in this respect were more marked than their differences. These things, however, are not what usually come to mind first when considering this period. It is often seen as a dark age, dominated by economic depression, unemployment, vicious class and racial conflict, and a sense of profound cultural malaise. Indeed, this was the case. Such features, however, were largely the product of a number of shorter-term factors. Mass political movements and nationalism in particular, although they had deep roots, were forced into prominence by wartime and post-war economic and political crises. Health policy in these years has to be seen in terms of deep, long-term factors and recent developments. The deep factors made for international similarities. Recent developments shaped health policy in particular ways in different nations. So distinctive were approaches to matters of health in Nazi Germany and Soviet Russia that they are most easily dealt with in separate sections. This does not mean they were not broadly similar to approaches found elsewhere. Both nations shared structuring assumptions about health and disease that informed action everywhere in the industrialized and industrializing world. To take concrete examples; hardly anyone – except a few Nazis – queried whether the hospital was the seat of the best medical attention, and that in laboratory science lay medicine's greatest promise.

There was a widespread view in the 1930s that ever since the Great War the world had lived in crisis. It is hard to deny that this perception was anything other than accurate. The war had brought financial disaster, high inflation, and a dislocation of world trade. The Wall Street crash of 1929 was followed by a catastrophic global slump. In Germany in 1932, 8 million of the country's 20 million workers were unemployed. A report of that year described 'hidden famine' among German workers (Prausnitz, 1933, p. 5). In the United States in 1933, one in four in the labour force was out of work. There was a general sense that unless steps, and many thought radical steps, were taken, the world or individual nations were destined for economic, social, and cultural disaster. Among the many responses engendered by this sense were frankly racial policies. These latter were transformations into concrete action of the prewar fears of degeneration and differential reproduction rates.

This section examines those matters covered by the terms 'public health' and 'welfare', but only in so far as they involved medical personnel or medical knowledge in some obvious way. It is not possible to do more than allude to the areas that were obviously important (perhaps the most important) determinants of health and disease, for example, diet, housing, or working conditions. In these latter, medicine usually figured as an element of debate, but generally had no major determining role in promoting change. What was meant by public health and who should be responsible for it, were highly contested in this period. In the case of welfare there is debate among historians about how far differences in national approaches are more important than similarities. No comprehensive account can be given here; examples are chosen from various countries to illustrate both contrast and identity in approaches.

In many countries towards the end of the Great War, concern with national health was soon converted into government reorganization. Austria formed ministries for social welfare and public health in June 1917. In April 1918, Poland established its Ministry of Public Health, Welfare and Labour Protection. The British formed a Ministry of Health with a Chief Medical Officer in 1919. Following suit, the French in 1920 formed a Ministry of Hygiene, [Public] Assistance and National Insurance in addition to a Conseil Supérieur de Natalité. A separate health ministry, chiefly concerned with preventive medicine, was formed in 1930. German attempts to establish a central ministry of health failed although the Weimar constitution made welfare work a formal state responsibility. Arrangements varied between states. In Prussia, for example, health matters were largely in the hands of the Ministry of Public Welfare established after the war. The Nazis dissolved Prussian autonomy, and the State Ministry of the Interior took over health issues. It was not until after World War II that America, in keeping with its distrust of federal government, formed a Department of Health.

Doctors, by and large, distrusted public-funded medical services. Everywhere they stuck out for certain rights or principles: financial independence, the right of patients to choose their medical advisor, and the right of doctors to charge patients directly. These rights or principles that doctors held dear were enshrined in codes of ethics, such as the Medical Charter adopted by the Confedédération des Syndicats Médicaux in France in 1928, the 'Ten Principles' of the AMA in 1934, and the Seven Principles introduced by the BMA in 1945. Doctors could be militant in the face of state medicine. In Germany, they organized strikes against socialist-supported Policlinics. In America, many of them opposed welfare measures, such as the maternity assistance provided by the Sheppard-Towner Act (see the following text), on the grounds that it was a government encroachment on individual liberties. The French medical profession fought attempts to introduce health insurance and successfully diluted the Social Insurance Law of 1928 with a Law of 1930 that gave physicians greater control over fees. Doctors were not the only professionals in health care opposed to state involvement. It was reported that in 1932 at the Second International Conference of Social Workers, some of the members expressed concern that under the influence of social insurance and social work 'the individual would become less inclined to rely upon himself, and would lean too much upon the helping hand of the State' (Prausnitz, 1933, p. 13). The spectre of socialized medicine in the Soviet Union was present in all resistance to state involvement west of the iron curtain. A striking example, however, indicates the penetration of government in this period. In Britain in 1920, the majority of the medical profession was engaged in some form of service for the state or for local authorities.

Various related issues were prominent in the welfare literature of all nations in this period. These roughly divide into two overlapping sorts; those concerned with maintaining a (present and future) fit, efficient working population, and those directed to managing the unproductive and possibly socially destructive. The principal concerns were the prevention and control of diseases; provision for medical attendance; maternal, infant and child health; industrial health; nutrition; 'social diseases' notably TB, VD, and alcohol abuse; and the care of the elderly and mentally disturbed. Permeating all these areas were eugenic and racial worries. As will be seen, now as then, these issues are not always easily distinguished. They were confronted in all countries and, broadly speaking, were addressed in similar ways. The difference in approaches between countries lay in the balance between the degree of involvement of voluntary agencies and the state.

America represented one extreme, Russia another. Most of Europe lay in between. Everywhere, education was promoted as an essential means to achieve a responsible and healthy citizenry.

Ideas about the preservation of health and the cure of disease in national populations as a whole were intimately bound up with ideas of participatory citizenship, whether the country concerned was a democracy or a dictatorship. Attempts to produce strong, well-integrated states were centred on the promotion, and sometimes enforcement, of what was seen as responsible individual behaviour. This was deemed to produce mental and physical health and socially beneficial action. 'Positive health' was almost a catch phrase in this era. Some groups of individuals were considered less rather than more capable of positive health and of behaving in a socially responsible manner. Everywhere, measures were taken to deal with such people (incarceration and extermination to name but two), but varied in intensity from country to country and decade to decade. In all places the underlying philosophy was one of the promotion of national *health* in every sense of the word (the synonym *strength* soon comes to mind). However, the idea of participatory citizenship had, in many countries, quite unforeseen consequences.

At first sight, interwar efforts to improve national health look like little more than an intensification of prewar approaches with the multiplication of laws, services, and welfare agencies. But something subtle was happening that cannot be pinned down to a historical moment. In 1914, the overall tone of welfare work, both voluntary and government-funded, harked far back to an older era of charitable care in which the wealthy carried out their social obligations and the poor, in turn, were expected to show gratitude. This tone changed slowly, almost imperceptibly, in the interwar years. A world that had existed for a very long time in the West was finally being buried. After World War II, there was a distinct sense that, for example, women had a right to expect reasonable antenatal care, qualified assistance in childbirth, and sufficient food for their children. To many, knowledge of and access to contraception seemed a legitimate right of an adult citizen. These sentiments had been created over the previous thirty years by left-wing parties, social investigators, trade unions, women's groups, lobbyists, political thinkers, journalists, and so forth. The examples just quoted refer mainly to women's issues, but the new attitude began to pervade post–World War I society in all its aspects. Characteristic of interwar welfare reform battles were not just struggles over how much provision for health should be made and by whom, but contests about the *rights* of citizens to such provision. In their very different ways, America, Nazi Germany, and Russia promoted vigorously the ideal of the responsible participating citizen.

The future of nations

EUGENICS AND RACE

Concern about differential reproduction rates, the spread of diseases deemed hereditary, and worries about the contamination of the population at large by genetically poor stock were widespread in the interwar years. Formally, such concerns were defined as eugenics; informally, they appeared in myriad discourses and practices centred on health by people who possibly never used the word 'eugenics'. Nonetheless, the term 'eugenics' appears so infrequently today it is hard to imagine that it was used repeatedly between the wars to designate *the* issue the world had to face. At the International Conference of Social Workers in 1932, eugenics was named the 'grander problem' to be solved if the world's current crises were surmounted (Prausnitz, 1933, p. 13). In all Western nations, bearers of disease or disease-producing traits were seen as a threat to the well-being of the whole (Fig. 3.6). Those with unsound heredity were seen as bearers of pathological threats, just as were sufferers from infectious disease. Concern about the effect of 'mental defectives', the 'feeble-minded', the insane, and so forth, on the future of a nation's stock, remained unabated in these years (it was widely held that the mentally retarded were both oversexed and irresponsible). Charity and welfare were sometimes blamed for fostering high reproduction rates among those deemed less able. The new science of psychology flourished within the eugenic framework, and the objects it had constructed before the war, such as intelligence, were widely tested and graded. When possible, the results were used to winnow the weak from the strong, the fit from the unfit, the able from the unable in many areas of life: industry, the armed forces, commerce, and the family. Obviously, not all advocates of psychological testing promoted it in the cause of eugenics.

Very often, concern about fitness to breed extended from individuals to 'races', seen as a sort of extended family. It should be noted that the term 'race' was often used indiscriminately in the interwar period to refer to ethnic groups, peoples, and nations. Sometimes it meant the human race. Jews, Celts and Gaels, 'the Poles', 'the Irish', the 'poor white trash' of the American South, let alone darker skinned or oriental peoples, were regularly regarded as races. Somewhere or other each of these groups,

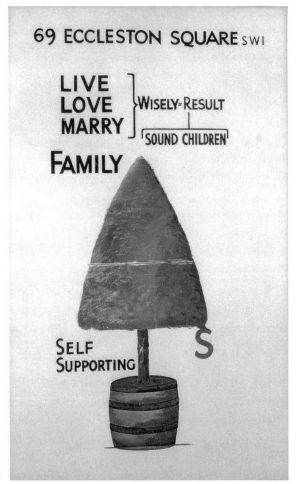

Fig. 3.6. Poster published by the Eugenics Society promoting 'wise' marriage for the sake of producing sound children, 1930s. *Source:* Eugenics Society Archives, Wellcome Library Archives and Manuscripts. *Credit:* Wellcome Library, London (L0030835); © The Galton Institute, London.

as a whole, was seen to be the bearer of undesirable pathological traits (witness 'Mongolism'). Some of these peoples, notably Jews, were sometimes seen as carriers of desirable traits. Thus, it was perfectly possible to worry about the eugenic threat of the individual imbecile while not caring at all about 'racial' intermarriage. The interwar years saw the intensive use of laboratory sciences, such as blood serotyping, and field sciences (e.g., anthropology) to distinguish the characteristics of the various 'races'.

Eugenic organizations existed worldwide. Russia had a Eugenic Society, formed in 1920. Japan, many of whose basic medical scientists had been trained in America and Germany, saw the formation of (at the minimum) five national eugenic societies and the establishment of at least four eugenic journals between the wars. Besides collecting data, eugenic societies debated how to promote their goals. Since the nineteenth century, increasing attention had been paid everywhere to defining, isolating, treating, and preventing disease in individuals for the good of the whole. Indeed, in certain circumstances, states curtailed individual freedoms in the perceived interests of the national welfare: for example, in compulsory vaccination against smallpox, the confinement of defectives and those with infection (symptom-free typhoid carriers were notorious cases, Ch. 2). Many eugenists held that through such things as education and tax incentives their ends could be attained. Most, however, saw no harm in putting the weak-minded in institutions. In Britain, 30,000 so-called mental defectives (not the insane) were institutionalized by World War II.

In the United States and Canada, besides segregation, immigration restrictions curbed the entry of ethnic groups deemed to be of low intelligence. Debating an act passed in the United States in 1924, a democratic congressman declared: 'The primary reason for the restriction of the alien stream . . . is the necessity for purifying and keeping pure the blood of America' (Kevles, 1986, p. 97). 'Blood' was a powerfully emotive term that ran through all eugenic rhetoric. 'There is power in the blood' ran an American hymn sung by Southern Protestants in the first half of the century (Larson, 1995, p. 5). Extreme hard-liners in the United States opted for sterilization, enforced if possible. 'Let us take stock of this rubbish,' wrote an Atlanta paediatrician of 'poor white trash' in the 1930s. 'Sterilize all individuals,' he went on, 'who are not physically, mentally or emotionally capable of reproducing normal offspring' (Larson, 1995, p. 1). Figures vary, but by one estimate 15,000 people had been sterilized under state laws in the United States by the late 1920s. California easily took the lead with 6,255 sterilizations by 1929. By 1932, twenty-seven states could legally practice sterilization. Habitual criminals, the feeble-minded, and the insane were the principal targets. Men had vasectomies, women had tubal ligation. The numbers of women increased markedly in comparison to men in the 1930s. Sterilization was usually carried out with the 'consent' of inmates or relatives. In practice, where consent began and coercion ended varied widely. Until the Nazis took the limelight, America was often looked to as the place in which a eugenic programme had made most progress. Referring to America's sterilization laws and the Immigration Restriction Act of 1924, the Bavarian Health Inspector Walter Schultze noted in 1932, that in the United States 'racial policy and thinking has become much more popular than in other countries.' Extreme racial hygienists expressed envy at the numbers of sterilizations in America, following the example of which, governments in Sweden, Denmark, and Finland enacted sterilization laws. The British were reluctant and did not follow the example set by some European countries. In Britain, many surgeons winced even at performing the operation on volunteers. In Japan, in 1940, a National Eugenics Law was passed which stipulated sterilization.

After the Great War, the rhetoric of racial hygiene in Germany still largely addressed the issue of how to discourage procreation by supposed inferiors. Concern was expressed about the relative lack of fecundity among the upper classes and the threat of feminists to the reproductive performance of the family. Weimar eugenists, however, were more parochial in their interests than their prewar compatriots. In 1918, Hermann W. Siemens (1891–1969), author of *What is Race Hygiene?* was warning of the consequences of the proliferation of the genetically unfit, one of which was the collapse of Germany in the face of an 'Asiatic triumph' (Proctor, 1992, p. 25). German eugenists worried more about the fatherland's struggle with its enemies in Europe and Russia than the general problem of the future of civilization. The Treaty of Versailles was economically stifling, but also left many Germans feeling dominated, as one said, by people 'culturally beneath them'. Militant racial hygiene policy did not fare well, however. The democratic parties in Germany at this time were strongly opposed to any act legalizing involuntary sterilization. Nonetheless, the sense of 'race' as synonymous with Nordic, Ayran, Semitic, and so forth was present although not pervasive. An indication of the complexity of positions acceptable at this time is given by Alfred Grotjahn (1869–1931), a leading figure in Weimar Germany's progressive health reform culture, a movement feared by the right as promoting proliferation of the poor. Grotjahn, a socialist, saw racial hygiene as an important constituent of social medicine and advocated compulsory sterilization. By and large, though, socialists were not prominent among the supporters of racial hygiene as the road to social betterment.

Nowhere in Europe did the strong eugenists have the sort of government support that would have been necessary for them to implement their prescriptions in full. The International Congress of Eugenics met in Rome in 1929 and Mussolini was asked to adopt eugenic measures. He showed no interest. Besides indifference there was also hostility to eugenics, particularly after Nazi enactments. A broad spectrum of liberals, socialists, feminists, Catholics, and many other strangely assorted bedfellows found eugenic intervention, although not necessarily eugenic ideals, unacceptable. Many geneticists felt it tarnished their discipline. The British biologist John Burdon Sanderson Haldane (1892–1964, son of John Scott Haldane) and the anthropologist and German-Jewish American immigrant Franz Boas (1858–1942) were probably the most famous academic critics of eugenics. In the 1930s, the very time that Nazi power was expanding, American researchers, notably Otto Klineberg (1899–1992), began to pile up statistics that denied a relation between race and IQ (this was well before the notion of IQ began to be questioned). By the late 1930s, eugenics was not considered a science in academic circles although eugenic ambitions were still widely shared.

WOMEN, BABIES, AND SCHOOLCHILDREN

In these years, government, voluntary, and professional attention to women and children intensified, largely on prewar lines. Medical measures, education, and welfare legislation remained the basis of intervention although national approaches varied greatly. Welfare legislation that had an effect on women and children was widespread in the interwar years. Before the war, many of the measures affecting women had been primarily directed at working males, but now women were more often specifically targeted although they were still affected by policies shaped to deal with other areas, for instance, declining populations, wage levels, and poverty in general. National health was influenced by many measures, such as the provision of maternity benefits. These latter were mainly prewar reforms, but their scope was extended (in Germany, e.g., to wives of insured husbands in 1924). In some countries national provision appeared for the first time, as in the Maternity and Infancy Act (popularly known as the Sheppard-Towner Act) passed in the United States in 1921. In 1929, it failed to secure further appropriations from Congress but it was reenacted in the Social Security Act of 1935. State child allowances were largely interwar innovations. Of the larger countries, France began the trend in 1932. Women's movements were very important driving forces behind these changes.

Antenatal care, rare in the extreme in 1914, became widespread, although not ubiquitous, in the wealthier countries. In 1942, 79.5 percent of women in England received prenatal care. Midwifery provision was on the agenda everywhere. The long-standing struggles between doctors and midwives for control of deliveries persisted, heightened by the ability of more people to pay because of insurance schemes and by the flooding of the private market with professionals during the Depression. Nutrition formed the focus for much government and private intervention. School milk and lunch programmes were initiated and extended. The lunch programme was particularly vigorously pursued in America during the Depression (an ironic by-product of reducing agricultural surplus). Medical and dental inspection and treatment of schoolchildren was extended, but the cursory and ritual nature of much inspection began to be questioned, notably in a four-year study of New York City between 1936–40 (the Astoria Health District Study).

The falling birth rate was another source of concern and legislation. It reached its all-time low in many European countries by the early 1930s. In 1933 it hit bottom in Sweden at 13.7 per thousand, England and Wales at 14.4, and Germany at 14.7. Policies encouraging births (pronatalism) in many countries frequently benefited women though not necessarily the birth rate. Nowhere was alarm over the declining birth rate greater than in France. It was falling before the war; the French lost 1.5 million soldiers during the war and the interwar years were seen at the time, as one historian records, as an age of 'acute crisis' (Reynolds, 1996, p. 21). Some blamed the lack of manpower for French capitulation to the Germans in World War II. Pro-natalist pressure resulted in a law of 1920 forbidding propaganda for birth control. Another in 1923 made the abortion laws stricter and prosecution more likely to result in conviction. Positive measures included paid maternity leave (1928), family allowances (1932), payments to mothers who nursed their own infants (1935), and first-birth premiums (1939). These various measures were the outcome of both reactionary and progressive agitation. Politically active women in France, whether Catholic or secular, conservative or radical, were virtually all supporters of the centrality of motherhood to maintaining a healthy society. Pronatalism notwithstanding, the French birth rate briefly fell below the death rate in 1938.

In the medical and public spheres, a falling birth rate was seen as an object of legitimate concern as was reproduction among undesirables. Sex in almost any guise, however, largely remained off the respectable agenda in this period which, broadly speaking, showed a commitment to the knowledge, practices, and values of the prewar years. Research on the physiology of sex was a reputable area of scientific activity. The oestrus cycle was described, and the principle male and female sex hormones were isolated. The marketing of them as extracts and synthetics (in women for conditions as diverse as asthma and menstrual dysfunction) was rarely perceived as an ethical pharmaceutical enterprise. Most doctors were in possession of no more information about sexual behaviour than anyone else. Sex was not part of the curriculum. Masturbation was still regarded as a cause of disease or certainly as mentally and physically enfeebling. Homosexuality remained deeply immoral. In complaints of infertility, the woman was usually assumed to be the culprit, although by the 1930s sperm examination was carried out in the few places that tendered to this problem (before this, 'living' sperm equalled fertility). Contraceptive information could not be obtained from doctors. It was outsiders, such as Marie Stopes (1880–1958) in Britain, who, in the face of much abuse, tried to make contraceptive information available. A cocktail of eugenics, paternalism, feminism, liberalism, and socialism was usually at work in such educational reformers. Many eugenists, though, disapproved of contraception on the grounds that it separated responsibility from passion and thus encouraged licentiousness and that the middle classes might use it and further reduce their rate of reproduction. Margaret Sanger (1879–1966), the American campaigner for contraception, however, saw it as eugenically important. She wrote, 'More children from the fit, less from the unfit – that is the chief issue of birth control' (Kevles, 1986, p. 90). The decline in the birth rate in these years was certainly assisted by withdrawal, the diaphragm, spermicidal creams and pessaries, the new 'rhythm method', and abstinence. Reported therapeutic abortions were rare in Protestant countries. In private clinics, money could buy most things. Illegal abortion was common and the results of it often devastating. It was estimated that England in 1936 as many as 20 percent of pregnancies ended in abortion although what proportion of this figure was illegal was anybody's guess.

Maternity care and state-supported medical provision for women and children expanded greatly in Britain. The Maternity and Child Welfare Act of 1918 provided grants-in-aid to public and private agencies. By this year, there were 3,038 health visitors in 154 towns. They were employed by both voluntary agencies and local authorities and sported a variety of qualifications. They both nursed the sick and acted as educators. These roles were gradually split. By 1933 there were over 6,000 such visitors and, after 1924, they had uniform qualifications from the Royal Sanitary Institute. Free or cheap meals and milk for mothers and babies became much more readily available. A Midwives Act of 1936 compelled local authorities to provide salaried, qualified midwives. Nevertheless, in some depressed areas such as the coal-mining valleys of South Wales, maternal mortality rose between 1922–3.

In Germany, in the 1920s, a low birth rate, illegitimacy (19 percent of births in Berlin in 1926) and high infant mortality all gave cause for concern. It was estimated that in the early 1920s there were 250,000 induced abortions a year and around 1 million in the last days of the Weimar Republic. Miscarriages and illegal abortions (many of which were associated with sepsis) were said by an observer in 1931 to be 'as numerous as normal births'. In the same year, the status of midwives in Germany was described by an English observer as 'unsatisfactory'. All required a diploma of competence after being in training for between nine and eighteen months. They were poorly paid and had no pensions. In Prussia, 90 percent of births were attended by midwives. In Berlin in 1931, three-quarters of the midwives were in private practice and nearly 60 percent of births took place in hospitals.

Rickets was common just after the war. In Dortmund in 1923, 43 percent of children between two and ten were reported as having rickets. In 1924, a Federal Child Welfare Act was passed in Germany recognizing that 'every child is entitled to education with a view to its physical, mental and moral well-being'. By 1926 there were over 5,000 infant welfare institutions controlled by communes or private welfare organizations. Public medical doctors, communal doctors, and welfare nurses staffed these institutions. Specially appointed doctors examined schoolchildren. In 1931 there were seventy-nine full-time school doctors in Berlin. Previously, this work had been in the hands of private practitioners and the medical profession resisted its transfer to the public arena.

Midwifery services varied enormously. These years saw the move to hospital and nursing home confinement that became almost *de rigeur* in many places after 1945. Besides the advocacy of the practice by obstetricians, the wealthy saw it as safe and modern, and for a poor woman it could provide a break from household drudgery. In reality, conditions in a hospital for those who could not pay could be stark and unfriendly. The midwifery service in the Netherlands was acknowledged to be among the best in the world. This no doubt contributed to the low maternal mortality in that country. Midwives attended 60 percent of confinements. They underwent three years of training and the national number was fixed at 900 (one per 8,000 of population). Two government schools of midwifery were free for students. Most midwives practised privately. Municipalities paid for the poorest mothers. In the 1930s the Mistress-Midwife at the Amsterdam school noted that because medical qualification was not restricted the country had a 'superfluity' of doctors (in addition to other graduates). So much so, she thought, that it was justifiable to use the term 'intellectual masses' of educated workers, the supply of which far exceeded demand. The delivery of babies had become an object of fierce competition. Describing child welfare and medical inspection of schoolchildren in The Netherlands in 1931, the distinguished British public health administrator Arthur Newsholme (1857–1943) noted that it was 'relatively little developed . . . in marked contrast to the important midwifery organization.' Nearby, in Denmark, midwifery was equally controlled, all potential midwives spending two years training at the one state centre. All deliveries, most of which were at home, were supervised by them unless there were complications. The comparatively excellent standard of care in the Netherlands and Scandinavia was seen in the maternal mortality figures of twenty-five per thousand in the 1920s. In the United States these were acknowledged to be shockingly high at eighty per thousand (a quarter of a million deaths in the decade).

The interwar years saw considerable erosion of the occupation of midwife, and the growth of hospital delivery in America. At the time of the Great War, midwifery was still a flourishing trade. Immigrants favoured midwives; hospital delivery by a private physician was expensive. Midwives might add cooking, cleaning, and supervising children to their services for relatively small fees. The training and licensing of midwives were immensely variable. What rendered the midwife extinct in America were those same forces of medical change at work everywhere, but which were quintessentially powerful in the United States: specialization, the rise of the hospital, a powerful private practice–orientated medical profession, and a weak public health sector. American obstetricians, creating their discipline as a modern, scientifically informed, and technologically prepared specialty, viewed childbirth as a medical event. 'Statistics are available,' said a professor of obstetrics in New York in 1922, 'to show that less than half of all pregnancies are normal' (Brickman, 1983, p. 82). The blame for obstetrical disasters was laid mainly at the door of the weakly organized occupation of midwifery but GPs without specialist training were also found culpable. Although a need for trained midwives was acknowledged by public health reformers and administrators, they were as much in thrall to modernization as obstetricians. Midwives were regarded as a temporary expedient until the expert physician was available to all. This was not a male medical conspiracy. American women who could afford hospital delivery by obstetricians increasingly chose what was presented as the most up-to-date and safest (and pain-free) form of childbirth. Almost everywhere, but notably in Germany and the United States, obstetric modernism was associated by some obstetricians and many women with 'Twilight Sleep' – the use of scopolamine to obliterate the consciousness of labour. Regarded with suspicion by some, it was later condemned as downright dangerous. Statistics bear out the picture of the midwife's decline in the United States. In New York City in 1909, 40 percent of births were attended by midwives and in 1933 only 8.5 percent. In 1935, 37 percent of births in the United States took place in hospital. In some parts of America, thousands of babies were delivered with no trained assistance.

Medical opposition to midwifery was often part of a broad conservative suspicion of public health reform. In 1925 the president of the AMA worried about the 'tendency . . . to make the treatment of the sick a function of society as a whole'. This tendency supposedly took away the individual's responsibilities and transferred them to the state. One of the doctors in *Arrowsmith* observed that 'sometimes I believe it'd be better for the general health situation if there weren't any public health departments at all, because they get a lot of people into the habit of going to free clinics instead of to private physicians, and cut down the earnings of the doctors and reduce their number, so there are less of us to keep a watchful eye on sickness'. Of the Sheppard-Towner bill of 1921, one physician, representing the American Gynecological Society, said that it 'will turn over an important part of [the work of physicians] . . . into the hands of nurses'. It would 'interpose a stumbling block to the progress of medicine' (Brickman, 1983, pp. 76–7).

Diseases and accidents

PREVENTION

By the interwar years, the control of epidemic disease had been routinized. Sanitary measures had been enacted and inspectorates established. The laboratory had been installed in the background as the authority that ensured the safety of the public at large, monitoring its material environment for living and chemical pathogens. Following the late-nineteenth-century lead, reformers emphasized the need for protective medical measures to be aimed at the individual. Vaccination, inspection, and education were advocated as the best means of guarding against epidemic and endemic diseases. During outbreaks, notification, identifying the causal agent, tracking suspects and carriers, isolation, and treatment were the first responses. Public health laboratories carried out tests for pathogens and searched for toxic substances, such as lead in water. They produced antisera and vaccines, although increasingly this work was taken over by the pharmaceutical industry. Arrangements varied. In Britain, a great deal of public health work was done freelance by hospital and university laboratories. In other

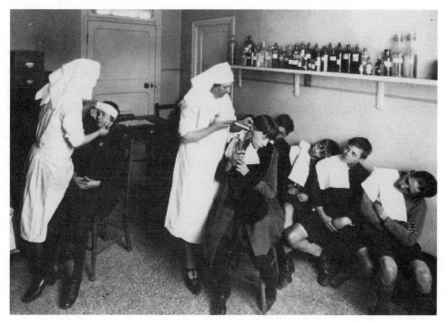

Fig. 3.7. In a typical day at Highgate New Town Clinic, north London, a nurse syringes a child's ear while others wait their turn. Another nurse bandages a patient's head, *c.* 1925. *Source:* Greater London Council photograph collection. *Credit:* London Metropolitan Archives.

places, such as the United States, local and central government laboratories did the work.

Increasingly, people were subject to routine inspections: when they were born, at school, at work, in the armed forces, and during pregnancy. Building on prewar precedents, public health clinics were established almost everywhere. They served whole communities or special populations, notably women and children. Created by central and local government and voluntary agencies and variously called 'dispensaries', 'policlinics', 'health centres', or simply 'clinics', they were usually separate from the regular curative medicine that was organized round a doctor's office or 'surgery'. They were staffed by public health doctors and nurses and, later, social workers of various sorts. Here, classes in health education could be given, babies could be weighed, children could be immunized and treated for nits, expectant mothers could be examined, nursing visits arranged, and so forth (Fig. 3.7). In the Weimar Republic, combined health, youth, and welfare offices were established. Between 1919 and 1923 in Prussia, 823 local authority and district clinics had been established. During World War I and after, health centres were founded across the United States. In 1930,

337

a subcommittee for the White House Conference on Child Health and Protection collected data from 1,511 major and minor health centres in the United States; 725 were privately run, 729 by county or municipal health departments, and a small number by hospitals, the Red Cross, TB associations, and so forth. They contained clinics (such as those for treating VD or ear, nose, and throat disorders), undertook nurse visiting, and child-welfare work. Some had laboratories.

Ever since the 1890s, long-term protection against disease by immunization had been held out as a real prospect. Active immunization against diphtheria (as opposed to passive serotherapy of the actual disease) had been experimented with before the war, but in the 1920s it was instituted on a large scale. America took the lead. In May 1933, the millionth New York City child was immunized against diphtheria by William Hallock Park (1863–1939), Professor of Bacteriology and Hygiene at New York University and Director of Hygiene services in the city. Deaths from diphtheria fell strikingly in New York. In 1926 there were 425 and in 1936 just 80. As noted, however, diphtheria mortality was falling everywhere in this period regardless of immunization, so any effect of the vaccine is difficult to gauge. Between 1941 and 1945 when the immunization rate dropped, Germany and German-occupied countries in Europe had a recrudescence of epidemic diphtheria. In 1939, Park reported that of 200,000 children, half were immunized and half had acted as 'controls'. Among these latter, cases of diphtheria were five times more frequent. It was not reported whether the 'controls' knew what was going on, but it seems unlikely that they did. The speed of adoption of mass immunization for diphtheria varied. In Britain, a national scheme was not fully instituted until 1942. Diphtheria immunization was not without risk. Deaths were reported. Problems were usually ascribed to improper preparation, storage, and administration of the vaccine.

Immunization against TB also began in these years. Bacille Calmette Guérin (BCG) was a strain of bovine TB developed in France during and before the Great War, and described as effective in protecting cattle and monkeys against TB. It was first given orally to humans in Paris in 1921. It was reported as harmless. Leon Calmette (1863–1933), one of the originators of the strain, began distributing the oral vaccine to doctors and midwives in 1924. Favourable and sceptical reports appeared. Mass vaccination was adopted in France. A severe outbreak of TB following vaccination in Lubeck, Germany, was attributed to accidental feeding of a virulent human strain. Intradermal immunization was introduced in Sweden in

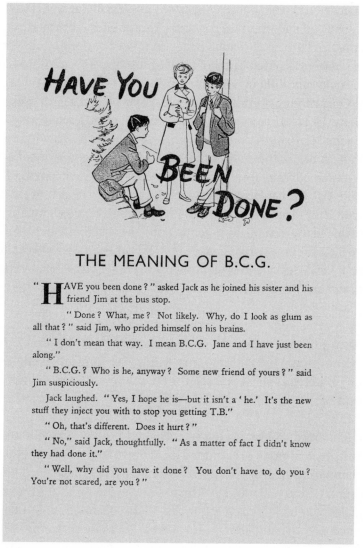

HAVE YOU BEEN DONE?

THE MEANING OF B.C.G.

"**H**AVE you been done?" asked Jack as he joined his sister and his friend Jim at the bus stop.

"Done? What, me? Not likely. Why, do I look as glum as all that?" said Jim, who prided himself on his brains.

"I don't mean that way. I mean B.C.G. Jane and I have just been along."

"B.C.G.? Who is he, anyway? Some new friend of yours?" said Jim suspiciously.

Jack laughed. "Yes, I hope he is—but it isn't a ' he.' It's the new stuff they inject you with to stop you getting T.B."

"Oh, that's different. Does it hurt?"

"No," said Jack, thoughtfully. "As a matter of fact I didn't know they had done it."

"Well, why did you have it done? You don't have to, do you? You're not scared, are you?"

Fig. 3.8. Leaflet issued by the Medical Women's Federation to promote BCG vaccination among school children, 1930s. *Source:* Medical Women's Federation Archive, Wellcome Library Archives and Manuscripts. *Credit:* Wellcome Library, London (L0027390).

1927 and the use of BCG became widespread in Scandinavia. Uptake was much more variable than with diphtheria immunization. Like diphtheria, TB incidence and mortality fell in these years. The role of BCG in these changes was contested at the time and still is (Fig. 3.8).

That education, propaganda even, was essential to improving the health of the population was never in question during this period. Quite what people needed to know, however, was not universally agreed. Health education by official agencies was particularly prominent in America and the Soviet Union. The term 'health education' used in any official capacity seems to have originated in the United States in 1919. A State Committee for Public Health Education was formed in Germany in 1919, and a Central Council for Health Education in England in 1927 (Rosen, 1958, p. 396). By 1922, there were sufficient people in the United States whose work touched on health education for them to form a separate section in the American Public Health Association. Voluntary and government agencies vied with each other for audiences. New media were used: moving film and radio. The U.S. Public Health Service began weekly health broadcasts in December 1921. Health museums and poster exhibitions flourished. Educators debated the best medium to use and how best to use it. In the case of film, the new documentary forms of the 1930s began to displace the older didactic styles. Films were used, probably to enormous effect, by the Nazis to promote racial hygiene.

TUBERCULOSIS, VENEREAL DISEASE, AND ALCOHOL

There were quite marked similarities within and between various countries in the management of TB and VD in these years. 'Control' (compulsory or voluntary), 'prevention', 'education', and 'treatment' were keywords. The aftermath of war saw a rise in TB levels in many places. In 1918 nearly 150,000 people died of TB in Germany, half as many again as in 1913. Eventually, almost everywhere, levels declined, but TB remained a menace. In Britain, in an attempt to counter it, the government established a system of free sanatoria and dispensaries for TB patients. In France, the Rockefeller Foundation's International Health Board was involved in TB control. It carried out a statistical survey, established dispensaries, and undertook a popular education campaign. In The Netherlands, there was no obligatory notification of TB and private initiatives predominated in its control with little central coordination. In 1931 there were thirty sanatoria with 4,800 beds (one to 2,800 persons) with patients making a contribution to the cost. By contrast, state intervention in TB control in Denmark was very evident. Respiratory TB was notifiable. In 1928, the country had seventy-one institutions (hospitals, sanatoria, etc.) devoted to TB cases. Most patients were paid for from insurance funds, but a great deal of government assistance was available including provision for the sufferer's family.

In Germany, notification of TB was obligatory in some states and not in others. Municipal arrangements were described in these years as 'very unequal'. The control of TB was in the hands of a Central Committee for the Prevention of Tuberculosis, a private body with a semiofficial character. Funds came from the Reich and, in Prussia, also from state-authorised lotteries. The committee was involved in education and the provision of sanatoria, of which there were 193 for adults and 382 for children in 1931. There were also TB dispensaries providing diagnostic facilities and carrying out social work. Whereas in Britain, institutional treatment was nearly always free to those in need, in Germany payment was through insurance, and the long duration of the disease frequently meant such funds were eaten up, the patient being left with no means to pay.

Organized American responses to TB and similar problems were notable for their voluntarism. The National Tuberculosis Association was the economic force behind the study and prevention of TB, giving money both to states and local affiliated groups. Similar societies included the American Social Hygiene Association, formed in 1914 from the amalgamation of the American Federation for Sex Hygiene and the American Vigilance Association. Societies focused on heart disease, diabetes, and infantile paralysis were formed between the wars.

World War I saw, relatively speaking, open debate about VD. Prostitution remained a key issue. In the United States, there was a militant anti-VD campaign. Behind this was concern about the likelihood of soldiers becoming infected. Educational materials warned that, 'A German bullet is cleaner than a whore'. Red-light districts in the United States were closed and officials used familiar analogies to legitimate such action. As one put it, 'To drain a red-light district and destroy thereby a breeding place of syphilis and gonorrhoea is as logical as it is to drain a swamp and thereby a breeding place of malaria and yellow fever'. So much had VD increased in Europe by the end of the war that contemporaries compared it to the Spanish 'flu of 1918'. In the 1920s and 1930s massive propaganda campaigns used older media and newer ones, such as radio and the cinema. Public lectures were given. In a college of domestic science in France in 1928, the lecturer warned the farm wives of the future 'to beware of butchers' hands, and in particular their spittle, of the hairdresser, of the servants' linen' (Quétel, 1990, p. 181). In some places, in spite of (or perhaps because of) the carefree image of the early 1920s, there was renewed reluctance to speak publicly about the issue. The educational film *Fit to Fight* that endorsed abstinence ('I wouldn't touch a whore with a ten-foot pole,' exclaims one character) was shown to American troops in the war, and was judged obscene in New York in 1919. A French physician advised men when dancing to 'put on their most fetching smile and caress the lady's neck, feeling at the same time for swollen glands under her skin . . . They should praise the bosom, but examine the skin for possible suspicious blotches' (Hays, 1998, pp. 259–60). Dance halls, the cinema or movies (the darkened venue as much as the film), and ice-cream parlours were all the foci of the wrath of moralists. In this respect, America, the home of some of the most puritanical attitudes in the West, was seen as the fount of European corruption (including sexual laxity).

Dispensaries were installed by local and central governments as the basis of diagnostic and therapeutic attack on the disease. In France, the *service annexes*, first established in 1916, were expanded in number so that by 1923 almost 200 were in operation. These small dispensaries offered free consultations and had laboratory facilities for diagnosis and monitoring treatment. As with TB, there was little in the way of a VD control policy in the Netherlands. There were a few free clinics including one in Rotterdam for sailors of any nationality. By contrast, the Danish state's concern with TB was also manifest in its attitudes to VD, citizens having the right to free treatment. Compulsion (with the help of the police) was also exercised among those unwilling to undergo therapy. In Britain, local authorities were obliged to establish clinics. A major campaign against VD was begun in the United States in the 1930s under the Surgeon-General, Thomas Parran (1892–1968). Eradicating the 'Shadow on the Land' as Parran called it, had been, he said, hindered by moralism. The campaign resulted in a National Venereal Disease Control Act of 1938 that provided federal grants to develop anti-VD programmes.

In many European countries, voluntary organisations or 'leagues' were established to eradicate VD, for example, the French National League against the Venereal Peril. Concern was international. Western European countries held a conference in Paris in 1920. World congresses followed. Venereal disease statistics are notoriously unreliable, but Belgium, where dispensaries were opened and vigorous propaganda pursued, seemed to have had singular success in reducing the incidence of syphilis.

The moral, economic, and medical campaign against alcohol retained much of its intensity between the wars, and in some countries dislike of drink was turned into legislation. This was most famously the case in the United States where prohibition began in 1920. The Scandinavian countries also cracked down on alcohol consumption at this time. In fact, in many places, following wartime decline in consumption, alcohol intake in the 1920s and 1930s remained well below pre-1914 levels. This was in part because wartime increases in the price of drink persisted and in many countries, such as Britain, enforced reductions in legal drinking hours more or less remained. Scientific and other studies continued to show links between alcohol intake and disease, individual and national efficiency, and madness. Alcohol was cited as a toxin that could damage the material that controlled heredity and could thus harm the race as a whole (the Nazis were particularly worried about this). Drunkenness, wrote Arthur Newsholme in 1927, is 'essentially a savage vice'. This observation suggested to him that 'absolute prohibition' was the necessary policy 'for savage races in which moral control cannot be expected' and also for 'the savage members of civilised communities'. In fact, tolerance for alcohol consumption actually increased in the late 1920s, and the United States and most other countries that had introduced severe antiliquor laws, repealed or moderated them.

THE HEALTH OF THE ECONOMY AND INDUSTRY

Unlike the end of the twentieth century, when the major industrial powers were becoming increasingly dependent on service industries, in the period considered here, the domestic production of coal, iron, steel, ships, military hardware, industrial plant, and so forth, was vital in many cases to national survival and certainly to international supremacy. Thus the health and efficiency of the workforce remained a subject of paramount importance in all Western countries. In regard to both health and disease, medical relations with industry were intimately entwined in wider political, economic, legal, and moral issues. Doctors obviously treated sick workers (or examined suspected malingerers) and this activity was tied to broader questions, such as the provision of compensation or disability pensions. Clinicians, epidemiologists, and laboratory researchers investigated industrial diseases and, once again, such investigations were tied to wider issues, such as working conditions.

Between the wars, industry and the economy continued to prove to be key areas where ideas from many disciplines were used interchangeably. Physiologists, economists, and social thinkers continued to share and swap ideas about the organization of the various bodies or systems they dealt with. For example, in the 1920s and 1930s, the economists of the Harvard 'Pareto Circle' used physiological ideas of regulation, integration, and coordination – the animal economy – to think about the monetary economy. From the 1930s onwards, the sociologist Talcott Parsons (1902–79), also at Harvard, argued that there were crucial similarities between biological organisms and societies. In *The Social System* of 1951, he claimed that both

343

were systems with their stability guaranteed by homeostasis (the concept formulated by the Harvard physiologist Walter Bradford Cannon, Ch. 3). It was also Parsons, originally trained as a biologist, who introduced the idea of the 'sick role' into medical sociology, a discipline he helped to make in the English-speaking world.

Interwar medical and biological investigators interested in occupations, studied the physiology and psychology of such matters as efficiency, skills, and aptitude, and advised on the conditions for optimizing these. The model of the body as a machine, or more specifically an engine to which the laws of conservation of energy could be usefully applied, was important in this connection (this did not preclude other models being used in other contexts). Before the Great War, the understanding of fatigue was given a role as a key to unlock the secret of industrial efficiency. Fatigue was conceived of as a physiological and psychological problem and also as a social pathology. It proved a useful concept for framing laboratory studies and for integrating them into wider debates about the body and society. Laboratory investigations of skill and aptitude were important, too, in mutually shaping them into technologies to maximize production. This approach was probably at its peak when applied to disability at the end of the Great War. Studies of fatigue and the development of aptitude tests for certain sorts of tasks continued throughout the 1920s when psychology began to replace physiology as the premier science of work. Psychologists shifted the emphasis from physical efficiency to the 'human factor', looking at such things as the happiness and attitude of the worker. The National Institute for Industrial Psychology, founded in Britain in 1921, took just such an approach.

An important interwar creation was the science of industrial hygiene that was, to some extent, developed by public health workers in response to the growth of the American chemical industry after the Great War when Germany no longer dominated the world market in this area. The science was first institutionalized at Harvard, mainly on the initiative of the dean of the medical school, David Edsall (1869–1945). Although a number of industrial diseases, such as lead poisoning, had long been recognized, Harvard workers took such conditions into the laboratory where they studied their detailed physiology. In doing so, they developed delicate measuring techniques and a physiology based on the concept of the sensitive balance of humans and environmental chemicals. In doing this, it has been argued, they were the creators of the ideas underlying the modern ecological concern that pollution, undetectable by the senses, is poisoning the environment (Sellers, 1997).

By the 1930s, many of the projects nurtured within industrial physiology were marginalized. The gross problems of recession, unemployment, labour relations, and industrial unrest made them look like a luxury. Eugenics was the one area in which scientific knowledge of the body and industrial production and national power were still mentioned in the same breath. The problems of the sick worker, industrial accidents, and diseases remained, of course. In general, these were managed by incorporating them into welfare systems. As studies demonstrated that accident and illness at work occurred in a regular fashion and that the risk of them could be assessed, so they were, like risks in other areas, increasingly incorporated into private and government insurance schemes. Any cost to industry was offset by price increases. This was, in the short term at least, a cheaper way of optimizing production than massive investment in the management and technology that would make work less dangerous.

Provision for sickness

BENEVOLENCE AND INSURANCE

Provision for orthodox medical care, especially treatment for those unable to pay the market price, increased everywhere in this period. Such provision was either free or by health insurance. Free services were directly funded by governments or voluntary agencies and were usually for the very poor or special groups, such as TB sufferers. In many nations, the idea of extensive state provision of welfare in the cause of a more organic society was promoted (for different reasons by both the right and left in politics). This was most notable in Weimar Germany where moves to comprehensive welfare were seen as a means to reintegrate a people fragmented and demoralized by war. Everywhere, health insurance became common, sometimes with, sometimes without government involvement. Some countries, such as Germany and Britain, built on prewar schemes. Others, such as France, introduced new systems based on legislation. In America, there was a massive increase in nongovernmental schemes. Insurance was by no means solely a commercial venture. Public insurance agencies, such as mutual or friendly societies, flourished. Almost everywhere, the result was increased cover for those already protected and the extension of cover to previously uninsured, vulnerable groups in the population. Whatever the form of provision there was consolidation of a long-term trend to provide welfare services for the whole population of nations and, in general, an increase in compulsion. Of course, in all countries, some groups remained sheltered by only the barest of provisions.

In Germany, after the dissolution of the monarchy and the establishment of the Weimar Republic, the Constitution of 1919 guaranteed various democratic rights and a comprehensive insurance system. Under the Social Democrats, between 1919–33, sickness insurance expanded. More groups, such as seamen (1927), were covered. In 1885 just under 10 percent of the population was compulsorily insured; by 1932 the number was one third. In 1914, 37 percent of dependants had some sort of cover. By 1925 the figure was 85 percent. Doctors, who had been opposed to the extension of insurance, came to regard it in the harsh economic climate of the late 1920s as the necessary evil that guaranteed their livelihood (reorganization under the Nazis is dealt with on (pp. 377–8)). The British figures tell a similar story. The 1911 Act originally protected about 15 million people out of a population of 45 million and by 1942, 25 million were covered. Dependants and children still remained outside the legislation. The act was far more important in that, as one author has observed, 'the insured person saw himself as receiving "free" medical care more as a right and less as a charity' (Abel-Smith, 1964, p. 248). In The Netherlands, nearly the entire wage-earning population belonged to societies of medical help, although responsibility for cover was left with the individual. Municipalities were responsible for the destitute. In general, health provision for nearly all health matters in the Netherlands was based on voluntarism with little government intervention. Perhaps because of the size and affluence of the country, the system worked comparatively well.

In spite of having supporters, compulsory health insurance legislation did not materialize in interwar America. The issue split interested parties of all sorts, but the overall mood in the years immediately following the British Act of 1911 was negative. Not surprisingly, many physicians were opposed to it, but so was the American Federation of Labour, a body with a large trade union membership. Business (including the insurance business) was generally antagonistic. A war against a nation that had invented compulsory health insurance, and the Russian Revolution, created enough anti-German and anti-Communist rhetoric to kill it. Medical costs rose considerably in America after the war; treatments were more expensive and doctors could command higher fees. On the insurance front, however, little happened in the 1920s. Franklin Delano Roosevelt took office in 1933 with the promise of a New Deal including a welfare safety net. In spite of the Depression, the climate was still too chilly for health insurance. The

Social Security Act of 1935 contained no provision for it even though measures had been considered. The act did contain maternity and child welfare provisions. In brief, in the United States, a vast patchwork of voluntary, industrial, state-assisted, and a myriad of other schemes, covered the citizen unable to pay in cash, but not so poor as to need the most basic state or charity assistance.

The French attempted to introduce a national medical insurance bill in 1920, prior to which time state programmes for medical care covered only 6 percent of the population, all indigent. Proponents of the bill, which was aimed at the labour force, applauded Lloyd George and the 1911 Insurance Act. One of them presented the bill as a means to 'protect the future of the [French] race, improve its health, bolster the quantity and quality of our manpower, spread the benefits of hygiene, and secure social peace.' Widely supported in some quarters but fiercely opposed by strange bedfellows (the Communist Party and the doctors), administrative delays held up the bill until 1928. It was finally implemented as a social insurance law in 1930, covering sickness, disability, and old age. Insurance was compulsory for low paid workers whose contributions were supplemented by employers and government. Another country that introduced health insurance between the wars was Japan, a nation that had rapidly industrialized at the beginning of the century. A law passed in 1922 went into effect in 1927 (a catastrophic earthquake partly caused the delay). The system was patterned on the German model. Insurance was compulsory for miners and factory workers. Japan underwent military expansion in the 1930s and, supported by the War Ministry, a National Insurance Law was passed in 1938 extending cover and basing it on the family.

THE HOME

Single-handed general practice remained the cornerstone of treatment by a medical professional throughout the interwar period. In many places, GPs did some sort of specialist work. Even in Britain, where this was unusual, GPs in the larger northern towns turned their hand to it. They had access to cottage hospitals and nursing homes where they carried out tonsillectomies and gave anaesthetics. In many countries, GPs welded together several elements to make a living. Besides their staple employment they worked as school doctors, factory inspectors, insurance doctors, public vaccinators, and so on. Private and insurance patients made up differing proportions of total patient numbers depending on where the GP was situated geographically and socially. Quality of practice varied hugely.

A significant development in interwar general practice that derived from the growth of specialization and ideas about improving efficiency was the move to group practice. Such moves were often part of broader attempts at reform of health policy. American doctors seemed to have experienced positively the specialist, group practice of war. They carried it home where conditions seemed amenable to its growth. Group practice flowered for a while. A practice might have up to ten specialists, each devoting time exclusively to, say, internal medicine, surgery, ear, nose, and throat conditions, and paediatrics. Other medical professionals and lay persons would be employed and there would be affiliation to a local hospital. In spite of such enthusiasm, group practice was not fully successful in the long run. Single-handed specialists and GPs were hostile and they accused group practices of commercialism and generating 'machine-like routine' (Stevens, 1998, p. 142).

Attempts were made to create group practices in Britain. Consultants tried it, but the ethos of clinical individualism did not work in its favour. An ambitious report of 1920 by a leading physician, Lord Dawson (1864–1945), suggested a radical shakeup of the primary heath care system with practitioners working as groups in publicly provided health centres. The Dawson Report sank with little trace. Although attempts to establish group practice and more broadly integrated health services were seen as efficient ways of optimizing health care in Britain, holist ideals were also at work. For example, Sir George Newman (1870–1948), Britain's first Chief Medical Officer appointed in 1919, took a broad view of the individual and environmental determinants of health and disease. Newman hoped to deliver modern, laboratory-based care in the service of what he described as Hippocratic preventive and therapeutic ideals. Newman planned to base general practice on health centres integrated with hospital and public health services. Doctors, he said, should be the custodians of the nation's moral health in addition to its physical one. They should be healers, not just of individuals but of the body politic. Such a view was widely shared in a Europe devastated by war. Newman's vision, like Dawson's, foundered on vested interests, economic ills, and professional suspicion of the state.

One failed British innovation in the provision of health care in this period merits mention. The Peckham Health Centre in south London, was a unique experiment whose components, however, were the familiar confidence in biological expertise, belief in 'positive health', and a search for holist solutions. The centre opened in 1926 and remained viable except for a couple of interruptions until 1950. Its founders were two doctors, George Scott

Williamson and Innes Pearse. Members paid subscriptions and in return received free health checks and the use of extensive recreational facilities. It was not a therapeutic institution. At the centre, individuals and families were supposed to grow physically and psychologically under the benevolent, but scientifically informed, eyes of Williams and Pearse.

Nurses probably saw more sick people at home in these years than doctors. The array of nursing services in existence, and the range of their employers, from patients to government, cannot be recounted here. Home nurses went under a variety of names in different countries: district nurses, visiting nurses, public health nurses, and so on. Before 1914, nurses outside hospitals cared for the sick and were expected to have some role in health education. After the war, these roles were increasingly differentiated. New positions, such as health visitor, were created. New interests, often stemming from psychiatry (notably Adolf Meyer's 'American school', (p. 285)), in psychological development, the community, 'dysfunctional families', behavioral disorders, and 'disturbances' of children and adolescents produced new occupations, such as the social worker, where knowledge and authority were based to some extent on medicine. Private nursing, an occupation usually hidden from view, was a large employer in these years. In America, so-called public health nursing was largely private nursing. A prewar creation, it continued to expand in the 1920s. In 1914 there were nearly 2,000 agencies hiring public health nurses, and by 1922 there were fifteen postgraduate schools teaching the subject. Public health nurses were ubiquitous: working for industry, department stores, insurance companies, hotels, school boards, milk and baby committees, and visiting nurse associations. But the rise of the hospital, the end of immigration, and the decline in infectious disease saw public health nurses relegated to an increasingly marginal role.

THE HOSPITAL

As before the Great War, hospital provision in these years mainly depended on a mixture of private and government-funded insurance schemes. In America, the prewar pattern was affirmed. The older, privately controlled voluntary hospitals remained legally under the control of trustees as charities. They were not profit-making companies. These hospitals constituted the élite of the American system. They often had links with universities and continued to appoint the cream of the medical profession, especially if they were white and male. Having gone through an economic crisis before the war, they solved their financial difficulties by taking in more and more paying patients who, for their part, increasingly perceived hospitals as places to get the best medical care. Thus, voluntary hospitals treated those who could pay and these people in turn subsidized the treatment of the poor who in turn 'paid' for their treatment by making themselves available for teaching and, less obviously, experiment. In 1922 in the United States, 65.2 percent of the income of such hospitals came from patients. The bulk of the remainder came from public sources and the rest from endowments, donations, and so forth. One consequence of these changes in the hospital population was that power shifted from trustees to doctors. Surgeons became particularly important in making purchasing decisions. Again, this was a change that had begun before World War I.

Paying patients in America could fund their beds through any one of a number of private insurance schemes. Individual private health insurance was rare in America before the 1930s because of high and unpredictable medical costs. To obviate this, insurers began to sell their policies through employers to large groups of workers. This strategy restricted insurance to the relatively healthy and reduced collection costs. In 1928, General Motors contracted with the Metropolitan Life Insurance Company to cover 180,000 employees. In the 1930s 'group hospitalization' was developed as the means of health insurance in America. Its history began in Dallas in 1929 when the Baylor University Hospital agreed to provide a stipulated amount of in-patient care per annum to various groups in return for an annual premium. Other individual hospitals followed suit, not least because the Depression now threatened income. The financing of the voluntary system was, as a book of 1932 declared, in 'crisis'. Later, citywide, then community-wide plans were developed. By 1937, the New York plan had 350,000 subscribers. By 1939 there were thirty-nine of these so-called 'Blue Cross' plans in operation with more than 6 million subscribers.

Municipal and county hospitals (public hospitals that relied on government appropriations rather than fees) in America during the interwar years continued to treat the poor, but received no paying patients. Length of stay was longer than in voluntary hospitals and patients had no choice of doctor. Religious, ethnic, and a small number of profit-making hospitals, all essentially private institutions, made up the remainder of American hospitals. These too expanded: by 1928 church-sponsored hospitals throughout the country numbered 841, with over 100,000 beds. Proportionately, black Americans were treated in a hospital less often than whites. In 1922 nearly a quarter of general hospitals reported that they limited their services to white patients. Mixed wards were rare. When blacks were admitted they were usually accommodated in separate wards, most often in the basement. Forty-two hospitals (1 percent) received only black patients.

In Britain, the prewar hospital system remained the basis of institutional care except that there was an administrative reorganization in 1929, and Poor Law hospitals were transferred to municipal authorities and developed as general hospitals. In this way, institutions that were once mainly devoted to long-term care became more like hospitals for the acutely sick. By 1934 there were 600 cottage hospitals in Britain staffed by GPs who were often criticized for poor surgical work. In spite of income from public authorities (e.g., the Ministry of Pensions), British voluntary hospitals faced economic collapse in the 1920s. For a start, the number of wounded servicemen in hospital gradually fell and hospitals lost the *per diem* payments that went with them. Central government was forced to make a once and for all payment to assist the hospitals. In the long run, two of the things that saved them were patients' fees and the fall in prices during the general economic crisis. Among the voluntary hospitals there remained a poor distribution of resources and overlap of specialist facilities. Attempts to integrate voluntary hospital services were relatively unsuccessful. Although treatment of the acutely ill was usually up-to-date, it was recognized that after-care services were wanting. As in America, members of the middle classes (some paying in full from their own pockets) increasingly filled the beds in these institutions. In London in 1911, patient payments constituted 8 percent of voluntary hospital income. In 1921 it was 33.9 percent and by 1939 it had risen to 39.4 percent (and nearly 60 percent in the provinces). Patients paid in various ways. The National Insurance Act made little immediate difference to the finances of voluntary hospitals except that the approved societies to which workers paid their fees were expected to make contributions to hospitals. Under so-called contributory schemes, patients paid a small amount each week into non-profit-making schemes (run by hospitals, employers, etc.) and received as a privilege, not a right, general hospital care. There was also a growth of private nursing homes.

In Germany, hospitals were chiefly national or municipal institutions. They were supported by taxation, assisted by payment according to means and by patients paying through insurance funds. In Berlin, about 65 percent of patients in public hospitals were partially paid for by insurance funds at a fixed rate of a few marks per day. The growth of insurance led to disputes about payment and many patients began to be sent to university clinics for an opinion. Exhaustive reports were increasingly required, usually with regard to industrial injury. Such work, said an American report of 1932, threatened to 'break down the strongest part of the clinical organization and teaching.' In Berlin, there were also Jewish, Catholic, and Evangelical voluntary hospitals. There were also private sanatoria.

In France, hospitals were largely public institutions. As noted, the war stretched the French hospital system to its limit and beyond. This was not simply a case of numbers. Many French surgeons, observing the example of American care at the front, insisted on using new technologies to manage the war-wounded. For financial reasons there was a reduction in return from charitable endowments after the war. Municipal authorities took up the shortfall. All of these factors induced the French into modernizing their hospitals. Institutions whose upkeep and management were once based on an ethos of charitable care were transformed into places that were seen as providing an essential service for the country's citizens. Hospitals took in new classes of patients despite the delay in the passage of the insurance bill. The state began to develop the guidelines of a national hospital policy. Subsidies were granted for certain services, notably, TB, radiology, and surgery. Region-centred urban hospitals were favoured over those in smaller cities. State-funded regional cancer research and treatment centres were established in ten large cities in 1923–4. Before 1928, a quarter of French *départements* (administrative areas) began to support hospitals and provide '*demi-assistance*' for admission to folk, such as artisans, small-holders, and shopkeepers, who had been impoverished by loss of savings during the war. In some areas, free hospital services were provided for classes that never before would have dreamed of entering such institutions. A bill passed in 1928 extended hospital insurance to a third of the population (13 million people). Over the next decade, legislative action ensured more and more people were covered. As in Britain and elsewhere, such legislation was a sign of profoundly changing social relations. Insurance was not charitable dependence. Care was becoming a right of citizens.

Special hospitals for particular groups of patients, such as children; or diseases, such as cancer, grew in these years. Across Europe and North America, asylum treatment for the mentally ill remained the norm. Indeed, increasing institutionalization characterized these years. In America, the state (public) asylum population increased from 159,000 beds in 1909 to 480,000 in 1940. Overcrowding, long stay and poor standards of care in public institutions were common everywhere even though in some places, notably America, psychiatry improved its professional status. In America, in 1946, an *exposé* in *Life* magazine compared conditions in state asylums to Belsen, the Nazi concentration camp.

Medicine in the Soviet Union

Russia has not, thus far in this volume, had a section to itself, but so profound were the new relations created between medicine and the state after the Revolution of 1917, that the marked contrasts and similarities between Soviet medicine and medicine elsewhere bear detailed attention. Broadly speaking, medicine in pre-Revolutionary Russian cities was like medicine in the rest of Europe because royalty, the aristocracy, merchants, and intellectuals often looked West for inspiration for reform. For example, a military hospital was established in Moscow in 1707, modelled on Greenwich Hospital in London. Russia had universities, two new ones being founded in the early nineteenth century at Kharkov and Kazan. In the second half of the nineteenth century, Russian medical science, especially physiology, and Russian medical scientists were at least as celebrated as those of Britain (although nothing compared with Germany).

What distinguished Tsarist Russia from the rest of Europe was that health care, like almost all education and science, was largely a state responsibility even before the revolution. It was hardly that the Tsarist regime cared more about the population's health than governments elsewhere – its budgets were pitiful – rather, it was a matter of power and control. Private practice, which was permitted, was difficult in such a poor country. In the second half of the nineteenth century, attempts were made to organize preventive and clinical medical services throughout the country. In 1864, the Zemstvo or local government was introduced. This was an elected district assembly. One of its functions was to administer medical provision and services devoted to health problems. Zemstvo medicine was a large-scale public service paid for by the people. Its remit included the management of district hospitals and asylums and the organization of practice. Many physicians worked in towns. Some went to the local Zemstva in the countryside searching for a venue where they could exercise professional independence while remaining state employees. Many, like Chekov, were idealists. In the countryside there were also *feldshers*. *Feldshers* were like modern Chinese 'bare-foot doctors' or the nineteenth-century French *officier-de-santé* (pp. 138, 212); basically trained, rural medical attendants. Prerevolutionary physicians were not, in general, opposed to state medicine, but they did want more autonomy and higher state expenditure on health. Unlike many of their American and European colleagues they were preponderantly left-liberal or socialist and in favour of involvement in preventive medicine. Their ideology led physicians to support the 1905 and the February 1917 revolutions (leading Russian psychiatrists linked insanity to conditions of life under the Tsarist regime).

Describing the history of medicine in the Soviet Union (most of the examples in this chapter will be taken from Soviet Russia) after the revolution is fraught with difficulty because of frequent and marked changes in policy. Many experiments in medical education, care, and prevention were tried and jettisoned. Soviet statistics must be treated with particular caution. Reports of what visitors considered the best in health care in the Soviet Union were based on limited and usually unrepresentative exposure. Two things, however, are striking about Soviet medicine. First, the *stated commitment* to deliver medicine (and especially preventive medicine) ultimately to *all* the people *equally* and in a manner that involved them in decision making. Nothing like this ideology could be found west of Minsk, even in nations where, in practice, far better medical attention could manifestly be delivered to large sections of the population. Second, and this can scarcely be stressed enough, Soviet *ideals* of the cognitive, professional, and material bases of good medicine put modernizers in capitalist countries in the shade. Experimental science, professional expertise, specialism, hospitals, and high technology properly used would, it was said, ensure the health of the people. The united force of science, technology, and the proletariat was proclaimed as irresistible. The glowing reports of travellers to the Soviet Union are worth noting, not only for what they often say about gullibility, but for the number of visitors (many far from pro-Communist) who saw the implementation of ideals and values that were often aired but infrequently implemented at home.

Almost immediately after 1917, major efforts were made to rebuild and transform the old public health system in Russia to deal with the effects of war and revolution. The Tsarist regime left two conflicting medical legacies. First, the official view that health and disease were the business of central, state-directed policy. This, the medical police approach, saw public health as properly being within the ambit of the ministry that oversaw general civil policing: the Ministry of the Interior. Second, was a reformist position that proposed that health matters be in the hands of scientifically educated, expert physicians to whom civil administrators should defer. Advocates of this approach regarded a ministry of health as the proper seat of medical policy making. These positions, of course, were detectable elsewhere in pre- and postwar Europe. Russian specialists dispute the extent to which the Tsarist system was built into the new regime.

The administrative apparatus of medical police crumbled with the collapse of the Ministry of the Interior. From the first, the Bolsheviks professed the cause of reason and science in medicine and public health, and stated that their medicine was a social medicine that would reject the individualistic, patient-centred practices of the capitalist West for a broader science of society. The hope that medicine would be part of a broad social science recalls similar aspirations being voiced in parts of the capitalist world. In 1918, in a statement about ultimate goals of policy, it was declared that health care was to be free, given by qualified professionals and accessible to all. Emphasis was to be placed on prevention by improving sanitation and living conditions. Such ideals were impossible to reconcile with the Bolshevik hard line that health care had to be prioritized by class.

Obviously, immense problems confronted the implementation of any new system: geography, postwar famine and epidemics (5 million cases of typhus between 1918–20), civil war (1918–1921), reconciling practical needs with ideological demands, and shortage of money. The party, trades unions, and women's and youth's organizations immediately united to teach cleanliness, distribute soap, and fight the louse. 'Either socialism will defeat the louse or the louse will defeat socialism,' said Lenin in 1919 (Fig. 3.9). During the 1920s the Soviets conducted an astonishing campaign for promoting public health. There was a fall in the incidence of infectious disease. Malaria control was an urgent priority. Planning began with two All-Russian congresses of bacteriologists and epidemiologists in 1921 and 1922. A programme of swamp drainage, land reclamation, and, after 1929, aerial spraying and (in the 1930s) individual treatment with new drugs was begun. The reported number of cases in the USSR during the 1920s fell from nearly 6 million to below 4 million. Smallpox vaccination had been made obligatory in 1919. The incidence of the disease fell although complete coverage of the population did not occur until the 1930s. The decline in epidemic disease in the 1920s also followed improvements in the agricultural sector and an increase in per capita food consumption.

Health expenditure, although rising in Russia in the early period (by a factor of close to three between 1923 and 1927), still left a health system recognized as seriously deficient. In 1928, just before the capitalist West was about to enter the Depression, a Five Year Plan, detailing a policy of rapid industrialization, was adopted in Russia. Much of the work for this plan, which resulted in a transformation of the economy, was carried out by prison camp labour. Collectivization of agriculture, often by forcible

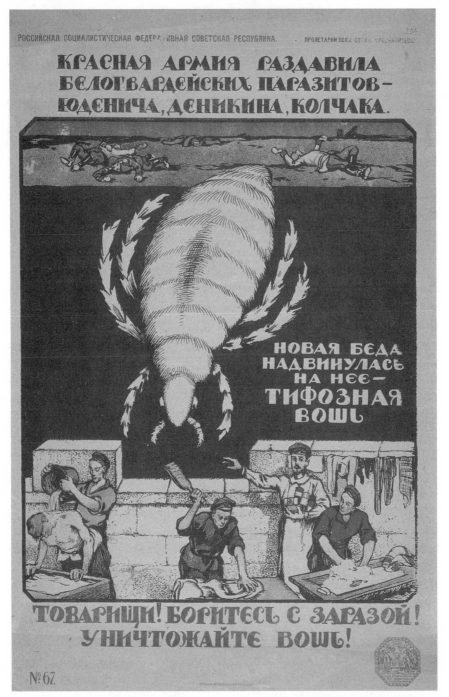

Fig. 3.9. Soviet poster warns that after the defeat of the White 'parasites', a new calamity threatens in the form of the typhus louse, against which the Red Army must fight by washing themselves and their clothes vigorously, 1921. *Source:* Lithograph, Wellcome Library Iconographic Collection. *Credit:* Wellcome Library, London (L0032770).

means, was also pushed through at breakneck speed. A period of intense suffering followed with declining living standards and a worsening of health conditions. Six million people were on food rations in 1930 and 40 million in 1932. In the latter year, there was severe famine especially in the Ukraine. Much that went on in the 1930s, including the suppression of opposition by deportation to Siberia, was hidden from outside (and inside) observers.

Health matters in the USSR were in the hands of republic-level commissariats. In the Russian Soviet Federative Socialist Republic (RSFSR), they were controlled by the Commissariat of Public Health (Narkomzdrav), created in 1918 and charged with unifying medical and sanitary affairs. Lenin's comrade-in arms, N. A. Semashko (1874–1949), was placed in charge. There was no single authority for the whole USSR (created in 1922). Below Narkomzdrav, were city and rural health departments of varying degrees of competence. Centralization of health care in Russia was backed by Lenin and won the day over much opposition, notably from the All-Russian Medical-Sanitary Workers Union (Vsmedikosantrud), formed in 1919. Representing *feldshers*, nurses, and other medical workers, Vsmedikosantrud called for extensive union participation in the management of health institutions. Narkomzdrav successfully called for the control of health care to be in the hands of 'specialists', that is, physicians, and for union participation to be confined, in Lenin's words, to 'energetic work'.

Besides political considerations, this approach was driven by attitudes to bourgeois science and expertise. The idea was to take what was good from bourgeois science, but to broaden it beyond the limitations set by bourgeois ideology and society. Bolsheviks, said Lenin, must learn 'humility and respect for the work of specialists in science and technology' (Weissman, 1990, p. 104). In Lenin's Russia, specialists in epidemiology, social medicine, and hygiene enjoyed unprecedented patronage. Science was accorded much more status than that of a luxury. It was, the party said, the essential means to house and feed the people, give them productive work, and make them healthy. In 1935 there were 932 research institutes in the Soviet Union employing 38,212 scientific workers. Institutes had several laboratories where related subjects were studied. For example, the Institute of Experimental Biology had departments of cytology, genetics, eugenics, zoopsychology, hydobiology, histology, and embryology. Narkomzdrav commanded thirty-four central research institutes.

While embracing bourgeois science, the Russians also attempted to develop a Bolshevik science with its own language, style of research, and form of knowledge. Bolshevik science was intended to expand bourgeois science beyond the limits set by mechanistic reasoning. The two sciences cohabited comfortably in the 1920s, but Stalinist science, as Bolshevik science became known, was pushed very hard in the 1930s. By the end of the decade, a massive, centralized, party-controlled, isolated science-making machine existed. The best known case history of a Stalinist science is that of Lysenkoism. T. D. Lysenko (1898–1976) developed a Lamarckian theory of inheritance that was favoured by the regime in the 1930s. Mendelian geneticists, many of whom had Western contacts, were persecuted. One by-product of this was the disappearance of eugenics in the Soviet Union.

The aim of creating a public medical system was principally to be met by a comprehensive state insurance system. From the start, funding the new system created problems, notably because of the conflict between ideals of universal egalitarian care and the special claim made by and on behalf of the proletariat. A bill of 1922 stipulated that certain sorts of workers (e.g., in state industries) were to be covered by social insurance. The proletariat was denominated the instrument of revolution and, historically, the special claims of workers had been recognized in attempts to introduce insurance during the Tsarist regime. After the revolution, workers argued for privileged medical services, a policy favoured by the Commissariat of Labour (Nakomtrud) that, until the 1930s, controlled social insurance. Narkomtrud's ideology was class-based and was orientated to funding, entitlement, and administration. Nakomtrud also supported strict control over physicians. On the other hand, Narkomzdrav, which controlled service provision, argued for a centralized system, more uniform care, and the professional autonomy of physicians. It subscribed to a more patient-orientated view of practice and supported the long-term value of medical science. Initially, Narkomzdrav's rather more egalitarian commitment prevailed, but by the 1930s Narkomtrud's perspective had triumphed and insured workers received medical services disproportionate to their number in the population as a whole. During the period of intense industrialization, the number of insured workers jumped rapidly from nearly 11 million in 1929 to over 22 million in 1932 (about 28 percent of the population). In 1933, the Commissariats of Labour were abolished and all their functions, including social insurance, were taken over by the trades unions. By this time, an extensive system of *ambulatoria* and polyclinics run by factory-based insurance organizations existed.

Agricultural workers on state farms were covered by social insurance (there were 2 million workers on 10,000 state farms in 1933). A variety of funds provided care for the noninsured, land-based worker. By the 1930s the majority of peasants worked on collective farms, of which there were 233,300 in 1933. Money earned from products sold to the state was distributed to members, but with part of it retained as 'invisible funds' that could be used for health work, such as the building of dispensaries and nurseries. Voluntary mutual aid funds were also established. In addition, there were state-supported health stations.

The potential conflict between Bolshevik respect for experts and the drive for unified state medicine was realized in attitudes to the medical profession. The Russian medical profession, although left-leaning, eyed Bolshevik reform with some circumspection. Sometimes it grumbled at aspects of state control (as it had done in the Tsarist era). Specifically, for example, there was resistance from obstetricians towards easily accessible abortion, and professors of clinical medicine opposed the new emphasis on prevention. Many physicians rejected the October Revolution but the government tolerated no opposition to it. Institutional bases of autonomous medical power, such as medical societies, were liquidated. During the civil war doctors were drafted. Narkomzdrav orders were backed by guns. Yet the new government also singled out doctors for special treatment among health workers. Attempts to equalize wages in the health sector were thwarted; doctors were guaranteed various privileges as were scientists. They were allowed a semiindependent section within Vesmedikosandtrud. By 1920, most physicians were in state service, either in the military or nationalized civilian health-care institutions, or they were unemployed. During the 1920s, private clinics and hospitals appeared in the larger cities (private practice was never effectively forbidden). In 1930, 5 percent of hospitals were in private hands. In Moscow, it was estimated that 17.5 percent of doctors were in private practice. In 1930, Narkomzdrat, with limited success, ordered the disbanding of private care.

Doctors increased in number. There were 33,000 doctors in the USSR in 1933 and over 80,000 ten years later, about half of estimated requirements. New medical faculties were opened. In 1913, there were thirteen medical schools in what would become the USSR. By 1924 there were thirty, and ten years later fourteen more had been added. Successful efforts were made to establish schools in distant republics, such as Irkutsk (Eastern Siberia). Barriers of admission by sex and race were abolished. In 1934, 75 percent of medical students were women, possibly because the more able among the men were entering the prestigious world of engineering. A great deal of experimentation with the content and form of the curriculum went on. Medical schools were eventually made into vocational institutions (e.g., engineering schools), divorced from universities. They were divided into three faculties to teach three sorts of doctors: practitioners of therapeutics and general prophylaxis, public health physicians, and specialists for the protection of mother and child. Methods of teaching based on teams of students were devised. Young graduates (there were no internships) were sent for three years of practice in rural districts. After this, a doctor might stay in the country or return to a city and apply for a job in a medical centre or work in a hospital and specialize. Exceptional students joined research institutes for three years, whereupon they could apply for a research position.

What the Russians called middle medical personnel: *feldshers*, midwives, medical nurses, nursery nurses, laboratory technicians, dentists, and pharmacists were critical workers in an area so vast. Most of these were trained in state technical schools: *technicums*. Reliance on them can be seen in the fact that in six years from 1927 to 1933, their numbers grew from 52,000 to 119,000. After the revolution, *feldshers* as a group were left to die out (ideologically speaking, only physicians were good enough). They were seen as a remnant of backwardness. This did not alleviate the shortage of doctors, and *technicums* were increased in number during the 1930s to train *feldshers*. Midwives were highly valued in post-revolutionary Russia. They underwent two years training on a course designed at The Institute for the Protection and Care of Motherhood in Moscow. By the 1930s, deliveries in cities were taking place in nursing homes. In the villages, the midwife's role extended to taking care of the newborn and organizing the local Soviet Committee for the Protection of Motherhood. Modern nursing as a secular profession was a new phenomenon in Russia. Regular schools of nursing attached to hospitals were created after the revolution. The typical Soviet physician received sufficient training to work at basic clinics in the city, which were set up on two grids. One, the 'open system', was based on residence; the other, the 'closed system', was based on occupation. In the open system, anyone could attend a neighbourhood clinic and be sent onto a more specialized facility. In the closed system, health centres were connected to industrial plants. Bigger centres might include a TB dispensary, day sanatorium, a VD clinic, dietetic clinic, dispensary, milk kitchen, and pharmacy. A showpiece dispensary in Kharkov (the 'Third Labour Polyclinic') had a diagnostic ward with ninety beds and physiotherapy wards. There was an X-ray department, chemical and bacteriological laboratories, and a large number of specialist clinical units, many devoted to women or children. The closed system was the source of a number of innovative public health practices, such as the provision of ergonomic exercises designed to compensate for the particular movements workers made at their plants.

In the countryside, where conditions were much more primitive, state authorities built on the foundations of Zemstvo medicine. By the 1930s, state farms had services comparable to those of the city. Conditions on collective farms were acknowledged as less satisfactory. Lack of personnel was one of the major problems. Physicians were extremely reluctant to work in the countryside. Much of the burden of care landed on *feldshers*. Obliged by the state to take part in the eradication of religion, they were often the object of hostility.

In theory at first, and later in practice, a feature of Soviet medicine that was commented on favourably by visitors (and envied by many who had no love of socialism), was the attempted abolition of the distinction between curative and preventive medicine. Prophylaxis figured large in all medical planning. In individual terms this appeared to observers as close inspection, from cradle to grave, of health-threatening times and circumstances (childhood, pregnancy, and the working environment). As in every other industrialized or industrializing nation, mother and child were accorded talismanic status. Russia and France vied for preeminence in this arena. In theory, women in the Soviet Union, were accorded equal rights with men. In the mid-1930s, over 39 percent of workers were women, apparently receiving the same wages as men. Special institutions, such as the Women's Consultation Bureau, were established, providing advice on menstruation, sexual intercourse, birth control, and related matters. Ideally, an expectant mother was examined at a bureau, given preferential treatment everywhere, seen once a month, and visited by a home inspector. Two months before confinement she could leave work on full wages. Between 1920 and 1936, a pregnant woman could legally decide to have an abortion. This liberty, in the eyes of most of the literate non-Soviet world, certified the evil nature of the Russian regime. By decree, abortions were free and had to be carried out by a doctor. Practical and ideological forces were at work here. Clandestine abortions were very frequent. Women were engaged in the production process. Stalin made abortion illegal when it served his purposes. The hope was that better maternity care would eventually obviate the need for abortion. In Moscow, a city of 2 million people in 1927, there were just over 53,000 births and 40,000 abortions. This was probably around the peak, after which numbers fell. During the period of easy access to abortion (largely a city phenomenon), the population of the Soviet Union continued to grow at about 3 million per annum.

Close supervision of the birth, feeding, weaning, and growth of children was praised and, if possible, practised in Russia. Certainly, in many cities, bureaus, nurseries, and other institutions paid great attention to milk provision, diet, and development generally. The assumption that scientific study of development was essential to successfully raising the nation's children was as important in Russia as anywhere else. The assumption was embedded in Moscow's State Scientific Research Institute for the Protection of Children and Adolescents. In the mid-1930s it had a staff of 130 scientific workers.

Seemingly rigorous laws relating to health (the needs of production could obviate them) also covered such things as factory building and inspection. Factories had committees on protection from hazards and on health that were created and run with extensive union involvement. Safety training was given prominence. The Russians took very seriously indeed the idea of a science of work that would identify conditions for maximum production by contented workers in safe surroundings, even though such conditions were usually far from being realized. Institutes for the study of occupational disease (in Moscow) and for hygiene of labour (in Leningrad) were established. Much research was done on toxic chemicals and diseases, such as silicosis. The clean, safe, model factories that visitors were allowed to see, such as the new metallurgy plants in Zaporozhye near the Crimea, stunned them. In 1937, the Swiss medical historian, Henry Sigerist (1891–1957), a social democrat who had been professor at Leipzig and six years earlier had emigrated to America, wrote of a visit to Russia: 'I shall always remember with deep emotion a day in 1935 spent in the Frezer Cutting Tool Plant, in Moscow, where I found pleasant surroundings, flowers everywhere, large well-ventilated and well lighted workshops with thousands of workers, men and women, mostly young people. The men were clean shaven, the women wore bright kerchiefs. All were busily engaged in work, while a woman's sweet voice sang, in German, through the loudspeaker, Schubert's song, "Du bist die Ruh', der Friede mild." And I could not help remembering other factories I had seen in the capitalist world. You come to realise what work can be, and what it must eventually become everywhere if there is to be a real civilisation' (Sigerist, 1937, p. 156).

Sanitation and the prevention of social disease were high on the Soviet agenda. A minimum of one sanitary physician was appointed for every 50,000 urban residents. Tuberculosis was targeted: a special department was organized within Narkomzdrav and a Tuberculosis Institute created in Moscow. Chairs in the subject were established in medical schools, and postgraduate courses begun. Dispensaries and sanatoria were founded that had, in 1937, 27,000 physicians. Tuberculosis dispensaries were sometimes large with a staff of up to twenty-five doctors. In the USSR, there were 750 dispensaries in 1936 (in Russia there were four in 1914). As in other things, rural areas of Russia suffered more from lack of provision than the towns. Dispensaries were centres for the control of TB in a district, carrying out studies of local epidemiology and social conditions, and providing diagnostic and therapeutic facilities. Although figures pronounced TB rates tumbling, Soviet health officials were well aware that their statistics were put to shame by those of most of Europe.

Antivenereal work was organized along much the same lines as action against TB. The dispensary was a fighting unit in the field. In 1936, the USSR had 1,476 of them. Patients were encouraged to visit through a system of secret identification. Treatment was made compulsory in 1927. Six months imprisonment could follow the knowing infection of a partner. Prostitution was attacked as a health problem (not a police matter). One attempted solution was the creation of *prophylactoria*, special institutions for women with VD, to live and work. These various measures along with contact tracing, education, and attempts to change attitudes towards shame, resulted in a claimed fall in incidence of gonorrhoea in the USSR from forty per ten thousand in 1914 to just over twenty in 1931.

Figures suggest that Narkomzdrav had some success in advancing to the goal of universally accessible, qualified care. In Russia, as everywhere else, hospital statistics were taken as the unquestioned demonstration of the success of a system of medical care. In 1913, it was estimated there were over 175,000 hospital beds (excluding mental hospitals) in what would become the USSR. In 1933, the number was said to be over 442,000. Maternity beds increased at the greatest rate. Hospital beds were utilized to capacity and maternity homes were overcrowded. Large hospitals, such as the Botkin Hospital in Moscow, which in the mid-1930s could accommodate 2,200 patients, were comparable to almost any similar institution found elsewhere.

Internationalism

International programmes and cooperation were both applauded as ideals and put into practice between the wars. Behind such activity lay humanitarian concerns, the hope of preventing future wars, downright self-interested protection against epidemics and doubtless many other stimuli.

Professional groups, charities, governments, and international agencies fostered collaboration. Straightforward emergency relief during disasters was the most visible form of cooperation. Relief from famine in the Soviet Union in 1921–3 was coordinated by the Norwegian Fridtjof Nansen (1861–1930), famed for his arctic explorations. Assistance to refugees, in a Europe of increasingly closed frontiers, was at the forefront of many relief programmes. Perhaps the most significant long-term effect of international work was to promote awareness of the vastly different ways in which health and disease statistics were returned, drugs prepared and standardized, and diagnoses established. Ideas of standardization and uniformity began to be elevated from the national to the international stage.

LEAGUE OF NATIONS

In 1919, no doubt partly because the fear of another war was so great and the possibility of it so likely, anything that could be done to avert it seemed worth trying. The League of Nations was formed in that year with forty-two members (not including the United States and Russia) 'to promote international co-operation'. The covenant stipulated that the league become involved in matters of health, and it soon did so. A great deal of its work was assisted by Rockefeller funds (even though the United States was not a member of the league). Most of the league's work centred on the prevention and cure of disease, medical education, public health, and standardization. However, abreast of international developments, ideas of promoting positive health began to creep into the agenda just before World War II.

In 1920, the Council of the League summoned a conference to draw up a scheme for dealing with international health matters. This conference was immediately faced with the spread of epidemics of typhus, relapsing fever, and cholera from Russia to Eastern Europe. On the conference's recommendation, an Epidemics Commission was set up that coordinated efforts to deal with the outbreaks and placed medical personnel and resources at the disposal of national authorities. The commission was then active in Greece in 1922 when, driven by advancing Turkish troops, 750,000 refugees arrived from Asia Minor carrying smallpox, cholera, and typhoid. A vaccination campaign was organized.

In 1923, the league formed a health organization (LNHO) with a health committee comprising specialists and public health officials who were to make policy. Epidemiology formed a major part of the organization's activity. An Epidemiological Intelligence Service was formed in Geneva, and an Eastern Epidemiological Intelligence Bureau was set up in Singapore in 1925. Ports in a vast eastern area (from Egypt and Vladivostok to Melbourne) kept the bureau informed telegraphically of epidemics, in order for quarantine measures to be recommended. The bureau undertook investigations into the efficacy of oral cholera vaccines. The Geneva Service standardized methods of compiling health statistics. Specific epidemiological enquiries pursued under the auspices of the organization in the 1920s, included investigations into cholera in India and Japan, cerebrospinal meningitis in Prussia, and health conditions in islands in the Southern Pacific.

The organization also had an educational programme for health workers. It published monographs on the public health arrangements of various countries and organized study tours for health workers. Such tours were inspired by political ideals. It was hoped, said the organization's literature that they would 'promote international co-operation and . . . establish contact between men engaged in similar work in different lands.' By 1930, 600 health officials had participated in this programme. International courses were organized in London and Paris in 1927.

Population movement and privation during the war had resulted in a recrudescence of malaria in Russia, the Balkans, Poland, and even Italy. A Malaria Commission was established in 1924 and carried out an enquiry. It recommended so-called *primary* measures: treatment of sufferers with quinine, tracking of cases, and instruction on means of prevention. Given the high price of quinine, the commission had clinical tests of mixtures of various alkaloids of cinchona bark carried out. Some of these were considered effective and cheaper. Malaria eradication and research programmes were widened in the 1920s to include, among other places, Corsica, Spain, and India. Education of health workers was considered imperative. Regular courses in malariology were set up in four European universities. A School of Malariology was opened in Rome in 1928. Engineers and agriculturists were taught land drainage and reclamation (Fig. 3.10). The Rockefeller Foundation, along with governments, subsidized students.

A commission was also appointed to study sleeping sickness in equatorial Africa. In the light of its work, representatives of relevant colonial ministries met in London in 1925 to discuss preventive measures. They agreed, among other things, on a passport for natives and standardization of registration. Specialists were sent to Entebbe on Lake Victoria in 1926–7, as a consequence of which, the commission recommended international agreements, supervision of native movement, and bush clearance. Another committee

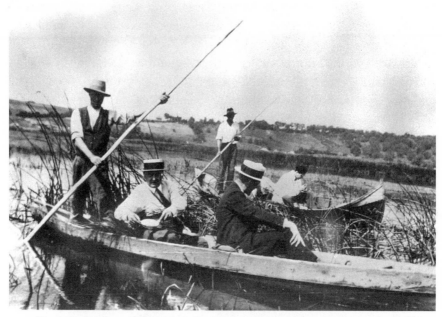

Fig. 3.10. Members of the Malaria Commission of the League of Nations collecting mosquito larvae on the Danube delta, 1929. *Source:* Wellcome Library Archives and Manuscripts. *Credit:* Wellcome Library, London (L0011626).

looked into the problem of the early diagnosis of leprosy, a scourge in South America, Eastern areas, and India (isolated cases also occurred in Scandinavia and the Baltic countries). The possibility of leprosy was frequently hidden by potential sufferers for fear of their being incarcerated in colonies.

In Europe, other diseases, preventive measures, and therapies were investigated; for example, BCG vaccination in Yugoslavia. An epidemiological study of the difference in death rate from cancer of the breast and of the uterus in Great Britain, Italy, and the Netherlands was undertaken. A clinical study of breast cancer showed that a third of women in these countries did not resort to surgery for breast cancer. Attempts were made to link racial types, blood groups, and cancer incidence, and to distinguish between the value of X-ray and radium treatments of cancer. A comparative enquiry was carried out into infant mortality in urban areas in Western Europe. When considered as a single group, stillbirths and children dying after premature labour comprised the largest number of deaths. Infantile diseases of the gut and respiratory tract came second. This study was seen at the time to indicate the inadequacy of prenatal and obstetrical care.

A great deal of the league's work centred on standardization, promoted through studies of vaccines, sera, and diagnostic testing. In 1925, a commission was set up to investigate nervous lesions in children who had been vaccinated against smallpox (postvaccinal encephalitis). Methods of lymph production and distribution were examined, but no blame could be allocated. Statistical evidence suggested that a first vaccination before the age of one reduced the incidence of sequelae. The health organization investigated the different methods of making the rabies vaccine in different countries and the comparative efficacy of the vaccines. Similar studies were carried out on the different standards in terms of units used to measure the efficacy of drugs and serums in different countries. A Permanent Standards Commission was established. Using the State Serum Institute in Copenhagen and public laboratories in other countries, the commission had some success in distributing drugs in standard units to commercial and government laboratories to be used as the basis for national and international uniformity of strength. Worldwide standards for insulin, digitalis, vitamins, and pituitary extract, among others, were determined in this way. Existing tests for syphilis were standardized in places as far apart as Montevideo and the Institut Pasteur in Paris. In the 1930s, with Rockefeller backing, the LNHO turned its attention increasingly to nutrition and the effects of poverty. It developed 'health indices' that took into account local factors, such as geography, population density, morbidity, insanity, and alcoholism.

ROCKEFELLER MEDICINE

The interwar years saw some expansion of Western medicine into countries where it had previously been only a small presence. Things changed relatively little in tropical countries. The most dramatic colonial upheavals and attempts to bring Western medicine to the whole population of new nations occurred largely after World War II. Creating new colonies in the old European style was no longer possible between the wars and the United States expressed no interest in doing so, but its economic interest in many places grew and with it Western medicine. The adoption of Western medicine throughout the world cannot be catalogued here, but the activities of the Rockefeller Foundation merit attention for two reasons. First, because of its scale, and second, because it attempted to solve national problems by applying what it saw as universal scientific solutions: in other words, American models. In 1913 the newly established Rockefeller Foundation had created its International Health Commission, which became a Board in 1916 and a Division in 1927. President of the foundation from 1917 was George E.

Vincent (1864–1961), who immediately launched a massive, integrated, global programme in public health and medical education. The League of Nations was an important conduit for the transport of Rockefeller policies. The successive heads of the foundation's international section were Wickcliffe Rose (1862–1931) and Colonel Frederick F. Russell (1870–1960), both strong leaders who had a huge influence on policy. The medical education division of the foundation was founded in 1919 and headed by Richard Pearce and has already been referred to (p. 297).

The scale of Rockefeller intervention is staggering. Practically every country in the world received some form of assistance although those with strong colonial governments were largely left alone. Assistance took two major forms. First, the financing of medical education, which largely involved encouraging medical schools to adopt the Johns Hopkins model. This was the principal form of aid in Europe and Australasia, but the rest of the world was encouraged to develop on these lines too. Rockefeller founded or helped promote modern schools in, for example, Beirut, Hong Kong, Singapore, Bangkok, and Beijing (Peking as it was then known in the West). Second, and of most relevance here, public health programmes were initiated and assisted.

The foundation's stated intentions behind its programmes were perfectly embodied in the form those programmes took. At the highest level the foundation always espoused the cause of human betterment through science and education. Disease was seen as *the* major obstacle to such improvement. Poverty, then, in Rockefeller thinking was largely a consequence than a cause of disease. This was evident in the justification of the hookworm programme in Mexico. The Mexican, freed of debilitating hookworm disease, would (it was said by a Rockefeller officer in 1925) have 'more money in his pocket with which to buy better food, better clothes, better homes and better schools. With better schools there will come enlightenment. Intelligence will displace ignorance, and with intelligence there will come a true social revolution' (Birn, 2000, p. 368). A contrast between this approach and the Russian route to such a goal was surely intended and would certainly have been made by readers at the time.

To a great extent, Rockefeller targeted diseases with relatively well-defined incidence, obvious injurious socioeconomic effects, and an aetiological agent that was known or whose mode of transmission was known. Diseases also had to be susceptible to laboratory investigation and eradicable by some combination of vaccines, straightforward public health measures, and education. Hookworm, yellow fever, and malaria roughly fulfilled these criteria. Leprosy and TB, in which there was clearly some extremely complicated relation to the socioeconomic causes of poverty, did not. Except for the slightly odd case of France, TB was never the focus of a major programme. The foundation consistently refused to get involved with TB in Mexico, a country to which it paid a great deal of attention and where a very successful yellow fever eradication programme had been organized. In Rockefeller strategy, the physician and scientist were favoured over the economist and urban planner as the agents of change. The technologies of the vaccine or the insecticide efficiently administered were seen as the most progressive of social forces.

The foundation was inflexible, obsessional almost, about the methods and standards it approved of and funded. Public health schools were supported by the foundation when they conformed to the model of the School of Public Health at the Johns Hopkins University. The foundation had funded this institution that opened in 1918 and trained public health experts who worked throughout the world. In the field, only the best qualified and up-to-date experts were countenanced and only the most scientific of methods. Organization was a high priority. The foundation aimed at a universal, stateless solution to public health matters. Not surprisingly, it ran into enormous local difficulties. On the one hand, Rockefeller intervention was seen as sinister American imperialism; on the other, it simply did not work because of ignorance of local practices. Problems were encountered with cultures that apparently shared enthusiasm for modern scientific approaches. The French TB programme looked, even to observers at the time, like a dialogue of the deaf. Rockefeller intransigence was well illustrated in Fiji. Sylvester M. Lambert (1882–1947) was a Rockefeller representative in the South Pacific islands that were ravaged by hookworm, yaws, and malaria, and where Western medical practitioners were few. Lambert campaigned to train local practitioners who would understand local customs and dispense public health advice. They would have been the equivalent of Russian *feldshers*. Lambert reported that his plan gave Pearce and the New York office 'almost physical nausea'. Pearce insisted that Rockefeller 'must stick to the policy of aiding only Class A schools'.

The question obviously arises; to what extent was the foundation an instrument American interests? The answer is that it was, but not in any obvious way. The name 'Rockefeller' was not held in high regard in many corners of American government nor by many members of the U.S. public. The Rockefeller Foundation was seen by some as anti-American; as a charitable device for furthering industrial strategies. A strike of mine workers in Colorado where the Rockefellers had interests, culminated in the 'Ludlow massacre' of 1914 – the 'Black Hole of Ludlow' – in which thirteen women and children were suffocated. Foundation employees saw themselves as furthering social progress by employing universal approaches of objective science. Nonetheless, these approaches, however universal they were proclaimed to be, were the modern American way of doing things and were seen as such both at home and abroad. American commercial and economic interests did, knowingly or not, follow Rockefeller enterprises. Sometimes, Rockefeller officials were more forthcoming than they knew about their policies. As one observed in 1917: 'Dispensaries and physicians have of late been peacefully penetrating areas of the Philippine islands and demonstrating the fact that for the purposes of placating primitive and suspicious peoples medicine has some advantages over machine guns.'

Between the wars, U.S. trade and investment made it the dominant power in Mexico, Central America, and the Caribbean. By 1945 its hegemony was secured throughout most of South America. Whereas many South American countries had remained neutral during World War I, almost the whole land mass eventually followed the lead of the United States after Pearl Harbour (1941). But even before American business showed up in the Southern American continent, Rockefeller money had been there paving the way, whether deliberately or not. A huge amount of foundation money was devoted to Central and South America in the 1920s. For example, using its usual approach, the foundation surveyed medical education in that continent and nearly $1,000,000 was invested in modernizing the medical school at the University of São Paulo in Brazil.

In Europe, Rockefeller officials walked a delicate tightrope between intervening in the affairs of nation-states and promoting peace and international collaboration by the alleviation of ill health. Political considerations and American interests were ever present, but not often crudely visible. Generosity did not flow equably. The Soviets were denied aid even for famine and typhus relief in 1921. Nonetheless, the foundation's stance in this matter looks like a recognition of the impossibility of running things in its own way rather than obvious anti-Communist dogma. In Europe, soon after the war, the international programme soon jettisoned short-term relief measures, such as its feeding programme, and turned to long-term strategies. A great deal of the foundation's energy was directed at modernizing public health in politically unstable areas, notably Poland and what it called Central (otherwise Eastern) Europe. Yugoslavia was a major beneficiary of this programme. A State School of Hygiene was established in Poland in

1926 on the model of the Johns Hopkins School of Public Health. This was half-funded by Rockefeller and half by the Polish State. Such intervention, whether designed as political or not, served American (and Western European interests). These regions were literally and metaphorically a *cordon sanitaire*. They were a buffer against invasions of both armed forces and epidemic diseases.

Everywhere, the principal Rockefeller strategy was to identify far-sighted institutions and individuals whose leadership, research, and teaching could be expected to follow American lines. The foundation granted fellowships, supported travel, created experts, arranged international meetings, and established institutes and clinics. A scheme for training statisticians began in the early 1920s, indicating the foundation's awareness of the importance of creating international uniformity as a road to political stability. The tropical medicine programme, which largely began by instituting prophylactic and therapeutic measures, increasingly incorporated laboratory investigations, especially at the Rockefeller Institute in New York, until then largely concerned with the diseases of industrial society. By the 1930s, work in the field was gradually losing out to laboratory-based viral research, which was seen as the cutting edge of progress.

With the formation of the foundation, the hookworm control programme of the Rockefeller Sanitary Commission that had been confined to the southern states of America, was translated onto a world stage. The programme, in the words of the foundation's historian, 'was extended to fifty-two countries in six continents, and to twenty-nine islands of the seas' (Fosdick, 1952, p. 33). The world of capital, in which Rockefeller had made his money, was soon found to be part of the problem (although it was not expressed that way). Migration of labour, especially from India, was identified as a major source of infection. Millions were examined and treated, many *en masse*. In conformity with Rockefeller policy, therapeutic incursions were always intended as partnerships with governments from which Rockefeller would gradually retreat.

After 1915, the prevention of yellow fever absorbed huge amounts of Rockefeller money. The offending mosquito carrier had been identified before the war (p. 228). The foundation created a commission under General William C. Gorgas (1854–1920), Chief Sanitary Officer of the United States Army in Cuba, which, in 1916, visited various South American countries. The commission concluded that the endemic centre of the disease was in Guayaquil in Equador. The plan to eliminate the fever from Guayaquil, and hence elsewhere, seemed to meet with success. Indeed, after 1919, no further cases occurred in Equador. Similar policies were effective elsewhere in South America except that, contrary to the view that eradication of the disease in its endemic centre was a sufficient prophylactic, it continued to make sporadic appearances. In 1925, a second commission was sent to West Africa. Four of the researchers died, including Hideyo Noguchi, discoverer (in 1913) of the spirochete in brains of individuals with tertiary syphilis. Towards the end of the decade, yellow fever broke out anew in South America, and the aetiological theory on which prevention was based, was put under the microscope. Fieldwork and research in laboratories in New York, West Africa, and Brazil resulted in a revised and much more complex causal theory that implicated several species of mosquitoes and jungle animals as carriers. The development of a vaccine in the foundation's New York laboratories was the high point of interwar work on yellow fever. In 1937, the laboratories of the Rockefeller's International Health Division (IHD) began production of the vaccine. In 1938, more than a million people were vaccinated. From 1942–6, 34 million doses of the agent were manufactured. Like so many modern vaccines, however, it seemed to arrive when the disease had been brought under control.

Malaria figured second only to yellow fever in the foundation's world programme. Originally, malaria control was confined to the southern states of America. In 1921, it was extended to Nicaragua, then to Brazil, and then to practically every malarious region in the world. The foundation supported training schools in, for instance, Athens and Karachi, granted fellowships and subsidized textbooks in a score of languages. It backed research into the natural history of the varieties of Anopheles mosquito and supported eradication programmes using a number of insecticides. During this period, malaria practically vanished from the United States, Italy, and Greece.

India supplies another case history of tension between the foundation and foreign government; in this case the, British one on the great subcontinent. Indian resentment at British control developed enormously between the wars, and by the late 1920s, Congress was demanding complete independence. Through repression and constitutional reform, Britain retained the upper hand. Increasingly during this period provincial governments were charged with public health administration, but lacked the financial wherewithal to handle it. Preventive medicine was largely for colonials. The foundation attempted to introduce disease control programmes, demonstration health units and the training of public health personnel. The diseases targeted were hookworm and malaria in the Madras presidency in the South, following discovery of the high levels of hookworm infestation in migrant labourers. In the opinion of historians, the foundation got nowhere. Government red tape and indifference stymied active public health measures. Beyond its specific projects, Rockefeller seemed to have no clear policy for India as a whole.

Western powers remained in control of almost the whole of southeast Asia during this period, many areas of which were rocked by anticolonial agitation. China, a republic in these years, remained in virtual anarchy with local warlords, central government, and other interest groups contending for power. In 1951, it was claimed that, since its establishment, the money the Rockefeller Foundation had expended on China was second only to that spent on the United States. From early on, investment in China was clearly seen by Rockefeller people as a means of promoting political stability in addition to being of medical benefit. 'If we wait till China becomes stable,' said one physician, 'we shall lose the greatest opportunity we have ever had of dealing with the nation.' China, of course, already had a tiny Western medical presence. Around 1914 there were over 300 Protestant mission hospitals. In 1919 there were 600 foreign physicians in China and 900 Chinese physicians trained in Western Medicine. Through fellowships, the foundation supported missionary medical education. Its major project, however, began in 1915 when it purchased a medical college from the London Missionary Society, which was made into the Peking Union Medical College (PMC). It was intended to be the 'Johns Hopkins of China'. Officially opened in 1921, it was any medical modernist's dream school and hospital, with its labs, technology, and bed provision. In conformity with Rockefeller strategy, the school was not intended to train run-of-the-mill doctors, but medical teachers and researchers. Some of Europe and America's medical luminaries, such as Walter Bradford Cannon, were visiting professors. The Japanese invasion of China and then World War II, eclipsed the school. In the 1920s, the Yale-educated James Y. C. Yen (1893–1990) organized a Mass Education Movement based on self-help and the combating of disease in China, by introducing Western knowledge and public health methods. Many of the small number of native Chinese who were educated in Western medicine, especially at PMC, were hostile to traditional Chinese medicine.

Nazi Germany

Dealing with Nazi Germany in a separate section immediately creates problems. It suggests that Nazi medicine was qualitatively so unlike Western medicine elsewhere that it needs to be put in historiographical quarantine. Separation is more a matter of narrative convenience because Nazi medicine and Fascism in general contained ideological and practical elements common to Western society at large in this period. That is, National Socialism does not need to be seen in all its aspects as something so alien that recourse to a unique explanation is required. There is good reason for dealing with Nazi medicine last, however, for the Fascists attempted to build a medicine that was based on assumptions that sometimes ran counter to those who held medical power elsewhere. Most striking about Nazi assumptions is how they were almost entirely opposite to those favoured by the Russian élite. A consideration of Fascism at the end of peacetime medicine also leads to the consideration of World War II.

Nazi medical ideals were intimately related to their ideas about race and their mythology of the authentic forms of historical German life. In the mid-1920s, many nations promoting ideas of fitness to breed, began to emphasize the importance of race as much as class or individual attainment. About twenty university institutes and a dozen or so journals devoted to the study of racial science and hygiene had been established in Germany even before the Nazis came to power. It was the primary subject of research at the prestigious Kaiser Wilhelm Institute for Anthropology in Berlin (1927–45), directed by Eugen Fischer (1874–1967), and at the Kaiser Wilhelm Institute for Genealogy in Munich (1919–45), directed by the psychiatrist Ernst Rüdin (1874–1952). In these places, Schutzstaffel (SS) physicians were trained to construct 'genetic registries', later used to round up Jews and gypsies. The largest centre for these sorts of studies was the Frankfurt Institute for Racial Hygiene, presided over by the physician and anthropologist Otmar von Verschuer and his assistant Joseph Mengele (the 'Angel of Death' at Auschwitz).

Biological and medical language was a very important constituent of the conservative, supremacist ideology of National Socialism. The Nazi state was to be an integrated organic one, in which individuals were to live in line with nature's dictates. Hitler insisted that the basis of law be 'healthy popular feeling'. The ideology of 'blood and soil' privileged the countryside with its invigorating open-air activities, simple life, and hardy peasant stock. Taking its cue from German Fascism, Nazi medicine was soaked in nationalist and holist doctrines. It was antispecialist and antitechnological. Nazis demanded the replacement of mechanistic thinking in science and medicine by an organic view. They praised the virtues of homeopathy and folk medicine over mass-produced chemicals, and condemned the separation of bedside and laboratory science. They touched a popular nerve. Natural health movements and alternative medicine were widely popular in Weimar Germany. The Nazi leadership denounced smoking and in some cases (Hitler himself) promoted vegetarianism. This was not just talk. Hospitals devoted to natural healing were established. Physical fitness (there was a Strength-through-Joy sports certificate) and the eating of whole-grain bread was promoted (sometimes demanded) with some success. Research on environmental toxins was supported. Potential genetic poisons were obviously of great interest, tobacco and alcohol in particular. Nazi ideologues permanently walked a tightrope between courting alternative medicine and keeping the doctors happy.

The National Socialist medical ideal was the GP; a broadly educated and experienced *family* doctor who was both an avuncular advisor and functionary, keeping an eye on the national health for the party. Nazi anti-modernist propaganda denounced the urban world as the seat of materialism, the diseases of civilization, atmospheric pollution, denervating modern inventions, and Jewry. The leader of the Nazi Physicians' League, Gerhard Wagner, expressed hatred for modern hospitals and polyclinics. In an organic (totally self-sufficient) world, the doctor, it was said, could practise an honest, uncomplicated medicine, treating individuals in their natural, supportive surroundings. Nazi medicine drew heavily on neo-Hippocratic writings, picturing the modern doctor working in the shadow of the Greek physician and using the body's natural healing powers (*vis medicatrix naturae*) to restore the patient's wholeness. Nationalism was also well served by the celebration of Paracelsus at this time. The medicine of that sixteenth-century doctor was praised for its simplicity and for being close to the people.

At least in the early years of the National Socialist regime, its medical spokesmen discounted specialism. Declared policy was to reduce the number of specialists and redistribute them. Postgraduate education was to include more generalist training. Specialist numbers initially fell by 40 percent when the Nazis came to power, although less for ideological reasons than for the fact that Jewish specialists were evicted from the profession. The antispecialist policy largely failed because of a reluctance of doctors to practise in the countryside. Indeed, one strand of Nazi ideology favoured specialists (just as another one created a romantic mythology of the machine). Surgeons, when pictured as masculine, practical, heroic individuals, were well accommodated in the Nazi martial ideology. The 'natural representatives of the master race usually turn to surgery', wrote one Nazi physician who considered that in surgery 'if anywhere, strong will and action are evidently still decisive' (Kater, 1989, p. 28).

Nazi's prided themselves on the masculine nature of their movement. An editorial in the journal of the Nazi Physicians' League of 1933 remarked that National Socialism was 'the most masculine movement to have appeared in centuries' (Proctor, 1992, p. 31). It was claimed that 'the heroic man of National Socialism and the organic fully developed racial man – these are one and the same' (Proctor, 1988, p. 237). Nazi policy was to take women out of the workplace and place them in the home. Makeup was frowned upon. Women were barred from certain professions. The proportion of women among German physicians grew, the regime waiving its quota because of preoccupations about medical reserves. The nursing force also increased from eighteen to twenty per ten thousand of population between 1932 and 1939. Women doctors faced massive discrimination once qualified (especially if they were married). Those committed to the movement *and* to emancipation developed a doctrine of the fitness of women for certain sorts of medical work because of innate female qualities.

Access to birth control was severely limited for German women. The government ideal was the four-child family. After December 1938, a mother of eight children was eligible for the gold Honour Cross of German Motherhood (bronze and silver were awarded to the slightly less fecund). The Nazis were not unusual in this, but it took ten babies to earn a gold medal in France. After 1938 in Germany, all public officials were required to marry or resign. Unmarried women were not considered citizens. The birth rate between 1933 and 1944 jumped from 14.7 per thousand to eighteen per thousand.

Not surprisingly, in an ideology centred on population and propagation, the Nazi doctor was expected to be especially skilled in obstetrics. Women were to give birth in the rural home not the urban hospital. The latter, as the seat of specialism and assisted labour, denoted modern perversions that corrupted traditional practices (pain in general was seen as a purifying experience). Nazi women, it was said, would welcome natural childbirth presided over by the GP. Racial hardiness and purity depended on it. Home delivery was vigorously promoted when Leonardo Conti (1900–45) became Reich health leader in 1939. His mother, a practising midwife, was made Reich director of midwifery. 'To be born in a hospital is bad,' said Conti junior in 1942, 'but childbirth in an everyday household is good' (Kater, 1989, p. 27). Dying at home was also advocated as the most natural end to life. As with so many things under National Socialism, rhetoric and reality were miles apart. Figures for institutionalized childbirth rose in the 1930s.

The health record of the Nazis was mixed. The official sickness rate rose. Tuberculosis and VD declined at first. There was a marked increase in diphtheria and scarlet fever. There was an increased incidence of industrial accidents, particularly among those engaged in the most physical of tasks, such as construction work. Demand for hospital beds grew faster than supply. Hospital building rates fell (the country was mobilizing for war). Broadly speaking, for most Germans who were not subject to discrimination, medical care before the war remained about the same or fell slightly below late Weimar levels. Factors beyond Nazi control, such as the Depression, did not help.

From the start of their regime in 1933, the Nazis showed their determination to bring about their preferred social order and to destroy any opposition. This was as true in medicine as anywhere else. They were not without help: physicians were Nazified sooner and more thoroughly than members of any other profession. At the time, this was a fact of which many doctors were proud. Medicine was an important metaphor within Fascist culture. One National Socialist doctor called Hitler 'the great physician of his people' (Kater, 1989, p. 4). In the universities, medical faculties were preeminent (the continuation of a Weimar development). The expulsion of Jewish staff of the faculties began in 1933 with a Law for the Reconstitution of the German Civil Service.

One of the first steps in the Nazi's dissolution of alternative power bases was the reorganization of social insurance. Sickness funds were largely in the hands of the unions and often administered by unpaid officers. The labour movement was jealous of this right and several times over the previous fifty years had fought off attempts to nullify it. Immediately after the trade unions were dismantled, a law was passed in May 1933 against self-governing structures in social insurance. Ostensibly reestablishing a professional civil service, the law purged 'nationally unreliable' and 'non-Ayran' persons from public service and had wide ramifications beyond medicine. It effectively disbarred honorary officials from trade union service. Government officials were appointed to run the sickness boards.

This purge was undertaken with another to disbar doctors (and dentists) in the 'nationally unreliable' and 'non-Ayran' categories, and also any who had engaged in communist activities, from holding a panel license (i.e., the right to insurance practice). There were 35,000 panel doctors in 1933. 'Non-Aryan' doctors, having settled in industrial areas, made up a significant number of doctors, especially panel doctors. In 1933 in Berlin (a city with a high proportion of Jews), over half of the 6,558 physicians were classified as non-Aryans. Nearly 60 percent of the 3,481 panel doctors fell in the same category. Jewish and socialist physicians were prominent in health reform programmes and in promoting local schemes, such as polyclinics. By the end of 1933, about 2,800 physicians had been excluded from insurance practice. The purge was welcomed by young Nazi physicians; the profession was overcrowded and there was a waiting list for panel practices. Between 1934 and 1938, nearly 6,000 Jewish doctors left Germany. Homosexual and politically active physicians got out too. The German Federation of Medical Associations gave the purge tacit approval. By 1935 the National-Socialist Physicians' Federation had 14,500 members. In 1938, Jews were effectively no longer allowed to be designated physicians. Among the myriad reasons for these actions, the least unsubtle were those of racial cleansing. Jewish physicians treated Jewish patients and, if the claims of medicine were to be believed, they prolonged the lives of many doubly contaminated by the overt diseases of the clinic and the more insidious disease of 'blood'. In spite of the expulsion of Jewish doctors, the numbers of practitioners slowly rose above Weimar levels. A great many doctors were employed by the Wehrmacht, the Sturmabteilung (SA), Hitler Youth and the SS. The net result was that in civilian practice the proportion of doctors fell (the same was true of nurses).

The explanations for the Nazi's intense racism cannot be fathomed merely by historical examination of biological and medical ideas, but it is important to see how these ideas were deep structural constituents of the National Socialist way of thinking. At Auschwitz, physicians described the gas chambers as the 'Great Hospital' where 'patients' received the 'Great Therapy' (Seidelman, 1992, p. 272). Two explicit assumptions underlay Nazi policies and practices with regard to health and disease. First, the Nazis *always* took the health of the state, metaphorically and materially, to be the highest good. It was far greater than the needs, rights, or demands of the individual (the needs of the ruling few perhaps excepted). Second, was the single-mindedness with which the Nazis identified racial purity with the 'blood' (literally and metaphorically) of people (in everyday parlance, the German people) of so-called pure Ayran (otherwise Nordic) descent. Any other 'blood' was regarded as polluting. For the Nazis, non-Aryan blood was a pathology-bearing substance Gerhard Wagner declared 'Judaism is disease incarnate' (Proctor, 1992, p. 36). Many individuals had previously taken such a line. The Nazis, however, ruled by dictatorship and made racial hygiene the key element of practical politics. Implementation of the new politics quickly followed the assumption of power.

Following its assault on the unions, in July 1933 the government passed the Law for the Prevention of Genetically Diseased Offspring. This law, based on United States legislation, permitted forcible sterilization of anyone with a disease designated genetic, such as feeble-mindedness, Huntington's chorea, schizophrenia, and severe alcoholism. Gerhard Wagner along with Heinrich Himmler and others drew up the list. Doctors were required to register all cases of genetic disease known to them. At least 350,000 people were sterilized under the law. Militants thought this a disgracefully modest number. Sterilization became big business. Companies designed and sold sterilization equipment. In women, X-rays, tubal ligation, and the new technique of injecting super-cooled carbon dioxide into the Fallopian tubes did the trick. In the year of the sterilization law, concentration camps were established by Goering and Himmler in Dachau for 'enemies of the state'. In 1935, the so-called Nuremberg Laws prohibited marriage or sexual relations between Jews and non-Jews. Prospective marital partners were to be examined by a physician to prevent 'racial pollution'.

The details of the Nazi's cleansing of this pollution need not be rehearsed here, but even an outline makes clear that they were under no illusion as to the size of the task necessary to produce what they deemed a healthy state. In 1937, the illegal sterilization of black children and gypsies began. In the same year 'Rhineland bastards' (children born after the occupation of the Rhineland by French Colonial troops from Africa) were sterilized. Most sterilizations came to an end in 1939 when the programme switched to euthanasia, murder, and genocide. In October of this year, Hitler issued an order allowing doctors to carry out mercy killings on the incurably sick. This was partly a practical policy bound up with the decision to go to war.

Euthanasia was widely debated everywhere and the Nazis were not the only ones to suggest the killing of what were called 'nature's mistakes' in an article in the *Journal of the American Psychiatric Association* (1942), which referred to retarded children (Proctor, 1992, p. 34). In Germany, the extermination of the mentally ill and retarded children by the use of lethal starvation and drugs was underway by 1940. Some 140,000 mental patients in Germany alone were killed by 1945. Polish and later Russian mental patients were systematically exterminated. When made public, and officially sanctioned in Germany, the policy had many supporters. Many parents wrote to hospitals requesting euthanasia for their children. At Haldemar psychiatric hospital, the 10,000th cremation was celebrated with beer for the whole staff (Proctor, 1992, p. 36). In January 1940, the first experiments were begun by physicians at Brandenburg Hospital to find a gas that would optimize mass killing. In 1941, experiments under the auspices of physicians were carried out on Zyklon B (hydrocyanic acid), using Russian prisoners at Auschwitz. Russians, who joined the war against Germany in 1941, had long been seen as a racial threat. In March 1942 death camps were erected in occupied territories and the mass gassing of Jews, Slavs, gypsies, and other 'racial enemies' began. The gas chambers of psychiatric hospitals in Germany were reinstalled at Auschwitz, Majdanek, and Treblinka. The scale of the slaughter that followed is now well known.

As is also well known, Nazi biological investigators used the opportunity of war to experiment on human beings. Before the war, experiments on unknowing adults and children were not uncommon (pp. 309–10), but with the Nazis the case seems to have been one of experiments forced on knowing (although by no means fully understanding), nonconsenting subjects. There seems to have been no precedent for this in the recent Western past. Studies were carried out on high-altitude decompression, the potability of sea water, the effects of sulphanilamide on gunshot wounds, the production of sterilty by X-rays, the efficacy of electroshock therapy, and many more things. Gynaecological 'investigations' were prominent. Studies on hypothermia (aimed at helping pilots ditched in the sea) were carried out at Dachau by military physicians from the physiology department at the University of Kiel. Political prisoners were immersed in vats of ice and freezing water. Later, experiments were conducted on men standing in cold night air who had freezing water poured over them. Many died. Some of the researchers who were involved refused to carry out orders.

World War II, 1939–45

THE WAR MACHINES

World War II began in 1939 as a European conflict and ended in 1945 with most nations in the world (three quarters of its population) being involved. Historians of medicine have written far less about World War II than about the Great War, so any account must have something of a fragmentary or unbalanced feel. This lack of detail in places probably does not prohibit some generalizations. Far less needs to be said about the Second World War than the First World War. The two wars can be painted on one canvas. The major powers created their modern war machines during the first global conflict, and in 1939 they wheeled them out again. Indeed, in one sense, they had never been put away. Civilian medicine between the wars was military medicine in waiting.

What *was* different about World War II was that it frequently blurred the distinction between combatant and noncombatant. Towards the end, it was fought out on virtually the whole of the enemies' territories. The use of the 'air raid' in Europe turned the war, at times, into one of attrition of civilians. Statistics are guesses: deaths totalled about 25 million military personal, 30 million civilians, and five million victims of the holocaust. Among these figures are at least 20 million Russians. Countries that had had negligible civilian casualties in the First World War counted their dead and wounded on a major scale in the Second World War. For example, about sixty thousand British civilians died of war-related causes, around a quarter of the number killed in the armed forces (figures vary). Approximately 190,000 civilians were wounded, most of whom had bomb-related injuries. Medicine at home was organized as part of a machine for ensuring survival, commitment to the war ends, and productivity, just as medicine at the front was. As one doctor, writing to the *British Medical Journal* in 1939 put it (in an observation that could have been made in any of the belligerent countries): the 'civilian population[s] must be treated as if they were combatant troops; they must be under authority' (Bourke, 1998, p. 226).

AT THE FRONT

Military medicine was, or was meant to be, a highly differentiated, hier-archically organized service industry, essential to an efficient fighting machine. In most armies, most men who went to war were inspected, vaccinated, and inoculated. On the best-organized fronts, sanitary measures were established to control infectious disease. Ideally, medical staff, including doctors, nurses, technicians, auxiliaries, and administrators, were arranged in teams. The hospital was at the apex of the system. Record keeping, as had been learned in civilian life, was essential to good, disciplined management. The aim of military medicine was to return men to the war fit to fight, or otherwise disposed of, so as not to interfere with the action. Venereal disease and psychiatric complaints occupied a great deal of medical work. Some military and civilian arenas, notably the prisoner of war camps in the Far East, such as Changi in Singapore, have medical histories that can be described using the usual parameters: mortality and morbidity rates, ratios of medical staff to patients, and so forth. However, the frequent extreme malnutrition, terrifying incidence of infectious disease, and the brutality of some prison camp personnel make their stories exceptional in some ways. Yet the organizational response of the interned to these conditions, based on military medical training, replicates the adaptability story that characterized Allied responses throughout the war.

Overall, Allied appreciation of the role that medicine could play in the war was greater than that of the Axis powers, and in consequence, Allied medical organization was superior. In the German army, the occasional persistence of older values that held sickness to be moral weakness probably cost it dearly. When medical services worked effectively they may well have turned the tide of a campaign, as British medicine possibly did in the Western Desert. Sickness rates among the British troops in this campaign were less than half those of the Wehrmacht. Good camp sanitation, the maintenance of sound hygiene among the troops, the medical policing of civilians and prophylactic measures, all played their part. British medical officers were probably treated more as equals by their combatant colleagues (possibly learning from the Great War) than were their German counterparts. In Burma, a wretchedly difficult campaign medically and militarily speaking, Lieutenant-General (later Field-Marshal Viscount) William Slim (1891–1970) recognized that medical success was far more than a medical matter. 'More than half the battle against disease', he declared, 'is fought not by doctors but by regimental officers.' 'Good doctors' were no use 'without good discipline' (Harrison, 2004, p. 194).

World War I was largely fought by stationary armies that organized a system of front-line medical management and distribution routes for the subsequent treatment of the sick and wounded. World War II was one of constant troop (and very often civilian) movement. Arrangements for evacuation and treatment, however, remained based on World War I models, but these generally required extensive modification. Aircraft evacuation of the wounded played a vital role in some theatres. Also, based on World War I experience, planners in all armies expected an action to produce a ratio of killed to wounded of something like one to four, and between 5 to 20 percent of troops injured. About 0.3 percent of troops were thought likely to report sick each day.

In the British army, the RAMC provided medical services. Each infantry battalion had a Medical Officer, a medical orderly and about twenty infantrymen. In April 1940, male doctors under forty-one were conscripted. A year later, the age was raised to forty-six and women doctors under thirty-one were included. By 1945 roughly a third of the nation's doctors were in uniform.

At the front were the Advanced and Field Dressing Stations. The CCS was the point of convergence of all casualties. The CCS was sited at the head of a railway, at the other end of which was a general hospital. Technical and organizational experiences in the Western Desert and North Africa seem to have been formative. Flexibility, mobility, and forward treatment became key phrases. Evacuation by aircraft (notably American aircraft in North Africa) was invaluable. Early unsatisfactory experiences with blood transfusion were turned into the production of a massive life-saving service. When there was rapid movement of the front line, mobile Field Surgical Teams were formed to act in forward areas (a development that captured the imagination of the press). Mobile Neurosurgical Units were formed permitting early closure of wounds. Operating conditions could vary enormously (in East Bengal the neurosurgical unit did all its operations at night, the heat was so intolerable). In North Africa there were relatively generous facilities for convalescence and rehabilitation. The four general hospitals 'provided facilities for massage, remedial mobility exercises, and weight exercises' (Harrison, 2004, p. 159).

The medical corps of the German army was organized by battalions, each one of which served an army in the field. A battalion usually had four companies, each controlling a field hospital. Stretcher bearers took casualties to a CCS. From there, serious cases went to a field hospital. Soldiers needing major surgery were sent to general hospitals that were usually set up in large towns. The medical department also had antigas, decontamination companies, and disinfestation platoons.

Combat injuries differed from those of the Great War. Bomb blasts, vehicle explosions and high-speed collisions, parachute jumping, and so on, tended to create simultaneous multiple injuries in the skeleton and viscera rather than the sort of damage accompanying a sniper's bullet. Burns to personnel trapped in aircraft and tanks were common. Surgery was far more successful than in the Great War. As operators recognized, this was not always because their techniques were much better. A number of factors were contributory. First, surgeons had, in the sulphonamides and then, after D-Day, penicillin, the systemic bacteriocides they had wished for in 1914–18. The overall death rate from wound infection among allied forces in the West was about 3 percent. Specialism was recognized and became the basis of organization. The orthopaedic surgeons did not reign supreme as they had done in the Great War. Plastic surgeons, such as Archibald MacIndoe (1900–60) at the East Grinstead Plastic Surgery Centre in England, developed their techniques and achieved worldwide recognition. Neurosurgeons also put their success down to prompt segregation of patients, a practice that began at Alamein in October 1942. Eventually, all head-wound cases were treated by neurosurgeons anywhere between ten to 1,000 miles from the front. In one Italian battle, one such unit of three operating teams performed 334 operations in sixteen consecutive days. There were specialist neurosurgical hospitals at home, notably the Military Hospital (Head injuries) in Oxford, and the Canadian hospital at Basingstoke. Death rates of 1 percent in head wounds were recorded by the British, Canadians, and Americans. Although limited, experience with heart wounds was to lay the technical basis and confidence for the huge growth of postwar cardiac surgery.

The *in vitro* antibacterial effect of the mould *Penicillium notatum* had been observed by Alexander Fleming (1881–1955) at St. Mary's Hospital, London in 1928. In 1936, using a Rockefeller Foundation grant to buy equipment, a group under Howard G. Florey (1898–1968) began work on antibiotic substances. In 1940, Florey, Ernst Chain (1906–79), and Norman G. Heatley (1911–2004) produced small amounts of penicillin from surface culture, and in 1941 carried out successful clinical tests. Attempts to interest a British pharmaceutical industry at war failed, and so Florey and Heatley travelled to America. In the United States, the Committee on Medical Research (CMR) had been formed in June 1941 to organize research on problems related to national defence. It organized work on, among other things, antimalarials, insecticides, blood and blood substitutes, and aviation medicine. The Chairman of CMR, Alfred N. Richards (1876–1966), was a professor of pharmacology at the University of Pennsylvania and extremely well connected to the American pharmaceutical industry. Richards used his government position and industrial connections to back clinical tests and large-scale production of penicillin. Small quantities were available by spring 1942. In Oxford, England, Florey and his group were also making small amounts. In 1943, groups of U.S. investigators were 'accredited' to use the antibiotic. Patients treated included the victims of burns after a fire at the Coconut Grove Nightclub in Boston. This was followed by a study of the use of penicillin in military orthopaedic cases at Bushnell General Hospital, Brigham, Utah. There was a further study at Halloran General Hospital, Staten Island, New York. Bushnell and Halloran were used as schools to teach penicillin therapy to medical officers. The aim of these studies was to convince the American army of penicillin's value, which they did. It was known that penicillin could be produced in reasonably large quantities by a fermentation process. So much interwar drug success had been based on synthesis, however, that the American government and the pharmaceutical industry, to no avail, invested hundreds of thousands of dollars in attempts to produce synthetic penicillin. The army, working on the 'bird in the hand' philosophy, backed fermentation. The first large supply, produced by the Merck Corporation, was delivered to Britain in May 1943.

The British army had been introduced to penicillin in 1942 when Florey offered the War Office a small quantity of the drug that he had prepared at Oxford. After some preliminary tests, more extensive assessments were carried out under Florey's supervision in Algiers in 1943 by the British neurosurgeon Hugh Cairns (1896–1952). Results in infected wounds were impressive – this was in injuries infested with maggots in hospitals thick with flies. The drug was tested in a variety of other spheres and was found to be effective in many conditions, but was notably successful in controlling gonorrhoea. It also transformed the treatment of burns. Penicillin, said Jefferson in 1947, made possible 'surgical methods which an older generation must have stigmatized as reckless, foolhardy, reprehensible.' By the close of the war, penicillin was being produced in quantities that exceeded military requirements.

The incidence of VD, as was foreseen by some, increased during the war both among servicemen and civilians. In Britain, it rose by 11.3 percent among servicemen, and a staggering 63 percent among women at home (illegitimate births rose too). The government increased the number of treatment centres and introduced compulsory treatment for women. The Health Education Council embarked on as public a campaign as it dared, including the use of radio. In the army, older attitudes were still present: either turning a blind eye or enforcing strict punishment. Nonetheless, punishment was not as severe as in the Great War. The army issued chemical prophylactics and condoms. The civilian world was less liberal and the Ministry of Health discouraged local authorities from distributing preventives. The wantonness and lack of moral discipline of Axis troops was denounced. The Japanese were vilified as sexually deviant. Psychiatrists discovered that British soldiers who contracted VD were more likely to be dependent and self-centred, the antithesis of the model citizen. Venereal disease rates did, of course, rise among the troops. With the end of the war in sight, figures peaked in a terribly dislocated Italy in 1945 (Fig. 3.11).

The management of VD was but one example of the expression of a new sensibility that was present in the British army throughout the war and was to have important consequences for expectations of medical care afterwards. The interwar years had seen the growth of a sense of the importance

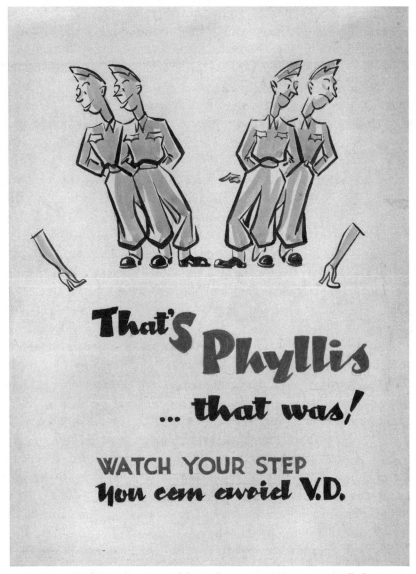

Fig. 3.11. British RAMC poster issued during the anti-VD campaign among Allied troops in Italy, 1943–4. *Source:* RAMC papers, Wellcome Library Archives and Manuscripts. *Credit:* Wellcome Library, London (L0025270).

of responsible citizenship to the running of democratic societies, and with it the claim that citizens in modern societies had basic rights to such things as health care, which should no longer be accepted as charity from the great and good. The army stressed the role of responsible citizenship through self-discipline in the control of VD. This was no longer (or not only) done by calling on a man's sense of Christian duty but by appealing to his under-standing of why promiscuity was harmful to modern democratic society. 'Guard against VD. Keep straight – keep sober. You owe it to yourself, your comrades, your efficiency,' said the posters. Those who did not conform to the code were, of course, not fit to live in civil society.

Military medicine was geared to produce efficiency. It had to attend to men who could not fight and return them to battle. If it could not do this, it had, as the U.S. army regulations put it, to see to 'the methodical dis-position of the sick and wounded so as to insure retention of effectiveness and to relieve the fighting forces of non-effectives' (Bourke, 1998, p. 226). In 1943, faced with escalating war neuroses, the U.S. army enlisted psy-chiatrists. Psychiatry was expected to play a major role in keeping men fit. Figures vary: in places, something like 50 percent of discharges were on psychiatric grounds. Military psychiatry identified fear and associated emotions as the greatest problem the soldier, and thus the army, had to face. Frank madness was of negligible concern. As an American psychiatrist put it in 1943, the state had to take heed of 'the knowledge which psychoana-lysts and psychiatrists have about anxiety, panic, aggression, submission, death, fears etc' (Bourke, 1998, p. 226). The categories of neurotic disorders in official classifications proliferated. The label 'anxiety neurosis' replaced the 'hysteria' of the Great War. The attention to fear was the product of mechanized slaughter refracted through a combination of factors. These included the medical experience of shell-shock; evolutionary and anthro-pological speculations on the emotions and the rise of civil society; the study of 'herd' psychology; the growth of holistic psychosomatic medicine; and research into the hormonal and nervous relations of mind and body as the physiological basis of behaviour.

Fear was identified as the root of behaviour that was dysfunctional in a military context. Men froze and could not pull the trigger. Frightened men panicked and wrecked discipline. They spread anxiety among their col-leagues. At every turn, psychiatrists were asked not to consider a man's per-sonal history, but the damage his behaviour would do to the unit. Whether your fear was acknowledged as genuine or you were branded a coward or a malingerer depended greatly on the needs of the platoon and the attitude of the psychiatrist. Psychiatrists could be frighteningly tough, enforcing discipline (it was their job) with threats of terrifying consequences (one American psychiatrist thought that men who had broken down in bat-tle should be sterilized). As usual, certain types of individual were held prone to inappropriate responses. Many psychiatrists thought of frightened soldiers as narcissistic, latent homosexuals. During air raids, Jews in Britain were said to lack the 'British tradition of conquering adversities, of bulldog endurance'.

HOME FRONT

In Britain, peacetime indices of civilian health saw no radical change during the war. The exception was the death rate among those over sixty-five that remained distinctly higher than prewar levels throughout the conflict. Infant mortality rose in England and Wales then fell below prewar levels. The death rate from TB did something similar. It initially rose (although not much), but by 1944 it had resumed its previous downward trend and was lower than in 1939. There were no devastating epidemics of childhood illnesses. There was a severe outbreak of measles in 1941 and 1942. The doctor–patient ratio rose so that by the end of the war in some areas there was one GP to 4,500 patients.

In spite of bombing and the disruption of civic amenities, there was no serious outbreak of infectious disease, such as typhoid. Water supplies were permanently chlorinated. Similarly, although tens of thousands sheltered underground during air raids there were no major epidemic consequences. There was a very nasty epidemic of meningitis in the winter of 1940–1. The death rate was 10 percent, the lowest fatality figure in the disease ever recorded, and was credited to the use of sulphonamides. Prophylactic tetanus inoculation was considered impractical, but the rescue services were instructed to administer the vaccine to all wounded civilians. There was no increase in the disease.

Developments in Britain merit some notice because of the creation after the war of the National Health Service (NHS), an institution of totemic significance for that country and a source of intrigue to the rest of the world. How far wartime arrangements rather than long-term changes were important to this development is debatable. World War II affected the British hospital system much like the Great War did the French one. It allowed modernizers to have their way. In 1938, an Emergency Medical Service (EMS) was established to provide, at home, casualty clearing facilities, base hospitals, and specialist hospitals, and to ensure that there were hospital beds for civilians and service personnel. The EMS formed a Public Health Laboratory Service and a regional Blood Transfusion Service. Blood transfusion was little used in the civilian world before 1945. By 1945 blood banks had been established and the procedure was incorporated into everyday hospital medicine along with the hard-earned knowledge that the use of blood products, such as sulpha drugs and vaccines, could be very dangerous. Under the EMS, 120 specialist centres had been established, those for orthopaedics and for skin diseases being the largest in number (twenty each). Anaesthetists and radiologists became recognized specialists. Laboratory services were made essential items in hospitals that had previously regarded them as a luxury. As in so many areas of modernization, America lay in the background. For example, America's Lease Lend Act of 1942 enabled British hospitals to acquire new equipment. Perhaps, in terms of future institutional arrangements, one of the significant features of the EMS was the incorporation of the voluntary hospitals into a single system of patient care, though not in terms of ownership and administration.

The problem with any account of the origins of the NHS is that one interest group or another will be offended by it. Civil servants, doctors, politicians, political parties, and various organizations have all claimed maximum credit. In the 1930s there was consensus that British health care provision was inadequate and in need of rationalizing. Apart from their haphazard location, the voluntary hospitals were not financially viable. In 1933, the BMA called for the extension of insurance to dependants and the Socialist Medical Association wanted a free comprehensive system of health care. There was wide agreement that preventive and curative medicine should be integrated. Britain, at this point, was no different from other nations. A comprehensive national insurance scheme was employed by most Western countries after World War II. From this perspective, in terms of delivery of care rather than ideological importance, the NHS was not a major innovation. In 1942, a committee chaired by William Beveridge (1879–1963) recommended a comprehensive social security system including a national health service. By the end of the war, Beveridge's propositions had been broadly agreed in principle. One sticking point was the role of the voluntary hospitals. When it came to power in 1945, one of the British Labour Party's specific contributions was its insistence that the voluntary hospitals be incorporated within the NHS. Its other was to compromise on a full-time salaried service for doctors.

1914–45, the legacy

As Chapter 4 will demonstrate, for some three decades after 1945, if measured by the hopes expressed by the public, the media, governments, and the commercial and industrial sectors, Western medicine enjoyed a wide and unprecedented faith in its power to deliver health to the developed nations

and perhaps the world as a whole. There were several concrete developments that immediately preceded and fostered this confidence, such as the
production of penicillin and streptomycin. But something much wider was
at work. The period 1914–45 saw increasing secularization and (before
World War II) a huge expansion in the supply of mass-produced goods,
which increasingly fell within the purchasing power of ordinary people.
In spite of the Depression, the healthy, materially satisfying life became a
real or tantalizing possibility for far more people in Western society than
ever before. To an unprecedented number of working-class people, the
post–World War II world delivered on this promise. In the 1970s, it was
recognized that after the war 'the world of developed capitalism . . . had
passed through an altogether exceptional phase of its history'. Observers
'looked for names to describe it: the "thirty glorious years" of the French (*les
trente glorieuses*); the quarter century Golden Age of the Anglo-Americans'
(Hobsbawm, 1996, p. 258).

The interwar years saw more than just a vision of widespread prosperity:
something else came with it. Among ordinary folk in the fragile and few
democracies of those days came subtle changes of attitude; changes that
were bound up with the right to vote. There dawned between the wars a
sense of the right to share in national prosperity in addition to the obligation to bear economic setbacks, a sense of rights to material comforts
and to health, and, related, a right to medical care. In the case of many
women, a there was sense of a right to control one's own reproduction.
Sometimes these sentiments were poorly vocalized, sometimes they were
well articulated. After the war, slowly in some places, rapidly in others,
these sentiments grew and flourished within the new economic climate,
and drove social change. Britons, for example, looked back from 1945 to
an era of charity, massively unequal wealth distribution, slums, and to the
privilege fed by the black market of the war years, and said 'Never again'
(Hennessy, 1992). In rather different ways, Germans and Americans did
something similar. The postwar world got what it asked for: roughly speaking, a medicine for democracy.

Chronological table for chapter 4: 1945–2000

Year	Medical and scientific events	Contemporary events	Nobel prize in physiology or medicine
1945	First electron micrograph of an intact cell published	End of hostilities, World War II: Europe, May 7; Pacific, August 14; Hiroshima destroyed by first nuclear fission bomb: August 6	Alexander Fleming, Ernst Chain, and Howard Florey 'for the discovery of penicillin and its curative effect in various infectious diseases'
1946	First randomised controlled clinical trial in United Kingdom of streptomycin in pulmonary tuberculosis (TB) by the Medical Research Council (MRC); Australian Act of Parliament creates the Australian National University and its medical research facility, the John Curtin School, in Canberra	First meeting of the United Nations; the first Soviet nuclear reactor is commissioned	Hermann Müller 'for the discovery of the production of mutations by means of X-ray irradiation'
1947		Dead Sea Scrolls discovered; first microwave cooker goes on sale in the United States	Carl Cori and Gerty Cori 'for their discovery of the course of the catalytic conversion of glycogen'; and Bernardo Houssay for his discovery 'of the part played by the hormone of the anterior pituitary lobe in the metabolism of sugar'

Year	Medical and scientific events	Contemporary events	Nobel prize in physiology or medicine
1948	National Health Service (NHS) begins in the United Kingdom		Paul Müller 'for his discovery of DDT as a contact poison against several arthropods'
1949	Nuremburg Code on human experimentation; cortisone found to be a useful treatment for rheumatoid arthritis	Germany split into east and west; North Atlantic Treaty Organization created as a common defence against the Soviet Union	Walter Hess 'for his discovery of the functional organization of the interbrain as a coordinator of the activities of the internal organs'; and Antonio Egas Moniz 'for his discovery of the therapeutic value of leucotomy in certain psychoses'
1950	First report of link between cigarette smoking and lung cancer published; chlorpromazine developed (R-P3276); cortisone introduced	Korean War starts	Edward Kendall, Tadeus Reichstein, and Philip Hench 'for their discoveries relating to the hormones of the adrenal cortex, their structure and biological effects'
1951	Rosalind Franklin produces sharp X-ray diffraction photographs of deoxyribonucleic acid (DNA)		Max Theiler 'for his discoveries concerning yellow fever and how to combat it'
1952	American Psychology Association introduces the first independent system for classifying mental disorders, called *The Diagnostic and Statistical Manual of Mental Disorders (DSM-I)*	Death of Joseph Stalin, leader of the USSR for thirty years	Selman Waksman 'for his discovery of streptomycin, the first antibiotic effective against tuberculosis'

Year	Medical and scientific events	Contemporary events	Nobel prize in physiology or medicine
1953	Watson and Crick publish the double helix structure of DNA; Gibbons develops the first cardiopulmonary bypass machine; Joseph Murray performs kidney transplant between identical twins in Boston, MA, United States	Queen Elizabeth II crowned; Sir Edmund Hillary and Tenzing Norgay reach the summit of Mount Everest; end of the Korean War	Hans Krebs for his discovery of the citric acid cycle; and Fritz Lipmann for his discovery of coenzyme A and its importance for intermediary metabolism
1954	Jonas Salk's trial of inactivated virus polio vaccine on one million six to nine year olds in the United States (published in 1955); chlorpromazine introduced in the United Kingdom causing dramatic fall of number of psychiatric inpatients		John Enders, Thomas Weller, and Frederick Robbins 'for their discovery of the ability of poliomyelitis viruses to grow in cultures of various types of tissue'
1955		Creation of the Warsaw Pact between the Soviet Union and the countries of Eastern Europe	Hugo Theorell 'for his discoveries concerning the nature and mode of action of oxidation enzymes'
1956	Chlorpromazine introduced in the United States causing first decline of psychiatric hospital patients in 175 years; pertussis vaccine and Salk poliomyelitis vaccine introduced in the United Kingdom	Hungarian uprising against Soviet domination, later crushed by Soviet invasion; Israeli, British, and French forces invade Egypt to prevent nationalization of the Suez Canal; transatlantic telephone cable in operation. U.K. Clean Air Act introduces smokeless zones	André Cournand, Werner Forssmann, and Dickinson Richards 'for their discoveries concerning heart catherization and pathological changes in the circulatory system'

Year	Medical and scientific events	Contemporary events	Nobel prize in physiology or medicine
1957	First 2-D ultrasound scanner built (patents registered in 1958) and published; Basil Hirschowitz, a gastroenterologist trained in Britain, unveils the first fully flexible, functional fiber-optic endoscope	Sputnik 1, the first artificial satellite in orbit, is launched by the Soviet Union, inaugurating the Space Age; Common Market established in Europe	Daniel Bovet 'for his discoveries relating to synthetic compounds that inhibit endogenous body substances, and especially their action on the vascular system and the skeletal muscles (i.e., antihistamines)'
1958	Bifocal contact lenses introduced; Ian Donald first uses ultrasound in obstetrics to examine the fetus		George Beadle and Edward Tatum 'for their discovery that genes act by regulating definite chemical events' and Joshua Lederberg 'for his discoveries concerning genetic recombination and the organization of the genetic material of bacteria'
1959	Jerome Lejeune identifies Down syndrome, named after John Langdon Down who first described the characteristics in 1866, as a chromosome anomaly of forty-seven, rather than forty-six, chromosomes		Severo Ochoa and Arthur Kornberg 'for their discovery of the mechanisms in the biological synthesis of ribonucleic acid and deoxyribonucleic acid'
1960	Librium first used in psychiatry as antianxiety medication (and first benzodiazepine); first laser was built in 1960 by Theodore Maiman		Frank Macfarlane Burnet and Peter Medawar 'for their discovery of acquired immunological tolerance'

Year	Medical and scientific events	Contemporary events	Nobel prize in physiology or medicine
1961	Albert Sabin's oral vaccine from live attenuated virus licensed in the United States; thalidomide (Distaval) removed from sale in United Kingdom by Distillers and U.S. Food and Drug Administration (FDA) delays its approval; total parenteral nutrition (feeding intravenously) becomes possible, allowing people with serious gastrointestinal disorders to avoid food and still be adequately nourished; Sydney Brenner, Francis Crick, and colleagues propose that DNA is coded in 'words', called 'codons', formed of three bases	Soviet cosmonaut Yury A. Gagarin makes the first manned space flight	Georg von Békésy 'for his discoveries of the physical mechanism of stimulation within the cochlea'
1962	Azathioprine, a derivative of 6-mercaptopurine, available as an immunosuppressant widely used for transplant recipients	Rachel Carson's Silent Spring; the Beatles' first single, Love Me Do released (Oct.)	Francis Crick, James Watson, and Maurice Wilkins 'for their discoveries concerning the molecular structure of nucleic acids and its significance for information transfer in living material'
1963		The Beatles' first number one hit, Please Please Me (Feb.); U.S. President John F Kennedy is assassinated	John Eccles, Alan Hodgkin, and Andrew Huxley 'for their discoveries concerning the ionic mechanisms involved in excitation and inhibition in the nerve cell membrane'

Year	Medical and scientific events	Contemporary events	Nobel prize in physiology or medicine
1964	Declaration of Helsinki guidelines for research workers on human experimentation; thalidomide found to reduce pain of leprosy; propranolol, the first clinically useful beta-receptor blocking drug, developed	Vietnam War starts	Konrad Bloch and Feodor Lynen 'for their discoveries concerning the mechanism and regulation of the cholesterol and fatty acid metabolism'
1965	Max Perutz and colleagues examine the structure of haemoglobin and begin to establish genetic defects – and hence medical conditions – associated with changes in DNA sequence; vaccine against measles become available in the United States		François Jacob, André Lwoff, and Jacques Monod 'for their discoveries concerning genetic control of enzyme and virus synthesis'
1966	French adopt brain inactivity as clinical definition of death; measles vaccine made available to U.K. general practitioners	Cultural Revolution, China; 116 children killed in school by the slippage of a rain-soaked colliery tip in Aberfan, Wales	Peyton Rous 'for his discovery of tumour-inducing viruses; and Charles Huggins for his discoveries concerning hormonal treatment of prostatic cancer'
1967	Breathalyser test analyses alcohol level in the breath, invented by Martin Wright of the National Institute for Medical Research (NIMR), London; Christiaan Barnard performs first human-to-human heart transplant in Cape Town, South Africa	The Six-day War between Israel and Egypt, June 5–10	Ragnar Granit, Haldan Keffer Hartline, and George Wald 'for their discoveries concerning the primary physiological and chemical visual processes in the eye'

Year	Medical and scientific events	Contemporary events	Nobel prize in physiology or medicine
1968	Structure of haemoglobin identified by Max Perutz using crystallography	Russian invasion of Czechoslovakia to crush reform movement known as Prague Spring; papal encyclical by Pope Paul VI against birth control by artificial means	Robert Holley, Har Gobind Khorana, and Marshall Nirenberg 'for their interpretation of the genetic code and its function in protein synthesis'
1969	Denton Cooley and colleagues insert first artificial heart	Neil Armstrong, commander of the Apollo 11 mission (United States), is the first man to set foot on the moon; the first computer network and predecessor of the Internet, the Advanced Research Project Association NETwork (ARPANET), is established; maiden flight of Concorde from Toulouse	Max Delbrück, Alfred Hershey, and Salvador Luria 'for their discoveries concerning the replication mechanism and the genetic structure of viruses'
1970	Lithium approved by U.S. FDA; Escherichia coli (E. coli) is identified as an important source of diarrhea; rubella vaccine introduced in the United Kingdom		Bernard Katz, Ulf Von Euler, and Julius Axelrod 'for their discoveries concerning neuro-transmitters and mechanism for their storage, release, and inactivation'
1971	Structure of insulin identified by Dorothy Hodgkin et al. using crystallography; United States introduces routine screening of blood products for hepatitis B antigen; U.S. Drug Abuse Council established; hepatitis B vaccine produced in the United States	Decimal currency introduced in the United Kingdom	Earl Sutherland Jr. 'for his discoveries concerning the mechanisms of hormone action'

Year	Medical and scientific events	Contemporary events	Nobel prize in physiology or medicine
1972	Computed axial tomography (also known as CAT) invented by Godfrey Hounsfield; U.K. National Blood Transfusion Service begins routine testing for hepatitis B; James Black discovers a new group of histamine receptors, H2-receptors	First e-mail sent; Watergate break-in, Washington, DC	Gerald Edelman and Rodney Porter 'for their discoveries concerning the chemical structure of antibodies'
1973		Britain joins the European Community; international oil crisis; Sydney Opera House opens	Karl von Frisch, Konrad Lorenz, and Nikolaas Tinbergen 'for their discoveries concerning individual and social behaviour patterns'
1974		Rather than be impeached, Richard Nixon became the first U.S. President to resign, August 9	Albert Claude, Christian De Duve, and George Palade 'for their discoveries concerning the structural and functional organization of the cell'
1975		Animal Liberation published by Australian philosopher, Peter Singer; last U.S. troops are evacuated from South Vietnam ending the Vietnam War	David Baltimore, Renato Dulbecco, and Howard Temin 'for their discoveries concerning the interaction between tumour viruses and the genetic material of the cell'
1976	National Institutes of Health (NIH) guidelines developed for study of recombinant DNA	Death of Mao Zedong (Tse-tung) and the fall of the 'gang of four', China	Baruch Blumberg and Carleton Gajdusek 'for their discoveries concerning new mechanisms for the origin and dissemination of infectious diseases'

Year	Medical and scientific events	Contemporary events	Nobel prize in physiology or medicine
1977	World Health Organization (WHO) announces that natural smallpox had been eliminated from the world's population	The Apple II is introduced as the first true 'personal computer', factory built, inexpensive and easy to learn and use; Elvis Presley dies age 42	Roger Guillemin and Andrew Schally 'for their discoveries concerning the peptide hormone production of the brain; and Rosalyn Yalow for 'the development of radioimmunoassays of peptide hormones'
1978	Louise Brown, the first baby conceived through in-vitro fertilization, born	Cardinal Karol Wojtyla elected as John Paul II, the first Polish Pope	Werner Arber, Daniel Nathans, and Hamilton Smith 'for the discovery of restriction enzymes and their application to problems of molecular genetics'
1979	NIH ethical criteria codified into written guidelines for research on human subjects; cyclosporine, an immunosuppressant antibiotic derived from a fungus, improves transplant results and reduces steroid use	Margaret Thatcher elected the first woman Prime Minister of the United Kingdom; Soviet Union invades Afghanistan	Alan Cormack and Godfrey Hounsfield 'for the development of computer assisted tomography'
1980	People for the Ethical Treatment of Animals (PETA), U.S. action group, founded; commercial production of human insulin through genetic engineering in bacterial cells (Eli Lilly and Co.)	Philips Electronics NV and Sony Corporation co-invent the compact disc; John Lennon shot dead in New York	Baruj Benacerraf, Jean Dausset, and George Snell 'for their discoveries concerning genetically determined structures on the cell surface that regulate immunological reactions,
1981	Acquired immune deficiency syndrome (AIDS) first described in the United States		Roger Sperry 'for his discoveries concerning the functional specialization of the cerebral hemispheres' and David Hubel and Torsten Wiesel 'for their discoveries concerning information processing in the visual system'

Year	Medical and scientific events	Contemporary events	Nobel prize in physiology or medicine
1982	Stanley Prusiner describes prions; gene for Factor IX [blood product] cloned	United Kingdom and Argentina go to war over the British territory of the Falkland Islands in the south Atlantic	Sune Bergström, Bengt Samuelsson, and John Vane 'for their discoveries concerning prostaglandins and related biologically active substances'
1983	Two British cases of haemophilia and AIDS reported; Helicobacter pylori, the bacterial cause of many peptic ulcers, discovered by Robin Warren and Barry Marshall		Barbara McClintock 'for her discovery of mobile genetic elements'
1984	Kary Mullis discovers polymerase chain reaction (PCR); human immunodeficiency virus (HIV) antibody screening tests available; a live lamb cloned from a sheep embryo cell in Cambridge, England, is first verified cloned mammal	Gas leak from Bhopal plant, near Calcutta, India, kills 8,000	Niels Jerne 'for theories concerning specificity in development and control of the immune system' and Georges Köhler and César Milstein 'for the discovery of the principle for production of monoclonal antibodies'
1985	Tests for HIV introduced in U.K. Blood Transfusion Service; bovine spongiform encephalopathy (BSE) first formally identified by Central Veterinary Laboratory, London		Michael Brown and Joseph Goldstein 'for their discoveries concerning the regulation of cholesterol metabolism'
1986	United Kingdom's Animal (Scientific Procedures) Act 1986; Wellcome Trust becomes major supporter of biomedical research	The term 'Internet' is used for the first time to describe the loose collection of networks that make up the ARPANET; accident at Chernobyl nuclear power plant, just north of Kiev, Ukraine	Stanley Cohen and Rita Levi-Montalcini 'for their discoveries of growth factors'

Year	Medical and scientific events	Contemporary events	Nobel prize in physiology or medicine
1987		CD-ROM introduced as a distribution medium for programs and data for the PC	Susumu Tonegawa 'for his discovery of the genetic principle for generation of antibody diversity'
1988	Fluvoxetine (Prozac) approved by FDA in 1988, the first selective serotonin reuptake inhibitor (SSRI)	Pan Am Flight 103 from London to New York City explodes over Lockerbie, Scotland, killing 259 aboard and 11 on the ground	James Black, Gertrude Elion, and George Hitchings 'for their discoveries of important principles for drug treatment'
1989	Alec Jeffreys coined the term 'DNA fingerprinting'; Human Genome Organisation (HUGO) founded	Berlin Wall brought down; massacre in Tiananmen Square, Beijing, China	Michael Bishop and Harold Varmus 'for their discovery of the cellular origin of retroviral oncogenes'
1990	Epidemiological surveillance of Creutzfeldt-Jakob disease (CJD) started in the United Kingdom to identify any changes in the occurrence after the epidemic of BSE in cattle	The Hubble Space Telescope is the first optical observatory to be placed into the Earth's orbit, which becomes functional in 1993 after astronauts repair its manufacturing flaws; Nelson Mandela released from prison; German reunification; Iraq invades Kuwait	Joseph Murray and Donnall Thomas 'for their discoveries concerning organ and cell transplantation in the treatment of human disease'
1991		The World Wide Web is born; UN attacks Iraq; USSR dissolved	Erwin Neher and Bert Sakmann 'for their discoveries concerning the function of single ion channels in cells'
1992	Wellcome Trust and Medical Research Council in the United Kingdom join forces in Human Genome Project		Edmond Fischer and Edwin Krebs 'for their discoveries concerning reversible protein phosphorylation as a biological regulatory mechanism'

Year	Medical and scientific events	Contemporary events	Nobel prize in physiology or medicine
1993		Flavr Savr tomatoes, genetically engineered for longer shelf life, sold in the United States	Richard Roberts and Phillip Sharp 'for their independent discoveries of split genes'
1994		Nelson Mandela becomes President of South Africa	Alfred Gilman and Martin Rodbell 'for their discovery of G-proteins and the role of these proteins in signal transduction in cells'
1995	Russia passes law to regulate claims of efficacy made for medicines		Edward Lewis, Christiane Nüsslein-Volhard, and Eric Wieschaus 'for their discoveries concerning the genetic control of early embryonic development'
1996	New variant Creutzfeldt-Jakob disease (nv CJD) first described in the United Kingdom, a disease that occurs in young people	The Taliban seize control of Kabul, Afghanistan, and implement a strict interpretation of Islamic law	Peter Doherty and Rolf Zinkernagel 'for their discoveries concerning the specificity of the cell mediated immune defence'
1997	Sequencing of E. coli genome; first mammal cloned from a fully differentiated cell, Dolly the sheep, at the Roslin Institute in Scotland		Stanley Prusiner 'for his discovery of prions, a new biological principle of infection'
1998	TB bacterium sequenced		Robert Furchgott, Louis Ignarro, and Ferid Murad 'for their discoveries concerning nitric oxide as a signalling molecule in the cardiovascular system'
1999	First human chromosome sequenced	Euro introduced in twelve European countries, with cash transactions remaining in local currency until 2002	Günter Blobel 'for the discovery that proteins have intrinsic signals that govern their transport and localization in the cell'

Year	Medical and scientific events	Contemporary events	Nobel prize in physiology or medicine
2000	Meningitis bacterium genome sequenced and 'working draft' of human genome sequence announced simultaneously in the United States and the United Kingdom, and Celera Genomics announced completion of their 'first assembly' of the genome		Arvid Carlsson, Paul Greengard, and Eric Kandel 'for their discoveries concerning signal transduction in the nervous system'

4 Medical enterprise and global response, 1945–2000

ANNE HARDY AND E. M. TANSEY

Overview

A new era for Western medicine opened with the return of peace in 1945. Throughout the West, states sought to implement enhanced welfare provisions with greater or less immediacy. As a discipline, orthodox medicine emerged from the war with its authority established; its practitioners, along with teachers, lawyers, and civil servants, among the core professional contributors to the modern world. In the fifty years that followed, the Western medical tradition, with its emphasis on science and education, and distinctive ways of thinking about the body, became widely influential even while certain features associated with that tradition disappeared. Notably, the strong awareness of the past that had been built in to medical education vanished. Doctors no longer read Hippocrates, Sydenham, or Paracelsus, no longer looked to the past to validate their own standing and authority within the community. The many specific medical traditions that had been created by various medical groups in the effort to establish their professional identity and credentials in a professionally competitive and insecure world (pp. 28–33) vanished. Medicine now had no need to look to its past for authority – the world of the laboratory, of medical research, of therapeutic power seemed to have arrived, and justified a multiplication of interests and specialties within the discipline. The holistic ideas that had permeated medicine in the interwar years were less replaced than washed away by a flood tide of innovation and experimentation. Driven by a newly dynamic research ethos, by a new conviction of therapeutic relevance, and by new welfare models, the scale of medical enterprise became increasingly vast, its organisation increasingly complex, and its approaches to knowledge and technologies increasingly reductionist. Even though, as Bynum noted previously (Ch. 2), new ideas and discoveries also encountered resistance from individuals and institutions – institutional drag – and took time to

405

alter the shape and practice of the institutions of medicine, the power of the administrative and organizational forces of modernism became increasingly apparent as the century moved to its close.

In the years after 1945, the therapeutic, organizational, and global reach of Western medicine extended to an unprecedented degree. The origins of some of these developments lay in the interwar years, but World War II also acted as a dynamic of change. Medicine and medical research had played a critical role in the conduct and outcome of the war: the development of penicillin by Howard Florey and his colleagues at Oxford, and the subsequent availability of the drug to Allied troops in the later stages of the fighting had, in particular, contributed to maintaining fighting power and to morale. As a result, Western governments began to fund medical research on an immense scale. Pharmaceutical companies too were galvanized into extensive research operations as new markets for medicines were created by social and organizational change. For some twenty years after the war, medicine appeared to be on an unending roll towards control over the mental and physical sources of human misery. The antibiotics, the steroids, and the new psychotropic drugs were the vanguard of a wide range of therapeutic discoveries that transformed the expectations of patients and boosted the prestige and authority of medicine. Governments developed or expanded patient access to medical treatment through state-managed or sponsored health systems. New international bodies such as the World Health Organisation (WHO), the World Bank, and the United Nations (UN) Food and Agriculture Organization, began to promote the adoption of Western medicine in the developing world. The health professions multiplied both in numbers of personnel and in specialized skills in response to medical innovation and social change. A popular culture of medicine came to pervade Western societies, driven by the new structures of provision and the new therapeutics, but also by the powerful new media of radio and television. For good or for ill, new standards of literacy and means of mass communication exercised an increasing influence on popular perceptions of medicine and of the medical profession.

The later twentieth century divides in the 1970s. Between 1945 and the early 1970s, Western society and Western medicine remained essentially buoyant, confident in the ideals of progress and prosperity, and the benefits of Western civilization. During these years the general prosperity of the West, and the maintenance of its lifestyles, had come to depend on fuel, more especially on oil. Industrial power, the internal combustion engine, and domestic heating and lighting systems, were all heavily dependent on oil for their functioning. In 1973, the world's major oil-producing countries declared a sharp price rise and announced their intention in the future to regulate production and increase prices in a concerted effort to conserve oil stocks. The immediate impact of this decision was a fuel crisis. In the longer term, the oil crisis brought inflation to the previously largely stable currencies of the West, and precipitated long-term economic instability and insecurity in Western economies. The effect of this changed financial climate on medicine was profound. Large modern hospitals became expensive to run and the costs of research and development escalated. Personnel became restless as the spending power of salaries was eroded by inflation. Even before economic pressure had entered the picture, there had been indications that patients were beginning to view modern medicine more critically. The thalidomide tragedy of the early 1960s led to increased stringency in the regulation of new drugs entering Western markets.

In the 1970s, the new suspicion of medical competence and medical probity increased as academics and interest groups began publicly to question medical authority. By 1980, moreover, the flood of new therapeutic innovation had begun to ease. Cures for such increasingly common medical conditions as cancer and Parkinsonism were perceived to be slow in coming. More sinisterly, old infections began to resurge and new ones emerged. Malaria, for which there had been hopes of control in the postwar years, once again looked to be outrunning medical ingenuity. The identification of human immunodeficiency virus/acquired immune deficiency syndrome (HIV/AIDS) in the early 1980s put an abrupt end to complacency about the potential for eradicating infectious diseases. By the end of the century, following the prolonged crisis over bovine spongiform encephalopathy (BSE), the appearance of the highly virulent *E coli* 0157 bacterium, and multiple drug-resistant strains of the common *Staphylococcus aureus* and of tuberculosis (TB), there was real alarm over the potential escalation of untreatable infections. The global experience of AIDS and of drug resistant TB notably served to highlight the growing disparity in available medical resources between the poor countries of the developing world and the wealthy developed states of the West. Although Western medicine had become widely influential in the developing world and was, in places, deeply engaged in the struggle to improve health and life chances among the world's poorest people, it became apparent that important drug treatments and medical technologies available in the affluent West were being denied to sick people in the neediest parts of the world.

Two central themes, therefore, run through this chapter. First, there is the paradoxical phenomenon of 'doing better and feeling worse' that developed in the West, despite increasingly successful and sophisticated medical treatments and enormous financial investment in medical research and welfare services. Second, the perception that the global distribution of medical resources increasingly favours the developed at the expense of the developing world. In the second half of the twentieth century, Western medicine moved from being powerful, purposeful, and progressive, towards a more uncertain identity; conscious of shortcomings, uneasy at the future, yet continuing, if less spectacularly, on an innovative therapeutic path. This chapter seeks to trace these developments, drawing on examples principally from the Anglo-American experience. The post-1945 world has as yet attracted little sustained attention from medical historians, and the problems of retrieving factual information and of drawing historical synthesis from an abundance of primary materials lie behind the narrower comparative focus of this chapter compared to its predecessors.

Medical research

The technology that helped to win the war also transformed the peace, and raised high social expectations on all fronts, especially with regard to health and the benefits that might accrue from scientific research. Technological advances permeated practically every area of medicine and medical research in the second half of the twentieth century. In the first two decades after the end of World War II, in the United States at least, consumer prosperity helped create and reinforce the optimism that medical advances, most notably those emanating from the pharmaceutical industry, would cure or prevent all ills.

Medical research affected almost every aspect of medical practice since the end of the war. It included work towards the deeper understanding of normal physiological processes; the development of therapies from pharmacological management to surgical interventions; diagnostic procedures ranging from blood tests to high-tech scanning equipment; and an impressive array of preventive strategies. After World War II, some of the divisions between basic and clinical research became much sharper than previously, due to factors that included the creation of specialized research institutes not necessarily associated with hospital facilities; new techniques and approaches to disease problems; and new ways of training research staff solely in laboratory methodologies without direct reference to clinical medicine.

As the twentieth century moved into its final quarter, the increasing disillusion with medicine's ability to provide the solutions to individual and societal problems was reflected by a growing disenchantment with medical research. Seemingly, research was increasingly expensive for decreasing returns, and its subject matter appeared to be esoteric and remote from immediate clinical needs. For the sake of convenience, the immediate sections following are divided into 'basic' and 'clinical' research, although Louis Pasteur's (1822–95) maxim must be remembered: 'There is only science, and the fruits of science'.

BASIC RESEARCH

Many scientists either returning to research labs after the World War II or starting their studies after deferment for military service, did so with new skills and interests generated in that conflict. For example, several had acquired experience with radar that aroused interest in using new electronic methods in laboratory investigations. The application of delicate recording and measurement techniques encouraged and furthered reductionist approaches to biological problems and led to some remarkable discoveries, such as the mechanisms by which nerves transmit impulses, for which the Nobel Prize in Physiology or Medicine was awarded in 1963 to (Sir) Alan Hodgkin (1914–98) and (Sir) Andrew Huxley (b. 1917) of the United Kingdom, and the Australian (Sir) John Eccles (1903–97). Such discoveries were not immediately translatable into clear-cut medical advances, even though the understanding of basic mechanisms would ultimately lead to detailed knowledge of their disruption in disease processes, thus facilitating the design and production of diagnostic and therapeutic strategies.

Another direct spin-off from the war, this time from nuclear research, was the availability of radioactive chemicals, limited to begin with, but more plentiful by the mid-1950s. Combined with paper chromatography that had been developed in the United Kingdom during the war, whereby small amounts of chemicals could be separated from each other and measured, biochemists had powerful new techniques to investigate the functioning of normal and abnormal cells. Using experimental animals, the work of Gerty Cori (1896–1957) and Carl Cori (1896–1984) (Nobel Laureates in 1947) in the United States and of (Sir) Hans Krebs (1900–81) (Nobel Laureate in 1953) in the United Kingdom, elegantly delineated the metabolic pathways later known as the 'Krebs cycle' and the 'Cori cycle' by which complex molecules, such as carbohydrates, are broken down to recyclable cellular components and the energy-rich compound adenosine triphosphate (ATP), the universal energy store of living organisms. The first electron micrograph of an intact cell had been published in March 1945 (Fig. 4.1), and after the war anatomists and histologists began to use electron microscopes routinely to reveal and investigate the ultrastructure of cells, thus providing detailed morphological and functional information about basic processes. Work such as this, elucidating both structural and functional details of tissues and cells, provided startling new ways of examining living organisms in the laboratory. It also heralded the beginning of the field of cell biology, which by the end of the twentieth century had merged with genetics and molecular biology to create a unified 'science of life'. At a direct practical level these new approaches to, and insights about, the detailed working of cells and tissues could be used to develop biochemical tests and diagnostic scans using radioactive 'tracers' that could be followed throughout the body with visualization techniques, such as X-rays.

Crystallographic modelling techniques blossomed in the late 1940s and early 1950s as the structures of complex macromolecules began to be determined. These included the structure of penicillin (1949 by Dorothy Hodgkin, 1910–94, Nobel Laureate in Chemistry, 1964); vitamin B12 (1957 by Dorothy Hodgkin); myoglobin (1958 by [Sir] John Kendrew, 1917–97, Nobel Laureate in Chemistry 1962); haemoglobin (1968 by Max Perutz, 1914–2002, Nobel Laureate in Chemistry 1962) and insulin (1971 by Dorothy Hodgkin and colleagues). These discoveries, perhaps regarded as esoteric and remote from practical medicine, permitted the deeper understanding of the modes of action of these compounds and greatly facilitated their synthetic manufacture.

One piece of basic research of clinical significance that went unrecognized and unacknowledged for many decades, finally came to fruition during the latter part of the twentieth century. In 1911 Peyton Rous (1879–1977) at the Rockefeller Institute in New York published his discovery that a virus caused cancer. He used the classical investigative techniques then at his disposal, by preparing an extract from a poultry sarcoma and injecting it into healthy chickens, where it produced further cancers. At the time, viruses were little understood and his work was not accepted. In was in the 1950s that the new generation of molecular biologists first used his virus as an investigative tool for studying cancer mechanisms. The virus was shown, unlike cancer inducers such as chemicals or radiation, to produce reliable, reproducible tumours in experimental animals and in newly

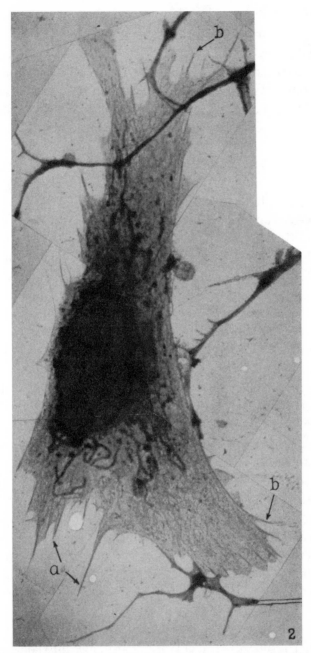

Fig. 4.1. Photomicrograph of a fibroblast-like cell, and nerve fibres cultured from chick embryo tissue. *Source*: Keith R. Porter, Albert Claude, and Ernest F. Fullam, 'A study of tissue culture cells by electron microscopy', *The Journal of Experimental Medicine*, 81 (1945), 233–46 (plate 10, Fig. 2). *Credit*: Reproduced from *The Journal of Experimental Medicine*, 81 (1945), 233–46, by copyright permission of the Rockefeller University Press.

411

developed tissue cultures, which permitted close examination and verifica-
tion of its actions. In the early 1960s, a gene was identified that produced
the protein that led to tumours and in 1966 Rous was honoured with the
Nobel Prize in physiology or medicine, three years after his son-in-law Alan
Hodgkin. Rous's basic research on virology was to have considerable and
unexpected importance later as the virus he had identified and studied so
extensively (subsequently called the 'Rous sarcoma virus') is of a class called
'retroviruses', the same group as the causative organism HIV of AIDS.

A major ethical issue that developed during this period was that of animal experimentation. Animal models for both normal physiological experiments and for pathological conditions had been broadly, but not universally, accepted as an integral part of biomedical research methodology by
World War I. This situation largely remained so until 1975, when the Australian philosopher, Peter Singer (b. 1946), published *Animal Liberation*,
which fuelled much controversy. Among other issues the book not only
questioned the morality of using living creatures as experimental subjects,
but also cast doubt on the validity of applying information obtained in this
way to the human condition. In the United Kingdom, which had passed the
oldest piece of legislation in the world about such work, the 1876 Cruelty to
Animals Act, the 1986 Animals (Scientific Procedures) Act was enacted.
Similar legislation followed in over twenty countries. In the United States,
the National Institutes of Health (NIH) issued a guide for the care and use of
laboratory animals, and in 1985 instigated its own programme of checking
animal facilities and researchers to ensure compliance with its guidelines.
The rise, during the final two decades of the twentieth century, of vociferous
opposition to the use of animals in any way (including for food or clothing), led to the formation of action groups such as People for the Ethical
Treatment of Animals (PETA) in the United States in 1980, and also organizations with an avowed agenda of terrorist activity, such as the Animal
Liberation Front (ALF). Some medical researchers, especially in the United
Kingdom, found themselves the focus of attacks that damaged their homes,
labs, and property.

MODERN GENETICS, GENETIC SCREENING, AND GENETIC ENGINEERING

In 1956, shortly after the end of World War II, Joe Hin Tijo (1918–2001)
and Albert Levan (b. 1905) announced that humans had forty-six chromosomes, and not forty-eight as previously thought. The association of
a forty-seventh with Down's syndrome was also made. During the next
twenty years or so, a number of linkages of conditions, such as haemophilia

and colour blindness, with specific chromosomes were identified. A sub-group of specialists – clinical geneticists –became an important part of the health care team, testing, diagnosing and counselling prospective parents about possible birth defects. By 1990 more than 600 chromosomal abnormalities had been described, which in some societies led to the aborting of affected fetuses, such as those suffering from Down's syndrome. Although chromosomes were understood to be composed of deoxyribonucleic acid (DNA), little more was known then. One of the most dramatic discoveries of the second half of the twentieth century was that announced in 1953 in Cambridge, United Kingdom, of a model (from crystallographic evidence) for the structure of DNA, by Francis Crick (1916–2004) and James Watson (b. 1928), for which they were awarded the Nobel Prize in Physiology or Medicine in 1962 (shared with Maurice Wilkins, 1916–2004). The theoretical implications, that a double helix of recurring units could explain cellular replication from generation to generation, were immediately obvious. The recognition of the possibilities of translating this knowledge into improvements in health care took a little longer. The regular use of DNA probes (i.e., radioactively labelled molecules that bind to target molecules or genes and can then be detected by an assay, such as autoradiography, thus indicating the presence or absence of the target) for the ante-natal diagnosis of genetic disorders (as opposed to the chromosomal abnormalities previously detectable) was developed from the 1980s onwards.

During the 1970s, the tools of molecular biology became increasingly important in the study of the basic processes of living organisms and in the examination of the underlying causes of disease. Progress in mapping the human chromosomes led to a deeper knowledge of genetic disorders, cancer, and ageing. In particular, the use of computers revolutionized the practice of science, especially in work on understanding the human genome. The Human Genome Project was initiated in the mid-1980s, building on work done at Cambridge, United Kingdom, by Frederick Sanger (b. 1918, Nobel Laureate 1958 and 1980) to 'decode', or analyse, the sequence of individual nucleotides making up the structure of DNA. The project was highly dependent on technology: high-speed automatic analysers, robotics, and sophisticated computing facilities. It was carried out by scientists in both the public and private sector; the International Human Genome Mapping Consortium financed by governments and charities from a number of countries, but principally the United States and the United Kingdom and with some input from Celera Genomics, a private American company.

413

Celera had established independent research in this area, with the declared intention of patenting gene fragments that might be of commercial use in the development of disease-specific therapies. In 2001, an announcement of the sequencing of the human genome gave hope that major benefits would accrue: improvements in the prevention, diagnosis, and management of infectious and genetic diseases, as well as other common killers or causes of chronic ill health, including cardiovascular diseases, cancer, diabetes, and mental illnesses. The analysis of those developments must await a further volume.

CLINICAL RESEARCH

Clinical research in the United Kingdom was handicapped to some extent by the lack of a centre of excellence. The Medical Research Council's (MRC) National Institute for Medical Research (NIMR) had not, despite initial decisions that it should, contained clinical facilities. Despite this, the MRC was associated with two major postwar advances in clinical medical research. The first was the development and introduction of the double-blind randomized control clinical trial, initially devised in 1946 in a trial of streptomycin, a new drug for the treatment of pulmonary TB. In the immediate postwar years the drug was in short supply and a trial was devised whereby one group of patients received the drug in comparison to another, control, group who were given the best accepted method of treatment then in use. Patients were randomly assigned to either treatment, and the results showed that in the streptomycin treated group 7 percent of patients died, compared with 27 percent in the control group, a highly significant finding in terms of the drug's efficacy. However, the organization and design of the trial was of even more significance, and it served as the model for many other such studies. This randomized model was further refined (called 'double-blind') so that neither doctor nor patient knew which was the test substance or which was the control (sometimes a placebo) until the completion of the trial.

The second advance was the development of epidemiological methods to investigate clinical conditions. In 1947, the same medical statistician, (Sir) Austin Bradford Hill (1897–1991), who had advised on the streptomycin trial, recruited a young physician (Sir) Richard Doll (b. 1912–2005) to assist in a study of lung cancer. An extensive survey finally showed, most unexpectedly and to some incredulity, that cigarette smoking was a causative factor. Almost simultaneously, results published in the United States by Ernst Wynder (1922–99) and Evarts Graham (1883–1957) also emphasized the carcinogenic effects of tobacco tar. Such studies highlighted the necessity of epidemiological research at a time when laboratory science was regarded as the gold standard of medical research.

In the United States, clinical research was specifically accommodated within the NIH's remit, initially by the provision of a 540-bed research hospital that opened in 1953 on the main campus in Bethesda, specifically designed to bring clinical care into close proximity with laboratory research. Physicians from each constituent institute were allowed to conduct research in addition to providing medical care in the hospital, and patients paid no fees once accepted into a research programme. Some of the research there impacted on health care throughout the world. For example, in the 1960s two NIH scientists collaborated on examining the problems of the hepatitis B infection that often occurred after transfusions during surgery, as a result of contaminated blood. Baruch Blumberg (b. 1925) and Harvey Alter (b. 1932) discovered a specific antigen that Blumberg went on to show was a surface protein of the hepatitis-B virus, and for which he received the Nobel Prize in Physiology or Medicine in 1976. The NIH blood bank became the first to screen all blood products for the presence of the antigen, a procedure that became routine in the United States in 1971.

The numbers of clinically qualified staff in medical research programmes declined during the latter part of the twentieth century. In the United States, the first staffing figures for the Hygienic Laboratory (the forerunner of the NIH) in 1909 show that 17 percent of the research staff were medically qualified; in 1986, the comparable figure was 8 percent. In the United Kingdom there has been a similar decline. During the first decades of the postwar period, much clinical research in the United Kingdom was funded on the 'dual-support' system, undertaken by University or National Health Service (NHS) staff, employed by their institutions to undertake core clinical or academic duties, with additional time allocated for research that was supported by additional funds from organizations such as the MRC. From the mid-1970s onwards, however, clinical workers everywhere were competing for decreasing research funds, at a time when it began to be difficult for medically qualified staff to receive adequate training in the necessary scientific disciplines, as the latter became increasingly sophisticated and specialized. As one commentator (Booth, 1993, p. 225) has explained, in earlier years aspiring clinical scientists would have studied physiology as undergraduates, and it was therefore relatively easy to undertake clinical research in say, cardiology, respiratory medicine, or gastro-enterology where research methods were often based on physiological techniques.

The emergence of molecular biology, in particular, demanded that clinical researchers not only needed to undertake advanced clinical training, but also acquire from scratch complicated research techniques in new fields. Several countries, including the United States, United Kingdom, and France, began to address this problem in the 1990s by establishing, *inter alia*, specialized training schemes and Clinical Research Centres. Whether these will be successful in revitalizing this area of medical research remains to be seen.

An important study of the relationship between basic and clinical research was published in 1976 by two Americans, the physiologist Julius Comroe (1911–84) and anaesthetist Robert Dripps (1911–73). They invited over a hundred colleagues to assess key advances in cardiovascular medicine, and then to analyse whether the underlying research leading to these advances was 'basic' or 'clinical' in original intention. Although their methodology was later severely criticized, they found that 40 percent of such work had been undertaken as curiosity-driven basic research and not carried out with any particular clinical intention.

However defined, medical research was a difficult concept to apply to the clinical care or observation of human subjects in the 1950s, when people were still reeling from revelations about Nazi atrocities conducted by doctors for the purposes of 'research'. The Nuremburg Code, which resulted from the trials of many of those responsible for such crimes, provided a ten-point guide to the ethical factors that should be considered when undertaking research on human subjects. The first point emphasised 'The voluntary consent of the subject is essential'. In 1964, the Declaration of Helsinki refined and developed the code to provide an extensive series of guidelines for research workers. However, they remained as guidelines, and the researchers Henry Beecher (1904–76) in the United States and Maurice Pappworth (1910–94) in the United Kingdom, attracted controversy and professional opprobrium in the 1970s by criticizing apparently respectable work that failed to meet these minimum requirements. From the 1960s onwards, all grantees from the NIH were required to satisfy basic ethical criteria. In 1979, these requirements were codified into written guidelines for research involving human subjects, and by the end of the twentieth century a computerized system monitored all such research in almost 5,000 American research institutions. By the 1990s, in the United Kingdom and many Western European countries, local ethical committees were established at hospitals and universities to scrutinize all project applications involving human subjects.

MEDICAL RESEARCH INSTITUTIONS

There was an enormous expansion in the provision of biomedical research institutes after World War II. In the United Kingdom, as in most Western countries, medical research was conducted in universities, hospitals and specialized institutes, and units financed either privately, by higher education central funding, or, most notably, by the MRC. Pharmaceutical companies also had their own research programmes largely directed towards the development of effective therapeutic compounds. Until World War II, the MRC (established in 1913 and known as the Medical Research Committee until 1922, p. 259), principally funded research by supporting the work of the NIMR, and providing research expenses and/or salaries awarded competitively to selected scientists in other establishments. Wartime needs led to the creation of specialized research groupings, such as the Physiological Research Laboratory at the Armoured Fighting Vehicles School (1941–6) and the Burns Research Unit in Glasgow (1942–52). Learning from, and adapting this experience of supporting a small group of researchers united around a common theme, the MRC, under the guidance of its secretary, Professor (Sir) Harold Himsworth (1905–93), began a programme of diversification that established 109 MRC Research Units around the United Kingdom (and one overseas in The Gambia) between 1945 and 1970 (Fig. 4.2). Units were initially created for the professional lifetime of their director, subject to regular review, which provided the MRC with research flexibility not easily available with fixed, long-term commitments. The subjects included both basic and clinical research problems and ranged in approach from population surveys to ultrastructure, from sociology to microorganisms, for example, the Epidemiological Research Unit (1960–90); the Unit for Research in Ophthalmological Genetics (1954–66); the Social and Public Health Sciences Unit (1968–present); and the Bilharzia Research Unit (1950–62).

Somewhat similarly, in the United States, the NIH devoted the war years to research problems directly related to military needs (e.g., vaccines against tropical diseases; treatments for burns and traumatic shock; and high altitude physiology). The cost of World War II had increased personal and estate taxes in the United States, which concomitantly increased charitable donations because tax-free dollars could be given to charity. Postwar, decreasing financial returns on such endowments, coupled with escalating research costs, hit some of the older charity-endowed foundations. Then in 1946, in the immediate postwar haze of medical optimism, federal funding arrangements for the NIH were expanded, and the programme grew from

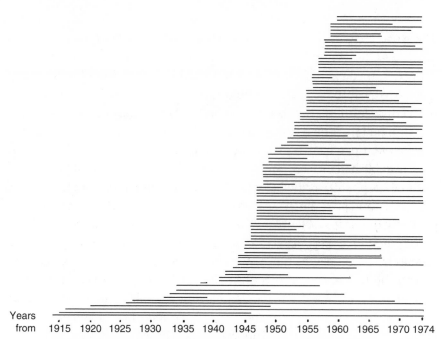

Years
from 1915 1920 1925 1930 1935 1940 1945 1950 1955 1960 1965 1970 1974

Fig. 4.2. MRC research establishments: the creation and lifespan of MRC Research Units 1913–60. *Source:* Adapted from data in A. L. Thomson. *Half a century of medical research,* Vol 2. *The programme of the Medical Research Council (United Kingdom),* London, Medical Research Council, London, 1975. Appendix C.

just over $8 million in 1947, to more than $1 billion in 1966. Associated with the growth in the grants programme was, as in the United Kingdom, enormous diversification in the array of work supported within the NIH framework of 'medical research': these included, for example, specialised research institutes on mental health, cardiac disease, and dental pathology. In 1948 the NIH became the National Institute(s) of Health and two major divisions were created: the National Microbiological Institute and the Experimental Biology and Medicine Institute. Gradually, however, administrators and researchers alike realized that organizing institutes to study disease processes rather than the physiological mechanisms indicated by such academic sounding titles, increased the chance of financial support from Congress. By 1960, there were ten components of the NIH, and by 1998 it comprised twenty-seven distinct institutes or research centres.

At the same time, some disadvantages of 'stand alone' institutes, especially in the training of new research staff, were exemplified by the decision of the Rockefeller Institute for Medical Research in New York to become a research university. Modelled somewhat on the founding philosophy of Johns Hopkins University (pp. 148–9), the Rockefeller's declared aim was to bring together research and scholarship in an environment that would provide future generations of scientists. In 1954, it received a charter to award degrees and in 1965 formally changed its title to the Rockefeller University. This revitalized the institute, bringing a regular fresh supply of graduate talent into its laboratories, a source not readily accessible to research institutes divorced from undergraduate and graduate teaching programmes. During this period, the university also began to accept outside charitable donations and government grants, in an attempt to diversify its sources of funding. Increasing competition for funds is illustrated by the fact that during the 1950s, over 1,200 new charitable foundations were established in the United States, although the proportionately large government input into medical research *per se* encouraged many such organizations to support other aspects of medicine. For example, both the Alfred P. Sloan Foundation and the Josiah Macy Jr. Foundation supported work within medical schools to increase representation of minority students.

Financial pressures also meant that during the latter part of the twentieth century several private institutes founded in the late nineteenth century had to adapt to changing pressures to grow, diversify, and seek new funding arrangements as their original endowments shrank. The Lister Institute in London (founded 1891), having failed to merge with the newly created MRC, was forced to close its original laboratory sites in the mid-1970s because of the lack of financial support, and to rebrand as a charity supporting research fellowships throughout the United Kingdom. Others survived by merging and expanding: in Sweden the Karolinska Institute (founded 1810) grew several times by absorbing, *inter alia*, the Institute of Physical Therapy (1960) and the Stockholm University of Health Sciences (1998). In contrast, the Pasteur Institute in Paris (founded 1888) came to rely almost entirely on external contributions and collaborations. This was largely the product of attempts by pressure groups and successive French governments to remove scientific research from traditional institutions, initiated by the prewar foundation of the Centre National de la Recherche Scientifique (CNRS) in 1939. Postwar Gaullist policy centralized scientific research as a tool to build national independence and prosperity, and subjected it to regular (usually five-year) planning reviews. Initially modelled on the Soviet Union, the promotion of science and technology in France by the end of the century followed that in the United States. Medicine was no exception: the specialized Institut National de la Santé et de la Recherche Médicale (INSERM) was founded in 1964 with a budget of FF 54 million. In 1971, INSERM created 'actions thématiques programmées', which prioritized fast developing, often multidisciplinary, areas. During the next three years, thirty-six such schemes were started and some subjects, most notably molecular biology, were fostered to a degree impossible in a single university. Increasing demands required increasing investment: at FF 246 billion, INSERM's 1974 budget was more than four times greater than that of ten years earlier.

In the United States the enormous growth in the NIH budgets slowed down in the final years of the 1960s. This was partly because of inflation in the American economy, and also the creation of new welfare programmes, such as Medicare and Medicaid, that competed for the 'health dollar' in Congress. Financial constraints stimulated considerable debates in the United States and elsewhere about the relative values of undirected research compared with goal-orientated, applied work. During the 1970s, the NIH initiated major projects in line with the latter approach, against cancer and heart disease, and in the following decade, AIDS too was subjected to this technique. The relative failure of this approach to deliver rapid therapeutic or preventive solutions led to a further policy reappraisal, with the consensus emerging that studying basic immunological and virological processes was an effective route to devise medical responses to disease.

One internationally important component of the NIH was the National Library of Medicine (NLM). Founded as the Library of the Surgeon-General in 1836, it became a constituent part of the NIH in 1968. One aspect of its work illustrates the exponential expansion of medical literature during the latter part of the twentieth century. In 1879, the library started an indexing and abstracting service called *Index Medicus*, published in annual volumes and including much, if not most, of the international medical literature. From its foundation until the late 1940s the volumes weighed approximately 2 kilograms (kg) per year. By the end of the 1970s each annual volume weighed 14 kg, despite being softbound, printed on thinner paper, in smaller font, and with narrower margins. By 2000, its electronic counterpart, Medline® abstracted nearly 4,000 journals and added over 400,000 references to its database each year. The problems caused by the growth of medical literature was epitomized in 1992 by the editor of the *Journal of the American Medical Association* (JAMA). He estimated that two million biomedical articles were published every year, and a diligent reader had but two options: to read two articles a day, knowing that within a year he would be sixty centuries behind; or to read 6,000 articles every day.

In line with developments elsewhere, Australia too reevaluated its medical research programme after World War II. There were four dedicated research institutes prewar, of which the Walter and Eliza Hall Institute in Melbourne was preeminent. Others were the Baker Institute, also in Melbourne, the Kanematsu Institute in Sydney, and the Institute of Medical and Veterinary Research in Adelaide. In 1946 an Act of Parliament created the Australian National University, to encourage talented native scholars to remain in the country. This included a dedicated medical research facility, the John Curtin School, in Canberra. The decision to set up a national research facility was indirectly associated with the discovery of penicillin. The Australian Howard Florey (1898–1968), Professor of Pathology at Oxford, who had been responsible for converting Alexander Fleming's laboratory observation into a commercial possibility, visited his native land in 1944 to survey medical research facilities. His report concluded that 'the research facilities in Australia fall far below the standards necessary in a civilized community . . .' (Fenner & Curtis, 2001, p. 4). Modelled on the MRC's NIMR in London, Florey proposed a central research institute, which coincided with the contemporary pressures to create a National University, and after much negotiation and discussion the two plans came together. Florey was not alone in his ideas. Macfarlane Burnet (1899–1985), the newly appointed director of the Walter and Eliza Hall Institute in Sydney (and Nobel Laureate in 1968 for his work on clonal selection of antibodies), also proposed that for Australia, 'one of the necessities is a central institute of medical research, concerned, like the National Institute of Medical Research at Hampstead or the Rockefeller [Institute] and a dozen other institutes in America, with fundamental rather than clinical studies'(Fenner & Curtis, 2001, p. 2). Initially, the resources for supporting the new university and its medical research were so meagre that temporary facilities were rented in Dunedin, Melbourne, and London.

In most countries, private endowments became increasingly important for medical research as the twentieth century approached its end, although in 1980 the NIH budget of $3.5 billion was still over twelve times greater than that of all private endowments. Several were disease related, such as cancer charities, or patient activated, such as Parkinson's Disease charities; others were wider in their philanthropic range. For example, the success of the Salk and Sabin vaccines (pp. 463–4) meant that the National Polio

Foundation in the United States changed both its focus and its name to become the March of Dimes Birth Defects Foundation. In Britain, the Nuffield Trust (established 1940) was especially important in supporting clinical projects during the 1960s to 1980s, while in 1991 the Nuffield Foundation (established 1943) founded a Council on Bioethics to consider ethical issues arising from advances in medicine and biology. The Wellcome Trust (established 1936) became a major supporter of biomedical research after 1986 when it diversified its investment portfolio, until that time solely dependent on one pharmaceutical company, the Wellcome Foundation. The MRC of Canada funded a substantial component of medical research, bolstered by some private funds, such as those in 1950 from the William Donner Foundation, which provided medical buildings and a research institute at McGill University. Several individual institutions, especially those associated with children, were increasingly well endowed to pursue research. These included the Great Ormond Street Hospital for Sick Children in London, which after heavy bombing during the war, raised funds by the sale of rubble in matchboxes. In 1987, the Wishing Well Appeal was launched to redevelop the entire hospital, and raised £54 million in just two years. In Toronto, the Hospital for Sick Children had assets, principally from donations, of over $65 million by 1965, and by the end of the 1990s its own foundation was awarding more than $3 million worth of grants annually to other universities and hospitals across Canada.

Health and disease

In many senses people in the west were healthier in the second half of the twentieth century than they had ever been before. Rising standards of living, the vastly greater access to health care, and the virtual disappearance of the common infectious diseases all contributed to very high levels of physical well-being. At one level, rising life expectancies (Table 4.1) and falling death rates (Table 4.2) continued established demographic trends, at another, there were shifts in the pattern of disease incidence and 'visibility'. The infectious diseases of childhood – so common before 1940 – were virtually eradicated by the introduction of new vaccines and extended immunization programmes. Poliomyelitis, which looked as if it might be a serious modern epidemic, was halted with the introduction of a vaccine in the mid-1950s. By the mid-1960s, TB had all but disappeared as a public health concern (Figs. 4.3 and 4.4). Following a worldwide eradication campaign, the WHO declared the ancient scourge of smallpox eradicated in 1977.

Table 4.1. *Life Expectancy at Birth, 1800–2000*

Country	1800	1820	1840	1860	1880	1900	1920	1940	1960	1980	2000
Australia									(1960–2) 70.97	74.45	79.75
England and Wales			41.27 (1841)	42.86	43.53	46.16	56.57	61.28	71.25	73.80	77.81
France						45.07	51.59	49.56	70.37	74.25	78.79
Germany									69.31 (West Germany)	73.45	78.08
Italy					32.85	41.75	45.88	57.63	69.21	74.03	79.13
Netherlands									73.35	75.77	78.11
Sweden	32.19	40.26	44.00	48.48	47.62	52.24	58.80	66.63	73.03	75.74	79.84
United States						47.3	54.1	62.9	69.82	73.74	76.62

Sources: Human Mortality Database. University of California, Berkeley (United States), and Max Planck Institute for Demographic Research (Germany). Available at www.mortality.org or www.humanmortality.de (data downloaded on February 25, 2004).
United States: 1900–1940 – *Historical Statistics of the United States, Colonial Times to 1970, Bicentennial Edition, Part 1,* U.S Bureau of the Census (Washington, DC, 1975).
Australia and all 2000 figures: U.S. Bureau of the Census, International Data Base (IDB).

Table 4.2. Death Rate per 1,000 Population, 1800–2000

Country	1800	1820	1840	1860	1880	1900	1920	1940	1960	1980	2000
Australia	–	–		20.9	14.6	11.7	10.5	9.8	8.6	7.4	7.12
England and Wales	–	–	22.9	21.2	20.5	18.2	12.4	14.4	11.5	11.7	United Kingdom 10.26
France	27.7 (1801)	25.4	23.7	21.4	22.9	21.9	17.2	18.0	11.3	10.2	9.07
Germany	–	24.4	26.5	23.2	26.0	22.1	15.1	12.7	11.6 / 13.6[a]	11.6 / 14.2[a]	10.1
Italy	–	–	–	30.9 (1862)	30.8	23.8	19.0	13.6	9.6	9.8	9.71
Netherlands	–	–	23.5	24.8	23.6	17.9	12.3	9.9	7.7	8.1	8.83
Sweden	31.4	24.5	20.4	17.7	18.1	16.8	13.3	11.4	10.0	11.0	10.47
United States	–	–				17.2	13.0	10.8	9.5	8.6	8.52

[a] West Germany / East Germany.

Sources: Europe: B R Mitchell, International Historical Statistics, Europe 1750–1993 (London: Macmillan Reference Ltd, 1998).
Australia: B R Mitchell, International Historical Statistics, Africa, Asia & Oceania 1750–1988 (New York: Stockton Press, 1995).
United States:1920–1960 – Historical Statistics of the United States, Colonial Times to 1970, Bicentennial Edition, Part 1, U.S Bureau of the Census. (Washington, DC. 1975).
1980 – U.S. Bureau of the Census, International Data Base (IDB)
All 2000 figures: U.S. Bureau of the Census, International Data Base (IDB).

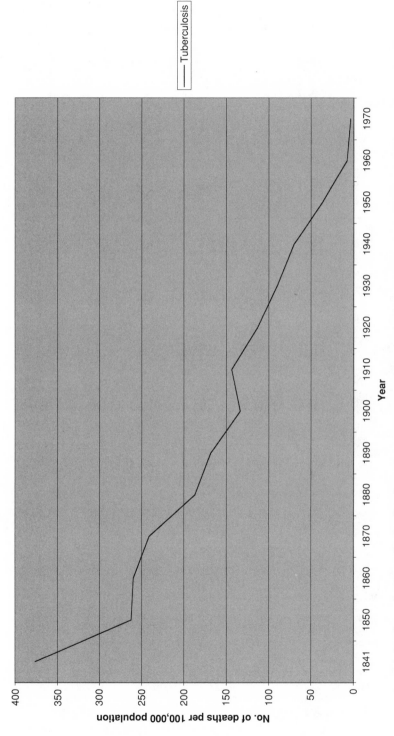

Fig. 4.3. Death rate for TB, England and Wales, 1841–1970. *Notes*: England and Wales pre-1900 data is for England; 1900 onwards is for England and Wales. TB (England and Wales): 1841–1900 = consumption/phthisis; 1910 onwards = TB (all forms) as in U.S. data. *Source: Annual Report of the Registrar General for England and Wales (Registrar General's Statistical Review of England and Wales)*.

425

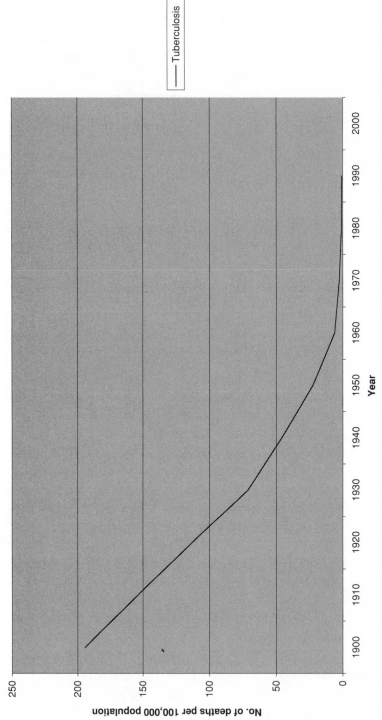

Fig. 4.4. Death rate for TB, United States, 1900–90. *Source: 1900–70 – Historical Statistics of the United States, Colonial Times to 1970, Bicentennial Edition, Part I, U.S. Bureau of the Census (Washington, DC, 1975). 1980 onwards – CDC (Center for Disease Control) NCHS (National Center for Health Statistics)* www.cdc.gov/nchs/datawh.htm.

The retreat of the infectious diseases did not mean a reduction in calls on medical expertise. Other conditions emerged or increased. In the 1940s, the conditions seen in doctors' surgeries did not include obesity, autism, depression, and anorexia nervosa; by the 1990s they did. The expansion of medical knowledge, and of public perceptions as to what constituted a health problem, combined to change the nature of disease concerns. Governments also helped to shape these concerns. In Britain, the MRC was sufficiently concerned by the rising trend of lung cancer deaths among men to commission research into its causes. Cancer, heart disease, diabetes, and the diseases of ageing, such as Parkinsonism and senile dementia (now more often called 'Alzheimer's Disease'), achieved a new prominence. These conditions, by and large, fell into the category described as 'chronic and degenerative' diseases. Unlike the acute infections, these generally affect older people. However, the downward trend in death rates and morbidity continued.

With the development of international communication networks by air, and the emergence of global travel as a fact of everyday life, Western countries found themselves by the 1980s, on the receiving end of re-infiltration of the old infections. Both immigrants and people travelling abroad for business or pleasure brought cases of malaria, TB, and typhoid into doctors' surgeries. Occasionally, such incursions could be frightening. In 1997, the outbreak of bubonic plague in India rang warning bells across the world. Occasional cases of the more alarming African infections, such as Lassa or Ebola fever, also made their way to the West, but did not succeed in generating outbreaks. The passage of infections from the developing to the developed world as a result of international travel repeated a pattern familiar from the recent past in developed countries, where the poor had been perceived, as they were, for example, by the Victorian novelist Charles Dickens, as a reservoir from which infections were passed on to the rich. Although the older infectious diseases, such as measles, typhoid, and TB, had been to a large extent overcome in the wealthy West, they continued to play a significant part as causes of death and debility in the developing world. Already noted in the 1960s, the disparity in levels of health and medical resources between the developed and the developing world grew more marked with time, becoming especially notable as the global epidemic of HIV/AIDS and treatments for that condition developed after 1980.

MORTALITY TRANSITIONS

Changes in the pattern of cause of death over time continued to be the subject of analysis and debate. The shift from infectious to chronic diseases as leading causes of death had been apparent already in the interwar period (Ch. 3), and from the 1950s it became clear that the old nineteenth-century pattern of dominance by the infectious diseases had vanished from the developed world. Even poliomyelitis, which briefly looked as if it might be a new plague, came under control following the introduction of vaccines in the mid-1950s. As the infectious diseases all but ceased to figure in the cause of death reports, chronic diseases and the diseases of ageing began to assume a new prominence in health and medical concerns. By the 1980s, a further shift had occurred with attention beginning to focus on the conditions now termed the 'diseases of affluence': Type 2 diabetes, heart disease, obesity, and cancer of the colorectal system. Where some historians, notably Thomas McKeown (1913–88), saw improved nutrition as leading to a reduction in death rates in the nineteenth century, ironically overnutrition increasingly seemed a contributor to the rise of a different set of diseases in the late twentieth century. In part, the change in pattern resulted from the greater longevity of Western populations, which led to higher numbers of surviving older people. Medical research and medical technologies, nonetheless, were also instrumental in indicting the behaviours associated with affluence and modern technology (notably the motor car, which led to severe reductions in exercise and physical fitness for many) as having a direct causal relationship with the 'diseases of affluence' and leading to new trajectories in significant causes of death.

The first of these new mortality trends to generate interest and investigation was the rise in deaths from lung cancer. Lung cancer had been a rare disease, but by the 1930s it was no longer possible to ascribe its rising incidence simply to improvements in diagnostic expertise and technology, such as X-rays, bronchoscopy, and open chest surgery. After World War II epidemiologists in both Britain and the United States began to inquire into the causes of lung cancer, using new statistical techniques, such as cohort, retrospective, and prospective studies. In 1950, two teams of researchers, Ernest Wynder and Evarts Graham in America, and (Sir) Austin Bradford Hill and (Sir) Richard Doll in England, almost simultaneously published independent results linking lung cancer to cigarette smoking. Further research confirmed these findings, and it became apparent that, because cigarette smoke is a weak carcinogen, the pathological impact of this new recreational drug (widely adopted only during the World War I) had taken some twenty years to produce a mortality effect. Lung cancer death rates continued to rise among men until the 1970s (Fig. 4.5) when they began to fall. The rise in rates among women began later. It had only gradually

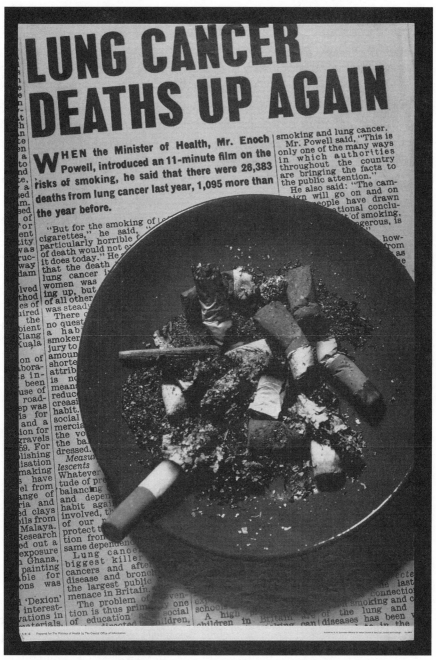

Fig. 4.5. British antismoking poster prepared for the Ministry of Health, 1960. *Source:* Lithograph after Reginald Mount and Eileen Evans, prepared for the Ministry of Health by the Central Office of Information, London. Wellcome Library Iconographic Collection. *Credit:* Wellcome Library, London (L0024898). Reproduced with permission of Her Majesty's Stationery Office.

become socially acceptable for women to smoke during the interwar years, and the later rise in the curve of lung cancer deaths among them reflected this delayed take-up of cigarette smoking.

Epidemiological studies also associated cigarette smoking with another significant postwar killer, coronary heart disease (CHD). By the end of the century, CHD was the commonest cause of death in Britain, the United States, and many other countries. Other causes were also involved, notably sedentary lifestyles and a high consumption of saturated fats of the type found in meat and dairy products. Nonetheless, as the antismoking message began to take effect, first in the United States, later in Britain, Australia, and to a lesser degree elsewhere, so CHD rates began to fall. The United States had the highest CHD rates worldwide in the 1950s, but by the late 1980s deaths had fallen by a quarter (Fig. 4.6). In countries where cigarette smoking did not decline, as in the USSR and Eastern Europe, death rates from both CHD and lung cancer remained high. By the end of the century, countries that had formerly been part of the USSR, such as Ukraine, Azerbaijan,

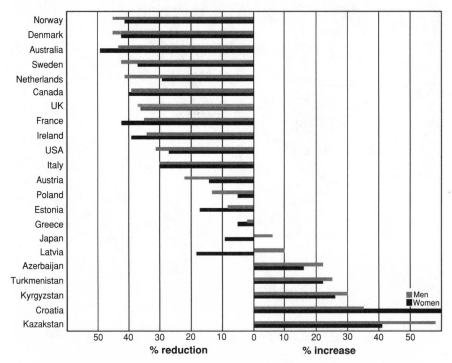

Fig. 4.6. Changes in death rates from CHD, men and women aged 35–74, between 1986 and 1996, selected countries. *Source:* Fig. 1.5b in Petersen, S. and Rayner, M. (2002), *Coronary Heart Disease Statistics*. British Heart Foundation: London, p. 26. *Credit:* Reproduced with permission of the BHF Health Promotion Research Group.

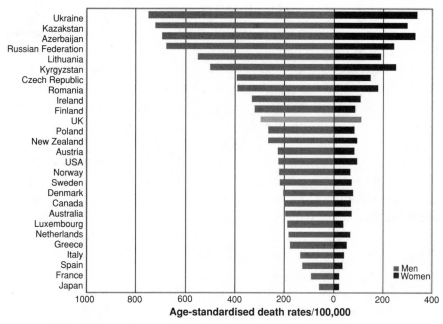

Fig. 4.7. Death rates from CHD, men and women aged 35–74, 1996, selected countries.
Source: Fig. 1.5a in Petersen, S. and Rayner, M. (2002), *Coronary Heart Disease Statistics*.
British Heart Foundation: London, p. 26. *Credit*: Reproduced with permission of the BHF
Health Promotion Research Group.

and the Russian Federation, were still recording the world's highest CHD death rates, at between 600 and 800 per 100,000 deaths for people ages thirty-five to seventy-four (Fig. 4.7).

Increasingly, however, CHD elsewhere was being associated with obesity and lifestyle. Beginning in America, but also notable in Australia and Britain, obesity was reaching epidemic proportions by the 1990s. By 2000, it was recorded that more than half of all Americans (some 97 million people) were either overweight or obese. The figures for Britain were similar; and in Australia the obesity rate was one in five. There were, of course, national and regional variations. In Western Europe, rates varied nationally from 10 to 25 percent; in the United States from 15 to 25 percent at the state level. Obesity in childhood was becoming an increasing concern, following the observation that overweight children generally became overweight adults. Nor was CHD the only medical problem associated with obesity. In the 1990s Type 2 diabetes increased rapidly in nearly all the states of America and in all age groups. The prevalence of diagnosed diabetes jumped by 33 percent nationally between 1990 and 1998, and by a worrying 70 percent among thirty to thirty-nine year olds.

Medical interest in CHD and obesity remained widely overshadowed by the popular attention given to the mythology and reality of cancer. In the 1980s, the epidemiologist Richard Doll pointed out that cancer had achieved public prominence because other diseases had been largely eliminated or reduced in fatality. Death rates from cancer, he noted, had scarcely changed between 1931–5 and 1981–4. Lung cancer, malignant melanoma, and cancers of the cervix and testes had alone registered increases in death rates. Although cancer ranked second to cardiovascular disease as a cause of death, it remained a feared killer, being associated with a painful and lingering illness and death in the popular imagination. In this sense, it was the most significant cause of death in the late twentieth century, and despite Doll's confidence, death rates increased. By 2003, a major WHO report on world cancer prevalence was predicting a 50 percent increase in cancer cases by 2020: the only area in which deaths were predicted to fall was northern Europe. The greatest cancer prevalence was in the developed world, from cancers linked to smoking and lifestyle – lung, colorectal, breast, and prostate – but also resulting from greater life expectancy. The report's authors singled out tobacco control as the single most effective way of reducing the toll of cancer, pointing to the effectiveness of the policy in Finland, and to the falling lung cancer rates among women in California, the most antismoking American state. Preventive measures, such as tobacco control, public education, and dietary advice, could, they suggested, do much to slow the increase.

Meanwhile, there were indications that the old infectious diseases might experience something of a resurgence as a problem for health and medicine in the developed countries. From the 1970s, economic, political, and social change began to recast these essentially prosperous, forward-looking societies. Inflation and industrial uncertainty, rising immigration from poor countries, and increasing rates of marriage breakdown and single motherhood, drug addiction, and homelessness, led to the reemergence of urban underclasses, notably in the great cities. From 1985, measles resurged in the United States, reaching a peak of 27,786 cases, with 100 deaths in 1990. The epidemic was worst in New York City, where it particularly hit the city's poor African American and Hispanic populations who also had little or no access to health care. In Russia, epidemic diphtheria reappeared following the collapse of Communism, social dislocation, and financial restriction on public health programmes.

Already in the 1970s there had been signs that TB was increasing among injecting drug users and the homeless in New York City. In the 1980s, however, TB was widely perceived by public health communities as a disease of the past; in that decade Bacille Calmette Guérin (BCG) immunization programmes were abandoned in Britain and the United States. The increase in deaths among these special groups gradually outweighed the continuing decline of the disease in the rest of American society, and from 1985 TB death rates began to rise once more. Urban poverty and rising HIV/AIDS incidence combined to produce an overall increase of more than 18 percent by 1991. The populations involved were mainly younger, African American, and urban. In Britain, a similar pattern emerged in the inner cities during the 1990s, with more than half of the newly reported cases being among immigrants and refugees. In London, detailed studies showed at least half of all patients to be unemployed, 5 percent with a history of homelessness, 7 percent being alcoholics, and 7 percent being HIV positive. The fall of Communism, bringing social and economic dislocation, war, and ethnic conflict, also resulted in escalating TB incidence in the former USSR and Eastern Europe after 1990. A significant feature of all these new TB surges was the presence of multidrug resistant strains of the disease.

EMERGING DISEASES

The reemergence of TB and acute childhood infections, and the appearance of multidrug resistant TB among socially deprived populations in the 1980s and 1990s, formed an ominous backdrop against which new infectious diseases emerged in the late twentieth century. While new diseases had appeared periodically in history, and become established or had disappeared, increasing public complacency about infectious disease in the years to 1980, the rise of the global communications industry, and the development of international medical research communities combined to give a new importance to such appearances. Some of the new diseases recognized may have existed before circumstance brought them to notice and they were identified clinically and scientifically. Legionnaires Disease, for example, a pneumonia generally transmitted through air-conditioning systems, was named in 1977 when an outbreak occurred among delegates to an American Legion convention in Philadelphia. Other new diseases were discovered to have resulted from changing local ecologies, from human incursions into new disease environments, species transfer, and genetic mutation. Increasingly, in the second half of the twentieth century, public health observers worried about the possibilities of a lethal airborne global epidemic on the pattern of the influenza epidemic of 1918.

433

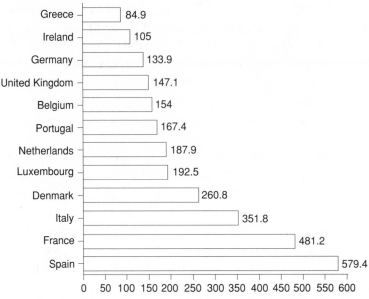

Fig. 4.8. Reported AIDS cases in Europe: cumulative rates per million population to December 1993. *Source:* Fig. 6.2, On the State of the Public Health. *Annual Report of the Chief Medical Officer of the Department of Health for the Year 1993* (HMSO, 1994, p. 143). *Credit:* Crown copyright material is reproduced with the permission of the Controller of HMSO and the Queen's Printer for Scotland. *Original Source:* European Centre for the Epidemiological Monitoring of AIDS.

The most spectacular and significant disease emergence of the late twentieth century was, however, that of HIV/AIDS in the early 1980s. A slow chronic disease resulting in immuno-deficiency and transmitted by infected body fluids, the disease syndrome was first recognized in the United States in 1981. The causal agent was identified amid much controversy in 1983. Apparently spreading by sexual transmission, through contaminated needles used by injecting drug users, and through infected blood products, HIV resulted in a worldwide epidemic. While its spread was limited in the developed world (Fig. 4.8), the disease was, by the 1990s, running out of control in the developing world, more especially in Africa and Southeast Asia. In 1990, the WHO estimates of the total cumulative number of HIV/AIDS cases was 1.2 million, of which 400,000 were infants and small children, mostly in sub-Saharan Africa. In the West, the disease rapidly became the focus of a massive international research effort into its nature, origins, progression, and treatment. Between 1980 and 2000, more money was spent in relative terms on research and drug development directed at HIV/AIDS than on any other disease in history. Early hopes for the development of a vaccine proved delusive because the virus mutated constantly. That characteristic also made it exceptionally drug resistant, although by the mid-1990s combined drug therapies were improving and prolonging the lives of AIDS patients in developed countries. The cost of these drugs put them beyond the reach of sufferers in the developing world; a situation that created resentments against Western drug companies.

HIV/AIDS proved a modern case study of reaction towards the emergence of a new lethal communicable chronic disease. The initial popular reaction to lay blame on the people of Haiti (where the disease was reputed to have originated) and gays (among whom it first manifested itself in the United States), met with stout responses from concerned communities; later suggestions that Africa was the cradle of the disease were also contested. The discovery of the causal organism proved a fruitful source of discord, with rival French and American research teams claiming credit. The role of the virus was disputed by another eminent scientist, Peter Duesberg (b. 1928), and his views acquired a minority following. In Britain, America, and elsewhere, compensation claims were fought by haemophiliacs who had been infected by blood products in the early stages of the epidemic. In the mid-1980s, Western governments launched vigorous educational campaigns aimed at limiting the spread of the disease. These were all but abandoned when it became apparent that no wildfire spread of infection into the general population was occurring. Western countries saw a surge of self-help organizations and charities dedicated to supporting AIDS patients and HIV positives, in addition to their friends and families. Many of these also aimed to influence national policies in respect of the disease. At the national level, voluntarism was especially strong in the United States. In Europe, policy developed in accordance with the ethos of individual states. In Britain, Switzerland, and the Netherlands, voluntary organizations helped shape policy. In France, Italy, and Eastern Europe they had little influence.

By the late 1990s, HIV was generally accepted in the scientific community as having originated in a simian immuno-deficiency virus. In several instances during the 1980s and 1990s, newsworthy disease outbreaks pointed up the connections between disease in humans, other animals, and the foods derived from them, and the way humans managed the environment. Salmonellosis in chickens and eggs, listeriosis in unpasteurised soft cheeses, *Eschirichia coli 0157* (*E. coli*) in undercooked minced beef, avian-borne West Nile virus, and Hong Kong chicken flu in 1997 were prominent examples. Notably, the later 1980s saw the emergence of BSE ('mad cow disease') in Britain, possibly as the result of using the brains of

435

scrapie-infected sheep in high-protein cattle feeds. Despite scientific analogies to scrapie, which had coexisted harmlessly with humans for centuries, and the insistence of leading British politicians that British beef was 'safe', there was great public concern over the possible transfer of the disease to humans through the food chain. In 1996, the National CJD Surveillance Unit (CJD: Creutzfeld Jacob disease, a distinct human spongiform encephalopathy) identified a previously unrecognized disease pattern, which they named new variant CJD (nv CJD). By contrast with the classic form, the variant occurred in relatively young people. Links were immediately made to BSE and the consumption of infected beef. Major food scares followed across the West, resulting in severe repercussions for the British beef industry, whose products were banned from European and American markets until it could be proven that the disease was under control. By 2003, however, the total number of cases of nvCJD remained very small and epidemiologists were revising the dire forecasts that they had made when the disease first appeared.

In the 1990s, several other well-publicized epidemic or potential epidemic emergencies occurred, including a major outbreak of *E. coli 0157* in Japan, bubonic plague in India, and a virulent avian influenza with the ability to transmit to man in Hong Kong. The last episode carried particularly worrying resonances for those anticipating another 1918 epidemic (pp. 249–50), and resulted in the mass culling of domestic poultry across Hong Kong. Despite the resources of twentieth-century medicine, no effective remedy for influenza had been developed, and new antivirals coming onto the market around the turn of the century promised no more than to shorten the duration of illness. Although vaccines were available, they had to be continuously calibrated to keep up with mutations in the virus, and there was no guarantee that sufficient vaccines could be manufactured to control any sudden appearance of a highly virulent strain. In the global culture of the 1990s, with hundreds of thousands of people travelling the world by air every day, the control of any virulent airborne virus represented a nightmare for national health organizations, epidemiologists, and the WHO alike. The nightmare scenario seemed about to break in spring 2003. A new and lethal type of pneumonia, dubbed Severe Acute Respiratory Syndrome (SARS) emerged in Guangdong province, China, in November 2002. By January 2003 the disease had taken hold, although the Chinese government suppressed information about the epidemic in the interests of 'social stability'. By early March, however, travellers from China had taken the disease to Hong Kong and Singapore, and by the middle of the month the WHO had issued an emergency travel alert. Within days, a worldwide scare was underway, fuelled by the reluctance of the Chinese authorities to admit the extent of their problem. By May, the disease had spread to some thirty countries, reportedly infecting some 5,500 persons and killing 375. Airlines began screening passengers before boarding, while the developed world debated preventive action. In the West, however, the disease showed little tendency to spread, and in early May the WHO was reporting that the disease had peaked everywhere except in China. In China, the disease continued to spread, and the situation was far from clear, although the authorities now began to take emergency measures. 'Is this the big one?', medical observers across the world were asking in March and April, but by May they had concluded with relief that it was not, as long as it did not mutate into a better transmitter.

Beginning during World War II, the global expansion of Western trade and industry permitted by new scientific methods and new communications systems, brought a new form of health hazard – the major industrial accident. Although occupational diseases and accidents associated with industry were far from being a new phenomenon, the scale on which these might occur was vastly enhanced after 1940. Presaged by the terrifying experiences of the effects of radiation on humans as a result of nuclear fallout after atom bombs were used on the Japanese cities of Hiroshima and Nagasaki at the end of the war, the last decades of the twentieth century offered a number of instances both of mega industrial accidents and of new occupational diseases. The former included a major gas leak from a container of methyl isocyanate at a factory in Bhopal operated by Union Carbide India Ltd, which killed almost 4,000 people and left more than 2,700 permanently disabled. By the end of the century the death toll had risen to over 14,000. Just two years later a nuclear reactor exploded at Chernobyl in the former Soviet Union (now Ukraine) that killed thirty people on the site, injured hundreds more, but was estimated to have exposed more than five million people to ionizing radiation from fallout of radioactive nucleotides, leading to a large increase in some cancers, especially thyroid cancers in children. Such large-scale accidents caused not only immediate acute medical emergencies, but long-term health problems caused by the contamination of air, food, and water supplies, and affected future generations because of induced genetic mutations. And it was not only such large-scale accidents: the careless discharge of industrial hazardous waste has been implicated in diseases, such as various types of cancer and chronic chest conditions. It is not only industry and wars that are responsible for pollution. Also important are the conditions that contribute significantly to changes in the environment and hence to changes in the patterns of diseases. Excessive use of insecticides both in agriculture and in public health for vector control is another source of significant environmental pollution. Excessive use of cars, some of which are not well maintained, is well known as a source of air pollution and its effect on developing lung cancer is well documented.

Medical practice

The nature of medical practice changed profoundly in the years after 1945, both in the hospitals and in the wider community. The great expansion in the therapeutic armoury, new medical technologies, rising patient demand, financial pressures, and the rise of specialist medicine all contributed to this change. The way in which new and expanding medical specialties were accommodated within new and existing frameworks of health care was especially influential in shaping national differences in medical organizations and determining how doctors and nurses practised. Thus in Britain, the structure of the NHS and the established practice of referral with general practitioners (GPs) acting as the gateway to hospital or specialist treatment, worked in favour of the survival of the GP in the local community. In America, by contrast, there was no referral system and doctors had every incentive to specialize. In 1963, some 70 percent of British doctors were in general practice against approximately 35 percent in the United States. Even in the hospital sector, the new technologies of emerging specialties effected institutional change: manpower and facilities needed to be concentrated if they were to be put to the best use. Specialist centres began to emerge, for example, for open heart surgery, oncology, and accidents and emergencies.

If the growth of specialism had been a hallmark of modernizing Western medicine since the nineteenth century, and had established itself in most developed countries (except Britain), during the interwar period (Ch. 3), improved technologies and expensive treatments brought a novel proliferation of medical specialities after 1945. It was a development that now also embraced Britain. Some of these new specialities were based almost wholly in the development of new medical instruments – diagnostic imaging, dialysis, and minimal access surgery are cases in point. The growth of the discipline of medical physics was a great stimulus to the development of new technologies. The growing expertise and professional ambitions of medical men was also a factor. Surgery, which before 1940 had been the province of generalists, fragmented into a range of specialized activities: brain surgery, heart surgery, paediatric surgery among them. Paediatrics similarly resolved into different components, including child psychiatry. Anaesthetics, which had often been practised by part-time generalists, now developed as a whole new professional subdiscipline, with specialized training and qualification, as did the new specialty of intensive care. Radiology, pathology, and the treatment of pain in specialist clinics followed a similar pattern. Cardiology emerged from general medicine, established itself in specialist units and departments, and gathered an array of skilled personnel in expert teams that included medical and nonmedical members. Teamwork also became an important feature of geriatrics as it began to establish itself as a specialty.

Specialism was the new face of medical practice by the later twentieth century. The numbers of specialists rose quickly in the immediate postwar period: in Britain, some 4,500 doctors described themselves as specialists in 1948; 7,000 did so by 1960. Increasingly, young doctors everywhere preferred to opt for a specialist career. Even in countries where general practice remained relatively popular, as in Britain, Canada, and France, it attracted fewer than half the new physicians coming into practice between 1960 and 1990 (Fig. 4.9). And as central governments increasingly sought to regulate the costs and quality of community medical practice after 1990, so the attractions of specialist and hospital practice grew.

HOSPITALS

The experience of World War II, and the consequences of the therapeutic revolution wrought significant changes in the public and political perception of hospitals. Despite the move to hospital medicine and expansion in hospital facilities that occurred in the interwar period (p. 269ff), most hospitals remained refuges for the chronic sick and the elderly before 1940. Drug treatments were simple and surgical procedures limited. Time spent in the hospital mostly involved bed rest and nursing care. But the phenomenal effort of medical provision engendered by the war brought modern blood transfusion methods, improved radiology and anaesthesia, antibiotics, and surgeons with specialized experience in, for example, trauma techniques, plastic surgery, and burns treatment. Hospitals became the locus of a whole new range of specialized medical procedures, some of which went on to establish new and distinct identities in specialist units and departments. Coronary care units, specialist respiratory disease clinics, premature baby

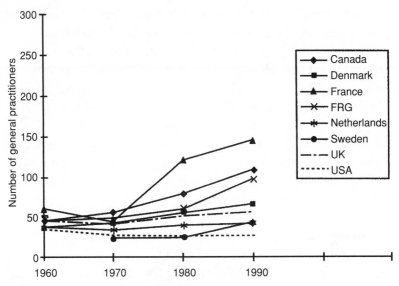

Fig. 4.9. Total number of GPs per 100,000 population, various countries, 1960–92.
Source: Fig. 11.2 in John Horder, 'Developments in other countries', in Irvine Loudon,
John Horder, and Charles Webster (eds.), *General Practice under the National Health Service
1948–1997*, London, Clarendon Press, 1998, p. 263. Original source: various, including
WHO statistics. *Credit*: Reproduced with permission of Oxford University Press and WHO.

units, and intensive care units were among the wide range of facilities that
emerged in association with hospital medicine in the 1960s. The chronic
sick and the elderly disappeared from the wards into specialist care homes,
to be replaced by patients whose hospital stays were increasingly curtailed
to the stages of acute treatment only (fast-tracking).

The effects of war were also felt in the availability and organization of hospital care. The provision of easily accessed hospital care was widely seen as
an entitlement for citizens of a modern postwar state: in Sweden, for example, new hospitals in every town are said to have symbolized the goodwill
and power of the welfare state. In America, the war-inspired mapping of
regional hospital services across the country influenced subsequent peacetime development: the 1946 Hill Burton Act initiated a major programme
of federal grants to help states in building local hospitals. In Britain, the
central supervision of hospital and ancillary facilities under the wartime
Emergency Medical Service (EMS) (p. 388) helped to shape the structure
of the new NHS. In 1948, most British hospitals were nationalized and
incorporated into a regionally based administration. Hospital building programmes became an integral part of social reconstruction programmes in
those European states that had been occupied by Germany during the war.

As symbols of modern scientific medicine, of medical progress, and of egalitarian modern social policies, hospitals reached their summit of eminence in the 1950s and 1960s. This symbolic identity was now reflected not only in the building of new hospitals, but in the modernist architecture that characterized them.

The medical preeminence of the modern hospital was especially notable in America. Here, the growth in hospital facilities and in-patient attendance rose sharply. Neither America's economy nor her domestic infrastructure had suffered the damage inflicted in Europe by five years of total war. Between 1946 and 1960, more than 1,000 new hospitals were built and the rate of hospital admissions doubled over prewar levels. Many of these new institutions were small, serving a local community and focusing on short-term care. By 1960, there were 5,000 short-term general hospitals in the United States against some 300 for long-stay care. In Europe, by contrast, the pattern varied. The Netherlands quickly initiated a hospital building programme after 1945, but in France hospital building was not considered until the second phase of postwar reconstruction after 1954. Britain did not launch a hospital building programme before the 1960s.

The postwar hospital building programmes did not necessarily produce an increase in the number of hospital beds available, although numbers generally kept step with population growth. The number of hospital beds per head of population expanded only slightly in Britain and the United States up to 1970; in France and Sweden the number continued to grow. Sweden, where the focus of treatment had traditionally lain in the hospital, had more general hospital beds per head of population than France, Britain, or America by the 1970s. In Eastern Europe, similarly, hospital provision remained generous, with the hospital at the centre of the care regime. Up to the fall of communism in the early 1990s, the socialist countries of central and Eastern Europe had some 20 percent more hospital beds than the countries of Western Europe. Even after 1990, when numbers of hospital beds did begin to fall in Eastern Europe, levels remained about twice as high as in the West, and in Russia the average length of stay remained high, at around fourteen days. In many former Soviet countries, women with uncomplicated deliveries, for example, would stay in hospital for seven days; in the West they would be discharged within twenty-four hours. Differing treatment regimes also raised the demand for hospital beds: TB, for instance, was treated by prolonged in-patient chemotherapy, whereas in Western Europe it would be managed on an out-patient basis.

For one group of patients in particular, the hospital became an increasingly rare experience. With the discovery of the psychotropic drugs, the traditional expedient of confining people with mental illness to institutions came to be seen increasingly as unnecessary and inhumane. In Britain, a movement for the care of such people in the community emerged in the 1960s. The number of patients in psychiatric hospitals was halved in most developed countries between the late 1950s and the late 1980s. Two phases have been discerned in this modern history of the asylum. In the 1950s and 1960s there was a 'benign' phase, when the mental hospitals opened their doors to release and resettle long-stay patients in the community. In most Western countries, the number of psychiatric hospitals was more than halved in the thirty years after 1960. This was followed by a 'radical' phase after 1970, when in response to financial pressures and the search for improved treatment options, the hospitals closed their doors and diverted patients to community-based services. The new phase emerged in the United States to be replicated elsewhere. Psychiatric hospitals 'the size of small towns' were scaled down or closed, the number of psychiatric in-patient beds falling dramatically between 1970 and 1990.

With the rising crisis in medical service expenditures, other patterns of hospital bed use also began to change. The pattern observed in post-1990 Russia replicated that occurring earlier elsewhere. Even in the 1960s, more patients were being processed through the hospital more quickly in Britain, as length of stay was cut back. The average length of stay for short-term patients fell from 14.5 days in 1961 to 10.2 in 1972. In the same period, for all patients, it fell from an average of 34.5 days to 24.2. Again, the pattern varied significantly by country and national medical cultures. By the 1980s, the average short stay was ten days in American hospitals against 24.6 in Sweden. In the 1980s and 1990s, further reductions were achieved with the development of day surgery – a direct and beneficial outcome of improved technologies. Ambulatory surgical services were developed in America, operated by 94 percent of community hospitals in 1987. At this date more than 40 percent of the operations being performed in America were done on an out-patient basis. European hospitals followed suit. By 1995, for example, 28 percent of German hospitals were offering day surgery. In France and the Netherlands, shorter hospital stays were achieved through a combination of technological progress, new drug treatments, and higher levels of community care.

This changing pattern of care, as well as the specific impact of new treatments, was reflected in hospital stay by specific cause. Cataract surgery, for example, had become almost entirely a day procedure by 1990. In the United States, the length of stay for heart attack victims fell from 19.7 days in 1964 to 10.6 in 1981; breast cancer stays from 10.5 days to 3.3; and normal births from 3.8 days to 1.9 days. As Rosemary Stevens has noted, hospitalization had become just one incident in the course of an illness, rather than being coterminous with the illness itself: 'the hospital seemed less a health centre than ever before, and more and more like a technical treatment station' (Stevens, 1999, p. 288).

The pruning of hospital patient care was accompanied by an increased concern for the quality and effectiveness of that care. From the later 1980s, state governments began to impose monitoring systems, with a view to evaluating value for money and enforcing accountability. In the process, the autonomy of hospital medicine began to be eroded, and public mistrust of the institutions emerged. In America, following the introduction of a disease-related reimbursement system, the federal government became increasingly involved in the standardization and regulation of hospital practice. From 1987, for example, organs for transplantation were distributed according to uniform federal criteria, and hospitals were obliged to identify potential organ donors to people in need of transplants. In Britain, government introduced a hospital ranking system under which hospital performance was assessed according to thirty-seven different criteria to obtain a star rating. Underachieving institutions – those with less than three stars, or none – risked the imposition of special government-appointed managers. Top-ranking three-starred hospitals were promised, in 2002, £1 million each to improve their services further. Well-intentioned as such measures might be, they were not necessarily productive. In Britain, it was reported that patient anxiety increased among those entering hospitals with low or zero ratings.

Patients increasingly had grounds to be anxious about entering the hospital in the later decades of the twentieth century. Although most such anxiety focused on anaesthetic accidents and mishaps in the operation itself, the real danger to patient health and life came from hospital infections. Overuse of antibiotics and the complexities of modern medical technology, both contributed to the return of the mid-nineteenth-century spectre of 'hospitalism'. The great problem was the emergence of antibiotic resistant strains of the bacteria causing wound infections, pneumonia, and gastro-enteritis. The classic wound infection bacterium, *Staphylococcus aureus*, had been totally susceptible to penicillin when the drug was introduced; by 1983 fewer than 10 percent of all cases could be cured by penicillin. Methicillin came to replace penicillin as the effective treatment of choice in the 1960s, but by the 1980s methicillin resistant strains of *S. aureus* (MRSA) were emerging, and during that decade outbreaks increased in size and frequency across the globe. In Britain in 1990, there were sixty-seven cases of MRSA and by 1999 there were 3,110. Already in 1993, only one drug, vancomycin, remained effective against these bacteria. Meanwhile, vancomycin-resistant strains of enterococci appeared after 1988, encouraged by hospital practices that allowed bacterial contamination of equipment, such as electronic thermometers, catheters and surgical instruments, intravenous lines, and mechanical ventilation.

HOSPICES AND PALLIATIVE CARE

As the hospitals were transformed into high-technology, acute short-stay institutions, so the problem remained of the care of the chronic sick and elderly who had previously found refuge there. In Britain and elsewhere, the concept of the nursing home developed during and after the war as a way of meeting these needs. Often privately run, but in some cases, notably in Scandinavia, state-provided, these homes offered a new type of care for frail patients. Increasingly, however, as the demographic pattern of Europe changed, as the proportion of elderly people in the population grew, and malignant and degenerative diseases, especially cancer, assumed greater prominence as causes of illness and death, so the management of terminally ill patients in great and continuous pain became an issue of care. The last decades of the twentieth century saw the emergence of a new type of care, one that focused on the management of pain. Partly deriving from the methods of a novel type of institution, the hospice, what became known as palliative care had become a widely recognised and practised medical care system by the end of the century.

Traditionally, and especially in the Christian countries of the West, pain had been viewed as redemptive, an affliction that must be accepted with stoicism. Medical opinion, moreover, generally considered pain as a diagnostic sign and warning of impending illness – a phenomenon that it might be dangerous to suppress. During World War II, however, the anaethesiologist John J. Bonica (b. 1917) developed the management of pain into a specialized skill and also a body of knowledge. Bonica thought that pain should be treated in new 'pain units' within hospitals and his ideas were influential. The first Pain Clinic was opened in Seattle in 1961, and 1974 saw the founding of the International Society for the Study of Pain. In the

1970s, pain units became a standard feature in hospitals concerned with the care of the terminally ill.

In a parallel development, the English doctor (Dame) Cecily Saunders (1918–2005) began investigating terminal pain and its relief as a result of her experiences at a special care unit run by the Irish Sisters of Charity, in the late 1950s. Although the word 'hospice' has a long history, its association with the care of malignant disease and the terminally ill dates from around 1900, when the Sisters of Charity began to found special care units. While the new attitudes to pain generated by Bonica's work helped to create a setting in which the idea of the hospice could flourish, Saunders's personal involvement with the problem of pain management was also highly influential. Saunders focused on the way in which drugs were used to control pain and set out 'cardinal rules' for their deployment: the symptoms troubling the patient were to be carefully assessed, as was the nature and severity of the pain. The regular giving of drugs was critical to Saunders's methods: her central concern was for the comfort of the patient. During the 1960s, she developed the concept of 'total pain', involving physical, social, spiritual, and psychological problems. In 1967 she opened St. Christopher's Hospice in Kent, where the control of pain, the alleviation of symptoms, and support for the patients' families were guiding principles. In the years after 1967, Saunders's writings and lecturing, and her travels in America and Europe, generated widespread interest in her methods and inspired the founding of hospices in other countries, for example, in Germany and Poland.

The expression 'palliative care' was not, however, coined by Saunders but was first used in Canada, with the opening of the Palliative Care Service at the Royal Victoria Hospital in Montreal in 1975. Developed in the hospital setting rather than in the hospice, palliative care had by the 1990s, become a wide-ranging field embracing many different institutions and aspects and types of care, including a new medical specialty, palliative medicine. The latter was defined in 1998 by the authoritative *Oxford Textbook of Palliative Medicine* as a medical specialty practised by doctors; palliative care, by contrast, was defined as 'the care offered by a team of doctors, nurses, therapists, social workers, clergy and volunteers' (p. 3). During the 1980s and 1990s, the concept of palliative care was developed and refined, partly under the guidance of the WHO, which by 1980 was becoming increasingly concerned about care for cancer patients. In 1982, WHO first drew attention to the problem of pain relief in cancer. By 1986, it had developed its own strategic approach to the problem (published in *Cancer Pain Relief*),

Country	Date	Type of service	Name of service
United Kingdom	1967	Inpatient hospice	St Christopher's Hospice
Sweden	1977	Home care service	Motala Hospital-based Home Care
Italy	1980	Home care programme	Pain Therapy Division of National Cancer Institute of Milan and Floriani Foundation
Germany	1983	Hospital inpatient unit	Palliate Care Unit, University Clinic, Cologne
Spain	1984	Palliative care unit within hospital medical oncology department	Medical Oncology Department, Valdicella Hospital, Santander
Belgium	1985	Palliative care unit; home care service	Unit de Soins Continus St Luc *and* Continuing Care, Brussels
The Netherlands	1991	Inpatient hospice	Johannes Hospice, Vleuten

Fig. 4.10. 'Founding' specialist hospice/palliative care services in seven European countries. *Source*: Fig. 2.1 in David Clark, Henk ten Have, and Rien Janssens, 'Palliative care service developments in seven European countries', in Henk ten Have and David Clark (eds.), *The Ethics of Palliative Care. European Perspectives*, Buckingham, Open University Press, 2002, p. 36. *Credit*: Reproduced with the kind permission of the Open University Press/McGraw-Hill Publishing Company.

and in 1990 extended this to include and promote palliative care. The revised WHO definition of palliative care issued in 2002 described it as 'an approach that improves quality of life of patients and their families facing the problems associated with life-threatening illness, through the prevention and relief of suffering by means of early identification and impeccable assessment and treatment of pain and other problems'.

The WHO's promotion of palliative care acted as a stimulus to its adoption in many countries, even if in voluntary and piecemeal fashion. If the WHO's concern was initially with cancer, the emergence of AIDS in the 1980s, and the spread of that epidemic in the industrialized countries through the 1980s and 1990s, added edge to the new interest in palliative care. In Western Europe, a decided development in care provision was detectable in the 1980s (Fig. 4.10), although in central and Eastern Europe it was not until after the fall of Communism that the tentative efforts of individuals began to expand into more systematic provision in the 1990s. In care terms, the new field continued to reflect Saunders's philosophy of caring for both the physical and spiritual needs of the patient and his or her family, but several different models developed for the delivery of such care. St. Christopher's had set an example of independent specialized institutional care; the Canadian model located this type of care in a specialized hospital setting. The first specialized palliative care service established in Europe, in Sweden in 1977, was a hospital-based home-care service. In this model, the patient remained at home, supported by a specialist care team on a twenty-four-hour basis. It was widely copied, for example in Italy and Belgium.

HOSPITAL NURSING

The role of the nurse in health care continued to be actively debated. Issues of education and professional status, and of the function and practice of nursing remained central to these debates. In many respects, these questions became more urgent as the impact of the new developments in therapeutics and medical technology began to be felt. The traditional work of the hospital nurse had been in tasks associated with diagnosis and treatment, and hospital nursing had meant providing patients with unfailing round-the-clock service. With the introduction of new technologies, increasing specialization, and, eventually, financial stringency, the role and responsibilities of the nurse both inside and outside the hospital began to change.

Inside the hospital, new tensions developed between the traditional supportive, caring model of nursing and the demands of new technology and new practices. Some nurses became technicians, for example, tending electronic monitoring equipment; others developed specialist skills as part of large medical teams in intensive care units, coronary care units, transplant surgery, and postoperative care (Fig. 4.11). At one level, nursing became less patient-centred and more mechanised. As national economies came under pressure after 1970, the spectrum of nursing requirements broadened further. In some cases, nursing practice moved closer to medicine. The 'nurse practitioner' with extended responsibilities in diagnosis and treatment first appeared in California in 1971, originally as a way of covering a shortage of doctors. By contrast, economies resulting from financial stringency resulted, in Britain, in trained nurses being required to fill in for depleted support staff in cleaning and cooking. As a result, both qualified and trainee nurses were said by 1987 to be leaving NHS employment 'in droves'.

Social change also contributed to altered perceptions of nursing outside the hospital, as wider employment opportunities opened to women. Already during World War II it was apparent that nursing was failing to attract young women contributors to the war effort. Openings in the Armed Forces were more seductive and there were also greater opportunities in clerical and support work. Reforms in education in the 1940s resulted in generations of increasingly well-educated young women, who began to consider their career options in the light of job satisfaction, material rewards, and social standing. By the 1970s, when, theoretically at least, few occupations remained closed to women, nursing no longer counted among the most popular career choices.

In these circumstances, new approaches to nursing began to emerge, as the profession tried to come to terms with the changing social and medical

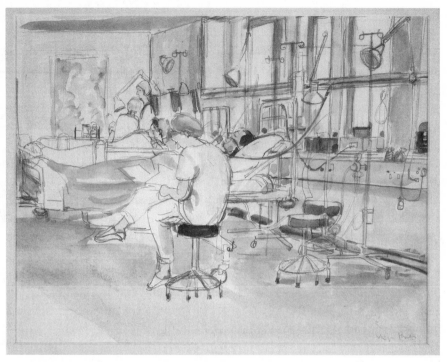

Fig. 4.11. A theatre nurse monitoring a patient in the recovery room after surgery, Chelsea and Westminster Hospital, London, 1995. *Source*: Pencil and watercolour drawing by Virginia Powell. Wellcome Library Iconographic Collection. *Credit*: Wellcome Library, London (L0028352).

environment. Much of the impetus for reexamining and revising the role of the nurse came from the United States, where academic nursing had become established in the interwar period. After 1945, American nursing analysts began to focus on nurse training as the key to professional change. Because of the variety of different skills and qualifications among nursing personnel, the professional status of the nurse was a central concern, and closely associated with this was the issue of professional autonomy, which was thought to influence the perception of a nurse's social standing. From 1948 onwards, repeated assessments of the state of nursing in America recommended higher education, professional training, and greater financial rewards as the keys to enhanced social standing. New models of nursing began to emerge, often influenced by concepts drawn from sociology and education.

Among the most influential of these new models was the concept of 'the nursing process' that emerged in America in the 1960s, and reached England through the Department of Nursing at Manchester University in the early 1970s. The core notion of this philosophy was that nursing was a process that should relate to the patient's problem. The taking of nursing histories, assessment of a patient's needs, construction of a nursing plan, and its subsequent evaluation were assumed to be viable independently of medical diagnosis. The approach responded actively to the patient and his or her condition; it rejected the traditional medical model of task-oriented nursing. The 1980s saw the introduction of the concept of 'primary nursing', which involves the delivery of care by individual nurses assigned to individual patients. By the 1990s, the work of the modern European nurse was seen to be based on patient-centred care and problem solving.

With the opening of employment and other markets as a result of European economic union in the 1970s, international communities began to take an interest in nursing standards. In 1977, the European Community issued two important directives that were significantly to influence attitudes towards nursing both inside and outside the community. The first aimed to secure the mutual recognition of nurse diplomas within the European Community; the second, to define the skills required of a general nurse. These were to have had at least ten years' general education, as well as a full-time training of three years with at least 4,600 hours of theoretical and practical instruction. Although the explicit aim of these directives was to facilitate workplace mobility and the harmonization of qualifications between countries, they soon achieved the status of international standards. Nonetheless, many countries, for example in Eastern Europe, were still far from achieving these standards. Meanwhile, the WHO also maintained a lively interest in nursing, and eventually developed its own guidelines for states wishing to revise national nursing regulations. The WHO model was formulated at the first European Conference on Nursing, held at Vienna in 1988. It envisaged nurses as responsible for providing a broad community-based service alongside their still-important role in the hospital sector; a service that would include life style counselling, the diagnosis of health problems, and home care for the elderly, sick, and frail.

These international models of modern nurse training and skills were widely debated, but international compliance remained sketchy. A wide range of nursing philosophies continued to exist in the developed world. In the former Soviet Union, medical models of nursing survived unscathed, and most doctors and nurses supported a traditional professional hierarchy with nursing dependent on and subordinate to medicine. In Finland, however, primary nursing had become the dominant model by the 1990s and, in Scandinavia generally, nursing had become a more or less comprehensive activity involving both health care and health promotion. Yet in certain circumstances, as in Swedish hospitals, the old model survived, and nurses remained formally subordinate to their medical colleagues.

The hospital, meanwhile, was gradually being displaced as the locus of nurse training. Separate nursing schools based in universities or institutes of higher education were becoming the norm. Here, the teaching was done by health care professionals rather than by doctors, as in the past, and as a result the traditional hospital-based training was reshaped to emphasize research, health care needs, and broad concepts of nursing. The nature of the training given in the different countries continued to vary, however. By 2000, all the countries covered by the WHO Regional Office for Europe required a nurse to undergo some three years' training, but the aims and nature of the training differed markedly. In Finland, for example, general nurse education had been replaced by specialist training in 1987. In France, the reforms of 1992 aimed to produce nurses trained in all aspects of nursing both inside and outside the hospital. In Britain, Project 2000 gave students eighteen months of general education, followed by training in one of four specialist areas (adult, child, mental health, and mental handicap). These efforts at the reform and reinvention of the popular image of nursing were, initially at least, of limited effect. In the early twenty-first century, nursing remained, in the view of WHO observers, a widely undervalued and underdeveloped profession, despite the unique functions that nurses had come to fulfil in modern health care systems.

MIDWIVES

If models of nursing multiplied and changed after 1945, the established model of the midwife as a practitioner who gives independent care to women in pregnancy and childbirth, changed less substantially. Midwives continued to offer such care, but the details of their practice were increasingly regulated by government and, increasingly, they found themselves practising in hospital, under the supervisory umbrella of GP or consultant care. By the 1990s, the professional dominance of the midwife over the birthing process had all but disappeared in many countries, as obstetrician-gynaecologists developed their specialty and asserted their right to manage births in a hospital setting. Since the introduction of the sulphonamide drugs against puerperal fever in 1935, deaths in childbirth had become rare in industrialized countries, and childbirth gradually became reconstituted as a dangerous, rather than a normal, process, with an emphasis on the risks involved for both mother and child. The processes of pregnancy and birth became subject to formal medical supervision and childbirth came to take place in hospital rather than in the home. Although this trend was already evident in Britain and America before World War II (pp. 331–36), it was only after 1970 that the pattern extended itself in the West. Home births attended by a midwife were the norm in Europe before 1970; after 1970 the rate of home deliveries dropped steadily. By the 1980s, it had become as difficult to arrange a home delivery as it had previously been to obtain a delivery bed in hospital.

As birth became medicalized, midwifery practice shifted from the home to the hospital. By 1980, for example, half of all Italian midwives worked in hospitals where they attended almost all births. Even in the Netherlands, which had a strong tradition of domiciliary midwifery, some 16 percent of practising midwives were employed by hospitals by 1984. Nevertheless, midwifery practice was to some extent sustained by local tradition and also by the critiques of modern medicine that began to emerge from the later 1960s. In Britain, where consultant-managed births were almost universal by 1970, a number of hospital authorities introduced 'GP Units' (General Practitioner Units) in the 1970s, where expectant mothers were cared for and delivered by midwives while under the supervisory care of their GP rather than a hospital consultant. This decade also saw the emergence of natural childbirth movements, whose emphasis on an ideal of nonmedicalized birth depended significantly on perceptions of the traditional skills of the midwife and on birth as a social rather than a medical process.

Significant differences remained in the provision, regulation, training, and practice of midwives in different countries. Numbers varied, for example, from 129.5 per thousand population in the Soviet Union to 11.4 per thousand in Ireland (Table 4.3). National regulations variously defined the responsibilities and powers of the midwife. In Norway, ante-natal care was the province of GPs; in Sweden, it was the province of midwives working independently in ante-natal clinics. In some countries, midwives could perform breech deliveries, in others these had to be performed by a doctor. In Turkey, midwives were not allowed to prescribe drugs, which had to be prescribed by a doctor. In some countries men were forbidden to become midwives, but in others, such as Denmark, the Netherlands, and Britain, midwifery practice was open to them. Training varied from four years to one year. In 1981, a WHO survey listed seven countries where midwives were obliged first to train as nurses, including Ireland, Norway, Portugal, Spain, and Sweden.

Table 4.3. *Midwives per 100,000 Population in Selected European Countries*

Country	Number per 100,000 Population[a]	Annual Percentage Change Since Early 1970s
Belgium	18.3	−4.9
Czechoslovakia	44.9	+0.6
Denmark	14.0	+6.2
Finland	17.1	−3.4
France	16.8	+1.1
Greece	34.5	+7.3
Hungary	25.7	+3.5
Ireland	11.4	−9.8
Italy	29.1	−1.5
Switzerland	22.4	−1.9
Turkey	31.2	−1.2
USSR	129.5	+1.1
United Kingdom	36.9	−0.4
Yugoslavia	35.2	+3.3

[a] Varies by country from 1980–4. In France and Greece, 1977.
Source: WHO (1986, unpublished data).
Copyright © 1990, From *Helpers in Childbirth, Midwifery Today* by Ann Oakley and Susanne Houd. Reproduced by permission of Routledge/Taylor & Francis Books, Inc and Ann Oakley.

Despite European Community and WHO ideals of greater integration in training and practice in midwifery as in nursing, the haphazard pattern of midwifery provision remained at the end of the twentieth century. Differing national patterns reflected variations in both the strength of specialist medicine and of the nursing profession, women's attitudes towards medical intervention, and the nature of national health care systems and the ways in which they were funded. In 1990, one analysis suggested that types of national health care system and the nature of their financing were critical to the nature of midwifery practice. In monopolistic systems, such as the British NHS, midwives appeared to retain control over uncomplicated deliveries. In pluralist systems, the midwife might be entitled by law to deliver uncomplicated births, but financial and other incentives ensured that physicians would seek to gain greater access to the management of pregnancy and childbirth.

FAMILY PRACTICE

The tides of change that swept across Western medical practice after 1945 did not leave untouched the work of doctors practising outside hospitals in the local community. The swift rise of medical specialism that characterized

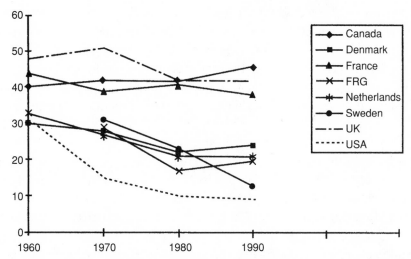

Fig. 4.12. General practitioners as a percentage of all physicians, various countries, 1960–90. *Source*: Fig. 11.3 in John Horder, 'Developments in other countries', in Irvine Loudon, John Horder, and Charles Webster (eds.), *General Practice under the National Health Service 1948–1997*, London, Clarendon Press, 1998, p. 263. Original source: W. J. Stephen, *An Analysis of Primary Medical Care*, Cambridge University Press, 1979; WHO, Regional Office for Europe, *Draft Profiles of General Practice*, Copenhagen, 1995; J. Fry and J. Horder, *Primary Care in an International Context*, London, Nuffield Provincial Hospitals Trust, 1994. *Credit*: Reproduced with permission of Oxford University Press, Cambridge University Press, WHO, and the Nuffield Trust.

the first years after the war had repercussions on family practice. Many doctors who became GPs had originally wanted to become specialists: a British survey taken in 1963 showed that half of all the GPs questioned had wanted to be specialists. As early as the 1950s, there were predictions that general practice would disappear, and in these years different patterns of practice in relation to specialism developed in the West (Fig. 4.12). Britain, Denmark, and the Netherlands retained a system in which the GP remained the patient's first port of call, the gateway to specialist treatment. In many other European countries including France, Germany, Belgium, and Switzerland, and in the United States and Canada, patients were free to consult specialists directly. By the 1990s, most German practitioners also had a specialist training, and continued in that role in community practice. Sweden initially created an essentially specialized service based in large health centres, but reversed that policy in 1968 when responsibility for the control of health and the social services was transferred to the provincial governments, bringing a new emphasis on primary care. In Eastern Europe, the traditional polyclinic, where both generalists and specialists were available to patients, remained the dominant model of practice up to the end of the Cold War in 1990. In the decade that followed, many east European countries began to look to Western models with a view to reforming and strengthening their own primary care systems.

Anxieties over the perceived threat of specialism to family practice led to new initiatives in support of that practice in the years around 1960. In Britain and the Netherlands, Colleges of General Practitioners established in the 1950s worked to reinforce the identity of general practice. Here was a greater emphasis in medical education on the training of GPs. More broadly, the International College of General Practice held its first annual conference in 1959. In the 1950s also, a new interest in family medicine as a specialty emerged in the United States. In the early 1960s, the WHO initiated a series of conferences and expert committees with the aim of defining and developing the role of the general physician. The definitions that resulted confirmed the model of the general physician as one with whom the patient had first contact, and who retained a continuing responsibility for comprehensive, personal, and family care. These characteristics distinguished the generalist from the specialist and provided a basis for training. The professional distance between general medicine and specialism was further emphasized with the introduction of the term 'primary care' in the early 1970s. The increasing contribution of other health professionals, notably nurses, to this level of medical care, was a central component of the primary care model, and this was extended in 1978, when the WHO Alma Ata Declaration employed the term 'primary health care' to extend the scope of the model into social services, such as housing and education.

Once again, the international definitions stressed the importance of education, training, research, and specific resources, if the role of the family practitioner was to be preserved and developed. As with the nurses, the role and identity of the general physician was continually debated in this period. Developments in the organization of medical care in the later decades of the twentieth century demonstrated that the enthusiasm for primary care continued to be difficult to preserve in the face of the pressures of modern medical practice. In Britain, during the early 1990s, increasing state control and fiscal restraints, together with the imposition of targets, for example for numbers of childhood immunizations provided and of women screened for cervical cancer, dismayed many GPs. In 1987, 12 percent of British GPs had reported feeling under pressure and continually short of time; by 1993 this had risen to 43 percent. By the end of the twentieth century, numbers of British GPs were taking early retirement and the country was beginning to face a serious shortage of entrants to general practice. At the same time, government initiated a drive to extend primary care in the community on cost grounds, as a less expensive alternative to hospital care.

Part of the pressure increasingly felt by 'traditional' family doctors lay in the changing pattern of the health problems they encountered in their surgeries. With the virtual disappearance of the common infectious diseases, primary care physicians increasingly found themselves involved in the long-term management of chronic diseases, such as diabetes and asthma, in the preventive work of detecting diseases, such as cancer in the early and treatable stages, and in succouring the social and psychological problems of their patients. A new spectrum of diseases appeared in primary care surgeries: autism, obesity, anorexia and bulimia, chronic fatigue syndrome, Alzheimer's disease, Parkinsonism, and drug abuse. Many of these involved long-term monitoring and sometimes fraught relationships with patients.

The business of prescribing for patients also became more complex. Where, before 1940, doctors had depended for their medications on a range of tinctures, tonics, and expectorants, of relatively small and benign effect in practice, the therapeutic revolution brought a vast new and powerful armoury within the doctor's reach. It also necessitated a great deal of additional work. Doctors now needed a large store of information about new drugs and treatments; they needed to be aware of potential side effects, and of potential adverse reactions caused by other medication patients were taking, or by preexisting conditions, such as high blood pressure. Moreover, the new, dynamic, commercial pharmaceutical industry was demanding of its clients. It was continually developing new products, about which it kept doctors informed by post and with visits from company representatives. Doctors needed to keep their knowledge of these products, and medical experience of their use, up to date.

New drugs and new technologies also helped to change the shape of primary medical practice. The introduction of the oral contraceptive pill in the early 1960s, for example, gave primary care doctors in many countries new responsibilities in family planning. The growth of travel and 'adventure' as leisure activities, as well as the globalization of the business community, brought new demands for access to a range of preventive treatments, from malaria pills to immunizations against typhoid, rabies, and yellow fever. The development of national screening programmes, for instance for cervical cancer, added further responsibilities. By the 1990s, physicians in many countries would be delegating some of these activities to practice nurses. At the same time, some old concerns diminished in significance. Except in the

Netherlands, there was a general move to locate childbirth in the hospital, where specialist services were readily to hand in emergencies. As a result, the traditional midwifery function of the GP was significantly reduced.

Primary care became increasingly professionalized. Not only did intending primary care physicians receive special training, but once in practice, their setting became specialized. In many countries, family doctors, still predominantly male, had traditionally practised from home, where one room was set aside as a surgery, and the doctor's wife frequently acted as receptionist and secretary. By the 1960s, doctors were moving into dedicated surgeries and employing receptionists. Doctors had often practised alone, or in partnership with one other colleague. In the 1950s and 1960s, this pattern began to change in some countries. In Britain and Sweden, group practice became the normal pattern in this period. By the 1990s, the health centre, a concept first introduced in the 1920s (p. 348), had become a common feature. In France, Germany, and the Netherlands, meanwhile, most family doctors continued to practise single-handed. Even in single-handed practices, however, doctors now generally acquired 'practice nurses'. In Sweden, where there was a shortage of trained GPs, 40 percent of primary care was being provided by nurses in 1984. By 2000, in Britain, there were proposals to increase significantly the medical responsibilities of nurses in general practice.

The delegation of tasks to nurses was one of several elements that began to distance patients from their doctors, and change the image and reality of primary care practice. Home visiting had been a hallmark of ordinary medical practice in the nineteenth and early twentieth centuries, but came under increasing pressure after 1945. In America, it had all but disappeared by the 1970s. In Britain, 22 percent of consultations took place in the patient's home in 1971; by 1990, only 10 percent did so. Some national traditions proved more resistant than others, however. In Belgium more than half of all GP consultations still occurred as home visits in the 1980s. Significant national differences also existed in the amount of consultation time given to patients. In the 1990s, consultation time ranged from an average of twenty-five minutes in Sweden to fourteen to fifteen minutes in the United States and Canada, and down to 8.5 minutes in Britain.

DOCTORS AND PATIENTS

The relationship between doctors and their patients changed subtly but significantly in the last decades of the twentieth century, in ways that affected the medical profession as a whole and attitudes towards orthodox medicine.

Neither medical authority nor patients' perceptions of their own role and identity are stable historical entities (Ch. 1). For some years after World War II, medicine was on a roll, its prestige higher and public confidence in it stronger than ever before. Governments had been convinced by the experience of war that medical research was a valuable investment. The introduction of the antibiotics and steroids, the availability of new immunizations against whooping cough and poliomyelitis, new psychotropic drugs, and the introduction of pioneering surgical techniques all forged a dynamic and successful picture of medical enterprise and power. Hospital building programmes and new social welfare measures reinforced a sense of medicine's positive contribution to an improving society, with new standards of living and of health and well-being. Before the mid-1960s, few questioned the purpose and benevolence of medicine and its practitioners.

During the 1960s, things began to change. This was partly the result of social developments and partly of the developments in medicine. New generations of better educated people, who had grown up free of the fear of sudden fatal infections in the age of antibiotics and immunizations, and of improved public services, began to question the ways in which these services were delivered and used. Expectations were rising, fuelled, perhaps, by modern media reporting of new medical techniques and treatments. Specific events were also influential in reshaping attitudes towards medicine and science – the thalidomide disaster (pp. 478–9), and the publication of Rachel Carson's *Silent Spring* (1962), documenting the destructive environmental impact of modern pesticide use, were cases in point. And although the 1960s were a decade of apparent economic prosperity, the escalating costs of the new medicine did not go unnoticed. Before 1960, medical advance had been achieved through new, relatively inexpensive drugs. After 1960, medical progress increasingly involved complicated procedures and complex technologies. In July 1969, Richard Nixon (1913–94), then President of the United States, sounded the first alarm, declaring that America faced a massive crisis in the uncontrolled expansion of medical care: 'Unless action is taken . . . we will have a breakdown in our medical system.' Yet such was the pressure of popular concern, that Nixon, nonetheless, funded the American 'cancer wars'.

A new sense of personal identity and self-worth among individuals was also to prove influential. The emergence of the women's liberation movement, for example, which was especially vocal in America, generated novel critiques of established institutions as male tools for the oppression of women. Gender aspects of the doctor-patient relationship began to come

457

under scrutiny. In 1971, the Boston Women's Health Collective published *Our Bodies Ourselves: A Health Book by and for Women*, which became an international best-seller. The book popularized the idea that women had the right to know about and to make decisions about, medical procedures that affected their bodies and their lives. In 1976 the influential sociologist, Ivan Illich (1926–2003), introduced many people to the concept of iatrogenic medicine with the publication of *The Limits to Medicine* (1976). Even before the feminist critique of medical practice became popular, there were signs of growing dissatisfaction with medical treatment in America. Medical malpractice suits had been unusual events before the late 1960s, but then began to rise. By the mid-1970s, the increasing frequency and severity of such claims had destabilized the American medical insurance market. Practitioners found themselves faced with new financial pressure for insurance cover. In 1982, an American obstetrician could expect to pay $10,900 for insurance against medical negligence claims; by 1986, the sum had risen to $30,000. Medical malpractice claims also began to rise in Britain in the 1970s, although at a significantly lower level than in the United States. A voluntary organization, Action for Victims of Medical Accidents, was formed in 1982 to provide preliminary advice and refer patients to solicitors. Between 1982 and 1986, some 3,000 people contacted the group, of whom 1,200 were referred to solicitors.

From the early 1970s, patients' rights became an issue in many countries, and the concept of a 'patient's charter', delineating patient rights and often setting out formal grievance procedures, was born. Several countries, including France, the Netherlands, and Britain composed such charters, although their provisions varied. In the United States, for example, some states, like New Jersey, gave their patient bills of rights the force of law. By contrast, the British (1991) set out ten rights and codified the standards a patient could expect to find within the NHS, but did not make them enforceable in law. The Nordic countries, as might be expected, were leaders in developing the principle of patients' rights. It was they who invented the hospital ombudsman to deal with individual complaints and to negotiate improved services on behalf of the public. In the event of failure, the ombudsman might be able to take a case to court, as in Finland, or to mediation, as in France and the Netherlands. The Nordic countries were also active in passing legislation to formalize relationships between doctors and patients. Norway's act, promulgated in 1999, included the right to choose a hospital, to have access to a specialist assessment within thirty days of referral, to obtain a second opinion, give informed consent, and complain.

The new public emphasis on patients' rights, and publicity surrounding medical malpractice stories, increasingly helped to undermine confidence in the medical profession in Britain, for example, during the 1990s. The number of new medical negligence claims rose by 72 percent between 1990 and 1998. In 2000, there were 23,000 outstanding medical negligence claims, at an estimated value of £3.9 billion. A survey for *General Practitioner* magazine showed that some 90 percent of doctors in the United Kingdom thought patients better informed than ten years previously. A majority considered that the modern technology of the Internet had increased the number of patients who self-diagnosed or asked for specific treatments. Of the doctors surveyed, nearly a third had faced a medical negligence claim and three-quarters thought patients more likely to question their advice than a decade ago. More specifically perhaps, a series of revelations at the turn of the century concerning the British mass-murderer GP, Harold Shipman (1946–2004) (who was convicted of doing away with 236 mostly elderly patients over a twenty-four-year period); apparently unacceptable practices in paediatric cardiology at the Bristol Royal Infirmary; and the preservation of dead children's organs without parental consent at the Alder Hey Hospital, Liverpool, led to an increase in patient complaints against doctors to the General Medical Council, from an average of fifty-eight a week in 1999 to eighty-six a week in 2000.

Medical education

The medical demands of World War II forced changes in medical education in most belligerent countries. In the United Kingdom, access increased as some medical schools opened their doors to women for the first time, and the course was shortened to satisfy the urgent need for medical personnel. These factors, and the expectation of postwar reorganization, led to the Goodenough Committee on Medical Education, which reported in 1944, just as the Normandy invasion was getting underway. This laid down guidelines for the training of doctors for the next forty years, which were implemented together with additional NHS legislation. In 1948, teaching hospitals became state hospitals; in London the independent hospital medical schools became independent corporate bodies; and the Postgraduate Medical Federation was established at Hammersmith Hospital, London, to enhance postqualification and professional training (p. 305). Medical education continued in two distinct phases: a preclinical scientific training of up to two years followed by clinical training of three years. Many medical

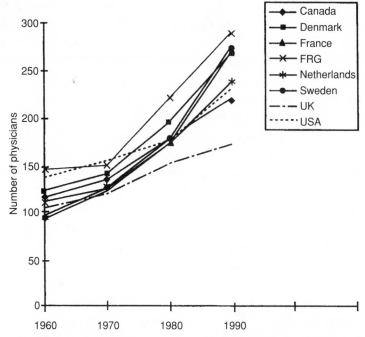

Fig. 4.13. Total number of physicians (i.e., total medically qualified personnel) per 100,000 population, various countries, 1960–90. *Source*: Fig. 11.1 in John Horder, 'Developments in other countries', in Irvine Loudon, John Horder, and Charles Webster (eds.), *General Practice under the National Health Service 1948–1997*, London, Clarendon Press, 1998, p. 262. *Original source*: Various including WHO statistics. *Credit*: Reproduced with permission of Oxford University Press and WHO.

schools also offered a one-year premedical training for students with no previous scientific background and in 1953 a preregistration year was introduced, during which the newly qualified doctor worked under supervision in approved medical and surgical posts. In most European countries, entry to medical school was at the usual university entrance age, normally the late teens, after a successful secondary education, and much basic and some postgraduate medical training was provided by the state. In North America, medicine became a graduate field of study and was privately funded (Fig. 4.13).

As in other countries, medical training in the Soviet Union had accelerated during the war, and in 1946 there were 144,000 physicians, compared with 130,000 in 1941. A major difference however, in contrast to many Western European countries, was the lengthening of the medical course, from five to six years in 1944, with the final year being devoted to the beginning of specialty training. It was not until 1955 that this was reversed, and specialization became completely postgraduate, as elsewhere. The organization of medicine was largely unchanged, with all doctors being trained and employed by the state. However, the country emerged from World War II with its medical infrastructure severely damaged. Almost 6,000 hospitals and dispensaries had been completely destroyed, and another 7,000 had been severely damaged. For medical and scientific institutes the comparable figures were 472 and 758. Physical reconstruction took the best part of the next three decades.

War and political upheaval meant that China too suffered much disruption of its medical education system. During the early decades of the twentieth century, the promotion of Western medicine was one of the planks of the modernist platform, the priority being to promote it as 'scientific' rather than 'foreign'. By 1949, there were fifty-six medical colleges and faculties in China teaching Western medicine, although practically all were operated by missionaries or foreign organizations like the Rockefeller Foundation. With the establishment of the People's Republic of China in 1949, an ambitious training programme of socialized medicine was instigated that focused on teaching doctors and other health personnel preventive medicine, and on integrating Western and traditional medical approaches. Western medical education became caught up in the Cultural Revolution from the mid-1960s to the mid-1970s: institutes were closed, academics were sent to the countryside, laboratories were converted to factories, and libraries were disbanded. It was not until 1975 that rebuilding and restructuring began, and by 1982 there were 116 medical colleges training 30,000 new students each year in Western medicine, traditional medicine, public health, and pharmacy. By then there were over half a million doctors trained in Western medicine in China (almost twice as many as traditionally trained practitioners). By the end of that decade medical education was the responsibility of a number of organizations: provincial health authorities supervised the majority, although only four of their ninety-six institutes taught Western medicine; and specific enterprises, including railways, coal mines, and the army all ran their own colleges. The Ministry of Public Health supervised thirteen 'core' institutes, eleven of which were in Western medicine. At the beginning of the 1990s there were ninety-two faculties teaching Western medicine although there were problems with large classes, out-of-date staff and resources, and passive students unused to interactive or Problem Based Learning (PBL). Major gaps were identified in molecular biology, immunology, virology, child development, and social and behavioural sciences, and with no major national resources with which to address these

461

deficiencies, staff with foreign-language skills were selected for specialist overseas training.

Expansion of higher education in the United Kingdom during the 1960s led to the founding of several new medical schools, and the rebuilding and reequipping of existing schools. By 1966 there were 2,500 places in the country (with nearly 30 percent occupied by women), which increased to around 3,800 during the early 1970s. Postgraduate education became a priority, and between 1960 and 1970, nearly 300 regional centres of post-graduate training were established in district general hospitals. Through-out this period, medical schools expanded the number of training places, which encouraged diversity in educational methods and approaches, espe-cially in newer medical schools, which were less restricted by the more conservative environments of long-established institutions.

A radical approach to medical education was taken in 1966 by McMaster University in Canada, which pioneered PBL. The McMaster model was followed and adopted by several new schools, including Southampton and Dundee (United Kingdom), Xochimilcho (Mexico), Newcastle (Australia), Maastricht (Netherlands), and Southern Illinois and New Mexico (United States). Other new medical schools were established, not only to add to the numbers of doctors, but especially to provide medical staff in remote areas, such as Tromsø in northern Norway.

Wholesale reform of medical education was proposed in the United States in 1984, with the publication of the Association of American Medical Colleges' *Physicians for the Twenty-first Century: General Professional Edu-cation of the Physician*, and in the United Kingdom (1993) in *Tomorrow's Doctors* produced by the General Medical Council. By and large, these reports advocated less didactic teaching and more emphasis on small group teaching, PBL, medical humanities, and communication skills. By the end of the period, evidence-based medicine was advocated as the new approach and students were taught to assess published accounts of the treatment of patients, trial data of therapies, and the appraisal of relevant literature. This contrasted with the academic approach taught fifty years earlier, that clinical problems could be solved by the intellectual application of basic scientific principles.

The translation of medical research into medical practice

PREVENTIVE MEDICINE

Before World War II, vaccines and antisera against some infectious diseases were in effective use, both kinds of preparations being used therapeutically and prophylactically. Wartime experiences, however, emphasized vaccines' use as preventives, and antisera were rapidly superceded as therapeutics by the arrival of the antibiotics. The rapid expansion of the pharmaceutical industry after the war encouraged considerable research and development of vaccines against the still common major infectious diseases, such as whooping cough, measles, polio, and smallpox. These advances were especially important for the prevention and treatment of viral-induced diseases because antitoxins and antibiotics were effective only against bacterial diseases. The science of virology was especially stimulated by technical advances, some begun before World War II, which came to fruition during or afterwards. Of particular note was the ultracentrifuge, which permitted minute viral particles to be separated; and the electron microscope, in which the structure of such particles could be identified and examined. Additionally, improved techniques of laboratory cultivation of viruses, which built on work during the 1930s on yellow fever virus, allowed strains to be kept and grown for laboratory experimentation, and, subsequently, for the commercial manufacture of vaccines.

Considerable progress was made during the 1950s, heralded by the award of the Nobel Prize in Physiology or Medicine (1951) to Max Theiler (1899–1972) for his work on developing a yellow fever vaccine. Particularly striking was work on poliomyelitis, as research during the decade spotlighted two competing views about vaccine development. On the one hand, Jonas Salk (1914–95) at the University of Pittsburg proposed an injectable vaccine made from inactivated 'killed' virus. On the other, Albert Sabin (1906–93) at the University of Cincinnati favoured an oral preparation of a vaccine made from live virus, artificially attenuated to make it harmless. Each technique had its advantages. Live attenuated virus had already been used to produce successful vaccines against smallpox and rabies, but took longer to produce than did a killed virus preparation. By 1955, the results of a large-scale trial of Salk vaccine in the United States declared it to be effective and it was immediately licensed for use. Several European countries, including the Netherlands and Denmark, subsequently began production in state-provided facilities. Despite this support for Salk's preparation, Sabin's vaccine continued to be tested, principally in countries outside the United States, including the Congo, Latin America, and the Soviet Union. Large-scale trials in the latter, involving more than 15 million people, confirmed the potency of the vaccine and stimulated the setting up of local production plants. By 1961, this vaccine too was licensed in the United States and the oral preparation gradually supplanted the Salk vaccine: its administration on a sugar lump was easier, cheaper, and more acceptable than Sabin's injectable preparation. It offered long-term immunity and the fact that it was a live, although attenuated, vaccine, meant that passive vaccination of the unvaccinated public by benign 'infection' was possible. In place of the sugar lump, the Chinese devised delivery by packing the vaccine in a dragee, a hollow sweet. By 1968, Salk's vaccine was no longer produced in the United States, although other countries continued to manufacture and administer it, and its low cost and long-term efficacy meant that the WHO subsidized its manufacture and distribution, especially in the developing world. Some countries, such as Denmark and Israel, continued to use both vaccines in combination, a strategy that proved particularly successful in high-risk areas, such as the Middle East.

Vaccination achieved its greatest success against smallpox. In 1958, the governing body of the WHO, the World Health Assembly, prompted by the Soviet Union, which had only just rejoined the organization, promoted a programme of global smallpox eradication. There were immediate technical difficulties, as many of the tropical countries where the disease was endemic, used a liquid vaccine that rapidly destabilized and became ineffective in hot climates. International reference centres to test and upgrade the vaccine were established, and by late 1977 the natural disease was finally eliminated from the world's human population (Figs. 4.14 and 4.15). The production of vaccines, whether by a commercial organization or government agency, raised a number of concerns by the latter part of the twentieth century. Vaccines were increasingly produced by specialized companies in dedicated factories. If such a firm ceased production for business reasons, or suffered contamination or breakdown, there was potential for a major public health disaster. Internationally, and especially in the United States, efforts were made to provide publicly owned vaccine production facilities, organizations that might use older, cheaper, production technology. These ideas did not receive widespread support and were strongly opposed by elements of the pharmaceutical industry.

DIAGNOSIS

During the final part of the twentieth century, the extensive technology that arose from biomedical research transformed the ability of the physician to diagnose the illnesses of his patients. Successful diagnosis, of course, did not guarantee effective therapy. In particular, disease processes could be examined in minute detail. These included the recognition of infectious agents,

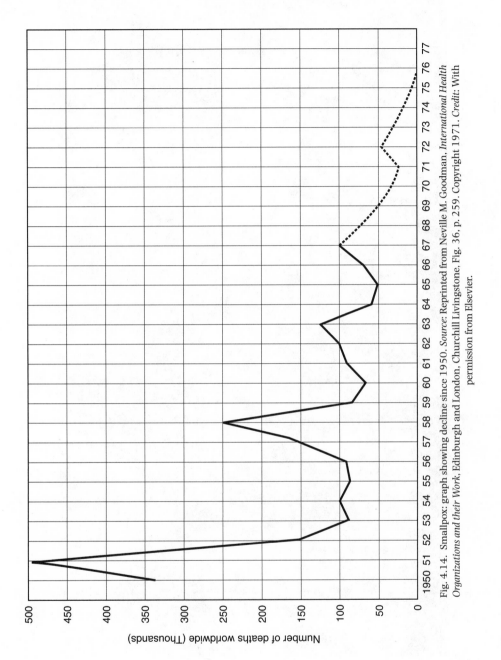

Fig. 4.14. Smallpox: graph showing decline since 1950. *Source:* Reprinted from Neville M. Goodman, *International Health Organizations and their Work*, Edinburgh and London, Churchill Livingstone, Fig. 36, p. 259. Copyright 1971. *Credit:* With permission from Elsevier.

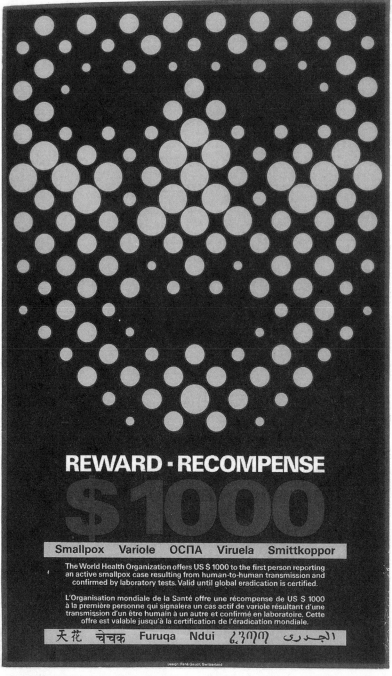

Fig. 4.15. WHO poster offering $1,000 reward to 'the first person reporting an active smallpox case resulting from human to human transmission and confirmed by laboratory tests.' The reward was valid until global eradication was confirmed in 1980. *Source*: Lithograph by René Gauch, c. 1960 for WHO. Wellcome Trust Iconographic Collection. *Credit*: Wellcome Library, London (L0023264). Reproduced with permission from the World Health Organization.

bacteria, viruses, and even smaller particles called 'prions', implicated in disease causation. Causative organisms or disturbed physiology could also be identified by traditional microscopical examination of biological materials, such as blood or stool samples. Increasingly, however, sophisticated biochemical tests became available for specific components of the infective organisms. Biochemical tests *inter alia*, for enzymes, hormones, and minerals facilitated the development of diagnostic tests to determine levels in body fluids. Radioimmunoassay, pioneered by Sol Berson (1918–72) and Rosalyn Yalow (b. 1921) (for which she shared the Nobel Prize in Physiology or Medicine in 1977) allowed very small amounts of hormones in the blood to be measured. Initially, blood and urine were the favoured fluids for examination: these enabled the definition of normal ranges of blood constituents (and concomitantly the definition of abnormal levels), either too low or too high, that might reflect a pathological condition. By the end of the century, sophisticated equipment to analyze minute traces of biological materials in faecal and breath tests (e.g., as in the 'breathalyser' that analyses alcohol levels in the breath) had become routine.

Technical and scientific advances in understanding, measuring, and manipulating biochemical reactions often depended upon improvements in equipment. In the 1960s, taking a blood sample involved the use of reusable needles and syringes, both being dipped in antiseptic and, perhaps (but more usually not), being autoclaved between uses. After a number of uses, needles would be resharpened on a grindstone apparatus, a process that could leave minute 'hooks' on the point, causing pain and tissue damage to the recipient of the needle as it was withdrawn. Advances in materials technology resulted in soft plastics that could be used for in-dwelling catheters and butterfly needles; disposable plastics for syringes; and disposable needles. These had a significant impact on diagnosis, as the regular taking of blood samples became a routine, nontraumatic part of the medical consultation; and preventive techniques and treatment became both safer, with less possibility of cross-infection, and more acceptable to both giver and receiver, as the potential for causing pain or damage was reduced. During the 1970s, the numbers of blood samples sent to clinical pathology labs in England increased from under 11 million in 1970 to over 18 million just eight years later (Fig. 4.16). In the Soviet Union, however, the supply of medical equipment suffered from the problems of production and distribution that afflicted all consumer goods. Prerevolutionary Russia relied heavily on imports, and while these decreased after the revolution, there was no build up of the relevant industries to correct the imbalance. Dedicated factories

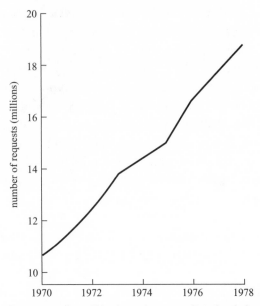

Fig. 4.16. Escalation in numbers of blood samples sent to clinical pathology laboratories in England, 1972–8. *Source*: Fig. 3 in Sir Christopher Booth, 'Technology and Medicine', *Proceedings of the Royal Society London*, B224 (1985), p. 271. Redrawn from Fig. 1 in Fleming, P. R. and Zilva, J. F. (1981) Work-loads in chemical pathology: too many tests? *Health Trends* 13 (2): 46–9. *Credit*: Reproduced with permission of The Royal Society and Sir Christopher Booth.

in Kharkov, Leningrad, and Moscow were established after World War II to supply medical equipment to much of the USSR, but quality was poor. From hypodermic needles to X-ray machines, autoclaves to knee hammers, complaints about shortages, breakages, and faults appeared in the medical press throughout the Soviet period.

As the genetic revolution got under way from the 1970s onwards, a particularly useful technique was the development of the Polymerase Chain Reaction (PCR) by Kary Mullis (b. 1944) who won the Nobel Prize in Chemistry in 1993. Basically, the technique 'amplifies' a molecule of DNA millions of times over, thus creating a measurable amount. This proved particularly successful in examining and identifying viruses: those causing Bell's palsy, Karposi's sarcoma, and human cervical cancer were all detected using this technique, as was the Coxsackie B virus implicated in causing childhood-onset diabetes. Polymerase Chain Reaction's (PCR) revolutionary use in diagnosis has been overshadowed, in the public mind at least, by its use in forensic pathology and criminal investigations, underpinning as it does the so-called 'DNA-fingerprinting' methodology.

Older technologies, such as auscultation, and stethoscopes, ophthalmo-scopes, and sphygmomanometers all continued to be used. X-rays, discovered at the end of the nineteenth century (p. 173), were used more cautiously than in earlier periods, as the dangers of excessive radiation exposure were recognized. Several refinements to the technique were made during the final decades of the twentieth century. These included the image intensifier (1955) that allowed moving X-ray pictures to be displayed and monitored using a TV camera, enabling the real-time analysis of blood vessels and the heart, which led to the subspecialty of angiography. In the 1960s, sonar techniques, developed during World War II for military purposes, especially for detecting submarines, were applied to medicine. The resultant ultrasound scanners allowed the functional examination of organs and, increasingly, after initial reluctance, the technique was also used to examine the fetus *in utero*. Medicine could now not just see within the body, but also examine the body within the body. Other advances included the invention of computerized tomography (CT, also known as CAT, computerized axial tomography) by (Sir) Godfrey Hounsfield (1919–2004, Nobel Laureate 1979), which used gamma rays and a rotary detector to produce detailed cross-sectional pictures of the body. During the same period, the knowledge that molecules resonate at different magnetic strengths and can therefore be distinguished from each other, was used to develop magnetic resonance imaging (MRI). Since the first introduction of these more sophisticated diagnostic techniques in the 1950s, numerous improvements and new applications have been made, and MRI has impacted on health systems worldwide. The initial research work done in British universities was patented through the British Technology Group, which eventually generated an income of £60 million for the United Kingdom. Much of the technical development was performed by physicists and engineers working in industrial laboratories, such as those of EMI or Thorn Electrical, although the high cost of research and development in this area forced many companies out of the field. In the 1980s, about fourteen companies manufactured scanners; by 2000 there were five. By 1996, there were over 10,000 machines in use, with Japan having eighteen scanners per million population; the United States had sixteen, Western Europe just below four, and with Britain having under three scanners per million. By the end of the period, the use of scanners had widened from their original diagnostic role, and both preventive and remedial procedures had evolved as equipment was becoming increasingly programmable to facilitate enhanced operational flexibility. The incursion of such specialized technical machinery into the clinical setting accelerated the coming to fruition of the field of medical physics that had started somewhat hesitantly with the discovery of X-rays at the end of the nineteenth century.

THERAPEUTICS

At the beginning of the twentieth century, the majority of medicines could offer little more than symptomatic relief. During the fifty years since the end of World War II, expectations of what medicinal drugs could achieve increased enormously. Knowledge of the mode of action of natural regulatory mechanisms in the body, such as neurotransmitters and hormones, facilitated the rational design of drugs modelled to enhance, decrease, or replace these endogenous mechanisms. More sophisticated drugs for the relief of pain and other symptoms were developed (e.g., analgesics, antihistamines, and antispasmodics), and were joined by drugs to cure and even prevent infectious diseases (e.g., antibiotics, vaccines, and acute medications). The long-term maintenance of degenerative disorders and complex chemotherapy regimes for cancers became possible (e.g., L-DOPA, beta-blockers, and chronic medications). By the end of the twentieth century, drugs were increasingly used illicitly or misused – for example, for pleasure (e.g., hallucinogenics) or to improve sexual or athletic performance (e.g., Viagra® or steroids). Drugs used in anaesthesia and antirejection drugs (e.g., neuromuscular blocking agents or cyclosporine) revolutionized parts of surgical practice. 'Nutraceuticals' (e.g., vitamins and minerals) were promoted to enhance health and well-being, and to rectify what were described as the rigours of modern Western lifestyles. Pills for the ill became pills for the well; and chemicals were developed to regulate reproduction (contraceptives and abortifacients on the one hand, fertility drugs on the other). *Inter alia*, new compounds against psychiatric and neurological diseases; cardiovascular and renal disorders; and digestive and muscoloskeletal complaints all appeared during the first three decades after the war. A vast industry grew to research, develop, and market these medications, and regulatory authorities instituted a variety of mechanisms to control the quality, cost, and use of medicines.

The postwar therapeutic revolution can be divided into two distinct phases. In the aftermath of the war, there was immediate optimism, fuelled not only by the publicity of the 'miracle drug', penicillin, but also in the United Kingdom and elsewhere by the extension of state-supported health services. No longer was access to medical care and products solely dependent on the family income. As more and more drugs for a widening array of complaints became available for an increasing number of patients, evidence accrued of unwanted, so-called side effects. The tragedy of thalidomide, which caused devastating malformations in fetuses of women prescribed the drug for pregnancy sickness, opened up a whole new chapter of drug regulation, both national and international. Towards the end of the twentieth century, growing awareness of environmental pollution coincided with concerns about drug safety and the dangers of indiscriminate use of powerful chemical and biological agents.

PENICILLIN AND ANTIBIOTICS

The discovery of sulphonamides in the 1930s heralded the postwar explosion of antibiotics typified by penicillin. Significantly, the first Nobel Prize for Physiology or Medicine of peacetime was awarded in 1945 to (Sir) Alexander Fleming (1881–1955), (Sir) Ernst Chain (1906–79), and (Lord) Howard Florey (1898–1968) for their work on penicillin. The story of its discovery is well known: the bacteriologist Fleming noted a bacterium-destroying mould, *Penicillium notatum*, in his London labs in 1928 and during World War II Chain and Florey, with other colleagues in Oxford, worked out techniques to extract the antibacterial agent, called penicillin, from the mould. Wartime needs for this powerful new drug to treat battlefield infections and venereal diseases (VD), most particularly syphilis, among the fighting forces, stimulated much industrial research (pp. 385–7). In the United Kingdom, six pharmaceutical companies joined the Therapeutic Research Corporation to collaborate in its production; in the United States, Merck, Squibb, and Pfizer, having received the *Penicillium* spores from England, all developed improved production techniques, and the drug was hailed almost immediately as a 'miracle drug' in British and Allied war propaganda. Before the introduction of the antibiotic, a simple accident, such as a prick from a rose thorn, could develop into a septic wound for which there was no cure. Penicillin, and its many derivatives, obtained either naturally or semisynthetically from moulds, increasingly brought about a sense of security and safety. Numerous outlets were suggested for the wonder drug – one venerealogist in the 1940s suggested that penicillin-impregnated lipstick would remove the potential danger of every kiss. As more companies became involved in its production and extraction techniques improved, the price of penicillin dropped dramatically; between 1943 and 1950 it fell by 90 percent. Similarly the price of the anti-TB drug streptomycin fell by the same percentage between 1948 and 1955.

The speed and ubiquity with which the antibiotics were incorporated into medical practice caused almost immediate problems with postwar black marketeering and adulteration, so dramatically portrayed in Graham Greene's *The Third Man* (1950). Very quickly doctors also realized that bacteria could rapidly mutate to become resistant to the drug. The widespread and indiscriminate use of antibiotics in medical and also veterinary practice (largely because they were extremely safe as well as initially highly effective drugs), rapidly stimulated the evolution and growth of resistant strains of bacteria, which in turn stimulated the drug industry to discover and manufacture new molecules to combat them. By the 1990s, a major medical concern was that organisms were increasingly resistant to most antibiotics, and one strain, a methicillin-resistant *Staphylococcus aurens* (MRSA), achieved notoriety as a 'super-bug', susceptible only to vancomycin, the antibiotic of last resort. Late in 2003, a vancomycin-resistant strain of *S. aureus* was reported.

Another approach to infectious diseases was to devise techniques to prevent transmission. An early postwar Nobel Prize for Physiology or Medicine was awarded to the Swiss Hermann Müller (1899–1965) in 1948, for his discovery of dichloro-diphenyl-trichloro-methylmethane (DDT) as an effective insecticide. During and immediately after the war, DDT had been used extensively to counter insect-borne diseases, most particularly typhus and, to a lesser extent, malaria. One estimate by the WHO is that the use of DDT in this way saved 25 million lives. Gradually, however, especially in the 1960s, the deleterious environmental effects of DDT on bird and fish reproduction, and its toxic accumulation in animal tissues, became known. Thus, at the end of the period, the perspective on DDT is completely different to that of fifty years earlier. Such environmental concerns, largely stimulated by the publication of Rachel Carson's *Silent Spring* (1962), became increasingly vociferous during the final decades of the twentieth century as the health dangers of, *inter alia*, industrial pollution, the accrual in the food chain of biologically active chemicals, such as steroids, and global warming all received widespread publicity.

DRUGS FOR MENTAL ILLNESS

The earliest astonishing breakthrough in postwar pharmaceutical development was that of drugs to treat mental illness, and modern psychopharmacology can be dated from the introduction of chlorpromazine in the early 1950s. Its unexpected success encouraged clinical, scientific, and industrial concerns to investigate further pharmacological therapies for psychiatric use, and created a lucrative medical marketplace. Chlorpromazine's psychoactive effects were noted almost by accident: the prewar discovery of histamine's role in allergy encouraged the development of antihistamine compounds, and one of these, a phenothiazine derivative called 'chlorpromazine' was seen to make patients drowsy. This 'drowsiness' was utilized therapeutically by a French surgeon Henri Laborit (1914–95) who used chlorpromazine to potentiate anaesthesia, and reported that it induced 'detachment' in his patients. This in turn attracted the attention of two Parisian psychiatrists, Jean Delay (1907–87) and Pierre Deniker (d. 1998), who used it to calm manic patients. News of their successes spread rapidly. Psychiatrists across Europe tried the new drug, and Heinz Lehmann (1911–99), a Francophone psychiatrist in Montreal, read their reports and accelerated its introduction into North America.

In the United Kingdom, chlorpromazine was introduced in 1954, and the number of in-patients in mental illness/handicap hospitals began to decline almost immediately. By 1990 there were 50 percent fewer psychiatric in-patient beds than in 1954 (Fig. 4.17). That decline was not solely due to drug therapy: the Mental Health Act of 1959 advocated the introduction of more benign social therapies such as open-door policies, although the introduction of a drug that calmed disturbed patients helped to create the climate that allowed patients to leave hospital care for local day-care centres. After chlorpromazine's introduction in the United States in 1956, the numbers of patients in psychiatric hospitals also began to drop for the first time in 175 years. The financial advantages of these policies to local health authorities and hospital boards must, however, not be overlooked.

Unlike developments in other therapeutic areas in the immediate postwar decades, those in psychopharmacology were almost entirely industry driven, as illustrated by reference to just two pharmaceutical companies: May & Baker, and Geigy. In the early 1950s, the United Kingdom firm May & Baker had a commercial relationship with Rhône-Poulenc, the French company that had developed chlorpromazine, which they marketed as Largactil. That success encouraged further company research into psychoactive drugs, and over the next few years, tranquillizers, hypnotics, and antidepressants all emerged from their laboratories. In the mid-1950s, about 1 million people in the United Kingdom were believed to be taking daily sedatives while one in seven Americans were believed to be taking barbiturates. By the late 1960s, every facet of life was becoming pharmaceuticalized, as the Rolling Stones recognized so acutely with their song 'Mother's Little Helper', which was a pill 'that gets you through your busy day'.

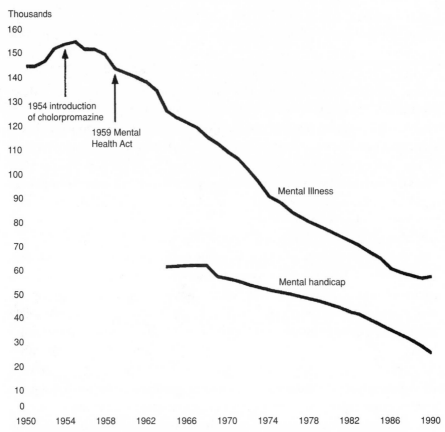

Fig. 4.17. Decline in psychiatric in-patients after the introduction of chlorpromazine (OHE): Title: Number of resident in-patients in mental illness/handicap hospitals and units, England, 1950–90. *Source:* Table 3.7, Section 3, 'Hospital Services' in Robert Chew, *Compendium of Health Statistics*, 8th edition, London, Office of Health Economics (OHE), 1992, p. 23. *Credit:* Reproduced with permission of the Office of Health Statistics.

The Swiss-based Geigy company started to investigate antihistamines in 1949. A compound with a powerful psychoactive stimulatory effect was discovered and initially tried on schizophrenic patients in the early 1950s, with disastrous results. Despite this apparent failure, the drug had demonstrated remarkable effects on mood, and the idea arose that if it caused unwanted arousal in schizophrenics, might it not produce a similar, wanted, effect in depressed patients? A trial was undertaken, with spectacularly successful results, and patients, their relatives and staff all remarked on a 'miracle cure' (Shorter, 1997, p. 261). Marketed as Tofranil, this was the first, and for many years the most frequently prescribed, tricyclic antidepressant.

474

An exception to industry-led innovation was the discovery in 1949 by the Australian psychiatrist John Cade (1912–80), that lithium had a quietening effect on manic patients. Lithium was not patentable and no drug company got involved in investigating or promoting it further. A Danish psychiatrist, Mogens Schou (b. 1918), carried out one of the first placebo-controlled, double-blind clinical trials in psychiatry, and his results emphasized the therapeutic possibilities of lithium. However, it was not until 1970 that the drug was finally approved by the Food and Drug Administration (FDA) of the United States, because there had been no powerful lobby to push for its acceptance and use, unlike other drugs that were promoted by commercial interests.

BRAIN CHEMISTRY AND TREATMENT OF OTHER DISORDERS

The accidental discovery and subsequent success of the psychoactive drugs encouraged focused research programmes into brain chemistry. Although pioneer work on the role of endogenous chemicals, such as neurotransmitters, hormones, and inflammatory mediators, had been performed before World War II, the therapeutic potential of these discoveries was reaped afterwards. A number of experimental approaches were taken: the anatomical distribution in the brain of neuroactive chemicals, such as acetylcholine and noradrenaline, was determined; experiments were performed on animals to assess the effect of applying these and related chemicals to precise sites in the nervous tissue; and examinations of the brain of animals and postmortem humans were undertaken to determine its chemical constituents in health and disease. In many ways the latter approach was the most interesting, revealing during the 1950s, two chemical substances that were to play important parts in the later development of psychoactive and neurologically important drugs. These chemicals were serotonin (also known as 5HT, 5-hydroxytryptamine) and dopamine. A considerable amount of basic neurochemical research work on these substances was undertaken in academic laboratories at the University of Bari and the Stazione Zoologica, Naples; the Cleveland Clinic, Ohio; the University of Edinburgh and the University of Lund, although their direct relevance to therapeutic strategies was not immediately recognized. Work on the chemistry and pharmacology of 5HT, in particular, was to lead to some powerful psychoactive drugs. By the late 1990s, 5HT had permeated popular culture and public awareness as 'the mood chemical' and was the major known substrate of drugs such as Prozac® (one of a class of antidepressants known as selective serotonin re-uptake inhibitors [SSRIs]), Ecstasy, and one of the mediators of the mechanisms whereby LSD induces psychedelic experiences.

Drugs that interfered with dopamine metabolism, on the other hand, were first developed in the 1950s and 1960s as antidepressants and antipsychotic agents. In the early 1960s it was discovered that a loss of over 80 percent of dopaminergic cells in part of the brain (the substantia nigra) was the primary deficit in Parkinson's disease. This led rapidly to an effective therapy (the oral administration of L-DOPA, a precursor molecule of dopamine), and in the United Kingdom the Parkinson's Disease Society was established in 1969 to campaign for the wide availability of the drug, which was not then provided by the NHS. Unfortunately, the problem of the drug's effectiveness 'wearing off' was soon discovered, and treatments for Parkinson's disease, both pharmaceutical and surgical, remain a high priority at the beginning of the twenty-first century. Surgical approaches included the transplantation of fetal brain cells into patients' brains, used sparingly and with limited success from the 1980s onwards, and stem cell implantation, first introduced experimentally at the beginning of the twenty-first century. Other degenerative diseases of old age, such as Alzheimer's disease, became important, almost urgent, targets for pharmaceutical research during the final years of the twentieth century, as life expectancy increased in most Western countries (Table 4.4).

The large-scale abuse, or unauthorized use, of medical products, became a growing problem by the final two decades of the period. Very largely it concerned psychotrophic substances, and the word 'abuse' covers a number of conditions, ranging from the use of illegal substances to overuse or dependence on prescription products. To some extent, it was a natural progression of earlier illegal drug use, but in particular it was fuelled by the ubiquitous availability of prescription and over-the-counter drugs by the 1960s. Heroin abuse surged in the United States during the 1960s, and by 1966 in the United Kingdom there were six times more heroin addicts than morphine addicts, as illicit drug use gained wider acceptance as part of the 'counterculture'. Work at the Rockefeller Hospital in New York in the late 1960s showed that an analgesic opiod drug, methadone, developed in Germany during World War II, could be used to replace heroin. It was not a cure for heroin addiction, as addicts still required a daily maintenance dose, but it permitted them to function normally. In 1971 the Drug Abuse Council was established in the United States to coordinate and direct programmes of research, treatment, and rehabilitation. Methadone, which as an oral preparation reduced the risk of contracting blood-borne viruses

Table 4.4. *Healthy Life Expectancy, The World Health Report, 2001*

Country	Total Population Life Expectancy at Birth
Australia	71.6
Belgium	69.7
Canada	69.9
China	63.2
Denmark	70.1
Finland	70.1
France	71.3
Germany	70.2
Greece	70.4
Hungary	61.8
India	51.4
Ireland	69.0
Italy	71.0
Netherlands	69.9
Norway	70.8
Portugal	66.8
Russian Federation	56.7
Spain	70.9
Sweden	71.8
Switzerland	72.8
Turkey	59.8
United Kingdom	69.6
United States	67.6

Source: WHO, *The World Health Report 2001*.

by those who shared injecting equipment, was increasingly accepted as a treatment for heroin addiction by drug treatment programmes around the world.

In other countries the problems were different. In Japan, for instance, metamphetamines became the drugs of choice in the 1970s, and remained so into the twenty-first century, although recreational solvent abuse became popular among teenagers. The almost impossibility of acquiring needles and syringes led to a high degree of sharing among intravenous drug users, although HIV infection, low throughout the country, was 0.1 percent in 1998. Hepatitis C, however, was high, often over 50 percent in clinic users tested in 1999, a figure enhanced by the raised hepatitis risk among people with tattoos.

THALIDOMIDE

Thalidomide first appeared in 1956, manufactured by Chemie Grünenthal in Germany, and licensed to and marketed by Distillers Company in the United Kingdom and the British Commonwealth. Toxicology tests showed the drug to be astonishingly 'safe', because it was impossible to find a dose high enough to kill a rat. It was promoted as the safest sedative on the market, and was particularly recommended for pregnant women suffering from nausea. Over the next few years, German obstetricians noted rare abnormalities in newborn infants, especially the condition of tetra-phocomelia, where the baby's arms and legs were so shortened that hands and feet were often attached directly to the trunk. At the same time, physicians and neurologists reported an increased incidence of peripheral neuritis in adult patients taking the sedative. The linkage between these cases and the use of thalidomide was not made.

In 1960 the Australian obstetrician William McBride (b. 1927), delivering deformed babies to mothers for whom he had prescribed thalidomide, suspected a causal link, although there were enormous difficulties replicating the teratogenic effects of the drug in laboratory animals. He published his observations in the *Lancet* in October 1961, but the pharmaceutical companies involved were intransigent and hostile to the suggestion that their product was responsible. Although the drug was rapidly withdrawn from the markets where it was then available, (e.g., the United Kingdom, Canada, Australia, and Germany), the provision of adequate compensation for the drug's victims remained an issue. Of considerable importance here were the journalists from the popular press, especially the 'Insight' team of the London *Sunday Times*, who uncovered and publicized the scandal and helped secure proper compensation for the victims, rather than the derisory sums initially offered. One estimate is that, worldwide, 40,000 people suffered from peripheral neuritis, and that between 8,000 and 12,000 damaged infants were born, 5,000 of whom lived to adulthood.

Thalidomide's story might have ended there, except for an unusual turn of events. Although the drug had been withdrawn, and had become a by-word for medical horror, a young doctor treating leprosy patients in Marseilles in 1964, desperate to lessen their anguish and pain, used some packets of thalidomide that had not yet been removed from the dispensary shelves. Not only did patients begin to feel better, but their lesions started to heal. This eventually led to new research on the discredited drug – could it be useful in other inflammatory conditions? For the first time, scientists began to investigate its mechanisms of action, and showed that thalidomide could modify some types of immune reactions, which suggested other therapeutic possibilities. Prescribed to men and to women over childbearing age, thalidomide was found to be useful for treating autoimmune conditions, such as multiple sclerosis and inflammatory bowel disease, and was also effective for patients with HIV. Examination of its action on cancer cells revealed that it could inhibit the proliferation of blood vessels (angiogenesis) associated with tumour development, thus effectively stopping or slowing down tumour growth. This finally provided the clue as to its devastating effects *in utero*, as it interfered with the blood supply to the developing limbs of the fetus. Historically, it was an important development. Reinvestigations of a drug, totally discredited in one context, revealed new therapeutic potential in completely unexpected areas.

DRUG SAFETY AND EFFICACY

A major issue of immediate concern in those countries affected by thalidomide was that of drug safety. Regulatory bodies were established, and appropriate, adequate, and effective testing procedures of new remedies were established in the laboratory and in the clinic. This was the first comprehensive drug safety legislation introduced in many Western countries. Concerns about drug safety came to the fore in the United Kingdom in the early 1960s, largely stimulated by the thalidomide tragedy. Before then, legislation had appeared in a rather piecemeal fashion. There had been revisions and updates of the Penicillin Act 1947, and the Dangerous Drugs Act 1951 and the Therapeutic Substances Act 1956 were both passed as consolidating legislation. By the time of thalidomide the United States already had a monitoring body, the FDA, although its (then) working methods and fraternization with the pharmaceutical industry made it a less effective instrument than it might have been, or was to become. In March 1961, the Richardson-Merrell pharmaceutical company of Cincinnati, Ohio, had millions of thalidomide tablets ready for the U.S. market when they confidently submitted the drug for FDA approval. A newly appointed member of staff, Dr. Frances Kelsey (b. 1914), was unhappy with the paucity of medical data and returned the application for amplification – the only delaying tactic open to her. Despite immense pressure from the drug company, its lawyers, and even some of her colleagues, to approve the application, Kelsey forced the company to resubmit half a dozen times. It was during this period that the drug was removed from the German market, and the FDA application too, was hurriedly withdrawn. The United States did not entirely escape the thalidomide tragedy, as some babies and adults were damaged during

Richardson-Merrell's testing procedures and by samples imported from Canada, but by and large, Kelsey's vigilance protected the world's largest market. It was not until the passing of the Safety of Medicines Act 1968, which established the Medicines Commission, that the United Kingdom finally acquired a unified legislative framework for medical drug control. The act regulated practically every aspect of the drugs trade, including the management of pharmacies and the labeling of drug containers, but in particular, providing regulations for mandatory clinical trials and animal testing

A number of additional problems and difficulties were increasingly recognized as many drugs, alone or in combination, were used for more patients and for long-term therapy. These included dosage levels (especially for long-term maintenance), patient compliance (as patients felt better they omitted their medication, thus falling ill again), and the placebo effect (when something apparently innocuous as a sugar pill could act as an effective medicine); and it was increasingly recognized that symptomatic improvements, however desirable, were not necessarily matched by an understanding and, perhaps, a successful treatment of the underlying disease mechanisms.

PHARMACEUTICAL INDUSTRY

World War II, and especially the need to produce penicillin in large quantities, stimulated United Kingdom companies to develop in-house research and development on a scale that only one such firm, Burroughs Wellcome & Co., had achieved in the first half of the century. In the United States, Switzerland, Germany, and France, pharmaceutical companies with a longer research tradition continued to flourish and all expanded internationally. Japan was the exception, developing its industrial base rather later, concentrating almost exclusively on the domestic market, and until the final years of the twentieth century, devoting little of its income to research, unlike companies in Europe and North America. In these countries during the 1950s, industrial research was principally directed towards finding compounds similar to those already shown to be effective, rather than towards understanding the underlying modes of action of such therapies. Most of the earlier effective drugs had been discovered by serendipity, either by empirical searches for new compounds or by testing established medicines for new effects. This latter route was more often taken by scientists working in drug companies who had access to a wide range of compounds that could be investigated for novel therapeutic effects, regardless of the mechanisms by which they caused their effects. By the 1960s, however, drugs began to be specifically 'designed', a process that relied on knowledge of the underlying pathological mechanisms and/or the molecular biology of other effective medicines and their receptor sites. Such techniques had been developed before World War II in bacteriological research, and were now applied more directly and systematically to all drug design. By and large these approaches, both empirical search and rational design, have been used in the discovery of most biologically active compounds, the latter being predominantly the prerogative of industrial concerns, especially in the final twenty to thirty years of the twentieth century.

An early example of drug development based on knowledge of endogenous cellular mechanisms, was work by (Sir) William Paton (1917–93) on a series of chemical compounds that blocked the effects of the natural mediator, acetylcholine. Although undertaken in an academic, not an industrial laboratory, his work led to the production of two life-saving drugs. One of these, decamethonium, the first of the neuromuscular blocking drugs, made a major impact in surgery as a muscle relaxant and in intensive care to permit artificial ventilation. The second, hexamethonium, was the first drug that specifically and safely lowered blood pressure. Working on similar principles during the late 1950s in the laboratories of Imperial Chemical Industries, (Sir) James Black (b. 1924, Nobel Laureate in 1988) developed propranolol, the first of the beta-blocker drugs to treat hypertension. Shortly afterwards, when working for Smith, Kline and French, Black devised a drug treatment for gastric ulcers, based on the same premise of blocking naturally occurring receptor sites.

By the end of the twentieth century the pharmaceutical business was a big, multinational industry. Companies that emerged from World War II were increasingly taken over or merged to create enormous conglomerates. Thus in the United Kingdom in the 1990s, the Wellcome Foundation (the successor of Burroughs Wellcome & Co.), merged with Glaxo, (originally Nathan & Sons) to form Glaxo Wellcome, which in turn merged with Smith Kline Beecham, itself an amalgamation of Smith, Kline and French with Beecham. In the United States, Upjohn merged with Pharmacia of Sweden; in Switzerland, Sandoz and Ciba joined forces. High research costs were a feature of all these companies. In 1965, it was estimated that sales of 'ethical' drugs (i.e., advertised only to medical professionals, not to the public) amounted to $4,210 million in the United States, of which $365 million was spent on research and development. In the United Kingdom, the comparable figures were £308 million and £13 million. Similar trends are reported for other Western European countries, such as Germany, Switzerland, and France.

In the Soviet Union, however, the situation was somewhat different. Before the Russian Revolution, approximately 59 percent of the total value of drugs used in Russia had been imported. By 1941 the lack of foreign currency and the dominant ideology of self-sufficiency meant that the percentage was practically zero. At the same time, the demands of heavy industry during the 1930s had left few resources available for the construction of medical facilities or the production of pharmaceuticals and medical equipment. Distribution problems further contributed to a paucity of drugs, and those that were available were of poor quality. The further destruction of industries and transport systems during World War II compounded the problems, and in 1946 a Ministry of the Medical Industry was established to improve production. It took over every manufacturing enterprise, laboratory, and institute, but problems of supply and quality remained. In a typical phrase of the time, the Minister of Health in 1951 suggested that 'sabotage' was responsible for major failings in the quality of Soviet medicines. An eye-witness from the mid-1950s reported the complete absence of sterile cotton and bandage gauze throughout the Crimea, and noted that not one pharmacy in the region had a complete range of the (limited number) of drugs officially available; and while in one shop penicillin could not be bought without a prescription, it was freely available next door, exhibited in the full glare of the sun. By the end of the 1950s there had been little improvement, and full responsibility for the supply of medicines reverted to the health ministry, which immediately created a Pharmaceutical Administration to try to remedy deficits.

By the 1960s, the Soviet Union had instigated a charge system for prescriptions, prompted by the same influences that caused the British NHS to introduce charges: ever-increasing costs. Shortages and poor quality continued to plague the system. In this, the situation with pharmaceuticals resembled the problems of supply and distribution experienced with other commodities within the Soviet economy, whether they were toilet rolls or sausages. The introduction of charges meant that pharmacies were required to show a profit, which initially led to black-market practices, drug substitutions, and accounting irregularities that seriously damaged pharmaceutical provision. The major difference from Western countries, however, was the lack of research investment in an industry that in the United States, the United Kingdom, Germany, and Switzerland was largely driven by innovation. By and large, the USSR copied Western products, usually without licensing agreements, and, in 1968 the USSR manufactured over 64 percent of all pharmaceutical products used in Comecon countries. Throughout this period, however, continuing difficulties with the production and distribution of products handicapped Soviet physicians to a serious extent.

During the Soviet period, doctors, like all other citizens, were unfamiliar with advertising. Medical journals did not carry advertising as there was no competition between state-supported industrial concerns, and there were no sponsored journals or events. This began to change with *perestroika*; and with the disintegration of the Soviet Union in 1990 and the transition to a market economy, physicians found themselves bombarded with information that they had no experience in dealing with or assessing. As in other areas, and in common with their fellow citizens, they took advertisements, sales claims, and promotions absolutely seriously. There was no regulation of advertising, and only in 1995 was a federal law passed to regulate the claims made for medicines. However, drug advertising regulations were far less stringent than elsewhere, and multinational companies consistently ignored their own internal regulations when operating in Russia. At the same time, counterfeit drugs flooded the Russian market, nearly 80 percent thought to be produced domestically, often by 'legitimate' manufacturers making extra profit from substandard goods.

China had had a similar history, importing Western drugs during the first part of the century, although these were available only to an urban élite. By the 1950s, the new government had little hard currency to buy foreign drugs and no indigenous industry had been developed. This prompted a unique fusion of Western and traditional medicine, as physicians were encouraged to use local substitutes for Western drugs, and pharmacologists started analysing the components of traditional remedies in terms of Western knowledge. By the end of the twentieth century this approach was of considerable interest to Western pharmaceutical manufacturers, as traditional medicines attracted growing attention, and sales, in the developed world.

In the United States and Western Europe, the speed of pharmaceutical innovation began to slow by the late 1960s; one estimate of the introduction of new drugs reveals that the figure dropped from over seventy per year to less than twenty in the 1970s. Many of these were not genuinely new therapeutic entities but derivatives of earlier compounds. Increased safety regulations, in the wake of the thalidomide tragedy, caused some of the difficulties. Extensive testing procedures in animals and humans delayed

Prescriptions items (millions)

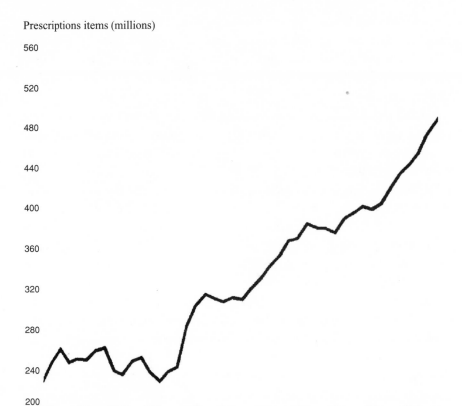

Fig. 4.18. Numbers of prescriptions dispensed in the United Kingdom since the start of the NHS (OHE): Title: NHS prescriptions dispensed by community pharmacies, United Kingdom, 1949–92 (92e is estimated). *Source:* Fig. 4.20, Section 4, 'The Pharmaceutical Services', in Robert Chew, *Compendium of Health Statistics*, 8th edition, London, Office of Health Economics, 1992, p. 61. *Credit:* Reproduced with permission of the Office of Health Statistics.

the appearance of some drugs on the market and prevented others. These increased costs reduced the numbers of compounds that might generate income. Earlier drugs, such as penicillin and chlorpromazine, had been used to treat patients within a matter of months of first manufacture. By 1978, the 'development time' of a new drug was calculated to be ten years, while research costs had increased from about £5 million per drug in the 1960s, to £25 million in the mid-1970s, and to £150 million in the mid-1990s. The increasing cost of drugs, and the demand and expectation for a prescription to be the result of a visit to the physician's surgery, led to enormously enhanced costs for the NHS in the United Kingdom (Fig. 4.18). In 1948 the annual drugs bill for the NHS was £13 million (27 p. per person) but by the year 2000 it had risen to £6,726 million (£112.81 per person)

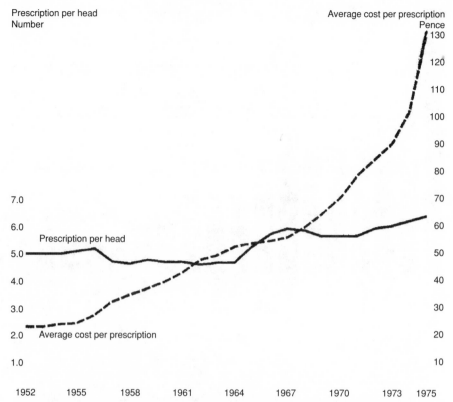

Fig. 4.19. Numbers of prescriptions per head of population per annum, and average cost per prescription, United Kingdom, 1952–75. *Source:* Table 4.7 in R. C. Chew and N. E. J. Wells, *Compendium of Health Statistics*, 2nd edition, London, Office of Health Economics, 1977, p. 23. *Credit:* Reproduced with permission of the Office of Health Statistics.

(Fig. 4.19). That scenario was, by and large, mirrored internationally (Fig. 4.20).

Many companies began to depend on just a few well-selling drugs for their pharmaceutical profits, and to diversify into other markets. In 1991, 53 percent of Glaxo's total sales were accounted for by just two drugs. Glaxo was unusual, compared with other major companies, in that pharmaceutical products comprised 100 percent of its output in 1994. Other companies relied considerably less on medicinals: Smith Kline Beecham (58 percent), Bayer (19 percent), and Ciba (33 percent).

Problems about the provision of modern pharmaceutical products for poorer nations remained unresolved by the year 2000. Although most of the world's population lived in developing countries they accounted, by the end of the period, for less than 20 percent of the pharmaceutical market.

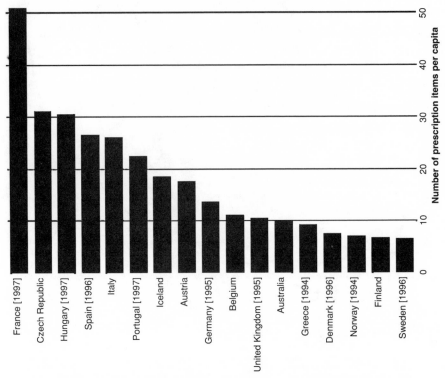

Fig. 4.20. Prescription items dispensed per capita in selected OECD (Organisation for Economic Co-operation and Development) countries, *c*. 1998. *Source:* Peter Yuen, *OHE Compendium of Health Statistics*, 13ᵗʰ edition, London, Office of Health Economics, 2001, Fig. 4.14. *Credit:* Reproduced with permission of the Office of Health Statistics.

The 1978 international conference in Primary Health Care, held at Alma Ata, recommended that essential drugs should be produced and distributed locally at the lowest feasible cost. 'Essential drugs' were deemed to include traditional remedies and cures. It was not until the final decades of the twentieth century that the pharmaceutical industry came under increasing attack because of various dubious activities in the developing world, including the sale and promotion of drugs that failed the more stringent safety regulations of the developed world; the failure to develop much-needed drugs against scourges such as malaria, which would not be major income providers given the poverty of those needing the treatment; and the aggressive marketing of expensive drugs for conditions treatable with cheaper medications. Some countries tried to circumvent the large multi-national companies by producing or importing cheaper copies of Western medicines. In South Africa, for example, a number of international pharmaceutical companies sued the government at the end of the 1990s to prevent the import of cheap drugs. Although the action was ultimately withdrawn, requests from developing nations that patents be set aside to allow them to buy or manufacture expensive Western drugs, particularly to treat AIDS, had still not been adequately addressed by the end of the twentieth century. Tellingly, the debates, campaigns, and negotiations associated with these issues were (and are) conducted within the remit, not of an international health authority but of the World Trade Organization (WTO), concerned with patents and industrial productivity.

SURGERY

Drug developments were obviously important in therapeutics, but also made a special impact in surgical practice. Anaesthetics, muscle relaxants, and immunosuppressants made possible surgery previously regarded as extremely risky and as absolutely last resort. These included safe cardiac- and neuro-surgery, and the final realization of the 'Brave New World' dream of transplant surgery. The last fifty years of the twentieth century saw the surgeon scale the heights as a popular medical hero, only to fall spectacularly from that preeminence after 1980. Like other areas of medicine, surgery underwent a transformation in the years after 1945. Before World War II, it had been assumed that surgery had reached its apogee, and that improvements in technique and operative skill were the most to be expected. The experience of the war, however, brought opportunities for surgical innovation and an enormous increase in confidence. Heart surgery, for example, had been recognized as a possibility, but had been accompanied by high death rates when attempted in the 1930s. During the war, surgeons, such as D. E. Harken (b. 1910) of the U.S. Military Hospital at Cirencester, England, successfully removed bullets and shrapnel from in and around the hearts of wounded soldiers. Returning to civilian practice, these men felt encouraged to apply their newly acquired expertise in the treatment of heart disease. Changes in the nature and scope of surgery can be illustrated by the example of cardiac surgery, which had seemed so impossible before the war. Indeed, the importance of this area of surgery increased almost exponentially as the incidence and death rates from heart disease climbed steadily in the developed world. By 1948, American surgeons had successfully operated for mitral stenosis – a common and debilitating narrowing of a heart valve. This achievement opened a key decade in the development of heart surgery in the 1950s. A critical development was of a machine to take over the function of the heart and lungs during operations, which was first introduced into routine surgery in the late 1950s, and enabled surgeons to work safely on parts of the cardiovascular system, especially the heart. In the late 1960s, a technique was developed whereby blocked coronary arteries could be replaced by lengths of peripheral vein, and twenty years later it was estimated that approximately 100,000 patients a year in the United States underwent this procedure. Implantable heart pacemakers became available after 1960, cutting death rates, and often enabling patients comfortably to live a near-normal life. During the 1960s, closed heart defibrillation and external cardiac massage were developed, again in the United States, and with these new techniques of monitoring and resuscitation, specialized coronary care units began to appear, the first being established at the Toronto General Hospital in 1963. By the twenty-first century, even developing countries were able to offer sophisticated heart surgery, if often to a limited clientele, while some 200,000 heart operations a year were being performed in the United States alone.

Another important development, with a high popular profile in the 1960s, was the emergence of transplant surgery. A successful kidney transplant had first been performed in 1953 by Joseph Murray (b. 1919, Nobel Laureate 1990) at the Peter Bent Brigham Hospital in Boston, Massachusetts between identical twins in whom there were no postoperative rejection complications because donor and recipient were genetically identical. The principal problem over the next decade or so was the immunological one of suppressing the normal immune reaction to alien tissue that led to rejection. An important contribution was made by the British zoologist (Sir) Peter Medawar (1915–87, Nobel Laureate 1960) who became interested in questions of graft rejection during World War II. The 60 percent burn injuries to a young airman whose plane crashed in a nearby garden set Medawar thinking about why skin grafts would not 'take' between genetically dissimilar individuals. Based completely in the laboratory (his first visit to a hospital ward being with Murray to see an early renal transplant patient), Medawar worked on the mechanisms and development of immunological tolerance, which influenced both Murray and two American pharmacologists, Hitchings and Elion. George Hitchings (1905–98, Nobel Laureate 1988) and Gertrude Elion (1918–99, Nobel Laureate 1988), working for Burroughs Wellcome & Co. at Tuckahoe in the United States, were looking at the effect of pyrimidine and purine molecules on cell growth. In 1951, they developed 6-mercaptopurine (6-MP) that caused remission in some leukaemias. The drug attracted the attention of a young physician, Robert Schwartz (b. 1928), working in William Dameshek's (1900–69) New England Medical Center. Wondering if this drug inhibited the immune reaction, Dameshek and Schwartz used it in transplant experiments in animals with considerable success. A British surgeon (Sir) Roy Calne (b. 1930) then in Boston, also worked with the transplant surgeons there and with the Burroughs Wellcome scientists, and subsequently showed that a 6-MP derivative, azathioprine, was particularly effective in suppressing the rejection of transplanted grafts. The drug was introduced into clinical practice and revolutionized renal transplant surgery, which became increasingly successful, and, concomitantly, increasingly routine. Hitchings and Elion shared the Nobel Prize for Physiology or Medicine (with Sir James Black) in 1988.

From the late 1970s, heart transplant surgery also became a routine therapy for heart failure patients. It depended on the successful resolution of a number of factors that came about in different times and in different places. Not only did surgical techniques in removing the donor heart and transplanting it into the recipient have to be developed, but basic immunology and intensive care nursing had to be understood and improved. Some key institutions led the way: Stanford University Medical Centre, United States; the Grote Schurr Hospital in Cape Town, South Africa; and the Papworth and National Heart Hospitals in the United Kingdom. The success of heart transplantation epitomizes the multidisciplinary approach and team work needed in the latter half of the twentieth century for the successful resolution of such problems – cardiologists, cardiac surgeons, immunologists and other basic scientists, and intensive care specialists who worked together to establish surgical routines, patient care, and long-term maintenance, moving from clinical need, into laboratory investigations, and then back to the bedside. At the beginning of the twentieth century it was estimated that one in three healthcare workers was a physician; at the end of the century the figure was one in fifteen, indicating an enormous increase in specialist technical staff employed in health care.

The first human to human heart transplant was performed by Christiaan Barnard (1922–2001) in Cape Town in December 1967. This was followed by surgery at Stanford University by Norman Shumway (b. 1923) in January 1968. After that, cardiac surgeons around the world attempted the operation and it became a symbol of national success, as country after county announced 'their' first transplant. None of these operations offered long-term success. The operation brought to the fore several other issues to be considered and overcome, including social and religious objections, and medical concerns at the operation: until that time no surgeon had faced the possibility of taking the beating heart out of a donor, even though that donor was legally dead. It was an emotional, ethical, intellectual, and technical challenge for many operating teams. The lack of success led to most surgeons abandoning the procedure.

There were enormous technical difficulties. The selection criteria for recipients had to be defined, laboratory tests had to be devised to assess rejection criteria from blood samples, and procedures had to be developed to assess rejection processes and to prevent and treat such responses. It was the underlying basic research, especially immunological work to understand and regulate rejection processes, that led to the successful development of transplantation as one of the most effective therapies for end-stage heart disease. Norman Shumway at Stanford and Richard Lower (b. 1929) at the Medical College of Virginia pioneered much of the necessary research during the 1970s. Cardiac surgeons were, however, slow to learn from the experiences of renal transplant surgery, and it was not until the late 1970s that azathioprine was introduced; and at the beginning of the next decade, an immunosupressant derived from a Norwegian fungus, cyclosporine, was successfully used for transplant patients. Cardiac transplantation was gradually reintroduced into the medical repertoire, initially at a limited number of specialized centres and without national and international attention, until it became a fairly routine procedure. By March 2000, over 55,000 heart transplants had been performed worldwide, by which time the one year survival rate was 81 percent with a patient half life (time of 50 percent survival) of 9.8 years.

Cardiac transplantation research contributed in numerous 'spinoff' ways to other projects. Mechanical support, electrical pacing techniques, mitral valve repair, coronary artery bypass grafting, cardiac patch repair, and cell transplantation all prospered because of research initiatives driven by the transplantation quest. Gradually, some of these began to emerge not only as alternatives to transplantation, but also as viable therapies for earlier stage cardiac disease. The research in basic immunology, and the development of tissue typing expertise and centres were important because they allowed clinicians to choose donors who, in theory at least, were a good match for the patient.

Transplant surgery quickly threw up new issues in medical ethics. As the procedures became routine, the numbers of patients for whom a transplant was desirable became problematic, more especially for patients with kidney problems, for whom supported life on dialysis was complex and wearying. Transplantation was costly, requiring trained staff, intensive nursing, and continued surveillance. Here, national patterns of patient

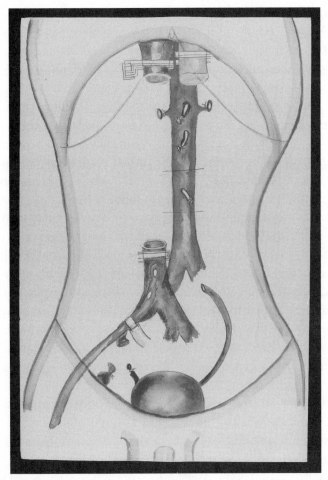

Fig. 4.21. An empty abdomen after removal of diseased viscera during a six-organ transplant, 1994. During the 1990s, procedures such as this sparked much controversy. *Source:* Watercolour drawing by Sir Roy Calne. Wellcome Library Iconographic Collection. *Credit:* Wellcome Library, London (L0024193).

care were significantly shaped by the nature of the health care system. In Britain, where transplant surgery, like all NHS care, was funded directly by the state, doctors began to ration scarce resources. Older patients had a reduced chance of being accepted for treatment because priority was given to those with longer potential life expectancy, and with greater current social responsibilities, such as the rearing of young children. In countries where health care was provided on an insurance basis, as in Germany, France, Italy, and elsewhere in Europe, such problems did not arise, as long as the supply of organs for transplant purposes held up. A more widespread

491

problem arose as a result of the development of improved systems for life support. At what point did it become permissible to remove organs for transplantation? In the early 1960s, it was agreed that once the brain stem failed, recovery becomes impossible. With this recognition, the development of specific criteria for brain death followed.

The success of organ transplants for the liver, kidney, and heart, created organ shortages for transplantation at a time when there were less than optimal prosthetic materials for the repair or replacement of diseased or destroyed human organs. Xenotransplantation, the use of animal organs and tissues, such as pig valves, was one commonly taken approach, although there was concern about infective organisms, especially pig viruses, jumping the species barrier. Worries such as these grew in the late 1990s in the light of theories, and some evidence, of such actions giving rise to serious diseases in humans, such as nv CJD and, as the twenty-first century began, SARS. However, organ shortages were acute and it was reckoned that by the end of the twentieth century about 15 percent of potential candidates awaiting transplant surgery in the United States died while on the waiting list due to the lack of suitable donors. Some techniques were devised to overcome these problems, such as transplantation from live related donors (e.g., kidney), or the splitting of donor organs, such as livers, which could be transplanted into multiple recipients. However, these efforts did not alleviate the need for transplantable organs, and considerable research ensued, especially from the 1990s, into the 'growing' of cells that could develop into the desired organ or tissue before implantation. Using cells taken from the ultimate recipient, this method overcame the problems of rejection. By the end of the twentieth century, however, only a few products had entered clinical trials, including skin and cartilage for the repair of joint defects. The promise of this technique, and the use of transplanted stem cells (with the potential to develop into any kind of tissue) to repair or replace diseased organs before a desperate need of transplantation was identified, remains to be assessed (Fig. 4.21).

Transplant surgery represented perhaps the most dramatic public face of late-twentieth-century surgery, but throughout the period surgery as an activity was characterized by multiple refinements and technological improvements. Ear, nose, and throat surgery was transformed by the introduction of the operating microscope in 1953, which made possible, for example, the correction of 'glue ear' in children, a common cause of deafness, by the insertion of grommets. Harold Hopkins' (1918–94) invention of fibre-optics after World War II rapidly improved the endoscopes, flexible tubes passed down the gastro-intestinal tract to observe the gut, initially used in diagnosis, but also stimulated the development of laparascopic surgical techniques. These allowed minimally invasive (so-called 'keyhole' surgery) to be performed for numerous conditions, notably the removal of kidney stones, the treatment of lumbar prolapse, cholecystectomies, and especially, but not exclusively, in gynaecological procedures, that just a few years earlier would have required extensive surgery and scarring, and involved increased care and hospital costs. It was in the 1970s that Patrick Steptoe (1913–88) in Oldham, England, first started using laparoscopy, an early step towards the success of the first in-vitro fertilization (IVF) programme. These procedures were significant in reducing the financial costs of surgery and hospitalization, and in establishing day surgery as a reality for many patients. By 2000, one-day stays for cataract operations and one-day hernia clinics had become commonplace. These developments also reduced the stress of surgery on patients, cutting death rates and postoperative complications.

As a result of the wartime emphasis on selected surgical specialties, such as reconstructive surgery, and the rapid postwar development in techniques and expertise, surgery as a medical discipline experienced a professional fragmentation unimagined in the prewar era of the general surgeon. Already in the 1960s, heart surgeons and brain surgeons had distinct popular identities, and by the 1990s cardiac surgery, and the medical assessment and treatment of heart conditions (cardiology), had become two separate specialties, generating new sets of subspecialties, such as interventional cardiology, pacing, cardiac imaging, and paediatric and fetal cardiology. Plastic surgery meanwhile, which had developed rapidly following innovations made during World War II, had extended its remit from the repair and reconstruction of accidental physical damage to the remodelling of physical features, such as breasts and noses, that their possessors found too large or too small, or otherwise wished to alter. With cosmetic surgery, as this became known, surgery entered the realm of consumer culture.

Engineering contributions to surgery included the development of nuclear magnetic resonance and CAT. Although devised and used principally for diagnostic use, such scanners were also used to assist surgeons to guide instruments to the operative or treatment site. They became increasingly used during the 1990s and were especially important for very delicate surgery, such as ablating minute areas of the brain without damaging adjacent tissue. Concomitant and complementary developments in robotic technology permitted surgeons to work very precisely within the body using minimally invasive techniques without the need for large incisions. In orthopaedic surgery, for example, robots could be used to shape the femur so that it fitted hip prostheses precisely; and in ophthalmology, robots began to be used to perform microsurgical operations. These procedures, at the very 'high-tech', resource-expensive end of the spectrum of Western medicine, required enormous integration between robotic engineers, information transfer technologists, and surgical specialists.

An operation that dominated much of a general surgeon's caseload for the two decades at the beginning of this period was vagotomy, the cutting of the vagus nerve to the stomach to reduce acid secretion, as a treatment for gastric ulcers. This was largely superseded by the discovery by (Sir) James Black of the H_2-receptor antagonists that effectively blocked the acid-secreting cells. Overnight, the surgical procedures became redundant and drug companies' profits soared as patients required long-term maintenance on the new drugs. In the early 1980s, an Australian physician, Barry Marshall (b. 1951, Nobel Laureate 2005), was alerted to the fact that stomach biopsies from ulcer patients routinely contained a bacillus later identified as *Helicobacter pylori*. Marshall performed a crucial self-experiment: he swallowed a culture of the bacteria, which had been taken from an ulcer patient. Developing ulcer symptoms, Marshall had the diagnosis confirmed by a colleague and then eradicated the symptoms and the ulcer with a dose of antibiotics. Although slow to gain acceptance, Marshall's work gradually influenced peptic ulcer treatment worldwide, and eradication of the causative bacteria became the treatment priority. Thus, the treatment of peptic ulcers since World War II shows a remarkable transition, from invasive surgical procedures to pharmaceutical therapies to alleviate the symptoms. Finally, at the end of the twentieth century, research using techniques familiar to scientists a hundred years earlier, found a causative organism for the disorder, which suggested yet a further therapeutic, and preventive, strategy.

BLOOD

The extraordinary development of late-twentieth-century surgery could never have occurred but for critical developments in the technology and organization of ancillary blood supply services that took place as a result of World War II. Many important modern treatments for malignant tumours, heart disease, and accidents, which involve serious blood loss for the patient, require the transfusion of whole blood into the patient to make good that loss. Although human blood transfusion had been technically possible since 1914, it was only with the enormous military and civilian challenge presented by World War II that national frameworks for blood collection, storage, and supply began to be put into place. Blood supply services developed in two directions: the banking of whole blood supplies for direct transfusion, and the plasma sector, which produced blood derivatives with therapeutic or diagnostic applications. These included clotting proteins, such as Factor VIII used in the management of haemophilia, and gamma globulins for the prevention of diseases, such as hepatitis, pertussis, and maternal/fetal rhesus incompatibility. After 1945, the demand for both whole blood and plasma escalated dramatically all over the world. In the United States, for example, the amount of whole blood collected rose from 1.2 million units in 1950 to 12 million by 1980. Additionally in that year, 5.7 million litres of source plasma were also collected.

Blood as a substance has its own mystique as the very staff of life. The universally accepted ideal is of a blood supply system that treats blood as a community responsibility. In such a system, the patient can rely on being supplied from a common stock, and donors are not paid. In practice, the systems that evolved varied from country to country. In general, blood became a community responsibility, but it also became a commodity, bought and sold in the marketplace. Most European systems were based on voluntary donation even though the donors usually received a 'payment' of some kind, from a cup of tea in Britain to a tax-free payment in Sweden. In America, however, commercial blood banks were established in the 1940s alongside the two main nonprofit blood service organizations, the American Red Cross and the American Association of Blood Banks. Paid 'volunteers' became a regular feature of the American system. Japan, which initially established a 'paid' donor system changed over to an almost entirely voluntary system in the mid-1960s.

The American commercial blood banks quickly attracted adverse publicity, being portrayed in the media as collecting among the poor and needy, drug addicts, and alcoholics, who were at high risk of transmitting hepatitis. Heightened publicity followed the publication in 1970 of *The Gift Relationship* by the English sociologist Richard Titmuss (1907–73), which was highly critical of the payment system. There was increasing concern over the potential for disease transfer. The ability of transfused blood to carry disease from donor to patient had become apparent already during the war when the rising incidence of hepatitis was linked to the increased use of blood transfusion. As contemporary observers then noted, the identification of the problem was complicated by the long incubation period of the disease. After 1945, the risks increased with the rapid growth of the industry. In 1978, the American Food and Drugs Agency required both blood banks and plasma collectors to label the source of their products as either 'paid' or 'volunteer'. As a result, 'volunteer' blood rapidly replaced 'paid' in the whole blood sector because no hospital wanted to be associated with the use of 'paid' blood from doubtful sources. Even volunteer blood was not invariably safe, however. Reliable tests for hepatitis B infection were introduced in the mid-1970s, but by the early 1980s it was apparent that another hepatitis strain, hepatitis C, existed. In 1984, some 180,000 transfused American patients were infected with hepatitis C, of whom about 1 percent died. The problem of blood-borne hepatitis was universal, but varied in significance between different countries because of the varying geographical distribution of the disease.

The vulnerability of patients dependent on blood and its products for their treatments, and the potential for blood to act as a transmitter of new or previously unidentified diseases, was driven home with the emergence of HIV/AIDS in the early 1980s. In many countries, numbers of patients transfused during surgery, and more particularly haemophiliacs dependent on Factor VIII, were infected because preventive action was not taken quickly enough after HIV had been discovered to be transmitted by blood early in 1982. In America, some 12,000 transfused patients and at least half the country's haemophiliacs – some 8,000 people – were infected.

As a result of America's worldwide dominance of the international plasma trade, further infections occurred worldwide. The American plasma derivatives industry obtained its supplies from a wide range of social settings, from colleges to prisons, the homosexual community being an important contributor. American blood supplies were, therefore, at high risk of other blood-transmissible diseases circulating in these communities. Whole blood did not, in general, cross national boundaries, but blood products were a highly mobile commodity. The European countries with the highest haemophiliac HIV infection rates were those that, like Germany, relied on imported blood products. In France, national pride in the purity of their blood led to tragedy when the French medical establishment, convinced of the probity of the national blood supply, failed to take action to prevent contamination with HIV-infected blood. In 1992, four French doctors were tried and convicted of failing to protect the nation's haemophiliacs. As with the thalidomide disaster and drug regulation in the 1960s, the 1980s HIV/blood disaster brought the restructuring and stricter regulation of blood banking procedures and protocols. Inevitably, national responses varied. Japan aimed to dispense with all imported blood products; France, Britain, and the United States established central coordinating bodies to supervise national practices.

Except in the world's poorest countries, national and international blood supplies became much safer as a result of the HIV/AIDS crisis. It was now widely recognized that blood is a dangerous commodity. A new test for hepatitis C was introduced in 1990. In the 1990s, however, other potential blood-borne threats emerged, or were perceived to emerge. In the United States, travel in and immigration from South America led to the importation of Chagas Disease, with the result that some blood centres began to reject donors who had travelled in Latin America. Similarly, the emergence of BSE in Britain, and its apparent association with CJD (Ch. 4), led to the rejection in both America and Australia of blood donors who had travelled in Britain.

WELFARE

A renewed impetus toward the implementation and extension of welfare provision was characteristic of the immediate postwar years in Europe. In Britain, and in German-occupied states such as Belgium and the Netherlands, the consolidation of medical services had begun in the early 1940s to meet the needs of war. As the war progressed, many governments committed themselves to far-reaching schemes for postwar reconstruction in the effort to maintain civilian morale. With the return of peace, these schemes were put into effect with greater or less immediacy. In Britain, the NHS became effective in 1948; in Sweden, the Sickness Insurance Act 1947 did not come into effect until January 1955. France did not fulfil even its basic wartime objectives before 1970. On the other side of the Atlantic, Canada's universal and comprehensive health insurance scheme was implemented in the mid-1960s.

A critical influence on many of these postwar developments was the report on Social Insurance and Allied Services produced for the British government in 1942 by the civil servant William Beveridge (1879–1963), which is commonly known as the Beveridge Report. As wartime discussions on the nature of postwar reconstruction developed in the context of peace, the Beveridge report offered guidelines if not a blue print for new forms of social provision and government responsibility. The report was essentially an attack on poverty, but Beveridge named 'five giants on the road to reconstruction': want, disease, ignorance, squalor, and idleness. Working on the basis that the state should provide security in return for service and financial contributions, Beveridge listed three factors essential to this

497

working contract: family allowances, a national health service, and high employment levels. In Britain, the Beveridge Report initiated the five programmes that lay at the heart of the postwar welfare state: social security, health, education, housing, and a policy of full employment.

The provision of health services proved, however, the most contentious part of Beveridge's vision of the welfare state empire. It was contentious because it threatened to impose state control over traditionally independent professions such as doctors, dentists, and nurses. These professions were used to self-regulation and professional autonomy. As Charles Webster has noted, doctors as a professional lobby opposed virtually every specific health care reform required to achieve a reasonably efficient and egalitarian application of medical advances. This was true in Britain and in many other states. In Britain, Anuerin Bevan (1879–1960), then Minister of Health, was locked in negotiation with the doctors' representatives right up to the Appointed Day, July 5, 1948, when the National Health Service Act was to come into force. In France, health legislation was only enacted after the country's constitution had been changed to prevent the political machinations of medical interest groups. Nor were medical lobbyists alone in attempting to influence national policies on health provision: trade unions, alternative practitioners, health service employees, insurance companies, pharmaceutical companies, and various businesses all had interests to safeguard or promote.

Partly as a result of the multiple negotiations that health service legislation provoked, the nature and pattern of state health care provision varies considerably among different countries. Influential also were differing national styles of social welfare, as had already been apparent in the interwar period, in the varying degree of voluntary and state involvement in welfare provision between different countries (pp. 323–7). Three basic models evolved. One was essentially a private health insurance system. This is the type that exists in the United States, which provides publicly funded health insurance only for special social groups, such as the elderly and the poor, and in Switzerland, where the state subsidizes private health insurance. A second model mixes public and private provision: this system prevails in most of Europe, in Belgium, France, Germany, and the Netherlands, for example. The third system is completely public, as in Britain, Canada, Sweden, Italy, and Spain. This guarantees medical care for all citizens through nationalized hospitals and publicly funded doctors.

These systems were put into place in the generally prosperous and optimistic years before 1970, and marked the culmination of the long-term

Table 4.5. *Private Health Expenditure per Capita (£ cash), 1960–97*

Country	1960	1970	1980	1990	1997
United States	40	92	268	932	1,333
Switzerland	7	26	161	502	606
Netherlands	9	10	126	293	387
Germany	8	22	106	277	381
Austria	4	16	107	221	373
Australia	15	24	126	261	365
Canada	25	35	82	269	352
France	9	17	85	243	333
Italy	2	6	47	192	331
Norway	3	5	69	199	299
Denmark	2	11	64	214	283
Finland	7	15	63	230	254
Greece	3	19	64	131	254
Ireland	2	6	41	145	225
Sweden	9	17	45	134	211
Portugal	–	4	26	87	161
Spain	1	6	28	104	144
United Kingdom	3	5	11	68	142
Turkey	–	3	16	21	20

Source: Peter Yuen, *OHE Compendium of Health Statistics*, 13 edition (London: Office of Health Economics, 2001), Table 2.24. Reproduced with permission of the Office of Health Statistics. *Original source:* OECD Health database

trend to provide welfare services for the whole national population. Even so, it quickly became apparent that, however constituted, such comprehensive services were neither cheap to run nor easily managed (Table 4.5). Nonetheless, public systems came under greater pressure. Expenditure on health as a percentage of Gross National Product (GNP) rose steadily in all countries (Fig. 4.22). In 1960, the largest spender, the United States, spent 5.3 percent of GNP on health. This had risen to 7.4 percent by 1971. The least expensive systems were run by Britain and Japan, costing 3.9 and 3 percent respectively in 1960. By 1971, both had risen to 5.2 percent. Several factors contributed to relentlessly rising costs. First, the proliferation of new medical specialities generated rising expenditures in equipment and personnel and a demand for adequate provision of space. New medical technologies were constantly being developed and applied in practice. Diagnostic technologies were a case in point, becoming increasingly sophisticated and expensive. Where X-rays, for example, had been the only

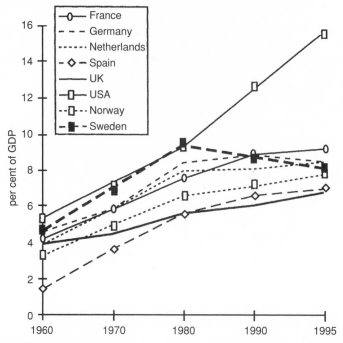

Fig. 4.22. Total health expenditure as a percentage of GDP, various countries, 1960–95. *Source:* Fig. C2 in Irvine Loudon, John Horder, and Charles Webster (eds.), *General Practice under the National Health Service 1948–1997*, London, Clarendon Press, 1998, p. 303. Original source: OHE, *Compendium of Health Statistics*, 9th edition, 1995, Table 2.3. *Credit:* Reproduced with permission of Oxford University Press and the Office of Health Statistics.

available diagnostic imaging technology in 1960, diagnostic ultrasound devices were becoming viable a few years later. In the year 2000 the MRI scanners installed worldwide were worth a total of more than £1.2 billion (p. 469). The number of drug treatments effective in treating a whole range of conditions spiralled. New surgical techniques added to the number of patients undergoing operations, in addition to adding to the cost of those operations. Second, patients were becoming more conscious of their own conditions and alert to the potential benefits of new medical treatments. Patient demand emerged for the first time as a serious influence on medical expenditures in the 1960s. Doctor demand, meanwhile, also rose as practitioners became familiar with new techniques. In Britain, for example, the number of GP requests for pathology tripled, and those for X-rays doubled between 1951 and 1968. A third, increasingly significant, factor driving up health expenditures was the changing age structure of Western populations. As death rates fell and life expectancies increased, the numbers of

Table 4.6. *Percentage of Population Age Sixty-Five and over in Selected Countries, 1890–1970*

Year	United States	Great Britain	France	Sweden
1890	3.9	4.5	8.3	7.7
1900	4.1	4.7	8.4	8.4
1910	4.3	5.2	8.6	8.4
1920	4.6	6.0	9.2	8.7
1930	5.4	7.4	9.6	9.2
1940	6.8	9.2	10.0	10.3
1950	8.1	10.9	10.3	10.3
1960	9.2	11.8	11.6	11.7
1970	9.9	12.5	12.1	13.8

Source: J. Rogers Hollingsworth, Jerald Hage, Robert A. Hanneman, *State Intervention in Medical Care. Consequences for Britain, France, Sweden, and the United States, 1890–1970*, (Ithaca & London: Cornell University Press, 1990, p. 47).

people over 65 rose steadily. In the United States, the elderly constituted 8.1 percent of the population in 1950, but 9.9 percent in 1970. In Britain, the figures were 10.9 and 12.5 percent respectively; in Sweden, 10.3 and 13.8 percent (Table 4.6).

Although these factors remained a constant pressure in driving medical costs upwards throughout this period, most states also experienced repeated short term 'crises' in welfare funding. These were invariably centred on the rapidly rising costs of medical services. Concerns over medical service expenditure were already growing in 1970, when the first oil price shock in 1973 precipitated one such crisis. At every point in the system, from the heating of hospitals and the feeding of hospital patients to the running of the doctor's car and the cost of drugs and implements, the costs of medical services escalated. From the mid-1970s, all countries began serious efforts of cost-containment in welfare provision, especially in respect of medical services. States everywhere began to extend their control over traditionally autonomous providers of medical care. Between 1976 and 1985, West Germany introduced patient cost-sharing schemes for such essentials as dentistry, prescription drugs, and hospital care. Hospital stays were limited for many illnesses, the number of prescription drugs available was reduced, and increases in medical salaries restricted. In Britain, government restructured the NHS administration with a view to greater efficiency in 1974 and again in 1982. In America, meanwhile, an ethos of free-market competition had already emerged, and had begun to replace government provision as the desirable model in reorganizing the health care system. This changing ethos was invigorated by the oil crisis and by 1980, American and Canadian hospitals, for example, had become obsessively concerned with management. Governments throughout the developed world were looking to cut health care costs by the 1980s. The last two decades of the twentieth century saw repeated efforts to maximise efficiency and so reduce the costs of health care. In most Western health care systems, the average length of a hospital stay fell dramatically, yet the number of patients coming into hospital rose markedly. Pharmaceutical costs were an obvious target area, and attempts were made to transfer drug costs to the consumer. Germany introduced the explicit rationing of pharmaceuticals, while Britain restricted the number of drugs that could be prescribed within the NHS. A restricted list of 600 drugs was issued in 1985 and this was extended in 1993. Budgets for specific sectors or providers also proved popular, and were perhaps one of the more effective cost-containment measures. These were introduced by Germany and Sweden during the 1980s and by Britain in the 1990s. Inevitably, some countries were more successful in the pursuit of cost containment than others. In Germany and Sweden, health care costs remained generally stable as a percentage of GNP, but they were among the very few nations who managed to reduce spending in real terms up to the mid-1990s. In the United States, by contrast, health expenditure had risen to 14.1 percent of GNP by 1991.

Inequalities in access to health care remained an issue for many countries notwithstanding the objective of comprehensive services. This situation partly reflected past patterns of national wealth distribution, as well as the personal preferences of medical professionals. Doctors everywhere preferred to practise in urban areas where there were more potential patients and access to them was easier. In France, in the 1970s there were more doctors in the north of the country than in the south, as well as more in towns. Some areas of the country, such as Brittany, had no physicians at all. Sweden, a highly urbanized country, had severe problems of health care delivery in the rural areas well into the 1980s. In England, where doctors had long favoured the south of the country over the north, a General Practitioner Committee was established under the NHS to regulate the geographical distribution of practices, and the 1960s saw an ambitious hospital building programme that sought to redress regional imbalances in hospital provision across the country. In America, the postwar hospital expansion programme favoured the politically important southern states, which were also relatively poor and underdeveloped. In the 1990s, however, 38 million citizens remained without health care cover in the United States.

As the reality of continuous financial crisis in the health services entered the political consciousness of both governments and their peoples from the 1980s, fresh tensions arose over the nature of health spending and the allocation of health benefits. The last decades of the century also saw increasing immigration of peoples from underdeveloped countries into the developed world, and added to the pressures on the welfare states. The dissolution of communist regimes across Europe after 1990 opened previously sealed borders and encouraged the movement of East European peoples out of economically deprived areas and into the wealthier countries, perceived as lands of economic opportunity. Issues of race were straining traditional ideas about welfare entitlement in Germany, France, the United Kingdom, and Scandinavia by 2000.

POPULATION AND FERTILITY

The years following World War II saw a marked shift in concerns over population and fertility from those prevailing before the war. Eugenics and falling birth rates (Table 4.7) were displaced by worries about global population increase, the threat of communism, and disparities in standards of living between different social classes. Between 1900 and 1950, the total world population increased from some 2,500 million to around 5,900 million. Africa, Asia, and Latin America contributed significantly to this increase, and the adverse effects of population pressure on the social and economic resources of these generally poor and underdeveloped areas was becoming apparent by 1950. At a time when the systems of colonial government, which maintained political control for over a century, were breaking down, the former colonial powers became anxious about the potential for political backlash as a result of imbalances between population and resources. The abrupt reversal of Soviet policy towards the West, and the inauguration of the Cold War in the 1940s, fuelled fears that deprived and discontented developing countries might turn to communism. Meanwhile, the postwar baby boom in the developed world brought fears for continued economic progress, and the standards of living of the comfortable classes.

Against this background, population control came to be seen as a prerequisite for solving the economic problems of the developing world and a justification for studying methods of birth control. For some, such as the American reformer Margaret Sanger (1879–1966), contraception

503

Table 4.7. Birth Rate per 1,000 Population, 1800–2000

Country	1800	1820	1840	1860	1880	1900	1920	1940	1960	1980	2000
Australia	–	–		42.6	35.2	26.7	25.5	17.9	22.4	15.3	13.01
England and Wales		–	32	34.3	34.2	28.7	25.5	14.1	17.1	13.2	United Kingdom 11.41
France	32.9 (1801)	31.7	27.9	26.2	24.6	21.3	21.4	13.6	17.9	14.9	13.12
Germany	–	39.9	36.4	36.4	37.6	35.6	25.9	20.1	17.4 / 17.0[a]	10.1 / 14.6[a]	9.18
Italy	–	–	–	38.0 (1862)	33.9	33.0	32.2	23.5	18.1	11.3	9.41
Netherlands	–	–	35.0	31.6	35.6	31.6	28.6	20.8	20.8	12.8	12.47
Sweden	28.7	33	31.4	34.8	29.4	27.0	23.6	15.1	13.7	11.7	10.14
United States	–	55.2	51.8	44.3	39.8	32.3	27.7	19.4	23.7	16.0	14.39

[a] West Germany / East Germany.

Sources: Europe: B R Mitchell, *International Historical Statistics, Europe 1750–1993* (London: Macmillan Reference Ltd. 1998).

Australia: B R Mitchell, *International Historical Statistics, Africa, Asia & Oceania 1750–1988* (New York: Stockton Press, 1995).

United States: 1920–1960 – *Historical Statistics of the United States, Colonial Times to 1970, Bicentennial Edition, Part 1, U.S Bureau of the Census,* (Washington, DC. 1975).

1980 – U.S. Bureau of the Census, International Data Base (IDB).

All 2000 figures: U.S. Bureau of the Census, International Data Base (IDB).

represented a means of easing the problems of poor Western families. Sanger's alliance with the wealthy women's rights reformer Kathleen McCormick (1875–1967) led directly, through the funding of crucial research, to the development of the oral contraceptive pill. In May 1960, the American Food and Drugs Agency approved the marketing of Enovid, the first of these pills. Within five years, the pill was the most popular form of birth control in the United States. In the decades that followed, the pill became a multimillion dollar business and was used by millions of women across the world. Nonetheless, it was by no means universally accepted as a contraceptive miracle. It proved most popular in Australia and New Zealand, and northern and Western Europe. In Japan, and in tropical Africa, India, and China, uptake of the pill among women of reproductive age was 5 percent or less in the 1980s. Indeed, in India and China, where governments were very actively involved in promoting family planning programmes, sterilization and intrauterine devices had become the dominant forms of contraception by the 1990s. In Russia, meanwhile, supply difficulties also prevented any significant take-up of the pill: abortion remained the principal method of fertility control into the twenty-first century.

Often credited with having triggered the revolution in sexual habits and moral attitudes that is perceived to have begun in the 1960s, the pill was less an originator of that revolution than a facilitator. The wider social changes that provided the historical context for its introduction had been initiated in the interwar period and accelerated by World War II. Moreover, the political and educational developments of the mid-twentieth century enhanced the material consciousness of working people, and perhaps especially of women, who began to feel that they had rights to control and to enjoy their own lives and bodies.

The development of the pill was also a product of the 1950s conviction that the application of science and technology to human problems represented progress and improvement in the human condition. Reaching the American market in the year before the first rumblings of the thalidomide disaster were heard, the pill was developed under the old loosely regulated system of drug production. As a drug, the pill was a novelty in that it was taken by healthy women. This had raised concerns from the beginning, and in clinical trials users had been found to experience a number of side effects, including nausea, breakthrough bleeding, and weight gain. The first reports of deaths from thrombosis among pill users came from Britain in 1961. By 1964, there were reports of a positive association with breast cancer. These reports marked the beginning of an enduring public and medical concern over, and research into, the effects of long-term pill use, punctuated by major scares when fresh epidemiological reports appeared to reinforce the nature and extent of risks.

The medical aspects of the pill were not the only source of trouble. It was rapidly apparent that social, cultural, political, and economic contexts were crucial determinants of its acceptance. Neither as a universal panacea for population problems, nor as a liberator of individual women, did the pill fulfil the expectations of its sponsors. The repeated health scares generated by medical reports on the pill served to discourage many women from continuing with it, or from taking it up in the first place. The official disapproval of the Catholic Church created a moral dilemma for millions of women across the globe. The emergence of new critiques of modern medicine, of new interpretations of feminism, and of new human rights perspectives on medical and other issues during the 1960s gave rise to pill-antagonistic attitudes. Feminists of the 1970s, for example, came to see the pill as a technology of male medical control; black civil-rights activists questioned it as a tool of genocide; and in India it was viewed as another form of Western oppression. Some governments feared its demographic consequences: such concerns prevented the marketing of the pill in Japan until 1999. Yet, although the pill by no means cornered the global contraceptive market, and failed as a tool for world population control, it did become the occasion for many governments to begin sponsorship of contraceptive services. Whereas in the past, contraception and its provision had been regarded very much as a matter for the individual and family, governments now began to facilitate access to contraceptive services. By 1993, nearly 90 percent of national governments were supporting family planning services.

Research on hormones also revolutionized the other side of the fertility coin in these years. Fertility drugs were introduced in 1960 and quickly achieved widespread use. However, their tendency to result in multiple pregnancies soon helped to turn infertility into a major issue. The IVF of human eggs had been envisaged since the 1930s, but it was only with the development of the technique of laparoscopy (which permitted the removal of eggs from healthy ovaries) around 1967 that this became possible. Even so, there were difficulties and disappointments before the first 'test-tube baby', Louise Brown, was born in England in 1978. Robert Edwards (b. 1925) and Patrick Steptoe (1913–88), who developed the successful technique, had previously failed in some twenty attempts to achieve a full-term pregnancy using IVF techniques over the previous decade. Once established, the technique became hugely popular. Initially developed as a treatment for women with blocked Fallopian tubes, it soon became apparent that IVF could be applied to other types of infertility, including male infertility resulting from low sperm counts. Within twenty years, an estimated 100,000 women a year were carrying IVF babies in Britain alone.

It has been suggested that the contraceptive pill transformed doctor-patient relations by stimulating women to demand a particular medical treatment from their doctors. It may also have encouraged women to seek to modify other features of their biological condition besides fertility, notably the consequences of the ending of their reproductive lives. The hormone oestrogen had been used to relieve symptoms of the menopause since the 1940s (hormone replacement therapy or HRT), but its popularity as a treatment greatly increased in the later 1960s. Between 1966 and 1973, the annual number of prescriptions for oestrogen almost doubled in the United States. Once again, however, epidemiological research threw up elements of risk. In 1975, evidence was published linking oestrogen use to an increased risk of endometrial cancer. Widespread media coverage followed and in the late 1970s the prescription rate plummeted. Meanwhile, patient package inserts describing the risks and possible side effects of the drugs had been introduced for both the pill and oestrogen. While helping to still criticism of the pharmaceutical companies, this development added a further layer of complication to the doctor-patient relationship. Women now began to question their doctor's judgment in suggesting that they accept the risks associated with taking these drugs.

CHILDREN

Political and medical anxieties about the health and fitness of babies and young children faded notably in the West after 1945 by comparison with the interwar period (Fig. 4.23). The pronatalist and eugenic concerns that had been so marked a feature of the interwar period (pp. 327–31) disappeared with a Western postwar baby boom. Death rates for babies and young children had been falling as part of the mortality transition since at least 1900 (earlier for young children). By 1940, infant mortality rates had generally fallen below fifty per thousand live births, and in the Netherlands and Sweden they were as low as thirty-nine per thousand (Table 4.8). By 2000, infant mortality rates averaged around six per thousand, being highest in Greece and Italy, and lowest in Sweden and Finland. These declines were achieved against a background of social change, in which young mothers increasingly assumed the care of their own infants, but decreasingly nurtured them at the breast. Before the 1960s, the decline of breast feeding

507

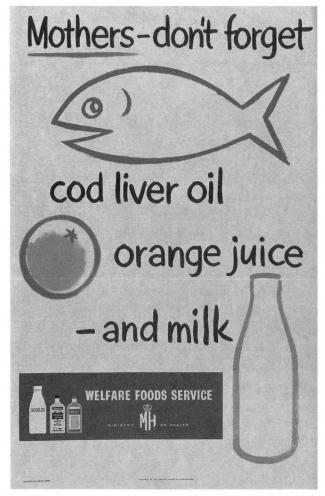

Fig. 4.23. British poster issued by the Ministry of Health reminding mothers that these vitamin-rich supplements were freely available to preschool children, 1963. *Source:* Lithograph for the Central Office of Information, HMSO, London. Wellcome Library Iconographic Collection. *Credit:* Wellcome Library, London (V0047908). Reproduced with permission of Her Majesty's Stationery Office.

was viewed as 'a fact of modern life', but as research into the relationship between the health and the feeding of infants and young children expanded, so this premise came to be questioned increasingly. The formation in the United States of La Leche International (1956), an organisation devoted to the promotion of breast feeding, heralded a wider movement that had spread to more than forty countries by the 1980s.

In the meanwhile, paediatrics, which had become well established in the interwar period as a specialty in Europe and America, though not

Table 4.8. Deaths of Infants under One Year per 1,000 Live Births, 1800–2000

Country	1800	1820	1840	1860	1880	1900	1920	1940	1960	1980	2000
Australia					117	100	69	40	20	11	5.04
England and Wales			154	148	153	154	80	57	22	12	United Kingdom 5.46
France			162	150	179	160	123	91	27	10	4.55
Germany			299	260	240	229	131	64	34 / 39[a]	13 / 12[a]	4.34
Italy					225	174	127	103	44	15	6.43
Netherlands			164	192	218	155	83	39	18	9	5.44
Sweden	240	163	146	124	121	99	63	39	17	7	2.99
United States							85.8	47	26	12.6	6.99

[a] West Germany / East Germany.

Sources: Europe: B R Mitchell, *International Historical Statistics, Europe 1750–1993* (London: Macmillan Reference Ltd. 1998).

Australia: B R Mitchell, *International Historical Statistics, Africa, Asia & Oceania 1750–1988* (New York: Stockton Press, 1995).

United States: 1920–1960 – *Historical Statistics of the United States, Colonial Times to 1970, Bicentennial Edition, Part 1*, U.S Bureau of the Census. (Washington, DC, 1975).

1980 – U.S. Bureau of the Census, International Data Base (IDB).

All 2000 figures: U.S. Bureau of the Census, International Data Base (IDB).

in Britain, expanded further. As a result of wartime evacuation and concerns over child welfare, the speciality acquired new legitimacy and political drive in Britain; and here, as elsewhere, began to develop its own subspecialties. A notable example was the emergence of neonatology, related to the dissemination of the technology of the incubator, but also to the observation that devoted nursing care greatly improved the survival chances of premature babies. Between 1960 and 1980, neonatal units became an integral feature of even the smallest general hospital. In the early years, efforts to sustain and nurture fragile babies were hampered by parental fatalism, but by the 1970s this had disappeared, to be replaced by a new popular sense of the value and human significance of even the most premature baby. Both the continuing decline in birth rates, and the reduced numbers of deaths among infants and children leading to an expectation of survival, helped to enhance the value of individual children within families.

The virtual disappearance of most of the acute infectious diseases of childhood made a significant contribution to improving general child health in this period. The promise of long-term protection against disease by immunization that had existed since the 1890s not only began to be fulfilled, but brought additional benefits. Although measles, whooping cough, and diphtheria had been declining as causes of death in the West since the nineteenth century (Figs. 4.24 and 4.25), the introduction of new immunizations, and of mass immunization campaigns, meant that the damaging sequelae, which could follow such infections, vanished as well. Indeed, the desirability of avoiding such damage to children's health was central to arguments in favour of the introduction of some of these vaccines. When the measles vaccine, for example, became available in the mid-1960s, many medical professionals resisted its general application on the grounds that measles was only a very rarely life-threatening illness. Proponents of the vaccine argued, however, that the morbidity associated with the disease was far from negligible, with severe bronchitis or pneumonia reported in thirty-eight per thousand cases; otitis media (infection in the ear drum) in twenty-five; and neurological disturbances in four. The case for the introduction of the German measles (rubella) vaccine was argued less on the risks to individual sufferers than on the danger of congenital malformations in utero, should women who had not been infected with the disease in childhood later develop it in early pregnancy.

With the great reduction in incidence and fatality of the infectious diseases of childhood, the experience of illness changed significantly for most Western children. On the one hand, most could expect to reach adulthood

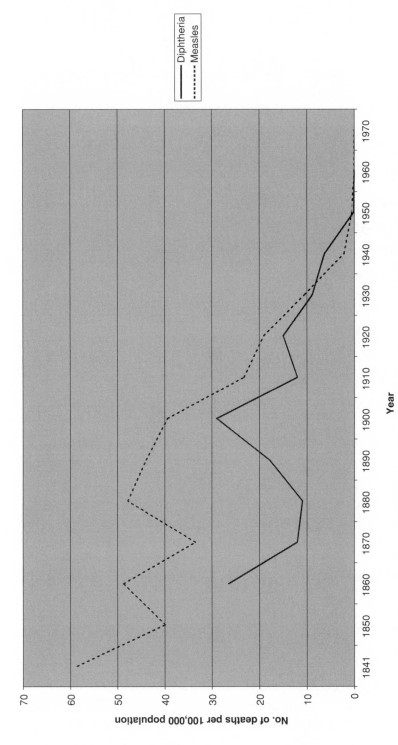

Fig. 4.24. Death rate for measles and diphtheria, England and Wales, 1841–1970. *Notes*: Diphtheria pre-1860 is classed with scarlet fever, therefore, no statistics, and from 1960 onwards is less than 0.05 per 100,000. *Source: Annual Report of the Registrar General for England and Wales (Registrar General's Statistical Review of England and Wales)*.

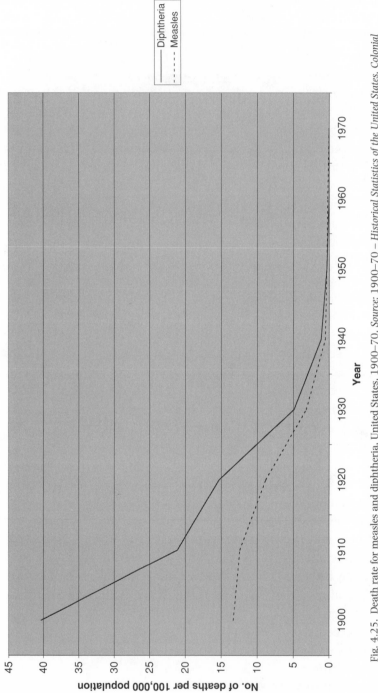

Fig. 4.25. Death rate for measles and diphtheria, United States, 1900–70. *Source*: 1900–70 – *Historical Statistics of the United States, Colonial Times to 1970, Bicentennial Edition, Part I*, U.S. Bureau of the Census (Washington, DC, 1975).

without serious illness, without significant experience of medical interventions, ill health, or hospital stay. On the other hand, for the relatively few who were unlucky enough to meet with dangerous accidents, or to develop serious illness, such as cancer, the hospital became the locus of treatment as never before. In this regard, the growing expertise and influence of the paediatricians brought a greater professional focus on the problems of sick children even as the general standards of child health improved dramatically.

As in other areas of health and medicine, however, old problems were soon replaced by new ones. Other issues emerged in child health, or assumed relatively greater significance. Although child guidance clinics had begun to appear in Britain and America before World War II, it had traditionally been customary for families to deny or conceal behavioural and psychiatric problems in young children. With the postwar extension of educational and welfare provision, and continuing reductions in family size (to the extent that populations were no longer maintaining their size in Germany and Italy by the 1980s), such problems began to concern families and social workers more acutely. Child psychiatry became a specialty in its own right, and new psychiatric and behavioural syndromes began to be identified in children. Already in the 1950s, behavioural problems and physical and mental impairments, such as cerebral palsy, were causing concern to public health officials and school authorities. Diagnosis of such problems increased in counterbalance to the reduction in physical ills. The term 'Attention deficit disorder', for example, was introduced in 1980 to describe restless and intractable childhood behaviour. By 1995, 2.5 million American children were being prescribed the drug Ritalin as a treatment for the condition, although it was still unclear that it was a real organic disorder. In 1954, Leo Kanner (1894–1981) identified autism, initially dubbed 'schizophrenia of childhood', as a distinct syndrome. By the mid-1960s, autism was attracting significant medical interest, and in the 1970s, media attention ensured its widespread publicity. Through the last decades of the twentieth century the numbers of children diagnosed as autistic mounted, although the diagnosis came to cover a much broader spectrum of behaviours than had originally been the case. Increasingly, the terminology used to describe physically and mentally dysfunctional children was modified and medicalized. The term 'spastic', for example, routinely used in the 1950s, had become unacceptable by the 1980s as affected families and support groups campaigned for the less insensitive labelling of such individuals.

In the meantime, the rise of living standards and changes in lifestyle also began to affect children's physical health. In these younger age groups too, the shifting pattern of mortality transition from infectious diseases to chronic and degenerative diseases was increasingly observed. Television, a declining emphasis on sport in education, and, by the 1970s, the widespread availability of preprepared foodstuffs with high fat content, such as burgers and pizza, all contributed to generate a new health problem. Obesity had been identified as a medical problem among adults in America and Britain after World War II, but by the 1980s had also become a common in children. Between 1980 and 2000, the number of overweight and obese American children (aged 15 and under) rose from 5 to 13 percent. By 2000, it was calculated that half of all British fifteen-year-olds were either obese (17 percent) or overweight. Type 2 diabetes, linked to obesity and generally known as 'late onset diabetes', had begun to appear in American adolescents in the 1990s; in 2003 the first British cases were diagnosed. Medical concern over childhood obesity had centred less on the child's immediate state of health than on the long-term implications for individual adult health in terms of heart disease, respiratory complications, and diabetes. It now seemed that childhood obesity intensified the risk of premature onset of chronic disease. The number of cases of Type I diabetes was also increasing as a result, it was thought, of the increased numbers of insulin-dependent diabetics surviving into adulthood and parenthood with a consequent rise in inherited susceptibility. Both medical advance and social change contributed significantly to a radical alteration in the pattern of childhood illness in the closing years of the twentieth century.

INTERNATIONAL ORGANISATIONS

The impetus to establish internationally funded organisations with the object of better world management, evident after World War I, was greatly strengthened by the experience of World War II. The interwar League of Nations was replaced by the UN. The primary purposes of the UN turned on the maintenance of international peace and security, but it also aimed to achieve international cooperation in solving economic, social, cultural, and humanitarian problems, and to encourage respect for human rights. In pursuit of these goals, a number of subsidiary organizations were set up in the 1940s and after that were to play highly influential roles in managing and responding to problems of international health. Key among these organizations were the Food and Agriculture Organization (FAO; 1945); the Children's Emergency Fund (UNICEF; later the UN Children's Fund; 1946), the World Bank (1946), and the World Health Organization (WHO; 1948). The FAO, with the goal of improving food supply and living standards across the world, and the World Bank, charged with raising the standards of living in developing countries, did not have direct responsibility for health issues but often became involved. In the global arena of international health intervention, the UN agencies rapidly outclassed existing players, such as the Rockefeller Foundation, the Red Cross, Save the Children Fund, and Oxfam.

At the heart of the increasingly complex web of health-concerned international organizations that developed after 1945, lay the WHO. The WHO's main purpose was the attainment by all peoples of the highest levels of health, and the twenty-two-point list of 'functions' laid out in its constitution gave it a wide spectrum of responsibilities. These ranged from acting as the directing and coordinating authority on international health work and assisting governments to strengthen health services, to the eradication of epidemics and other diseases, health research, and the development of informed public opinion on health among all peoples. Inevitably, some 'functions' received more attention than others, although the organization continued to develop new initiatives as fresh challenges arose.

Perhaps the most high-profile programmes run by the WHO were those focused on specific disease eradication, notably the successful smallpox eradication programme (1967–80), and the poliomyelitis eradication programme (1988). Since 1955, WHO has continually been engaged in a bitter struggle to control malaria. After significant ups and downs in this field, the organization refocused its efforts in 1998, with the new 'Roll Back Malaria' programme, designed to work towards malaria eradication through local district health systems in targeted endemic and epidemic areas.

The WHO's engagement with the major communicable diseases affecting humanity was underscored by its efforts towards controlling HIV infection, which from 1986 centred on helping the establishment of national AIDS programmes. When, for example, HIV was discovered to be spreading rapidly through India around 1990, the WHO and the World Bank jointly mustered $120 million for an aggressive education programme. As the relentless global spread of the disease became apparent through the 1990s, the UN drew together six of its aid organizations in the cosponsored Joint United Nations Programme on HIV/AIDS (UNAIDS). Within this framework WHO worked with UNICEF, the UN Development Programme (UNDP), the UN Population Fund (UNFPA), UNESCO, and the World Bank (and later the UN Drug Control Programme and the International Labour Organization [ILO]) to orchestrate and strengthen the efforts of all the different organizations involved with HIV/AIDS. Indeed, AIDS had provided the catalyst for several such organizations to expand their interest in health care work. In the 1980s, for example, some 1.5 percent of the World Bank's lending had been directed to health; by 1995, that expenditure had risen to 5.5 percent. In that year, more than 10 percent of the bank's $1.2 billion lending for health projects was devoted to AIDS prevention and treatment.

The high-profile disease eradication programmes were only one aspect of the WHO's international concerns, however. The organization's headquarters were in Geneva, but its administration was divided into six major geographical regions (Fig. 4.26). Both centre and regions engaged in a wide range of other activities and initiatives in response to both global and local concerns. These included, for example, the coordination of training standards for nurses and primary care doctors; an international network of influenza surveillance centres; research into diarrhoeal diseases, cancer, and psychiatric disorders and diagnoses; a campaign to establish an international code governing the marketing of breast-milk substitutes; the compilation of the international Codex Alimentarius, setting uniform technical standards for additives and colours for foodstuffs; and the investigation of the health consequences of the Chernobyl nuclear accident of 1986 (Ch. 4).

A notable collaborator in many of WHO's programmes was UNICEF. Initially established to help child victims of World War II, UNICEF was, from 1953, particularly concerned with the nutrition and health care of children in developing countries. Prominent among joint WHO and UNICEF programmes were those on childhood immunization. In 1978, the two organizations declared their goal of 'Health for All by the Year 2000', a major plank of which was immunization against malaria, diphtheria, whooping cough (pertussis), tetanus, poliomyelitis, and TB, all of which specially affected children under five in the developing world. The achievement of the aim proved far from easy, however. The global polio eradication campaign, for instance, was struggling badly by the intended completion date of 2000. Commitments made in 1988 to sponsor further research into the disease and its vaccines had not been honoured. By 2002, the intended completion date for polio eradication had been deferred to 2007, and powerful figures within the campaign were expressing doubts whether the goal of eradication could, in fact, ever be achieved.

Cooperation between the different international agencies did not preclude tension and rivalry both between and within them. These were apparent in, for example, the history of the Children's Vaccine Initiative, which

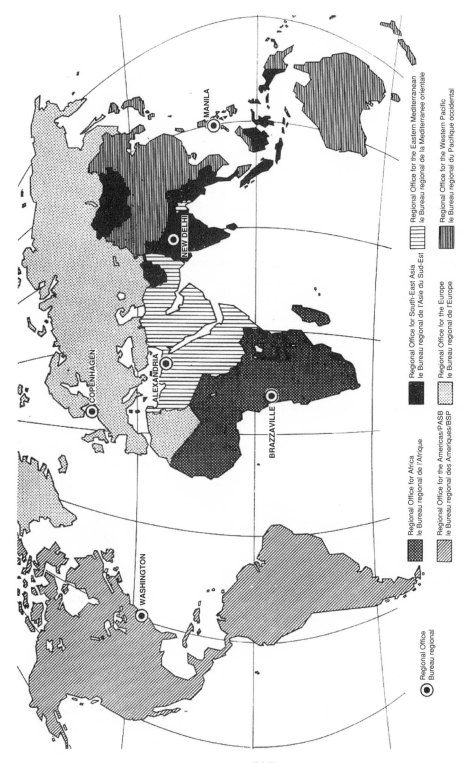

Fig. 4.26. WHO regional offices. *Source:* Reprinted from Neville Goodman. *International Health Organizations and their Work*, Edinburgh and London, Churchill Livingstone, Fig. 31, p. 215. Copyright 1971. *Credit:* With permission from Elsevier.

517

in the early 1990s aimed to develop new and improved vaccines for the developing world. The WHO, in particular, had a reputation as a highly 'turf-conscious' organization, intensely hierarchical, and set in its own cultural ethos. It was regarded as inefficient – 'a bureaucratic quagmire' – by critics, who included the World Bank, the Rockefeller Foundation, and UNDP. Another critic observed the organization's increasing politicization, noting that the appointment of staff in the six regions independently of the central office in Geneva had resulted in inferior appointments, making it 'a shadow of what it once was' (Muraskin, 1998, p. 51). It was also noted that the WHO's policy emphasis tended to follow the interests of the Director-General, leading, for example, to the neglect of TB control programmes for most of the 1980s and 1990s. Tensions also existed within the organization between 'the North' and 'the South', which differed in their assessments of the relative importance of various initiatives. Moreover, WHO member countries, represented in the World Health Assembly (the WHO's governing body), also attempted to influence and politicize policy choices and the distribution of aid. This trend may have been exacerbated by the enhanced representation of Communist bloc countries after China joined the organization in 1973.

The implementation of policy in the field was always problematic for the international organizations. Money granted for specific programmes often found its way into the pockets of local politicians, bureaucrats, and industrialists rather than funding the desired improvements. Local preferences often proved to be, for example, expensive Western-style hospitals rather than clinics offering family planning, prenatal, care and immunization programmes. Despite WHO and World Bank support for health infrastructure projects, such as local clinics and improvements in water supply and sanitation, funding continued to drain away to the hospitals. Some failures were due to a lack of understanding of local cultures and traditions: in the 1980s, the World Bank tried to establish in Bangladesh a corps of local health workers trained to give advice. As they were not provided with drugs and the means of treatment, the local population continued to seek help from the traditional healers who could and did provide remedies. Nonetheless, WHO initiatives did achieve some spectacular successes, most notably the smallpox eradication programme, which in 1977 resulted in the elimination of this exceedingly unpleasant disease. Following on from its experience with smallpox, WHO successfully deployed local community health workers in immunization and epidemic emergency duties in Southeast Asia and elsewhere.

The complexities of implementing health programmes in the field meant that WHO and UNICEF did not achieve the target of 'Health for All' by the year 2000. Significantly too, while the international organizations laboured with poverty, disease, and ill health in 'the South', 'the North' failed to heed the call, considering that it could not apply to the developed countries. As the world entered the twenty-first century, rising levels of urban poverty, homelessness, immigration, and infectious disease in the West, as well as the emergence of new communicable diseases, called into question the practice of setting such target dates.

WESTERN MEDICINE AND THE DEVELOPING WORLD

Medicine came to play a growing and increasingly complex part in the evolving relationship between the industrialized countries and the developing world. After World War II, the West's determination to establish what it perceived as a better world order was paralleled, in many post-colonial countries, by a sense that Western aid was compensation for colonial rule. The number of organizations involved in development and assistance programmes for the developing world proliferated, from the UN organizations, through individual governments, to nongovernmental organizations (NGOs). For the first two decades after the war, international effort was primarily directed towards the economic development of the world's poorer countries; health improvements, it was thought, would logically follow on improved economic performance and rising living standards. The NGOs, meanwhile, concentrated their work on emergency aid – on disaster and famine relief – while WHO similarly focused on what seemed to be the immediate crisis: the vast problems of communicable disease in the developing world. At this time, the control and eradication of specific diseases dominated WHO policy, rather than the wider problems of provision of health services and of general health and well-being.

This approach was partly the result of the recent spectacular developments in modern medicine, which encouraged both Western agencies and developing world governments to think in terms of the obvious icons of that new medicine: physicians and surgeons, hospitals, medicines and pharmaceuticals, medical technologies, and disease eradication programmes. Some developing countries sought cheaper and more flexible options: Ethiopia, for example, began training auxiliary physicians in four-year hygiene degrees, and by 1968 had staffed sixty-eight health centres providing basic health care facilities across the country. Others preferred the Western model: although some parts of India, for example, adopted a low-cost model; the country had 106 medical colleges training Western-style doctors by 1979, and, in the All India Institute of Medical Sciences, an impressive centre of sophisticated modern medical care.

Many of these initiatives resulted in the provision of modern hospitals in urban areas at the expense of lower key health services in rural ones: in Tanzania circa 1980, where 14 percent of the population lived in towns, urban hospitals accounted for 60 percent of the country's entire health budget, a figure that would have provided for fifty-three low-budget dispensaries. In Bangladesh, similarly, three-quarters of the health budget was spent on curative services, including specialized orthopaedic, cardiovascular, and eye units, in urban areas containing 8 percent of the country's population. In some cases, hospital investment proved misguided: in 1960s Somalia, both the European Economic Community (now the European Union [EU]) and the USSR built hospitals when there were no nursing staff available, and little popular support for their use. As one observer noted in 1985, thirty years after the foundation of WHO, the developing world still lacked an infrastructure that could 'put health care truly on the map' (Brockington, 1985, p. 57). This remains the case twenty years later.

The health care systems of the developing world thus remained highly diverse and, for the most part, extensively dependent on private care, self-help, and traditional healers. Local financial and political circumstances were important in determining the level and type of care provided under government initiatives, although a basic model of a publicly funded network of facilities was generally followed. Major urban hospitals, smaller district hospitals, rural health centres, and a network of local postings, often staffed by part-timers, peripatetic professionals, and ancillary workers or volunteers, described the general picture, but it was subject to great local variation. Inequalities in Western-style health care provision between urban and rural areas were often extreme, and into the 1990s traditional healers continued to provide basic health care for up to 90 percent of the rural populations of Africa and South Asia, and directly or indirectly for 80 percent of the world's population. In Malawi, in the late 1980s, for example, there were fewer than 150 qualified doctors for a population of 8 million people, but some 5,000 traditional medical practitioners.

The fragmentary nature of health infrastructures over vast tracts of the globe cannot be laid at WHO's door, partly because WHO's remit was never prescriptive: the organization fulfilled an essentially advisory and educational function, only intervening at the request of and with the consent of, national governments with all local costs and staff being provided and paid for by the government concerned. Moreover, the appeal of modern medicine was, both in the West and elsewhere, almost mythic in the 1950s and 1960s; and both governments and donors preferred 'visible' projects. It took time before it was realized that the building up of public health infrastructures, with special attention to primary health care, was essential if any long-term reduction in illness was to be achieved.

During the 1970s, there was a shift towards this perspective as the new emphasis on universal rights to health care began to emerge. In 1978, WHO and UNICEF convened an international conference on primary health care at Alma Ata, which set the ambitious target of 'Health for All by the Year 2000'. Primary health care, defined as accessible care within communities, with community participation, and at a locally affordable cost, was seen to be the crucial element in achieving this goal. Primary care did not, in fact, mean medical care, but care based on homes and families, provided according to need, culturally acceptable, and with an emphasis on health education. The involvement of the community in the planning process was thought critical. This meant a move away from the central modern hospital and physician-based medical care towards less technologically sophisticated, locally accessible facilities, usually staffed by less highly trained professionals. By 2000, however, many of the poorest countries in the world still lacked welfare systems, local difficulties of finance and trained manpower proving an effective barrier to the implementation of health care schemes. In India, for example, where primary care had been adopted as a national health policy in 1983, there was no community participation in building up services, and despite a massive expansion in primary care facilities, their effectiveness was undercut by inadequate supplies and managerial problems. In general, it remained true that the poorer the country, the lower the qualitative and quantitative standard of health care.

The influence and impact of modern Western medicine in the developing world was initially, perhaps, most obvious in the disease control and eradication programmes developed under WHO's aegis. In general, indeed, the medical history of modern developing countries cannot be written without repeated reference to the work of the WHO across a wide range of fields. Communicable diseases were, however, recognized to be a very significant source of premature death, poverty, and misery in the developing world and were from the beginning a central objective of WHO's mission. Within five years of its foundation, for example, WHO was working to control TB in twenty-eight countries, using tuberculin testing and BCG vaccination. Diethylcarbamazine was used effectively to bring filariasis under control in

South west Asia, DDT to eradicate typhus from Afghanistan, and penicillin to control yaws in Thailand. The notably successful smallpox eradication campaign, completed by 1980, was followed by childhood immunization programmes against measles, whooping cough, tetanus, and poliomyelitis, although the success of these was more variable. In India, for example, just 42 percent of children had been immunized in 2001.

It soon became clear, too, that the world's disease ecology was not static, but shifted, not only according to apparently random patterns of virulence, but also with human activity. The building of the great dam at Aswan in Egypt in the 1960s, for example, which covers an area of 5,000 kilometres, led to an upsurge in schistosomiasis infections, as intermediate host snails colonized the new water resource. Similar situations developed in Zambia, Zimbabwe, Nigeria, and Ghana. In the years after 1970, both new and old infectious diseases represented a continuing challenge to world health. The AIDS/HIV epidemic that began in the early 1980s, offered a sobering lesson in the potential impact of new infections, and on the vulnerability of the world's poorest nations. In the twenty years after 1981, more than 20 million lives were lost to AIDS, and tens of millions more people came to live with HIV; 95 percent of these cases occurred in the developing world.

HIV also offered an opportunity to other infections, and in its wake came an upsurge in the ancient scourge of TB. In 1993, WHO declared TB a global emergency, with an estimated 8 million new infections and 3 million deaths a year worldwide. The year 1995 saw the introduction of a new strategy in the fight against TB: directly observed treatment with short course (chemotherapy) (DOTS). Five key elements characterized this: government commitment to sustained TB control; sputum smear microscopy services; the supply of drugs; surveillance and monitoring systems; and the highly effective use of trained observers in the administration of treatment. In many respects, it was a successful strategy, producing cure rates of up to 95 percent in even the poorest countries. In Peru, for example, a decade of DOTS strategy led to the successful treatment of 91 percent of cases, and a fall in the incidence of new cases. Despite WHO's best efforts, however, the annual toll of new cases globally remained the same in 2003 as it had been in 1993, although recorded deaths were down to 2 million a year. At that time, the worst TB problem lay in India, where the disease presented a stiffer challenge than AIDS, with some 4.5 million active cases, 400,000 deaths and 1.8 million new infections a year. Indeed, WHO's predictions for TB were gloomy: a billion newly infected cases by 2020, of whom 70 million would die. The worst problems were in Eastern Europe, with 250,000 new cases a year, Southeast Asia (3 million) and sub-Saharan Africa (2 million). And, as in the industrializing West during the nineteenth century, the bulk of these infections were in socially and economically valuable young adults.

One of the biggest challenges over the years to WHO's mission to control disease came from malaria. In the 1950s, there were some 250 million cases of malaria every year, with 2.5 million deaths. New therapeutic drugs and the new insecticides Dieldrin and DDT were, however, a cheap and effective combination against the disease, and encouraged the hope that it might quickly be eradicated. In 1955, the World Health Assembly launched a global eradication campaign, with the aim of stopping transmission and eliminating infection within a limited period, so that when the programme ended there would be no resumption of transmission. By the mid-1960s it was evident that the campaign was in difficulties. In 1969 the World Health Assembly was obliged to acknowledge that malaria control could not be achieved in a time-limited operation: the ecological complexity surrounding the disease was too great. The resilience of both the malaria parasite and the host mosquitoes were becoming clear, the former evolving resistance to previously effective drugs, the latter to insecticides.

Although in 1970 some 40 percent of populations previously living in malaria endemic areas had been relieved of the infection, the picture began to deteriorate soon after. By the 1990s, the optimism of the 1950s was recognized as hopelessly misplaced. Malaria had moved back into many areas and some of these areas, where the relatively benign vivax form had previously prevailed, had been recolonized by the much more dangerous falciparum malaria. In many parts of Asia and sub-Saharan Africa, falciparum malaria became resistant to a significant range of drugs, and that resistance spread across the world with alarming speed. By 2000, estimates were of at least 300 million cases of acute malarial illness each year, with 1 million deaths: 71 percent of these deaths were in children aged under five and 90 percent of them occurred in Africa. It was in this context that a new and more tightly focused initiative was launched for the twenty-first century, the 1998 'Roll Back Malaria' programme. Adopting a philosophy similar to that of DOTS, this aimed to work through local health systems in specific endemic and epidemic areas.

From the 1970s, in fact, WHO was developing a more environmental awareness of the contexts and sources of human disease. Just as the primary health care initiative was directed at providing health care infrastructures in developing countries, so the designation of 1981–90 as the International

Drinking Water and Sanitation Decade reflected the awareness of the importance of sanitary infrastructures for public health. The goal of this 'decade' was to achieve adequate water and sanitation for all, in recognition of the continuing devastating toll of diarrhoeal disease on poor populations and especially on small children. That this objective was problematic was also recognized because the problem was not static: because of population growth, it was calculated that some 2 billion people would require basic facilities by 1990. In India, meanwhile, where 80 percent of the urban population had access to potable water, only 10 percent of the rural population did so. In Bangladesh, just 6 percent of households had basic sanitation facilities, and in North Yemen only 4 percent had access to clean piped water.

A feature of this campaign was that it aimed not simply to implement the filtration and chlorination plants, and flush toilets and water-carried wastes universal in the industrialized world, but to develop other methods, such as dry conservancy, which were more appropriate to local circumstances (and more affordable), and to involve the people of local communities in their organization. A number of such new methods were developed; improved water supplies were delivered to more than 800 million people, and improved sanitation to some 750 million. In this respect, the decade was one of considerable achievement. Population growth ensured, however, that the original goal remained unattained. By 1990, 1.1 billion people were without access to better water and 2.4 billion had no access to any form of sanitation. A decade later, Vision 21, the Water Supply and Sanitation Collaborative Council, was created to take the struggle forward, with the aim of achieving universal access by 2025. The scale of the problem remained daunting, however. In India, for example, only 31 percent of the rural population had access to potable water in 2003 and just 0.5 percent to basic sanitary facilities.

Clean water supplies and effective sanitation were of basic importance to human health and survival in the developing world, as they had been in the industrial cities of the West in the nineteenth century. Although life expectancies in the developing world rose from forty years in 1950 to fifty-five in the 1990s, and death rates fell in virtually all developing countries at the same time, the picture varied between countries. In 1990, for example, expectation of life at birth in Mali was forty-five years, but was seventy-six in Hong Kong. Except in the newly industrialized countries, such as Costa Rica, Jamaica, and the 'tiger economies' of Southeast Asia (Hong Kong, Singapore, South Korea, and Taiwan), few could expect to

Table 4.9. *Expectation of Life at Birth and Infant Mortality in European Union Countries, c. 1995–6*

Country	Year	Life Expectancy		Infant Mortality Rate per 1,000 Live Births
		Males	Females	
Austria	1996	74.1	80.4	5.1
Belgium	1992	73.1	79.9	8.2
Denmark	1996	73.1	78.4	5.6
Finland	1995	72.9	80.4	4.0
France	1994	74.4	82.8	5.9
Germany	1995	73.4	80.0	5.3
Greece	1996	74.9	81.2	7.3
Ireland	1993	72.6	78.2	6.1
Italy	1993	74.6	81.1	7.1
Luxembourg	1996	73.3	80.9	4.4
Netherlands	1995	74.7	80.6	5.5
Portugal	1996	71.2	78.6	6.9
Spain	1995	74.4	81.8	5.5
Sweden	1995	76.3	81.8	4.0
United Kingdom	1995	74.1	79.5	6.2
EU average	1995–96	74.1	80.7	6.0

Source: Table A.11, On the State of the Public Health. Annual Report of the Chief Medical Officer of the Department of Health for the year 1997 (HMSO, 1998, p. 280).
Crown copyright material is reproduced with the permission of the Controller of HMSO and the Queen's Printer for Scotland.

live into their sixties. Significantly, most of the world's poor countries still suffered very high levels of infant and child mortality into the 1990s. Thus in India, infant mortality rates fell from 146 per 1,000 live births in 1947 to 68 per 1,000 in 2003, compared to a European average of six in the mid-1990s (Table 4.9). A very considerable factor in this infant mortality was diarrhoeal disease, which still accounted for at least 2.2 million deaths a year worldwide in 2000.

Issues of infant mortality and child health coexisted uncomfortably with wider questions of population growth, fertility, and women's health. Political, cultural, religious, and ethical beliefs made these last questions a policy minefield for both UN agencies and NGOs. So much was already apparent before WHO began work, involvement in fertility issues having been ruled out of court by its temporary predecessor. It was agreed only that WHO might offer family planning advice to those who asked for it. Many argued that economic development would do more to ensure the means to feed the burgeoning world population than population control programmes, while the traditional societies remained opposed to the concept of family planning. In the early postwar decades, attention therefore focused on maternal and child health, with a view to helping mothers ensure the survival of their children. Repeated famines and high infant mortality as well as soaring population figures helped to keep the issue alive, however. In 1967, the UNFPA was created, with a view to easing this contentious question away from WHO and UNICEF. Financial contributions from national governments were voluntary, enabling countries opposed to family planning to refuse contributions. In 1968, however, the Teheran Conference on Human Rights adopted 'birth spacing' as such a right.

With the creation of UNFPA, the health of mothers became an increasing cause of concern. Thus, the agency began to examine the health risks associated with unwanted and unintended pregnancies, and campaigned to strengthen the social position of women through education, family planning advice, and the development of appropriate contraceptives. The importance of women's education and social status was illustrated in the Indian state of Kerala, where high literacy rates and relatively high social status among women was associated with death rates that were significantly lower than in states where women were not so privileged. By the 1990s, UNFPA's approach to the issues of women's health was increasingly radical, as in the campaign against female genital mutilation, which was estimated to affect between 85 and 114 million women. In the twenty-first century, however, the problems of women's health and welfare in the developing world remained immense. In India, only one in three women received an antenatal checkup during pregnancy, and 136,000 women died of pregnancy-related causes each year, more than anywhere else in the world. Maternal mortality rates remained highest in sub-Saharan Africa, however, at 9.2 per thousand live births, compared to 5.1 in Southeast Asia, and 0.24 in Europe. Just thirteen developing countries accounted for 70 percent of all maternal deaths. At this time it was estimated that 350 million couples worldwide were still without access to effective or affordable family planning services, and fertility rates continued to be highest in the poorest countries.

At the same time as the development community began moving to take action against the problems of infant mortality and maternal health in the 1970s, anxieties were beginning to surface over the health impact of Western lifestyles and commercial enterprise on the world's poor. An early instance of this concern centred on the marketing of commercial baby milk formula, notably by the Swiss company Nestlé. Because artificial feeding has been highly correlated with infant diarrhoea, this became a controversial issue in the 1970s, attracting activists from many Western countries and a flood of reports, films, investigations, demonstrations, boycotts, and international meetings. The outcome in 1981 was the adoption by the World Health Assembly of an unprecedented International Code of Marketing of Breast Milk Substitutes. Despite further action by Nestlé, which in 1982 funded an independent Infant Formula Audit Commission to investigate complaints raised by concerned individuals or groups relating to its marketing activities in infant feeding, the issue refused to go away. Activist groups, such as the International Baby Food Action Network, continued to monitor the marketing of infant formula products and to organize boycotts against manufacturers, including Nestlé, into the 1990s.

The baby milk campaign represented just one facet of a growing realization of the damage Western commercial interests were inflicting on health in the developing world. Once again, the emergence of specific health concerns in the West translated into related concerns for the rest of the world's population at WHO and elsewhere. Thus, as Western anti-cigarette-smoking campaigns began to gather momentum in the 1970s, tobacco manufacturers increasingly turned their attention to the marketing of their products in the developing world. Already in 1978, the WHO Expert Committee on Smoking Control warned that in the absence of resolute government action, the probability was that a smoking epidemic would affect the developing world within a decade, and that a major avoidable public health problem would be inflicted on the countries least able to withstand it. Only five years later, another expert committee stated that these predictions were coming true. In Bangladesh, for example, cigarette consumption had more than doubled in ten years and lung cancer had become the third commonest cancer among males.

The smoking issue was multifaceted. Increases in cancer and respiratory disease generally were a recognized health consequence of smoking, but observers also pointed to the likely impact on infant and child health: expenditure on cigarettes in households where money for food was already marginal would reduce the nutritional status of young children. The daily smoking of just five cigarettes in a poor Bangladeshi household, it was calculated, might lead to a monthly dietary deficit of 8,000 calories. By the 1980s, however, tobacco dependency, including traditional, non-cigarette-related use, was said to affect at least half of all adult men in the developing world. Most became addicted while still in their teens: in China a quarter of men were addicted by the age of eighteen, in India a third by the age of twenty. And the problem escalated. In 2001, Chinese students were reported to begin smoking on average at the age of ten years and seven months. By the 1990s, cancer and heart disease – the classic Western 'lifestyle' diseases – were entrenched in many non-Western countries; although neoplasms and diseases of the circulatory system were the leading causes of death in the West, more than half of all deaths attributed to them occurred in developing countries. By the twenty-first century, moreover, it was becoming apparent that cigarette smoking also affected TB mortality: it was reported from the Indian state of Tamil Nadu that smokers were four times as likely to become ill with TB as nonsmokers. In India as a whole, half of all TB deaths were in men aged between thirty and sixty who smoked.

The international effort to limit the damage brought about by smoking was hampered both by slow recognition in a world dominated by glossy Western advertising and westernized ambitions, and by the economics of the tobacco trade, which provided valuable cash crops in many poor countries. Even so basic a preventive measure as health warnings on cigarette packets was slow to reach the developing world. Thailand was an honourable exception, implementing the measure in 1974 and strengthening it in 1997; but across vast tracts of Asia, including China, Malaysia, Indonesia, Taiwan, the Philippines, and Vietnam, such warnings were only introduced in the 1990s. By 2000, however, anxiety was reaching a crisis point in the global health community, with the recognition that tobacco killed 4.9 million people every year. In May 2003, the World Health Assembly adopted the WHO Framework Convention on Tobacco Control, which was signed by twenty-eight countries and the EU at the first opportunity. Signatories to the convention undertook to implement, periodically update, and review comprehensive national tobacco control policies. It was recognized that price and tax measures were an effective means of reducing consumption, especially among the young, but also that other measures were important. In China, for example, a significant reduction in teenage smoking had been achieved since 1996 in Beijing, after the local authority banned smoking in public places, and withheld student loans and grants-in-aid to university and college students who smoked, and the State Administration of Industry and Commerce banned tobacco advertising on the mass media.

The activities of multinational companies also aroused international concern in respect of another area, that of the supply of medicines. Already in the 1980s, the multinational pharmaceutical companies were being criticized for unethical behaviour in promoting the sales of expensive curative medicines to the poor in developing countries, in taking advantage of weak drug-control agencies in those countries, and in failing to undertake major initiatives in developing new drugs specifically for developing world markets and specifically targeted at tropical diseases. Despite the vast problems of illness and ill health in the developing world, the great bulk of drugs supplied to the world market were consumed by the world's richest countries. As the then Director General of WHO, Halfdan Mahler (b. 1923) remarked in 1981, 'The public health services of the 67 poorest developing countries, excluding China, spend less in total than the rich countries spend on tranquillizers' (Melrose, 1982, p. 16). Although countries, such as India and Brazil, were developing their own pharmaceutical industries, supplying generic and much cheaper medicines to domestic and developing world markets, most developing countries had little or no manufacturing capacity, and forty-five of the poorest nations, mostly in Africa, were entirely dependent on imported finished drugs. Moreover, the generic drugs were opposed by both the major Western pharmaceutical companies and by doctors, who claimed that brand-name drugs were intrinsically superior.

With the emergence of the global AIDS epidemic in the 1990s, however, the availability and price of drugs became an increasingly bitter issue. By the end of the decade, when there were 25 million HIV infected people in Africa alone, and when effective antiretroviral drugs that significantly prolonged and improved quality of life for HIV victims had become available, discontent with the policies of the multinationals escalated. A number of NGOs, notably the medical aid agency, Médecins sans Frontières (Doctors without Borders), initiated a campaign to open up developing country access to generic drugs. Following a number of high-profile court cases, including the suing for infringement of WTO rules on patent protection of the South African government by forty pharmaceutical companies in 2001, members of the WTO agreed in September 2003 to allow poor countries to import cheap generic copies of patented drugs. Restrictions placed on the colour, size, and shape of such products were widely criticized, however, because they would raise the production costs of manufacturers and, therefore, prices. Then, in October 2003, the South African Competition Commission found two multinational pharmaceutical companies, GlaxoSmithKline and Boehringer, guilty of charging excessive prices for antiretrovirals and of abusing their patents in such a way as to restrict access to these drugs.

This decision, which was in keeping with WTO policies, was welcomed by Médecins sans Frontières as clearing away patent barriers to access and opening up the availability of generic medicines.

On the issue of drug costs, as with so many questions of health service provision, the social and economic situation of the great majority of developing countries was a critical factor. Most of their populations remained agricultural, living in rural areas, dependent on cash crops and without a self-sufficient, and efficient, agricultural base. For the most part, they did not undergo industrialization, and their continuing poverty compared to the industrialized nations sustained a sense of postcolonial dependency on the wealthy West.

Medicine and the media

From small beginnings in the first half of the twentieth century, medicine's relationship with the media became, in the second half of that century, increasingly 'complex, multifaceted and crucial' (Lederer and Rogers, 2000, p. 501). Perhaps the most critical development was the introduction of television, which brought real and fictionalized medical procedures and personalities into the daily lives of millions of viewers by the early 1960s. Television, and the older media of printed word, radio, and film, reflected and fostered changing social attitudes towards medicine and its practitioners. In the first years after the war, medical establishments in both Britain and America were firmly in control of the ways in which medicine was presented in the media, assisted by existing film censorship regulations. In 1955, the American Physician Advisory Committee on Television, Radio and Motion Pictures was established to review the way in which scripts presented medicine and medical issues. In general, the media at this time offered a largely appreciative and uncritical picture of the profession and its activities. The hugely successful television series, 'Dr. Kildare' and 'Dr. Finlay's Casebook', for example, played a significant part in favourably shaping public perceptions of hospital medicine and hospital doctors, and of family doctors, in both Britain and America for most of the 1950s and 1960s. In Britain, 'Emergency Ward 10' was also thought to have helped nurse recruitment.

Although many doctors initially opposed the televising of medicine, arguing that greater popular familiarity with medicine and disease would increase hypochondria, others appreciated the educational potential of television in particular. In Britain, Dr. Charles Fletcher (1911–96) became the first presenter of the path-breaking series 'Your Life in Their Hands' (1958). It was a programme that presented an operation or other medical procedure, such as brain surgery or the latest methods of cancer treatment, for public information. In Fletcher's view, 'every doctor should now be willing to collaborate with the media today in public education about what medicine has to offer in the prevention and cure of disease' (Karpf, 1988, p. 7). At first, therefore, medical influence ensured a medical perspective on the profession's activities and manipulated the media into making its own contribution to the 1950s myth of the invincible progress of modern medicine. But the tensions inherent in this control were also apparent. The British Medical Association's (BMA's) popular magazine, *Family Doctor*, for example, was not allowed to carry advertisements for the Family Planning Association. When in 1959, moving with the times, the journal printed articles on 'Marrying with a baby on the way' and 'Is chastity outmoded', the BMA ensured that the entire stock was ceremonially pulped.

Medical events and social change produced a more critical media attitude towards medicine, as towards other professional and 'establishment' groups, during the 1960s. The thalidomide tragedy opened the eyes of many to the darker side of drug development and modernizing medicine. A new 'consumer' perspective developed, with interest shifting from the provision of services to the nature and quality of the services provided. Media interests in medicine followed this trend in producing more critical portrayals of medicine and its practitioners. Where the 1948 film 'The Snake Pit', for example, had cast the psychiatrist as compassionate hero, later productions such as 'King of Hearts' (1968) and 'One Flew Over the Cuckoo's Nest' (1975) took a more critical approach to psychiatry. The television series 'M*A*S*H', screened in the United States between 1972 and 1982, played up the military surgeons' resort to comedy as a morale booster in the face of endless operations on wounded soldiers and civilians in war-torn Korea. By the 1990s, filmmakers were producing portrayals of medical men that would have greatly dismayed the medical establishments of the 1950s, such as the cannibalistic Dr. Hannibal Lecter in 'Silence of the Lambs' (1991), and its sequel, 'Hannibal' (2001).

Nor was it only doctors who came in for adverse media attention. In a slightly different scenario, the nursing profession, now struggling to achieve new models of nurse function and practice, and a new professional authority battled for many years against the entrenched popular stereotype of the Nightingale nurse, the doctor's handmaiden. The image had been reinforced and glamorized by the popular early serials, such as

'Dr. Kildare', and persisted despite social change and the efforts of the new feminists into at least the late 1970s. The popular image of nursing was increasingly seen as a problem by nursing professionals, who also deplored the emergence of other popular media stereotypes, the nurse as sex object (Chief Nurse 'Hot Lips' Houlihan in 'M*A*S*H'), and the nurse/matron as battleaxe, as in the British comedy film, 'Carry on Nurse'. As economic stringency began to bite in the 1980s, such images were increasingly felt to have a destructive effect both on nurse recruitment and on the retention of individual nurses within the profession.

The media not only reflected new social trends, but helped to create them. Two examples from Britain illustrate the point. In 1980, the British Broadcasting Association's annual Reith Lectures were given by Ian Kennedy (b. 1941), who suggested that the relationship between doctors and patients should be reshaped, with patients taking greater responsibility for their own lives by questioning the power of their medical attendants. This has been widely perceived as marking a watershed in the British public's perception of medicine, provoking the growth of more critical responses to medicine and its practitioners. Later that year, the popular investigatory programme 'Panorama' looked at the issue of brain death. The focus of the programme was on four American patients who had been declared brain dead but later recovered, however, the differences between British and American practice in this regard were not revealed; none of the patients met the British medical criteria for the certification of brain death. Although the BBC had been warned of potential serious damage to public willingness to allow organs to be used for transplantation, and that patients would die as a result, the programme was screened. The transplant programme remained stationary for the next two years, and in the words of historian Geoffrey Rivett, 'In a single night, *Panorama* virtually destroyed trust between television and the medical profession' (Rivett, 1998, p. 296).

A new realism crept into television depictions of medicine and its practitioners from the 1980s. Beginning with the serial 'St. Elsewhere' (1982–8) and continuing with 'ER' (1990s) and others, medical men and women ceased to be model professionals and became people with tangled personal and professional lives. The strains and stresses of medicine in practice were increasingly highlighted, as were the shortcomings of medicine and modern medical facilities. Other medical realities were positively distorted in the interests of high drama, and could reinforce unrealistic popular expectations. In 1995, an analysis published in the *New England Journal of Medicine* of the success rates of cardiopulmonary resuscitation in three popular television serials, concluded that the survival rates presented there were significantly higher than those achieved in contemporary medical experience.

Newspaper interest in medicine followed much the same trajectory as that of film and television, although with something of a time lag. Scare stories about medical problems and procedures had long been popular press material, but before *c.* 1990 the reporting of new medical developments in the British broadsheet press, for example, remained generally balanced and informed. A decline in broadsheet standards set in during the last decade of the century, and biases in reporting became increasingly apparent. This was notably the case in the reporting of, for example, the supposed links between the measles, mumps, and rubella (MMR) vaccine and autism, in the debate over genetically modified foodstuffs, and in the persistent reporting of doubtful epidemiological studies purporting to show that the consumption of various foodstuffs caused cancer. For all that disease, health, and medicine have attracted occasional coverage since newspapers were invented, it was only after World War II that they became a major subject for the Western media. If cholera was headline news, if Pasteur became a media phenomenon, if appendicitis was popularized by Edward VII's operation, these were transient sensations compared to the near saturation coverage of medical achievements, medical scandals, and medical politics in the press, in addition to the romanticization and fictionalization of the medical world depicted on screen, achieved in recent decades. The post-1945 media obsession with medicine and its practitioners in fact and in fiction testifies to the central role that medicine plays in modern Western culture and society.

Afterword

In the twenty-first century, the Western medical tradition, now more than 2,000 years old, retains its specific identity. Despite a radical transformation in the last half of the twentieth century, the tradition continues to be recognizable in the form of the clinical encounter by its emphasis on science, the sorts of medical education it relies on, and its distinctive view of the human body. There has certainly been change, but continuities remain. The future of the tradition may at times seem uncertain, its ability to deliver human expectations and fulfil human hopes doubtful, its authority in question, yet it will have successes, too. New therapeutic routes, such as gene therapy, may take decades of development before successful treatments can be realized. Old and existing medical conundrums, such as malaria and HIV, may remain unresolved. Human expectations of medicine and its practitioners will change. New medical problems will become apparent while some old ones will decline in importance. As medicine changes and develops further in the twenty-first century, new perspectives and new priorities for historical study will also emerge. The Western medical tradition, with its deep historic roots, remains a powerful force in the organization and conceptualization of medical practice across the world.

Bibliographical essays

Chapter 1

Indispensable to understanding the period is Volume One of K. Marx, *Das Kapital*. For a graphic insight into the social realities of the period, this should be supplemented by F. Engels, *The Condition of the Working Class in England*, Moscow, Progress Publishers, 1973. Eric Hobsbawm, *The Age of Revolutions*, London, Weidenfeld and Nicholson, 1962, provides an unsurpassed overview of the core dynamics of the decades between 1789 and 1848. There are a number of introductions to the notoriously difficult thought of Michel Foucault. None of these can, however, substitute for a direct reading of his works. Of most obvious relevance is: *The Birth of the Clinic: An Archaeology of Medical Perception*, London, Tavistock, 1973.

A more than adequate account of the 'medical history' of the first half of the nineteenth century, as well as later developments, is found in C. Lawrence, *Medicine in the Making of Modern Britain, 1700–1920*, London, Routledge, 1994. There is also W. F. Bynum, *Science and the Practice of Medicine in the Nineteenth Century*, Cambridge University Press, 1994. A somewhat problematic, but nonetheless useful framework for understanding the changing relations between patient and doctor is provided by: N. D. Jewson, 'The disappearance of the sick-man from medical cosmology, 1770–1870', *Sociology*, 10 (1976), 225–44. I. Waddington, *The Medical Profession in the Industrial Revolution*, Dublin, Gill and Macmillan, 1984, deals with the reorganization of practice in Britain at the institutional and political level. Provocative claims about the relations between medical politics and medical theory are found in A. Desmond, *The Politics of Evolution: Morphology, Medicine, and Reform in Radical London*, University of Chicago Press, 1989.

It is instructive to compare and contrast Foucault's account of French medicine at the turn of the nineteenth century with the more traditional historiography of E. H. Ackerknecht, *Medicine at the Paris Hospital, 1794–1848*, Baltimore, Johns Hopkins University Press, 1967. For an attempt to review the issues see the essays in C. Hannaway and A. La Berge (eds.),

Constructing Paris Medicine, Amsterdam, Rodopi, 1998. The eighteenth-century background to the transformations of the revolutionary era is considered in T. Gelfand, *Professionalizing Modern Medicine: Paris Surgeons and Medical Science and Institutions in the 18th Century*, Westport, CT, Greenwood Press, 1980. The impact of the military exigencies of the period is stressed in D. M. Vess, *Medical Revolution in France, 1789–1796*, Gainesville, University Presses of Florida, 1975.

The best modern treatment of Laennec is J. Duffin, *To See with a Better Eye: a Life of R. T. H. Laennec*, Princeton, Princeton University Press, 1998. On Broussais see J.-F. *Braunstein Broussais et le matérialisme: médecine et philosophie au XIXe siècle*, Paris, Méridiens Klincksieck, 1986.

The American context is best approached through J. H. Warner, *The Therapeutic Perspective: Medical Practice, Knowledge, and Identity in America, 1820–1885*, Cambridge, MA, Harvard University Press, 1986; idem, *Against the Spirit of System: The French Impulse in Nineteenth-Century American Medicine*, Princeton, Princeton University Press, 1998.

It is more difficult to find a satisfactory overall account of the highly fragmented German scene. But see E. Lesky, *The Vienna Medical School of the 19th Century*, Baltimore, Johns Hopkins University Press, 1976; A. M. Tuchman, *Science, Medicine, and the State in Germany: The Case of Baden, 1815–1871*, New York, Oxford University Press, 1993.

The expansion of medicine into a public sphere may be examined through C. Hamlin, *Public Health and Social Justice in the Age of Chadwick: Britain, 1800–1854*, Cambridge University Press, 1998; Ann F. La Berge, *Mission and Method: The Early Nineteenth-Century French Public Health Movement*, Cambridge University Press, 1992. The wider context of nineteenth-century developments is considered in D. Porter, *Health, Civilization, and the State: A History of Public Health from Ancient to Modern Times*, London, Routledge, 1999. Stimulating historiographical insights are to be found in M. Poovey, *Making a Social Body: British Cultural Formation, 1830–1864*, University of Chicago Press, 1995.

Chapter 2

The period before World War I is now a historical memory, and there is a reasonable synthetic and monographic literature on health, medicine, and disease in the second half of the nineteenth century. There are several reference books and general volumes that I have used on a regular basis, and their inclusion here does not mean that specific portions of them are not relevant to later discussions. For general treatment of many of the themes of this section see W. F. Bynum and Roy Porter, eds., *The Companion Encyclopedia of the History of Medicine*, 2 vols., London and New York, Routledge, 1993. Both Colin Blakemore and Sheila Jennett, eds., *The Oxford Companion to the Body*, Oxford, Oxford University Press, 2001, and Stephen Lock et al., eds., *The Oxford Illustrated Companion to Medicine*, 3rd ed., Oxford, Oxford University Press, 2001, have very helpful historical coverage. W. F. Bynum, *Science and the Practice of Medicine in the Nineteenth Century*, Cambridge, Cambridge University Press, 1994, inevitably covers much of the material contained in this chapter. It also has a full bibliographical essay. Two of the other co-authors of the present volume have written monographs that deal with the British dimension: Anne Hardy, *Health and Medicine in Britain since 1860*, Basingstoke, Palgrave, 2001; and Christopher Lawrence, *Medicine in the Making of Modern Britain, 1700–1920*, London, Routledge, 1994. The various meanings and uses of science for nineteenth-century clinicians have been subtly analysed in several works by John Harley Warner. His *Against the Spirit of System, The French Impulse in Nineteenth-Century American Medicine*, Princeton, Princeton University Press, 1998, looks at the influence of French clinical science on America. His 'The fall and rise of professional mystery: epistemology, authority and the emergence of laboratory medicine in nineteenth-century America', in Andrew Cunningham and Perry Williams (eds.), *The Laboratory Revolution in Medicine*, Cambridge, Cambridge University Press, 1992, focuses more specifically on the relation between clinicians and scientists.

MEDICAL SCIENCE

A large number of books and articles have looked at aspects of nineteenth-century medical science. An old-fashioned survey of physiology is K. E. Rothschuh, *History of Physiology*, trans. G. B. Risse, New York, Krieger, 1973. The collection of essays edited by F. L. Holmes and William Coleman, *The Investigative Enterprise*, Berkeley, University of California Press, 1988, contains much thoughtful analysis, mostly on continental themes. Helmholtz is well served in the introduction and translated collection of his writings, Russell Kahl, *Selected Writings of Hermann von Helmholtz*, Middletown, CT, Wesleyan University Press, 1971. Claude Bernard has attracted his own special literature. The older biography by J. E. D. and E. H. Olmsted, *Claude Bernard and the Experimental Method in Medicine*, New York, Schuman, 1952, is still useful. F. L. Holmes, *Claude Bernard and Animal Chemistry*. Cambridge, MA, Harvard University Press, 1974, scrutinizes his early career, and William Coleman, 'The cognitive basis of the discipline: Claude Bernard on physiology', *Isis,* 76 (1984), 49–70 provides a more recent assessment. Bernard's *An Introduction to the Study of Experimental Medicine* (1865), New York, Dover, 1957, remains in print and is a rewarding classic of medical science.

The development of experimental physiology in Britain is the subject of Gerald Geison, *Michael Foster and the Cambridge School of Physiology,* Princeton, Princeton University Press, 1978. The emotive debate about animal experimentation is best approached through R. D. French, *Antivivisection and Medical Science in Victorian Society,* Princeton, Princeton University Press, 1975, and the collection of essays in Nicholaas Rupke, (ed.), *Vivisection in Historical Perspective,* London, Routledge, 1987. Harriet Ritvo, *The Animal Estate: The English and Other Creatures in the Victorian Age,* Cambridge, MA, Harvard University Press, 1987, offers a wider cultural perspective.

W. Bruce Fye, *The Development of American Physiology,* Baltimore, Johns Hopkins University Press, 1987, offers a survey of the American physiological scene, with emphasis on interactions between physiology and clinical medicine during the period. What was called 'physiological medicine', mostly in Germany, was based on the clinical approach advocated by Wunderlich, the background for which can be appreciated through Georges Canguilhem, *On the Normal and the Pathological,* trans. C. R. Fawcett, Dordrecht, Reidel, 1978.

Esmond R. Long, *A History of Pathology,* New York, Dover, 1965, remains an excellent introduction to the ideas and practises of pathologists. Among nineteenth-century exponents of the discipline, none has received more historical attention than Rudolf Virchow. Erwin Ackerknecht, *Rudolf Virchow, Doctor, Statesman, Anthropologist,* Madison, University of Wisconsin Press, 1953, does justice to the various facets of Virchow's life. Leland J. Rather, *Disease, Life, and Man, Selected Essays by Rudolf Virchow,* Stanford, Stanford University Press, 1971, makes several key essays available in English. An even more ambitious translation project was Rudolf Virchow, *Collected Essays on Public Health and Epidemiology,* edited and introduced by L. J. Rather, 2 vols., Canton, ME, Science History Publications, 1985. Ian F. McNeely, *'Medicine on a Grand Scale': Rudolf Virchow, Liberalism and the Public Health,* London, Wellcome Trust Centre for the History of Medicine at University College London, 2002, puts Virchow's medical politics in their liberal context.

Much has been written about bacteriology and the coming of germ theory within medicine. William Bulloch. *The History of Bacteriology*, London, Oxford University Press, 1938, written long ago by a leading bacteriologist, remains an excellent source for ideas and techniques. Michael Worboys, *Spreading Germs, Disease Theories and Medical Practice in Britain, 1865–1900*, Cambridge and New York, Cambridge University Press, 2000, is a full and subtle study of a country that was largely a backwater in the field.

The literature on Pasteur is enormous. Gerald Geison's article on him in the *Dictionary of Scientific Biography* is virtually a monograph itself, and provides a sensitive examination of the development of his thought. Geison's *The Private Science of Louis Pasteur*, Princeton, Princeton University Press, 1995, rather controversially looks at the relationship between Pasteur's public science and the science as revealed in his laboratory notebooks. A recent biography, more in the traditional hagiographical mould, is Patrice Debré, *Louis Pasteur*, trans. Elborg Forster, Baltimore, Johns Hopkins University Press, 1998. There are many popular biographies of this saint of experimental medicine. Bruno Lateur, *The Pasteurization of France*, trans. A. S. Smith and J. Law, Cambridge, MA, Harvard University Press, 1988, looks at the wider social history of Pasteur's legacy.

Koch, too, has had a full press. A good biography in English is Thomas D. Brock, *Robert Koch, A Life in Medicine and Bacteriology*, Madison, University of Wisconsin Press, 1988. Several articles by Christoph Gradmann look at specific aspects of his research career, especially his work on tuberculosis and tuberculin. Typhoid and the chequered history of Typhoid Mary are the subject of Judith Leavitt's fine monograph, *Typhoid Mary, Captive to the Public's Health*, Boston, Beacon Press, 1996. Anne Hardy, *The Epidemic Streets, Infectious Disease and the Rise of Preventive Medicine 1856–1900*, Oxford, Clarendon Press, 1993, is a rich study, based on London and with a full chapter on typhoid.

Arthur M. Silverstein, *A History of Immunology*, San Diego, Academic Press, 1989, is an excellent survey of this complicated field. Silverstein has recently published a study of Paul Ehrlich, *Paul Ehrlich's Receptor Immunology. The Magnificent Obsession*, San Diego, Academic Press, 2002. The biography of Elie Metchnikoff by Alfred I. Tauber, *Metchnikoff and the Origins of Immunology: From Metaphor to Theory*, New York, Oxford University Press, 1991, is comprehensive and stimulating. A sophisticated reading of another aspect of early immunology is provided by Pauline Mazumdar,

Species and Specificity: An Interpretation of the History of Immunology, Cambridge, Cambridge University Press, 1995.

MEDICAL INSTITUTIONS

An outstanding recent book on medical education is Thomas N. Bonner, *Becoming a Physician, Medical Education in Great Britain, France, Germany and the United States, 1750–1945*, New York, Oxford University Press, 1995. Although Bonner's monograph is not overtly comparative, his sensitive discussions of education in four different cultures allow comparisons to be made. Bonner earlier wrote a monograph on the medical education of women: *To the Ends of the Earth: Women's Search for Education in Medicine*, Cambridge, MA, Harvard University Press, 1992. Two excellent monographs on the United States are William G. Rothstein, *American Medical Schools and the Practice of Medicine*, New York, Oxford University Press, 1987, and Kenneth M. Ludmerer, *Learning to Heal, The Development of American Medical Education*, New York, Basic Books, 1985. The collection of essays edited by Ronald L. Numbers, *The Education of American Physicians*, Berkeley, University of California Press, 1980, has good material on more specialized aspects of medical training, such as anatomy, pathology, and internal medicine. French medical education after the decline of the early nineteenth century is best approached through work on the French universities, including Harry Paul, *From Knowledge to Power: The Rise of the Science Empire in France, 1860–1939*, Cambridge, Cambridge University Press, 1985, and George Weisz, *The Emergence of Modern Universities in France, 1863–1914*, Princeton, Princeton University Press, 1983. For Germany, see Arleen Marcia Tuchman, *Science, Medicine and the State in Germany, The Case of Baden, 1815–1871*, New York, Oxford University Press, 1993; Charles E. McClelland, *The German Experience of Professionalization*, Cambridge, Cambridge University Press, 1991, and Geoffrey Cocks and Konrad H. Jarausch (eds.), *German Professions, 1800–1950*, New York, Oxford University Press, 1990. Abraham Flexner's surveys and monographs still make compelling reading: *Medical Education in the United States and Canada*, New York, Carnegie Foundation, 1910; *Medical Education in Europe*, New York, Carnegie Foundation, 1912; and *Medical Education: A Comparative Study*, New York, Macmillan, 1925.

Guenter B. Risse, *Mending Bodies, Saving Souls*, New York, Oxford University Press, 1999, is an outstanding history of hospitals from antiquity to the recent past. Three large chapters on the nineteenth century look at both care and teaching in a number of major hospitals, including the introduction of antiseptic and aseptic surgery. The older book by John D. Thompson and Grace Goldin, *The Hospital: A Social and Architectural History*, New Haven, Yale University Press, 1975 is still an excellent source. Charles Rosenberg, *The Care of Strangers: The Rise of America's Hospital System*, New York, Basic Books, 1987, is a wonderfully stimulating study of the American scene. Hospitals in London are dealt with in Geoffrey Rivett, *The Development of the London Hospital System, 1823–1982*, London, King Edward's Hospital Fund for London, 1986; and Keir Waddington, *Charity and the London Hospitals, 1850–1898*, Woodbridge, Royal Historical Society, 2000. The collection of essays edited by Lindsay Granshaw and Roy Porter, *The Hospital in History*, London Routledge, 1989, is still useful. There are many monographs on individual hospitals. Owen H. Wangensteen and Sarah D. Wangensteen, *The Rise of Surgery, From Empiric Craft to Scientific Discipline*, Folkestone, Kent, Dawsons, 1978, is triumphalist in its orientation, but useful in its information. More sober is Ann Daley, *Women under the Knife, A History of Surgery*, London, Hutchinson Radius, 1991.

The literature on nursing has become extensive. Excellent monographs include Susan Reverby, *Ordered to Care, The Dilemma of American Nursing 1850–1945*, Cambridge, Cambridge University Press, 1987; Monica Baly, *Florence Nightingale and the Nursing Legacy*, London, Routledge, 1986; and Anne Summers, *Angels and Citizens, British Women as Military Nurses, 1854–1914*, London, Routledge, 1988.

There are full accounts of the funding and founding of the Institut Pasteur in the literature on him cited in the preceding text. See also, Paul Weindling, 'Scientific élites and laboratory organisation in *fin de siècle* Paris and Berlin: the Pasteur Institute and Robert Koch's Institute for Infectious Diseases compared', in Cunningham and Williams, *op. cit.*, 170–88. Harriett Chick, et al., *War on Disease: A History of the Lister Institute*, London, André Deutsch, 1971 and George Corner, *A History of the Rockefeller Institute, 1901–1953*, New York, Rockefeller Institute Press, 1964, are straightforward insiders' histories of these two research institutes.

DISEASE AND DISEASES

Arthur L. Caplan, H. Tristram Engelhardt, Jr., and James J. McCartney (eds.), *Concepts of Health and Disease, Interdisciplinary Perspectives*, Reading, MA, Addison-Wesley, 1981, is a good collection of essays on health and disease. The collection edited by Charles Rosenberg and Janet Golden, (eds.), *Framing Disease, Essays in Cultural History*, New Brunswick, Rutgers University

Press, 1992, provides a series of historical models that have been very influential.

Stanley Joel Reiser, *Medicine and the Reign of Technology*, Cambridge, Cambridge University Press, 1978, is the standard history of physical diagnosis. It has an extensive bibliography. George Rosen placed the ophthalmoscope at the centre of his analysis of specialization in medicine and surgery: *The Specialization of Medicine with Special Reference to Ophthalmology*, New York, Froben Press, 1944. More recently, historians are less convinced by technology-driven models. See, for example, the articles by Christopher Lawrence and Joel Howell in W. F. Bynum, Christopher Lawrence, and Vivian Nutton (eds.), *The Emergence of Modern Cardiology*, *Medical History*, Supplement No. 5, 1985. For debates about the use of the speculum, see Ornella Moscucci, *The Science of Woman. Gynaecology and Gender in England, 1800–1929*, Cambridge, Cambridge University Press, 1990. The development of diagnostic techniques in haematology is discussed in Maxwell M. Wintrobe (ed.), *Blood, Pure and Eloquent*, New York, McGraw-Hill Book Company, 1980. X-rays feature centrally in Joel Howell, *Technology in the Hospital: Transforming Patient Care in the Early Twentieth Century*, Baltimore, Johns Hopkins University Press, 1995.

There is an extensive body of literature on tuberculosis. A good general history is Thomas Dormandy, *The White Death, A History of Tuberculosis*, London, Hambledon, 1999. F. B Smith, *The Retreat of Tuberculosis, 1850–1950*, London, Croom Helm, 1988, deals with the disease in England. David S. Barnes, *The Making of a Social Disease: Tuberculosis in Nineteenth-Century France*, Cambridge, MA, Harvard University Press, 1995, sensitively deals with the disease in France. Sheila Rothman, *Living in the Shadow*, New York, Basic Books, 1994, poignantly evokes the experiences of American tuberculous patients. Arthur Ransome's optimistic predictions about the continuing decline of tuberculosis are contained in his *Researches on Tuberculosis*, London, Smith, Elder & Co., 1898.

A superb clinical history of syphilology (and dermatology) is John Thorne Crissey and Lawrence Charles Parish, *The Dermatology and Syphilology of the Nineteenth Century*, New York, Praeger, 1981. Claude Quétel, *History of Syphilis*, trans. Judith Braddock and Brian Pike, Oxford, Polity Press, 1990, is rich on French material. Alan Brandt, *No Magic Bullet, A Social History of Venereal Disease in the United States since 1880*, New York, Oxford University Press, 1985, is sound on attitudes in America.

L. J. Rather, *The Genesis of Cancer*, Baltimore, Johns Hopkins University Press, 1978, is an excellent analysis of the pathological theories of the disease from antiquity to the late nineteenth century. Jacob Wolff, *The Science of Cancerous Disease from Earliest Times to the Present*, originally published in 1907, trans. Barbara Ayoub, Canton, ME, Watson Publishing, 1989, is both a period piece and a wonderful introduction to an earlier world. James T. Patterson, *The Dread Disease: Cancer and Modern American Culture*, Cambridge, MA, Harvard University Press, 1989, is better on social concerns than clinical aspects. William S. Bainbridge, *The Cancer Problem*, New York, Macmillan, 1914, is a comprehensive summary of the disease on the eve of the Great War.

Disease prevention and public health have attracted much historical scholarship. A superb international study is Peter Baldwin, *Contagion and the State in Europe, 1830–1930*, Cambridge, Cambridge University Press, 1999. The essays in Dorothy Porter (ed.), *The History of Public Health and the Modern State*, Amsterdam, Rodopi, 1994, are of high standard and look at the subject in a dozen countries worldwide. Although the first cholera pandemic has the most extensive literature, there is excellent work on later pandemics, such as Richard J. Evans, *Death in Hamburg, Society and Politics in the Cholera Years, 1830–1910*, Oxford, Oxford University Press, 1987, and Frank Snowden, *Naples in the Time of Cholera, 1884–1911*, Cambridge, Cambridge University Press, 1995. John Snow's researches on cholera during the 1848 and 1854 epidemics has been adequately appreciated historically; he has now been the subject of a full and carefully researched biography, Peter Vinten-Johansen et al., *Cholera, Chloroform and the Science of Medicine, A Life of John Snow*, New York, Oxford University Press, 2003. Two other major post Chadwickian figures, John Simon and Arthur Newsholme, have also been analysed in first-rate biographical studies: Royston Lambert, *Sir John Simon 1816–1904 and English Social Administration*, London, MacGibbon and Kee, 1963; and John M. Eyler, *Sir Arthur Newsholme and State Medicine, 1885–1935*, Cambridge, Cambridge University Press, 1997.

French public health can be approached through the essay by Matthew Ramsey, 'Public health in France' in the D. Porter volume, cited above, pp. 45–118; and the monographs of Jean-Pierre Goubert, *The Conquest of Water, The Advent of Health in the Industrial Age*, trans. Andrew Wilson, Princeton, Princeton University Press, 1989; Martha Lee Hildreth, *Doctors, Bureaucrats, and the Public Health in France, 1888–1902*, New York, Garland, 1987; and Jack D. Ellis, *The Physician-Legislators of France: Medicine and Politics in the Early Third Republic, 1870–1914*, Cambridge, Cambridge University Press, 1990. Both the essay by Elizabeth Fee in the D. Porter volume (above) and John Duffy, *The Sanitarians, A History of American Public Health*, Urbana, University of Illinois Press, 1990, introduce the American dimension.

The history of psychiatry possesses an extensive literature. Roy Porter, *Madness: A Brief History*, Oxford, Oxford University Press, 2001, provides a racy overview, with emphasis on Britain. Edward Shorter, *A History of Psychiatry*, New York, John Wiley, 1997, surveys the subject from the late eighteenth century to the recent past. For Britain, the best analysis is Andrew Scull, *The Most Solitary of Afflictions*, New Haven, Yale University Press, 1993. For France, Jan Goldstein, *Console and Classify: The French Psychiatric Profession in the Nineteenth Century*, Cambridge, Cambridge University Press, 1987, remains the standard source. Gerald Grub, *The Mad Among Us: A History of the Care of America's Mentally Ill*, New York, Free Press, 1994, examines the United States. Janet Oppenheim's *'Shattered Nerves': Doctors, Patients and Depression in Victorian England*, New York: Oxford University Press, 1991, is a sensitive study on the neuroses, with much good material on women, as is Elaine Showalter's *The Female Malady: Women, Madness and English Culture, 1830–1980*, New York, Pantheon Books, 1985. Mark Micale, *Approaching Hysteria: Disease and Its Interpretations*, Princeton, Princeton University Press, 1995, is particularly rich on the French scene. Peter Gay, *Freud: A Life for our Times*, London, Dent, 1988, is a full and sensitive biography by a leading cultural historian. G. E. Berrios and Roy Porter (eds.), *A History of Clinical Psychiatry*, London, Athlone Press, 1995, offers a series of essays on many psychiatric disorders, divided into social and clinical approaches.

MEDICINE AND SOCIETY

Patients have become much more central to medical history, although much of the pioneering work was done by Roy and Dorothy Porter on earlier centuries. Rothman's work, above, is an excellent introduction to the nineteenth-century patient. This account of Emily Gosse's last illness is taken from several works: Edmund Gosse, *Father and Son*, Harmondsworth, Penguin, 1986 (originally published in 1907); Edmund Gosse, *The Life of Philip Henry Gosse, F. R. S*, London, Kegan Paul, 1890; Ann Thwaite, *Glimpses of the Wonderful. The Life of Philip Henry Gosse*, London, Faber and Faber, 2002; and L. R. Croft, 'Edmund Gosse and the "new and fantastic cure" for breast cancer', *Medical History* 38 (1994), 143–59. Pat Jalland's rich investigation of the lives of middle-class women in Britain is in *Women, Marriage and Politics, 1860–1914*, Oxford, Oxford University Press, 1986.

The essays in Robert Baker (ed.), *The Codification of Medical Morality, Vol. Two: Anglo-American Medical Ethics and Medical Jurisprudence in the Nineteenth Century*, Dordrecht, Kluwer, 1995, discuss the formulation of ethics and etiquette codes in the century. Russell G. Smith, *Medical Discipline: The Professional Conduct Jurisdiction of the General Medical Council, 1858–1990*, Oxford, Clarendon Press, 1994, analyses the central British regulatory body.

Matthew Ramsey's outstanding essay, 'The politics of professional monopoly in nineteenth-century medicine: the French model and its rivals', in Gerald Geison (ed.), *Professions and the French State, 1700–1900*, Philadelphia, University of Pennsylvania Press, 1984, is a brilliant account of licensing and monopoly considerations within medicine. William G. Rothstein, *American Physicians in the Nineteenth Century, From Sects to Science*, Baltimore, Johns Hopkins University Press, 1972, is good on the relations between 'regulars' and their sectarian rivals. John Harley Warner, *The Therapeutic Perspective, Medical Practice, Knowledge and Identity in America, 1825–1885*, Cambridge, MA, Harvard University Press, 1986, offers a subtle reading of these same relationships, based on extensive archival work.

Anne Digby, *Making a Medical Living, Doctors and Patients in the English Market for Medicine, 1720–1911*, Cambridge, Cambridge University Press, 1994, is a pioneering examination of the nuances of medical practice in Britain. David Green, *Working-Class Patients and the Medical Establishment: Self-Help in Britain from the Mid-Nineteenth Century to 1948*, New York, St Martin's Press, 1985, examines the growth of contract practice. E. P. Hennock, *British Social Reform and German Precedents. The Case of Social Insurance, 1880–1914*, Oxford: Clarendon Press, 1987, compares the British and German experiments with state-organized health care.

Paul Greenhalgh, *Ephemeral Vistas*, Manchester, Manchester University Press, 1988, evokes the round of international World's Fairs, beginning with the Great Exhibition of 1851. Norman Howard-Jones, *The Scientific Background of the International Sanitary Conferences, 1851–1938*, Geneva, World Health Organization, 1975, provides a sound discussion of these meetings. I have also drawn on my own article, 'Policing hearts of darkness: Aspects of the international sanitary conferences', *History and Philosophy of the Life Sciences*, 15 (1993), 421–34. Table 2.1 is taken from my article. Sir Joseph Fayrer's account is retold in his autobiography, *Recollections of My Life*, Edinburgh, William Blackwood, 1900. Table 2.2 is constructed from Fielding H. Garrison, *An Introduction to the History of Medicine*, 4th ed., Philadelphia, Saunders, 1929, p. 789.

The medical policing of American borders is the subject of Alan M. Kraut, *Silent Travellers, Germs, Genes, and the "Immigrant Menace"*, New York, Basic Books, 1994; and Howard Markel, *Quarantine! East European Jewish Immigrants and the New York City Epidemics of 1892*, Baltimore, Johns Hopkins University Press, 1997.

DOCTORS AND THE STATE

Two collections of essays offer up-to-date perspectives on war and medicine: Roger Cooter, Mark Harrison, and Steve Sturdy (eds.), *War, Medicine and Modernity*, Stroud, Sutton, 1998; and Mark Harrison and Steve Sturdy (eds.), *Medicine and Modern Warfare*, Amsterdam, Rodopi, 1999. There is now a large literature on tropical and imperial medicine. For India, see Mark Harrison, *Public Health in British India, Anglo-Indian Preventive Medicine, 1859–1914*, Cambridge, Cambridge University Press, 1994, and David Arnold, *Science, Technology and Medicine in Colonial India*, Cambridge, Cambridge University Press, 2000. Roy Macleod and Milton Lewis (eds.), *Disease, Medicine and Empire*, London, Routledge, 1988; David Arnold (ed.), *Imperial Medicine and Indigenous Societies*, Manchester, Manchester University Press, 1988; and David Arnold (ed.), *Warm Climates and Western Medicine*, Amsterdam, Rodopi, 1996, contain essays on a variety of topics. W. F. Bynum and Caroline Overy (eds.), *The Beast in the Mosquito: The Correspondence of Ronald Ross and Patrick Manson*, Amsterdam, Rodopi, 1998, provides insight into the discovery of the mode of transmission of the malaria parasite. The case for quinine is made by Daniel Headrick, *The Tools of Empire, Technology and European Imperialism in the Nineteenth Century*, New York, Oxford University Press, 1981. The relationships between the military and tropical medicine have been explored by Philip Curtin in several books and articles, including *Disease and Empire, The Health of European Troops in the Conquest of Africa*, Cambridge, Cambridge University Press, 1998. For the French experience, see Michael A. Osborne, *Nature, the Exotic and the Science of French Colonialism*, Bloomington, Indiana University Press, 1994.

Chapter 3

Literature on this period is patchy. In general, the United States is best served and perhaps Britain is served next best. Many of the works described in the bibliographical essays of the final section of this volume also cover the period 1914–45. To avoid duplication they will only occasionally be cited here. See also the references to this chapter, not all the works cited are duplicated here. In general, the social historical literature for this period is much more extensive than the literature on the history of medical science and clinical practice. Much of the best material is to be found in articles in learned journals rather than in books. There is no single volume that provides comprehensive coverage of this period alone, nor indeed is there one for any particular country.

HEALTH AND DISEASE

For disease see J. N. Hays, *The Burdens of Disease: Epidemics and Human Response in Western History*, New Brunswick, NJ, Rutgers University Press, 1998. On nutrition see Harmke Kamminga and Andrew Cunningham (eds.), *The Science and Culture of Nutrition, 1840–1940*, Amsterdam, Rodopi, 1995. For Britain, an important contribution to debates about health is Charles Webster, 'Healthy or hungry thirties', *History Workshop*, 13 (1982), 110–29.

WORLD WAR I

World War I has been quite well served by historians. See the relevant essays in Roger Cooter, Mark Harrison, and Steve Sturdy (eds.), *War, Medicine and Modernity*, Stroud, Sutton, 1998; and Roger Cooter, Mark Harrison, and Steve Sturdy (eds.), *Medicine and Modern Warfare*, Amsterdam, Rodopi, 1999. On the front from the British side see Ian R. Whitehead, *Doctors in the Great War*, London, Leo Cooper 1999; and John Laffin, *Surgeons in the Field*, London, Dent, 1970. On the German side see Derek S. Linton, 'The obscure object of knowledge: German military medicine confronts gas gangrene during World War 1', *Bulletin of the History of Medicine*, 74 (2000), 291–316. There are essays on psychiatry and the Great War in Mark S. Micale and Paul Lerner (eds.), *Traumatic Pasts: History, Psychiatry, and Trauma in the Modern Age, 1870–1930*, Cambridge, Cambridge University Press, 2001. On shell shock see Ben Shephard, *A War of Nerves*, London, Jonathan Cape, 2000. On nursing see Lyn MacDonald, *The Roses of No Man's Land*, London, Penguin Books, 1983; and Margaret R. Higonnet (ed.), *Nurses at the Front, Writing the Wounds of the Great War*, Boston, Northeastern University Press, 2001. On rehabilitation see Matthew Price, 'Bodies and Souls: The Rehabilitation of Maimed Soldiers in France and Germany during the First World War', Ph.D. thesis, Stanford University, 1998 and David A. Gerber (ed.), *Disabled Veterans in History*, Anne Arbor, University of Michigan Press, 2000. An important study that explores the wider ways in which the war was exploited is Nancy K. Bristow, *Making Men Moral: Social Engineering during the Great War*, New York, New York University Press, 1996.

MEDICAL EDUCATION AND THE MEDICAL PROFESSION

Some of the best sources still remain documents of the time. For Europe, see Abraham Flexner, *Medical Education: A Comparative Study*, New York, Macmillan, 1925. For America, *The Final Report of the Commission on Medical Education*, New York, Office of the Director of Study, 1932. More modern are the works of Stevens, cited in the bibliographical essay for Chapter 4. For academic medicine in Britain see George Graham, 'The formation of the medical and surgical professorial units in the London teaching hospitals', *Annals of Science*, 26 (1970), 1–22. The medical profession in Germany is dealt with in a wider context in Geoffrey Cocks and Konrad H. Jarausch (eds.), *German Professions, 1800–1950*. New York, Oxford University Press, 1990; and Charles E. McClelland, *The German Experience of Professionalization: Modern Learned Professions and their Organizations from the Early Nineteenth Century to the Hitler Era*, Cambridge, Cambridge University Press, 1991.

MEDICAL ORGANIZATION AND CARE

Contemporary accounts are valuable; for instance, the many surveys made by Arthur Newsholme, of which there are too many to cite here. A most useful comparative study is Howard M. Leichter, *A Comparative Approach to Policy Analysis. Health Care Policy in Four Nations*, Cambridge, Cambridge University Press, 1979. For more recent works on America see the studies by Stevens cited in the bibliographical essay for Chapter 4. For France, see Patrice Pinell, 'Cancer policy and the health system in France: "Big medicine" challenges the conception and organization of medical practice', *Social History of Medicine*, 4 (1991), 75–101; Timothy B. Smith, 'The social transformation of hospitals and the rise of medical insurance in France, 1914–1943', *The Historical Journal*, 41 (1998), 1055–87. On Germany, see Peter Rosenberg, 'The origin and development of compulsory health insurance in Germany' and Stephan Leibfried and Florian Tennstedt, 'Health-insurance policy and Brerufsverbote in the Nazi takeover' in Donald W. Light and Alexander Schuller (eds.), *Political Values and Health Care: The German Experience*, Cambridge MA, The MIT Press, 1976, pp. 105–26; 127–84.

NURSING

See the works cited in the bibliographical essay for Chapter 4 and in addition to Darwin H. Stapleton and Cathryne A. Welch (eds.), *Critical Issues in American Nursing in the Twentieth Century: Perspectives and Case Studies*, Guilderland, NY, The Foundation, 1994; Celia Davies (ed.), *Rewriting Nursing History*, London, Croom Helm, 1980; Christopher Maggs (ed.), *Nursing History: The State of the Art*, London, Wolfeboro, NH, Croom Helm, 1987.

THE MEDICAL SCIENCES AND CLINICAL PRACTICE

As noted, these subjects are poorly served for these years perhaps because the triumphalism preceding the Great War and the years succeeding 1945 have attracted so much attention. For an overview, see Christopher Lawrence, 'Clinical research' in John Kriege and Dominic Pestre (eds.), *Science in the Twentieth Century*, Amsterdam, Harwood, 1997, pp. 439–59. On biochemistry see Robert E. Kohler, *From Medical Chemistry to Biochemistry: The Making of a Biomedical Discipline*, Cambridge, Cambridge University Press, 1982. For endocrinology, a useful guide is Victor Cornelius Medvei, *The History of Clinical Endocrinology*, Casterton Hall, Carnforth, Lancashire, The Parthenon Publishing Group, 1993. On bacteriology see W. D. Foster, *A Short History of History of Clinical Pathology*, E. & S. Livingstone Ltd., Edinburgh, 1961 and idem, *A History of Medical Bacteriology and Immunology*, London, Heinemann Medical, 1970. For virology, a useful guide is Ton van Helvoort, 'History of virus research in the twentieth century: The problem of conceptual continuity', *History of Science*, 32 (1994), 185–235. On clinical science see A. McGehee Harvey, *Science at the Bedside. Clinical Research in American Medicine*, Baltimore, The Johns Hopkins University Press, 1981. On specific work, see Michael Bliss, *The Discovery of Insulin*, Basingstoke, Macmillan, 1987. Biographies are valuable sources, for instance, Saul Benison, A. Clifford Barger and Elin L. Wolfe, *Walter B. Cannon: The Life and Times of a Young Scientist*, Cambridge, MA, The Belknap Press, 1987; Elin L. Wolfe, A. Clifford Barger, and Saul Benison, *Walter B. Cannon: Science and Society*, Cambridge, MA, Boston Medical Library, 2000. On practice and the growth of technology, specific studies include Joel D. Howell, *Technology in the Hospital, Transforming Patient Care in the Early Twentieth Century*, Baltimore and London, The John Hopkins University Press, 1995. Howell is a good guide to the literature on the managerial changes in hospital medicine in this period. See also Keith Wailoo, *Drawing Blood*, Baltimore, The Johns Hopkins University Press, 1997. For holistic approaches and sometimes conservative reactions to modern medicine, see the essays collected in Christopher Lawrence and George Weisz (eds.), *Greater than the Parts: The Holist Turn in Biomedicine 1920–1950*, New York, Oxford University Press, 1998. On Germany, see Carsten Timmermann, 'Constitutional medicine, neoromanticism, and the politics of antimechanism in interwar Germany', *Bulletin of the History of Medicine*, 75 (2001), 717–39. On human experimentation, see Susan S Lederer, *Subjected to Science: Human Experimentation in America before the Second World War*, Baltimore, The Johns Hopkins University Press, 1995.

SPECIALIZATION

A subject that has not received the attention it deserves. For general accounts of Britain and America, see Rosemary Stevens, *Medical Practice in Modern England, The Impact of Specialization and State Medicine*, New Haven and London, Yale University Press, 1966; idem, *American Medicine and the Public Interest. A History of Specialization*, Berkeley, University of California Press, 1998. There are many older anecdotal histories, but for modern studies in this period see, for example, Roger Cooter, *Surgery and Society in Peace and War: Orthopaedics and the Organization of Modern Medicine, 1880–1948*, Houndmills, Basingstoke, Macmillan, 1993. On cardiology see Christopher Lawrence, 'Moderns and ancients: The new cardiology in Britain 1800–1930', in W. F. Bynum, Christopher Lawrence, and V. Nutton (eds.), *The Emergence of Modern Cardiology, Medical History*, Supplement 5, 1985, pp. 1–33. On hydrology see George Weisz, 'Spas, mineral waters and hydrological science in twentieth-century France', *Isis*, 92 (2001), 450–83. A still valuable study of the creation of neurosurgery is John F. Fulton, *Harvey Cushing: A Biography*, Springfield, IL, Charles C. Thomas, 1946.

PUBLIC HEALTH

There is a mass of literature, most of it cited in the bibliography for Chapter 4. As a starting point, see the essays in Dorothy Porter (ed.), *The History of Public Health and the Modern State*, Amsterdam, Rodopi, 1994. On Germany see Manfred Berg and Geoffrey Cocks, *Medicine and Modernity, Public Health and Medical Care in the Nineteenth- and Twentieth-Century Germany*, New York, Syndicate of the University of Cambridge, 1997. On occupational health, see Paul Weindling, (ed.), *The Social History of Occupational Health*, London, Croom Helm, 1985; and on the gradual inclusion of accident claims into ordinary insurance see Steve Sturdy, 'The industrial body' in Roger Cooter and John Pickstone (eds.), *Medicine in the Twentieth Century*,

Amsterdam, Harwood, 2000, pp. 217–34. Although largely concerned with the world before 1914, Anson Rabinbach's *The Human Motor: Energy, Fatigue and the Origins of Modernity*, Berkeley, University of California Press, 1992, is an important text for understanding models of the body used in industrial physiological research between the wars.

PHARMACEUTICAL INDUSTRY

Articles particularly pertaining to this period include John E. Lesch, 'Chemistry and biomedicine in an industrial setting: The invention of the sulfa drugs' in Seymour H. Mauskopf (ed.) *Chemical Sciences in the Modern World*, Philadelphia, University of Pennsylvania Press, 1993, pp. 158–215; David Greenwood, 'Conflicts of interest: The genesis of synthetic antimalarial agents in peace and war', *Journal of Antimicrobial Chemotherapy*, 36 (1995), 857–72. An excellent account of the American pharmaceutical industry and academic medicine is John P. Swann, *Academic Scientists and the Pharmaceutical Industry: Cooperative Research in Twentieth-Century America*, Baltimore, Johns Hopkins University Press, 1988. On the British industry, see Jonathan Liebenau, 'The rise of the British pharmaceutical industry', *British Medical Journal*, 301 (1990), 724–8.

INTERNATIONALISM AND THE ROCKEFELLER FOUNDATION

The literature on these subjects is quite large, particularly on the latter. See Paul Weindling (ed.), *International Health Organisations and Movements, 1918–1939*, Cambridge, Cambridge University Press, 1995. For a contemporary account see, League of Nations, *Health Organisation*, Geneva, Information Section, 1931. There is a mass of literature on the Rockefeller Foundation. For an insider's view see Raymond B. Fosdick, *The Story of the Rockefeller Foundation*, New York, Harper and Brothers, 1952. There are many specific studies of Rockefeller interventions; for a guide to public health see Ilana Löwy and Patrick Zylberman, 'Medicine as a social instrument: Rockefeller Foundation, 1913–45', *Studies in History and Philosophy of Biological and Biomedical Sciences*, 31 (2000), 365–79. The volume is a special issue devoted to 'The Rockefeller Foundation and the Biomedical Sciences'.

SOVIET MEDICINE

There is a great deal of literature from the 1930s, much of it rose-tinted, on Soviet medicine, for example, Arthur Newsholme and John Adams Kingbury, *Red Medicine, Socialized Health in Soviet Russia*, London, William

Heinemann, 1934 and Henry E. Sigerist, *Socialised Medicine in the Soviet Union*, London, Victor Gollancz Ltd, 1937. An older but useful source is Gordon Hyde, *The Soviet Health Service. A Historical and Comparative Study*, London, Lawrence and Wishart, 1974. Modern literature in English is scarce. See the essays in Susan Gross Solomon and John F. Hutchinson (eds.), *Health and Society in Soviet Russia*, Bloomington, Indiana University Press, 1990. On Russian science see Nikolai Krementsov, *Stalinist Science*, Princeton, Princeton University Press, 1997.

EUGENICS AND THE RACIAL STATE

Not surprisingly, there is a large literature on eugenics and Nazi medicine. For a broad view of the background the best source is J. Andrew Mendelsohn, 'Medicine and the making of bodily inequality in twentieth-century Europe' in Jean- Paul Gaudillère and Ilana Löwy (eds.), *Heredity and Infection: The History of Disease Transmission*, London and New York, Routledge, 2001, pp. 21–79. For eugenics in Britain and America, see Daniel Kevles, *In the Name of Eugenics: Genetics and the Uses of Human Heredity*, Harmondsworth, England, Penguin Books, 1986 and Philip R. Reilly, *The Surgical Solution: A History of Involuntary Sterilization in the United States*, Johns Hopkins University Press, Baltimore, 1991. In France, pronatalism is dealt with in Siân Reynolds, *France between the Wars: Gender and Politics*, London, Routledge, 1996. For Germany before Fascism, see Paul Weindling, *Health, Race and German Politics between National Unification and Nazism 1870–1945*, Cambridge, Cambridge University Press, 1989. Medicine in general under the Nazis is dealt with in Michael Kater, *Doctors under Hitler*, Chapel Hill, The University of North Carolina Press, 1989. Racial policy in Nazi Germany is dealt with in Robert N. Proctor, *Racial Hygiene: Medicine under the Nazis*, Cambridge MA, Harvard University Press, 1998 and Michael Burleigh, *Death and Deliverance: "Euthanasia" in Germany c. 1900–1945*, Cambridge, Cambridge University Press, 1994. See also the essays in Arthur L. Caplan, *When Medicine Went Mad: Bioethics and the Holocaust*, Totowa, NJ, Humana Press, 1992.

WORLD WAR II

Although, for some, a relatively recent memory, World War II has been less well served by historians than the Great War. There are official histories. For the British, see Sir Arthur Salusbury and W. Franklin Mellor, *Medical Services in War: The Principal Medical Lessons of the Second World War, Based on the Official Medical Histories of the United Kingdom, Canada,*

Australia, New Zealand and India, London, H. M. S. O., 1968. Of modern studies, Mark Harrison's *Medicine and Victory: British Military Medicine in the Second World War*, Oxford, Oxford University Press, 2004 is invaluable. See also the essays in Cooter, Harrison, and Sturdy cited in the preceding text. Not surprisingly, the literature on penicillin is huge. For a start see Trevor I. Williams, *Howard Florey, Penicillin and After*, Oxford, Oxford University Press, 1984 and Roland W. Clark, *The Life of Ernst Chain: Penicillin and Beyond*, London, Weidenfeld and Nicolson, 1985. On penicillin in war surgery (and on making a surgical career in the interwar years), see G. J. Fraenkel, *Hugh Cairns: First Nuffield Professor of Surgery University of Oxford*, Oxford, Oxford University Press, 1991.

Chapter 4

There is no satisfactory general overview of the history of Western medicine after 1945. R. Cooter and J. Pickstone, *Medicine in the Twentieth Century*, Amsterdam, Harwood, 2000, offers only patchy coverage, some contributors confining their attention to the first half of the century. Exceptions include the chapters on 'The reproductive body', N. Pfeffer, pp. 277–90, 'Supported lives', J. Stanton, pp. 601–15, and 'Medicine, technology and industry', S. Blume, pp. 171–85. J. Le Fanu, *The Rise and Fall of Modern Medicine*, London, Little, Brown, 1999, contains accounts of twelve significant advances in medical treatment. Single country overviews are rare, but for England and Wales see V. Berridge, *Health and Society in Britain since 1939*, New York and Oxford, Cambridge University Press, 1999, and the concluding chapters of H. Jones, *Health and Society in Twentieth Century Britain*, London and New York, Longman, 1994 and A. Hardy, *Health and Medicine in Britain since 1860*, Basingstoke, Hampshire, Macmillan, 2000. G. Rivett, *From Cradle to Grave: Fifty Years of the National Health Service*, London, King's Fund, 1998, provides brief details of advances in, for example, surgery, cardiology, and drug treatments. Rivett's Web site, www.nhshistory.com, is a searchable collection of up-to-date information of events since 1998 based on the contemporary chapter of that book. *History of Western Biomedicine* is a gateway hosted by the Karolinska Institute at www.mic.ki.se/West.html, which provides access to a variety of specialist Web sites including several in the twentieth century; Michael Warren's Web site, 'A Chronology of State Medicine, Public Health, Welfare and Related Services in Britain: 1066–1999', www.chronology.org.uk/, includes an extensive section on the twentieth century. Eyewitness accounts and reviews of several developments in late-twentieth-century medicine are published as *Wellcome Witnesses to Twentieth Century Medicine,* series eds. E. M. Tansey, D. A. Christie, and L. A. Reynolds, also freely available at www.ucl.ac.uk/histmed/witnesses.html.

In general, however, accounts of many medical, health, and welfare developments during the second half of the twentieth century are still to be written.

MEDICAL RESEARCH

A thoughtful overview of medical research by a distinguished practitioner is D. Weatherall, *Science and the Quiet Art: Medical Research and Patient Care,* Oxford, Oxford University Press, 1995. There are several general subject histories that take the Plato to NATO survey approach, and thus include some, often limited, material on twentieth-century work. The few texts devoted to postwar research include S. de Chadarevian, *Designs for Life: Molecular Biology after World War II,* Cambridge, Cambridge University Press, 2002 and M. Morange, *A History of Molecular Biology,* Cambridge, MA, Harvard University Press, 1990. In addition to biographies and autobiographies of individual scientists, useful collected biographies include D. M. Fox, M. Meldrum, and I. Reznak, (eds.) *Nobel Laureates in Medicine or Physiology: A Biographical Dictionary,* New York, Garland Publishing, 1990, and additional material on Chemistry Laureates can be found at www.nobel.se/chemistry/index.html; and Physiology or Medicine Laureates at www.nobel.se/medicine/index.html.

Areas of controversy and difficulty raised by Rachel Carson's *Silent Spring,* Boston, Houghton Mifflin, 1962 [environmental pollution] and P. Singer *Animal Liberation: A New Ethics for our Treatment of Animals,* New York, New York Review, 1975 [animal experimentation], started debates and discussion that have continued into the twenty-first century. E. M. Tansey, 'The dustbin of history, and why so much modern medicine should end up there,' *Lancet* 354, 1999, 811–12, highlights some of the problems associated with the explosion in biomedical publishing in the latter half of the twentieth century.

Web sites and official histories of research organizations can be found by searching under the name of the organization, although again, coverage of the second half of the twentieth century is patchy. Histories of major bodies include F. Fenner and D. Curtis, *The John Curtin School of Medical Research: The First Fifty Years, 1948–1998,* Gundaroo, Brolga Press, 2001; E. Hanson, *The Rockefeller University Achievements: A Century of Science for the*

Benefit of Humankind 1901–2001, New York, Rockefeller University Press, 2000; A. L. Thomson *Half a Century of Medical Research,* Vol. 1. *Origins and Policy of the Medical Research Council*, London, Medical Research Council, 1973; Vol 2. *The Programme of the Medical Research Council (UK)*, London, Medical Research Council, London, 1975. The National Institutes of Health (NIH) maintain their own History Office and an historical resources Web site at http://history.nih.gov; INSERM's history can be reviewed at http://infodoc.inserm.fr/histoire. Several of these sources consider funding issues, which were also examined by J. H. Comroe and R. D. Dripps, 'Scientific basis for the support of biomedical science,' *Science* 192, 1976, 105–11.

Clinical research is specifically considered by Christopher Booth's 'Clinical research' in W. F. Bynum and R. Porter (eds.), *Companion Encyclopedia of the History of Medicine*, vol. 1, London and New York, Routledge, 1993, 205–29.

HEALTH AND DISEASE

Changing disease patterns are discussed in R. Doll, 'Major epidemics of the 20th century: From coronary thrombosis to AIDS', *Journal of the Royal Statistical Society* Series A, 150, 1987, 373–95. The problems of emerging diseases, including tuberculosis, multidrug-resistant infections and HIV, are also powerfully depicted in L. Garrett, *The Coming Plague: Newly Emerging Diseases in a World out of Balance*, New York, Farrar, Straus and Giroux, 1994, and are further assessed in J. Whitman (ed.), *The Politics of Emerging and Resurgent Infectious Diseases*, Basingstoke, Hampshire, Macmillan Press, 2000, which includes essays on international law in the control of emerging infectious diseases, the political causes of the current tuberculosis epidemic, challenges to WHO, and HIV/AIDS. On HIV/AIDS see E. Fee and D. M. Fox (eds.), *AIDS. The Making of a Chronic Disease*, Berkeley, University of California Press, 1992. These essays cover a range of aspects from political and media coverage through blood transfusion to women, gays, drug users, and Third World infections; see also V. Berridge, *AIDS in the UK. The Making of a Policy 1981–94*, New York, Oxford University Press, 1996. On tuberculosis see M. Gandy and A. Zumla (eds.), *The Return of the White Plague: Global Poverty and the New Tuberculosis*, London, Verso, 2003; on mad cow disease see S. C. Ratzen (ed.), *The Mad Cow Crisis; Health and the Public Good*, London, UCL Press, 1998, and M. Schwartz, *How the Cows Turned Mad*, English translation, Berkeley, University of California Press, 2003.

MEDICAL PRACTICE

Late-twentieth-century medical practice is discussed in the concluding chapters of P. Starr, *The Social Transformation of American Medicine*, New York, Basic Books, 1982, in E. Shorter, *Doctors and Their Patients: A Social History*, New Brunswick, NJ, and London, Transaction Publishers, 1991, and in I. Loudon et al. (eds.), *General Practice under the National Health Service 1948–1997*, London, Clarendon Press, 1998, which includes a comparative survey of practice in Europe. F. Mullan, *Big Doctoring in America: Profiles in Primary Care*, Berkeley and London, University of California Press, 2002, examines the revival of primary care in America in the later twentieth century.

HOSPITALS

R. Stevens, *In Sickness and in Wealth. American Hospitals in the Twentieth Century*, Baltimore and London, Johns Hopkins University Press, 1999, provides a detailed account of the complex developments in America; M. McKee and J. Healy (eds.), *Hospitals in a Changing Europe*, Buckingham, Open University Press, 2002, discusses the postwar situation in Europe.

NURSING

The postwar modernization of nursing is described in J. Fulton, *An Evolving Profession*, Manchester, Open College, 1996. P. Allan and M. Jolley's (eds.), *Nursing, Midwifery and Health Visiting since 1900*, London, Faber & Faber, 1982, includes a number of pertinent essays, notably I. S. Palmer, 'The growth of nursing in the United States of America'. Recent European nursing history is covered in Chapter 2 of J. Salvage and S. Heijnen (eds.), *Nursing in Europe. A Resource for Better Health*, Copenhagen, WHO, 1997, which is also useful on current issues in nursing; sections on nursing in G. Rivett, *From Cradle to Grave* (1998) describe the situation in England.

MIDWIFERY

The transformation of modern midwifery practice is discussed in R. G. Devries and R. Barroso, 'Midwives among the machines. Recreating midwifery in the late twentieth century' in H. Marland and A. M. Rafferty (eds.), *Midwives, Society and Childbirth*, London, Routledge, 1997. Historical insights into European midwifery practice and legislation can be found in A. Oakley and S. Houd, *Helpers in Childbirth. Midwifery Today*, New York and London, Hemisphere, 1990; on American midwifery see the closing pages of J. B. Litoff, *American Midwives 1860 to the Present*, Westport, CT,

Greenwood Press, 1978, and E. DeClerq, 'The transformation of American midwifery, 1975 to 1998', *American Journal of Public Health* 82, 1992, 680–4.

PALLIATIVE CARE

The best overview of the development of palliative care, and of Cecily Saunders's role, is H. ten Have and D. Clark (eds.), *The Ethics of Palliative Care: European Perspectives*, Buckingham, Open University Press, 2002, together with D. Clark and M. Wright, *Facing Death. Transitions in End of Life Care. Hospice and Related Developments in Eastern Europe*, Buckingham, Open University Press, 2003.

MEDICAL EDUCATION

Histories of medical education include those for the United States: Association of American Medical Colleges, *Physicians for the Twenty-First Century: Report of the Project Panel on the General Professional Education of the Physician and College Preparation for Medicine*, Washington, DC, Association of American Medical Colleges, 1984; for China, J. Z. Bowers et al. (eds.) *Science and Medicine in Twentieth Century China: Research And Education*, Ann Arbor, Center for Chinese Studies, the University of Michigan, 1988; and for the United Kingdom, the General Medical Council, *Tomorrow's Doctors: Recommendations on Undergraduate Medical Education*, London, General Medical Council, 1993. M. G. Field, *Doctor and Patient in Soviet Russia*, Cambridge, MA, Harvard University Press, 1957, provides a detailed account of immediate postwar Russian medicine and medical education.

TECHNOLOGY AND MEDICINE

Discussions of the development and impact of medical technology are included in several of the works already mentioned, including D. Weatherall (Oxford, Oxford University Press, 1995), Le Fanu (London, Little, Brown, 1999), and some of the essays in Cooter and Pickstone (Amsterdam, Harwood, 2000). Specific accounts are rendered by Sir Christopher Booth 'Technology and medicine', *Proceedings of the Royal Society London* B, 224, 1985, 267–85; and by the contributors to J. Stanton (ed.) *Innovations in Health and Medicine: Diffusion and Resistance in the Twentieth Century*, London and New York, Routledge, 2002. Chemical diagnostic techniques are included in the essays edited by C. Reinhardt, *Chemical Sciences in the 20th Century: Bridging Boundaries*, Weinheim and Chichester, Wiley-VCH, 2001; and those in Peter Morris (ed.), *From Classical to Modern Chemistry: The*

Instrumental Revolution, Cambridge, Royal Society of Chemistry in association with the Science Museum, 2002, especially 'Impact of instrumentation on biomedical and environmental sciences', pp. 251–332. The development of the biotechnology industry is assessed by both R. Bud, *The Uses of Life: A History of Biotechnology*, Cambridge and New York, Cambridge University Press, 1993, and a detailed account by an insider is C. Robbins-Roth, *From Alchemy to IPO: The Business of Biotechnology*, Cambridge, MA, Perseus, 2000, and P. Rabinau, *Making PCR: A Story of Biotechnology*, Chicago and London, University of Chicago Press, 1996.

DRUGS AND THE PHARMACEUTICAL INDUSTRY

M. Weatherall, *In Search of a Cure: A History of Pharmaceutical Discovery*, Oxford and New York, Oxford University Press, 1990, includes some post-World War II material on antibiotics, cancer drugs, and psychotrophics. Jordan Goodman's chapter, 'Pharmaceutical industry', pp. 141–54, in Cooter and Pickstone is also useful. J. Le Fanu, (London, Little, Brown, 1999) provides case studies of several drugs, including penicillin, cortisone, streptomycin, and chlorpromazine. The introduction of the latter, the first psychoactive drug, is detailed in J. P. Swazey, *Chlorpromazine in Psychiatry: A Study of Therapeutic Innovation*, Cambridge, MA, MIT Press, 1974, a topic developed in E. Shorter, *A History of Psychiatry: From the Era of the Asylum to the Age of Prozac*, New York, John Wiley, 1997. Other histories of individual drugs include R. Vos, *Drugs Looking for Diseases: Innovative Drug Research and the Development of the Beta Blockers and the Calcium Antagonists*, Dordrecht and London, Kluwer Academic Publishers, 1991. The essays in J. Lindenmann and W-D Schleunig (eds.), *Interferon: The Dawn of Recombinant Protein Drugs*, Berlin and London, Springer, 1999, examine the discovery, use, and impact of interferon, and J. Goodman and V. Walsh's *The Story of Taxol: Nature and Politics in the Pursuit of an Anti-Cancer Drug*, Cambridge and New York, Cambridge University Press, 2001, examines the discovery, development, and deployment of an anticancer drug. There are numerous histories of individual drug companies, many of them produced as celebratory or anniversary volumes. Useful volumes include J. Slinn, *A History of May & Baker 1834–1984*, Cambridge, Hobsons, 1984; an account of the Glaxo company [after 1962] by E. Jones, *The Business of Medicine*, London, Profile, 2001; and L. Galambos and J. E. Sewell, *Networks of Innovation*, Cambridge and New York, Cambridge University Press, 1995, which examines vaccine development at Merck, Sharp and Dohme, and

Mulford. Discussions of national and international aspects of the industry and its regulation include an examination of the peculiar failure of the industry in Japan in L. G. Thomas, *The Japanese Pharmaceutical Industry: The New Drug Lag and the Failure of Industrial Policy*, Cheltenham, Edward Elgar, 2001. Bill Inman's *Don't Tell the Patient: Behind the Drug Safety Net*, Los Angeles and Bishops Waltham, Highland Park Productions, 1999, discusses drug safety; Harry Marks's *The Progress of Experiment: Science and Therapeutic Reform in the United States 1900–1990*, Cambridge, Cambridge University Press, 1997, includes detailed analyses of the development of clinical trials. The James Lind Web site at http://www.jameslindlibrary.org/ documents the evolution of clinical trials, with an emphasis on twentieth-century material. Particular problems for prescribers in parts of the former Soviet Union are articulated in V. Vlassov et al., 'Do drug advertisements in Russian medical journals provide essential information for safe prescribing?' *Western Journal of Medicine*, 174, 2001, 391–4. A variety of historical material relating to the development of polio vaccines can be found in the Hauck Center for the Albert Sabin archives at http://sabin.uc.edu and in the Web site of The Time 100 Polls: Virologist Jonas Salk at www.time.com/time/time100/scientist/profile/salk.html.

Histories of drug addictions and problems include a broad-ranging account by T. Carnwath and I. Smith, *Heroin Century*, London, Routledge, 2002; H. B. Spear, (J. Mott, ed.) *Heroin Addiction Care and Control: The British System 1916–1984*, London, Drug Scope, 2002, provides an insider account of the development of drug treatment policy written by a former Chief Inspector of the Home Office Drugs Branch of the United Kingdom; R. Brynner and T. Stephens, *Dark Remedy: The Impact of Thalidomide and Its Revival as a Vital Medicine*, Cambridge, MA, Perseus Publishing, 2001.

SURGERY

Developments in surgery must be gleaned from a variety of sources: useful here are C. Lawrence and T. Treasure, 'Surgeons' in R. Cooter and J. Pickstone (eds.), *Medicine in the Twentieth Century*, Amsterdam, Harwood Academic; Abingdon, Marston, 2000, 653–70, selected essays in J. Le Fanu, *The Rise and Fall of Modern Medicine*, London, Little Brown, 1999 and the sections on surgery in G. Rivett, *From Cradle to Grave*, London, King's Fund, 1998. A specific case study that includes detailed discussion of the development and diffusion of the relevant methodology and technology is Thomas Schlich, *Surgery, Science and Industry: A Revolution in Fracture Care,*

1950s–1990s, Basingstoke, Hampshire, Palgrave, 2002. On blood see D. Starr, *Blood. An Epic History of Medicine and Commerce*, New York, Alfred A. Knopf, 1998, and A. W. Drake et al., *The American Blood Supply*, Cambridge, MA, MIT Press, 1982.

WELFARE

Welfare states and medical systems are variously described and discussed in E. Immergut, *Health Politics. Interests and Institutions in Western Europe*, Cambridge, Cambridge University Press, 1992. Detailed accounts of different countries may be found in I. Douglas-Wilson and G. McLachlan (eds.), *Health Service Prospects. An International Survey*, London, Lancet, Nuffield Provincial Hospitals Trust, 1973, J. Blaupain et al., *National Health Insurance and Health Resources. The European Experience*, Cambridge, MA, Harvard University Press, 1978, and M. W. Raffel (ed.), *Comparative Health Systems. Descriptive Analyses of Fourteen National Health Systems*, University Park, Pennsylvania State University Press, 1984. These resumes can be updated from A. Dixon and E. Mossialos, *Health Care Systems in Eight Countries: Trends and Challenges*, London, European Observatory on Health Care Systems, 2002; efforts to meet post-1970 financial stringency are described in E. Mossialos and J. Le Grand (eds.), *Health Care and Cost Containment in the European Union*, Aldershot, Hampshire, Ashgate, 1999. Also on this subject, J. A. Morone and J. M. Goggin, 'Health policies in Europe: Welfare states in a market era', *Journal of Health Politics, Policy and Law*, 20, 1995, 557–69; and D. Wilsford, 'States facing interests: Struggles over health care policy in advanced industrial democracies', ibid., 571–613. J. Rogers Hollingsworth et al., *State Intervention in Medical Care*, Ithaca and London, Cornell University Press, 1990, offers historical comparisons of the performance of medical systems in Britain, France, Sweden, and the United States across the twentieth century. There are as yet few individual country studies; notable exceptions are, on Britain, C. Webster, *The National Health Services since the War*, vol. 1, London, HMSO, 1994, vol. 2, HMSO, 1996; on Sweden, A. J. Heidenheimer and N. Elvander (eds.), *The Shaping of the Swedish Health System*, London, Croom Helm, 1980; and N. F. Christiansen and K. Petersen, 'The Nordic welfare states: A historical reappraisal', *Scandinavian Journal of History*, Special issue, 26, 2001, 153–6. On the American health care system, see M. W. Raffel and N. K. Raffel, *The US Health System. Origins and Functions*, New York, Wiley, 3rd ed., 1989, which covers the topic into the 1980s.

POPULATION AND FERTILITY

Issues of population and fertility, and the modern history of birth control are covered by E. Watkins, *On the Pill. A Social History of Oral Contraceptives 1950–1970*, Baltimore and London, Johns Hopkins University Press, 1998, which focuses mainly on America, and L. Marks, *Sexual Chemistry*, New Haven and London, Yale University Press, 2002, which has a broader global perspective.

INTERNATIONAL ORGANIZATIONS AND THE DEVELOPING WORLD

The principles and structure of the United Nations and its agencies are set out in B. Broms, *The United Nations*, United Nations, Helsinki, 1990. N. M. Goodman, *International Health Organisations and their work*, Edinburgh, Churchill Livingstone, 2nd ed., 1971, describes the organisation and early work of WHO to 1970, with shorter accounts of related agencies. W. Muraskin, *The Politics of International Health: the Children's Vaccine Initiative*, Albany, State University New York Press, 1998, offers a critical account of WHO's activities and an insight into the political complexities of development programmes, as does S. Lee, 'WHO and the developing world: the contest for ideology,' in A. Cunningham and B. Andrews (eds.), *Western Medicine as Contested Knowledge*, Manchester and New York, Manchester University Press, 1997, 24–45. C. Caulfield, *Masters of Illusion: The World Bank and the Poverty of Nations*, London, Macmillan, 1997, is a popular critique of the bank's activities. J. Power, (ed.), *Vision of Hope. The Fiftieth Anniversary of the United Nations*, London, Regency Corporation Ltd, 1995, is a variable insider's account, which provides useful information on the UN agencies' work for women and children in developing countries. F. Brockington, *The Health of the Developing World*, Lewes, Sussex, Book Guild, 1985, is a solid general account of demographic and disease patterns, with an interesting perspective (Ch. 4) on the WHO's involvement. D. R. Phillips, *Health and Health Care in the Third World*, Harlow, Herts., Longman Scientific and Technical, 1990, is a partly historical, partly social studies analysis of health care provision, which usefully draws on examples from a wide range of countries. D. Melrose, *Bitter Pills. Medicines and the Third World*, Oxford, Oxfam, 1982, is a wide-ranging examination of the subject, critical of the role played by Western commercial interest. On malaria, see S. Litsios, 'Malaria control, the Cold war, and the postwar reorganisation of international assistance' *Medical Anthropology*, 17, 1997, 255–78, and R. Packard, 'Malaria dreams: postwar visions of health and development in the Third World', *Medical Anthropology*, 17, 1997, 279–96. The official account of the eradication of smallpox is F. Fenner et al., *Smallpox and Its Eradication*, Geneva, WHO, 1988, but see also S. Bhattacharya, *Expunging Variola: The Control and Eradication of Smallpox in India, 1947–1977*, New Delhi and London, Orient Longman, India and Sangam Books, UK, forthcoming June 2006, and S. Bhattacharya, 'Uncertain advances: a review of the final phases of the smallpox eradication programme in India, 1960–1980' *American Journal of Public Health*, 94, 2004, 1875–83. There is no historical account of the recent history of tuberculosis in the developing world. On the baby milk controversy, see J. Dobbing, *Infant Feeding. Anatomy of a Controversy 1973–1984*, Berlin and London, Leiden, Springer-Verlag, 1988.

MEDICINE AND THE MEDIA

The subject of medicine and the media is examined in the British context by A. Karpf, *Doctoring the Media*, London, Routledge, 1988, and more broadly by S. Lederer and N. Rogers, 'Media', in R. Cooter and J. Pickstone (eds.), *Medicine in the Twentieth Century*, Amsterdam, Harwood Academic; Abingdon, Marston, 2000, 487–502.

General bibliography

GENERAL HISTORIES OF MEDICINE

Berridge, V. *Health and Society in Britain since 1939*, New York and Oxford, Cambridge University Press, 1999.

Blakemore, C. and Jennett, S. (eds.) *The Oxford Companion to the Body*, Oxford, Oxford University Press, 2001.

Brockliss, L. and Jones, C. *The Medical World of Early Modern France*, Oxford, Clarendon Press, 1997.

Bynum, W. F. *Science and the Practice of Medicine in the Nineteenth Century*, Cambridge, Cambridge University Press, 1994.

Bynum, W. F. and Porter, R. (eds.) *The Companion Encyclopedia of the History of Medicine*, 2 vols., London and New York, Routledge, 1993.

Cooter, R. and Pickstone, J. *Medicine in the Twentieth Century*, Amsterdam, Harwood, 2000.

Desmond, A. *The Politics of Evolution: Morphology, Medicine, and Reform in Radical London*, University of Chicago Press, 1989.

Duffin, J. *History of Medicine: A Scandalously Short History*, Toronto and London, University of Toronto Press, 1999.

Hardy, A. *Health and Medicine in Britain since 1860*, Basingstoke, Hampshire, Macmillan, 2001.

Horder, Thomas, *Health and a Day*, London, J. M. Dent and Sons Ltd., 1937.

Jacyna, L. S. *Philosophic Whigs: Medicine, Science, and Citizenship in Edinburgh, 1789–1848*, London, Routledge, 1994.

Jones, H. *Health and Society in Twentieth Century Britain*, London and New York, Longman, 1994.

Karolinska Institute. *History of Western Biomedicine*, www.mic.ki.se/West.html.

Lawrence, C. *Medicine in the Making of Modern Britain, 1700–1920*, London, Routledge, 1994.

Le Fanu, J. *The Rise and Fall of Modern Medicine*, London, Little, Brown, 1999.

Lock, S. et al. (eds.) *The Oxford Illustrated Companion to Medicine*, 3rd ed., Oxford, Oxford University Press, 2001.

Loudon I. (ed.) *Western Medicine: An Illustrated History*, Oxford, Oxford University Press, 1997.

Porter, R. (ed.) *The Cambridge Illustrated History of Medicine*, Cambridge and New York, Cambridge University Press, 1996.

Tansey, E. M., Christie, D. A., and Reynolds, L. A. (series eds.) *Wellcome Witnesses to Twentieth Century Medicine*, London, Wellcome Trust Centre for the History of Medicine; also freely available at www.ucl.ac.uk/histmed/witnesses.html

Waddington, I. *The Medical Profession in the Industrial Revolution*, Dublin, Gill and Macmillan, 1984.

GENERAL HISTORICAL BACKGROUND

Berg, M. *The Age of Manufactures: Industry, Innovation and Work in Britain: 1700–1820*, London, Fontana, 1985.

Carson, R. *Silent Spring*, Boston, Houghton Mifflin, 1962.

Daunton, M. J. *Progress and Poverty: An Economic and Social History of Britain 1700–1850*, Oxford University Press, 1995.

Elias, N. *The Civilizing Process*, Oxford, Oxford University Press, 1994.

Eliot, G. *Middlemarch* (1871–2), Oxford, Oxford University Press, 1988.

Engels, F. *The Condition of the Working Class in England*, Moscow, Progress Publishers, 1973.

Greenhalgh, P. *Ephemeral Vistas*, Manchester, Manchester University Press, 1988.

Hennessy, P. *Never Again: Britain 1945–51*, London, Jonathan Cape, 1992.

Hobsbawm, E. *The Age of Revolutions: Europe 1789–1848*, London, Abacus, 2002.

Hobsbawm, E. *The Age of Extremes. A History of the World, 1914–1991*, New York, Vintage Books, 1996.

Hobsbawm, E. and Ranger, T. (eds.) *The Invention of Tradition*, Cambridge University Press, 1983.

Hudson, P. *The Industrial Revolution*, London, Edward Arnold, 1992.

Marx, K. *Das Kapital (Capital)*, ed. Engels F, etc., 3 vols, vol. 1 trans. by S. Moore and E. Aveling; vols. 2 and 3 trans by E. Untermann, Chicago, Charles H. Kerr & Co., 1915.

Olson, R. *The Emergence of the Social Sciences 1642–1792: Twayne's Studies in Intellectual and Cultural History*, Boston, Twayne Publishers, 1993.

Perkin, H. *The Origins of Modern English Society 1780–1880*, London, Routledge, 1969.

Reynolds, R. *France between the Wars: Gender and Politics*, London, Routledge, 1996.

HEALTH AND DISEASE

Bainbridge, W. S. *The Cancer Problem*, New York, Macmillan, 1914.

Barnes, D. S. *The Making of a Social Disease: Tuberculosis in Nineteenth-Century France*, Cambridge, MA, Harvard University Press, 1995.

Berridge, V. *AIDS in the UK. The Making of a Policy 1981–94*, New York, Oxford University Press, 1996.

Brandt, A. *No Magic Bullet, A Social History of Venereal Disease in the United States since 1880*, New York, Oxford University Press, 1985.

Caplan, A. L., Tristram Engelhardt, H. Jr., and McCartney, J. J. (eds.) *Concepts of Health and Disease, Interdisciplinary Perspectives*, Reading, MA, Addison-Wesley, 1981.

Crissey, J. T. and Parish, L. C. *The Dermatology and Syphilology of the Nineteenth Century*, New York, Praeger, 1981.

Doll, R. 'Major Epidemics of the 20th Century: From Coronary Thrombosis to AIDS', *Journal of the Royal Statistical Society* Series A, 150 (1987), 373–95.

Dormandy, T. *The White Death, A History of Tuberculosis*, London, Hambledon, 1999.

Evans, R. J. *Death in Hamburg, Society and Politics in the Cholera Years, 1830–1910*, Oxford, Oxford University Press, 1987.

Fee, E. and Fox, D. M. (eds.) *AIDS: The Making of a Chronic Disease*, Berkeley, University of California Press, 1992.

Gandy, M. and Zumla, A. (eds.) *The Return of the White Plague: Global Poverty and the New Tuberculosis*, London, Verso, 2003.

Garrett, L. *The Coming Plague: Newly Emerging Diseases in a World Out of Balance*, New York, Farrar, Straus and Giroux, 1994.

Greenwood, M. *Epidemics and Crowd-Diseases: An Introduction to the Study of Epidemiology*, London, Williams and Norgate, 1935.

Hays, J. N. *The Burdens of Disease: Epidemics and Human Response in Western History*, New Brunswick, NJ, Rutgers University Press, 1998.

Kamminga, H. and Cunningham, A. (eds.) *The Science and Culture of Nutrition, 1840–1940*, Amsterdam, Rodopi, 1995.

Leavitt, J. *Typhoid Mary, Captive to the Public's Health*, Boston, Beacon Press, 1996.

Patterson, J. T. *The Dread Disease: Cancer and Modern American Culture*, Cambridge, MA, Harvard University Press, 1989.

Pinell, P. 'Cancer Policy and the Health System in France: "Big Medicine" Challenges the Conception and Organization of Medical Practice', *Social History of Medicine*, 4 (1991), 75–101.

Quétel, C. *History of Syphilis*, trans. Braddock, J. and Pike, B., Oxford, Polity Press, 1990.

Ransome, A. *Researches on Tuberculosis*, London, Smith, Elder & Co., 1898.

Rather, L. J. *The Genesis of Cancer*, Baltimore, Johns Hopkins University Press, 1978.

Ratzen, S. C. (ed.) *The Mad Cow Crisis: Health and the Public Good*, London, UCL Press, 1998.

Rosenberg, C. and Golden, J. (eds.) *Framing Disease, Essays in Cultural History*, New Brunswick, NJ, Rutgers University Press, 1992.

Rothman, S. *Living in the Shadow*, New York, Basic Books, 1994.

Schwartz, M. *How the Cows Turned Mad*, trans. Schneider, E. Berkeley, University of California Press, 2003.

Smith, F. B. *The Retreat of Tuberculosis, 1850–1950*, London, Croom Helm, 1988.

Snowden, F. *Naples in the Time of Cholera, 1884–1911*, Cambridge, Cambridge University Press, 1995.

Webster, C. 'Healthy or Hungry Thirties', *History Workshop*, 13 (1982), 110–29.

Whitman, J. (ed.) *The Politics of Emerging and Resurgent Infectious Diseases*, Basingstoke, Hampshire, Macmillan Press, 2000.

Wolff, J. *The Science of Cancerous Disease from Earliest Times to the Present*, originally published in 1907, trans. Ayoub, B., Canton, ME, Watson Publishing, 1989.

Worboys, M. *Spreading Germs, Disease Theories and Medical Practice in Britain, 1865–1900*, Cambridge and New York, Cambridge University Press, 2000.

PATIENTS, DOCTORS, AND MEDICAL PRACTICE

Cooter, R. 'Dichotomy and Denial: Mesmerism, Medicine and Harriet Martineau', in Benjamin, M. (ed.) Science and Sensibility: Gender and Scientific Enquiry, 1780–1945, Oxford, Basil Blackwell, 1991, pp. 144–73.

Croft, L. R. 'Edmund Gosse and the "New and Fantastic Cure" for Breast Cancer', *Medical History*, 38 (1994), 143–59.

Digby, A. *Making a Medical Living, Doctors and Patients in the English Market for Medicine, 1720–1911*, Cambridge, Cambridge University Press, 1994.

Gelfand, T. 'The History of the Medical Profession', in Bynum, W. F. and Porter, R. (eds.) Companion Encyclopaedia of the History of Medicine, vol 2, London, Routledge, 1993, pp. 1119–50.

Green, D. *Working-Class Patients and the Medical Establishment: Self-Help in Britain from the Mid-Nineteenth Century to 1948*, New York, St. Martin's Press, 1985.

Jacyna, L. S. (ed.) *A Tale of Three Cities: The Correspondence of William Sharpey and Allen Thomson*, London, Wellcome Institute for the History of Medicine, 1989.

Jalland, P. *Women, Marriage and Politics, 1860–1914*, Oxford, Oxford University Press, 1986.

Jewson, N. D. 'The Disappearance of the Sick-Man from Medical Sosmology, 1770–1870', *Sociology*, 10 (1976), 225–44.

Jewson, N. D. 'Medical Knowledge and the Patronage System in 18th Century England', *Sociology*, 8 (1974), 369–85.

Lawrence, C. and Macdonald, F. *Sambrook Court: The Letters of J. C. Lettsom at the Medical Society of London*, London, Wellcome Trust Centre for the History of Medicine, 2003.

Lawrence, C. and Weisz, G. (eds.) *Greater than the Parts: The Holist Turn in Biomedicine 1920–1950*, New York, Oxford University Press, 1998.

Lederer, S. S. *Subjected to Science: Human Experimentation in America before the Second World War*, Baltimore, Johns Hopkins University Press, 1995.

Loudon, I. et al. (eds.) *General Practice under the National Health Service 1948–1997*, London, Clarendon Press, 1998.

Loudon, I. *Medical Care and the General Practitioner, 1750–1850*, Oxford University Press, 1987.

Macmichael, W. *The Gold-Headed Cane*, New York, P. B. Hoeber, 1925.

Mullan, F. *Big Doctoring in America: Profiles in Primary Care*, Berkeley and London, University of California Press, 2002.

Ramsey, M. *Professional and Popular Medicine in France, 1770–1830: the Social World of Medical Practice*, Cambridge, Cambridge University Press, 1988.

Ramsey, M. 'The Politics of Professional Monopoly in Nineteenth-Century Medicine: The French Model and Its Rivals', in Geison, G. (ed.) *Professions and the French State, 1700–1900*, Philadelphia, University of Pennsylvania Press, 1984.

Rothstein, W. G. *American Physicians in the Nineteenth Century, From Sects to Science*, Baltimore, Johns Hopkins University Press, 1972.

Shapin, S. 'The Politics of Observation: Cerebral Anatomy and Social Interests in the Edinburgh Phrenology Disputes', *Sociological Review Monographs*, 27 (1979), 139–78.

Shorter, E. *Doctors and Their Patients: A Social History*, New Brunswick, NJ and London, Transaction Publishers, 1991.

Starr, P. *The Social Transformation of American Medicine*, New York, Basic Books, 1982.

Warner, J. H. *The Therapeutic Perspective, Medical Practice, Knowledge and Identity in America, 1825–1885*, Cambridge, MA, Harvard University Press, 1986.

Weiner, D. B. *The Citizen-Patient in Revolutionary and Imperial Paris*, Baltimore, Johns Hopkins University Press, 1993.

Winter, A. *Mesmerized: Powers of Mind in Victorian Britain*, University of Chicago Press, 1998.

MEDICAL SPECIALIZATION

Bynum, W. F., Lawrence, C., and Nutton, V. (eds.) *The Emergence of Modern Cardiology*, *Medical History*, Supplement No. 5, 1985.

Cooter, R. *Surgery and Society in Peace and War: Orthopaedics and the Organization of Modern Medicine, 1880–1948*, Houndmills, Basingstoke, Macmillan, 1993.

Moscucci, O. *The Science of Woman. Gynaecology and Gender in England, 1800–1929*, Cambridge, Cambridge University Press, 1990.

Rosen, G. *The Specialization of Medicine with Special Reference to Ophthalmology*, New York, Froben Press, 1944.

Stevens, R. *American Medicine and the Public Interest. A History of Specialization*, Berkeley, University of California Press, 1998.

Stevens, R. *Medical Practice in Modern England. The Impact of Specialization and State Medicine*, New Haven, Yale University Press, 1966.

Weisz, G. 'Spas, Mineral Waters and Hydrological Science in Twentieth-Century France', *Isis*, 92 (2001), 450–83.

PSYCHIATRY

Berrios, G. E. and Porter, R. (eds.) *A History of Clinical Psychiatry*, London, Athlone Press, 1995.

Goldstein, J. *Console and Classify: The French Psychiatric Profession in the Nineteenth Century*, Cambridge, Cambridge University Press, 1987.

Grub, G. *The Mad Among Us: A History of the Care of America's Mentally Ill*, New York, Free Press, 1994.

Micale, M. S. and Lerner, P. (eds.) *Traumatic Pasts: History, Psychiatry, and Trauma in the Modern Age, 1870–1930*, Cambridge, Cambridge University Press, 2001.

Micale, M. *Approaching Hysteria: Disease and Its Interpretations*, Princeton, Princeton University Press, 1995.

Oppenheim, J. 'Shattered Nerves': Doctors, Patients and Depression in Victorian England, New York, Oxford University Press, 1991.

Porter, R. *Madness: A Brief History*, Oxford, Oxford University Press, 2001.

Schwartz, J. *Cassandra's Daughter: A History of Psychoanalysis in Europe and America*, London, Allen Lane, the Penguin Press, 1999.

Scull, A. *The Most Solitary of Afflictions*, New Haven, Yale University Press, 1993.

Shorter, E. *A History of Psychiatry: From the Era of the Asylum to the Age of Prozac*, New York, John Wiley, 1997.

Showalter, E. *The Female Malady: Women, Madness and English Culture, 1830–1980*, New York, Pantheon Books, 1985.

SURGERY, ANAESTHETICS, AND BLOOD

Daley, A. *Women under the Knife, A History of Surgery*, London, Hutchinson Radius, 1991.

Drake, A. W. et al. *The American Blood Supply*, Cambridge, MA, MIT Press, 1982.

Lawrence, C. 'Anaesthesia in the Age of Reform', *The History of Anaesthesia Proceedings*, 20 (1997), 11–16.

Lawrence, C. and Treasure, T. 'Surgeons' in Cooter R. and Pickstone J. (eds), *Medicine in the Twentieth Century*, Amsterdam, Harwood Academic; Abingdon, Marston, 2000, pp. 653–70.

Pressman, J. D. *Last Resort: Psychosurgery and the Limits of Medicine*, Cambridge, Cambridge University Press, 1998.

Schlich, T. *Surgery, Science and Industry: A Revolution in Fracture Care, 1950s–1990s*, Basingstoke, Hampshire, Palgrave, 2002.

Starr, D. *Blood. An Epic History of Medicine and Commerce*, New York, Alfred A. Knopf, 1998.

Temkin, O. 'The Role of Surgery in the Rise of Modern Medical Thought', *Bulletin of the History of Medicine*, 25 (1951), 248–59.

Wangensteen, O. H. and Wangensteen, S. D. *The Rise of Surgery, From Empiric Craft to Scientific Discipline*, Folkestone, Kent, Dawsons, 1978.

TECHNOLOGY AND MEDICINE

Booth, C. 'Technology and Medicine', *Proceedings of the Royal Society London* B, 224 (1985), 267–85.

Bud, R. *The Uses of Life: A History of Biotechnology*, Cambridge and New York, Cambridge University Press, 1993.

Howell, J. *Technology in the Hospital: Transforming Patient Care in the early Twentieth Century*, Baltimore, Johns Hopkins University Press, 1995.

Morris, P. (ed.) *From Classical to Modern Chemistry: The Instrumental Revolution*, Cambridge, Royal Society of Chemistry in association with the Science Museum, 2002.

Rabinau, P. *Making PCR: A Story of Biotechnology*, Chicago, IL and London, University of Chicago Press, 1996.

Reinhardt, C. *Chemical Sciences in the 20th Century: Bridging Boundaries*, Weinheim and Chichester, Wiley-VCH, 2001.

Reiser, S. J. *Medicine and the Reign of Technology*, Cambridge, Cambridge University Press, 1978.

Robbins-Roth, C. *From Alchemy to IPO: The Business of Biotechnology*, Cambridge, MA, Perseus, 2000.

Stanton, J. (ed.) *Innovations in Health and Medicine: Diffusion and Resistance in the Twentieth Century*, London and New York, Routledge, 2002.

Wailoo, K. *Drawing Blood*, Baltimore, Johns Hopkins University Press, 1997.

Weisz, G. 'The Posthumous Laennec: Creating a Modern Medical Hero, 1826–1870', *Bulletin of the History of Medicine*, 61 (1987), 541–62.

Wintrobe, M. M. (ed.) Blood, Pure and Eloquent, New York, McGraw-Hill Book Company, 1980.

MEDICAL AND LABORATORY RESEARCH

Albury, W. R. 'Experiment and Explanation in the Physiology of Bichat and Magendie', *Studies in the History of Biology*, 1 (1977), 47–131.

Berliner, H. S. *A System of Scientific Medicine: Philanthropic Foundations in the Flexner Era*, New York, Tavistock, 1985.

Bernard, C. *An Introduction to the Study of Experimental Medicine*, trans. Green, H. C. from first English ed., 1865, New York, Dover, 1957.

Booth, C. 'Clinical Research', in Bynum, W. F. and Porter, R. (eds.) Companion Encyclopedia of the History of Medicine, vol. 1, London and New York, Routledge, 1993, pp. 205–29.

Canguilhem, G. *On the Normal and the Pathological*, trans. Fawcett, C. R., Dordrecht, Reidel, 1978.

de Chadarevian, S. *Designs for Life: Molecular Biology after World War II*, Cambridge, Cambridge University Press, 2002.

Chick, H. et al. *War on Disease: A History of the Lister Institute*, London, André Deutsch, 1971.

Coleman, W. 'Prussian pedagogy: Purkyne at Breslau, 1823–1839', in Coleman, W. and Holmes, F. L. (eds.) The Investigative Enterprise: Experimental Physiology in Nineteenth-Century Medicine, Berkeley, University of California Press, 1988.

Coleman, W. 'The Cognitive Basis of the Discipline: Claude Bernard on Physiology', *Isis*, 76 (1984), 49–70.

Comroe, J. H. and Dripps, R. D. 'Scientific Basis for the Support of Biomedical Science,' *Science*, 192 (1976), 105–11.

Cunningham, A. and Williams, P. (eds.) *The Laboratory Revolution in Medicine*, Cambridge, Cambridge University Press, 1992.

Fenner, F. and Curtis, D. *The John Curtin School of Medical Research: The First Fifty Years, 1948–1998*, Gundaroo, Brolga Press, 2001.

Fox, D. M., Meldrum, M. and Reznak, I. (eds.) *Nobel Laureates in Medicine or Physiology: A Biographical Dictionary*, New York, Garland Publishing, 1990.

Geison, G. *The Private Science of Louis Pasteur*, Princeton, Princeton University Press, 1995.

Haigh, E. 'The Roots of the Vitalism of Xavier Bichat', *Bulletin of the History of Medicine*, 49 (1975), 72–86.

Haigh, E. *Xavier Bichat and the Medical Theory of the Eighteenth Century*, London, Wellcome Institute for the History of Medicine, 1984.

Harvey, A. Mc. *Science at the Bedside. Clinical Research in American Medicine*, Baltimore, Johns Hopkins University Press, 1981.

Holmes, F. L. and Coleman, W. *The Investigative Enterprise*, Berkeley, University of California Press, 1988.

INSERM, http://infodoc.inserm.fr/histoire

Kahl, R. *Selected Writings of Hermann von Helmholtz*, Middletown, CT, Wesleyan University Press, 1971.

Kriege, J. and Pestre, D. (eds.) *Science in the Twentieth Century*, Amsterdam, Harwood, 1997.

Lateur, B. *The Pasteurization of France*, trans. Smith, A. S. and Law, J., Cambridge, MA, Harvard University Press, 1988.

McNeely, I. F. 'Medicine on a Grand Scale': Rudolf Virchow, Liberalism and the Public Health, London, Wellcome Trust Centre for the History of Medicine, 2002.

Nobel Laureates (Chemistry), www.nobel.se/chemistry/index.html

Nobel Laureates (Physiology or Medicine), http://www.nobel.se/medicine/index.html

Rather, L. J. *Disease, Life, and Man, Selected Essays by Rudolf Virchow*, Stanford, Stanford University Press, 1971.

Tansey, E. M. 'The Dustbin of History, and Why So Much Modern Medicine Should End up There,' *Lancet*, 354 (1999), 811–12.

Thomson, A. L. *Half a Century of Medical Research*, Vol. 1, *Origins and Policy of the Medical Research Council*, London, Medical Research Council, 1973; Vol 2, *The Programme of The Medical Research Council (UK)*, London, Medical Research Council, 1975.

Tuchman, A. M. 'From the Lecture to the Laboratory: The Institutionalisation of Scientific Medicine at the University of Heidelberg', in Coleman, W. and Holmes, F. L. (eds.) The Investigative Enterprise: Experimental Physiology in Nineteenth-Century Medicine, Berkeley, University of California Press, 1988, pp. 65–92.

Turner, R. S. 'The Growth of Professional Research in Prussia', *Historical Studies in the Physical Sciences*, 3 (1971), 137–82.

van Helvoort, T. 'History of Virus Research in the Twentieth Century: The Problem of Conceptual Continuity', *History of Science*, 32 (1994), 185–235.

Warner, J. H. 'The Idea of Science in English Medicine: The "Decline of Science" and the Rhetoric of Reform, 1815–45,' in French, R. and Wear, A. (eds.) British Medicine in an Age of Reform, London, Routledge, 1991, pp. 136–64.

Warner, J. H. 'Science in Medicine', *Osiris* 2nd ser. 2nd series, 1 (1985), 37–58.

Weatherall, D. *Science and the Quiet Art: Medical Research and Patient Care*, Oxford, Oxford University Press, 1995.

RESEARCH DISCIPLINES

Bulloch, W. *The History of Bacteriology*, London, Oxford University Press, 1938.

Coleman, W. and Holmes, F. L. (eds.) *The Investigative Enterprise: Experimental Physiology in Nineteenth-Century Medicine*, Berkeley, University of California Press, 1988.

Foster, W. D. *A Short History of History of Clinical Pathology*, E. & S. Livingstone Ltd., Edinburgh, 1961.

Foster, W. D. *A History of Medical Bacteriology and Immunology*, London, Heinemann Medical, 1970.

Fye, W. B. *The Development of American Physiology*, Baltimore, Johns Hopkins University Press, 1987.

Geison, G. *Michael Foster and the Cambridge School of Physiology*, Princeton, Princeton University Press, 1978.

Jacyna, L. S. '"A Host of Experienced Microscopists": The Establishment of Histology in Nineteenth-Century Edinburgh', *Bulletin of the History of Medicine*, 75 (2001), 225–53.

Kohler, R. E. *From Medical Chemistry to Biochemistry: The Making of a Biomedical Discipline*, Cambridge, Cambridge University Press, 1982.

Lesch, J. E. *Science and Medicine in France: The Emergence of Experimental Physiology, 1790–1855*, Cambridge, MA, Harvard University Press, 1984.

Long, E. R. *A History of Pathology*, New York, Dover, 1965.

Maulitz, R. C. *Morbid Appearances: the Anatomy of Pathology in the Early Nineteenth Century*, Cambridge, Cambridge University Press, 1987.

Mazumdar, P. *Species and Specificity: An Interpretation of the History of Immunology*, Cambridge, Cambridge University Press, 1995.

Medvei, V. C. *The History of Clinical Endocrinology*, Casterton Hall, Carnforth, Lancashire, The Parthenon Publishing Group, 1993.

Morange, M. *A History of Molecular Biology*, Cambridge, MA, Harvard University Press, 1990.

National Institutes of Health, http://history.nih.gov

Olson, R. *The Emergence of the Social Sciences 1642–1792: Twayne's Studies in Intellectual and Cultural History*, Boston, Twayne Publishers, 1993.

Rothschuh, K. E. *History of Physiology*, trans. Risse, G. B., New York, Krieger, 1973.

Silverstein, A. M. *A History of Immunology*, San Diego, Academic Press, 1989.

VIVISECTION AND ANIMALS IN MEDICAL RESEARCH

Bell, C. 'Second Part of the Paper on the Nerves of the Orbit', *Phil. Trans.*, 113 (1823), 289–307.

Elliot, P. 'Vivisection and the Emergence of Experimental Physiology in Nineteenth-Century France', in Rupke, N. A. (ed.) Vivisection in Historical Perspective, London, Croom Helm, 1990.

French, R. D. *Antivivisection and Medical Science in Victorian Society*, Princeton, Princeton University Press, 1975.

Ritvo, H. *The Animal Estate: The English and other Creatures in the Victorian Age*, Cambridge, MA, Harvard University Press, 1987.

Singer, P. *Animal Liberation: A New Ethics for our Treatment of Animals*, New York, New York Review, 1975.

DRUGS AND THE PHARMACEUTICAL INDUSTRY

Bliss, M. *The Discovery of Insulin*, Basingstoke, Macmillan, 1987.

Brynner, R. and Stephens, T. *Dark Remedy: The Impact of Thalidomide and Its Revival as a Vital Medicine*, Cambridge, MA, Perseus Publishing, 2001.

Carnwath, T. and Smith, I. *Heroin Century*, London, Routledge, 2002.

Galambos, L. and Sewell, J. E. *Networks of Innovation*, Cambridge and New York, Cambridge University Press, 1995.

Goodman, J. and Walsh, V. *The Story of Taxol: Nature and Politics in the Pursuit of an Anti-Cancer Drug*, Cambridge and New York, Cambridge University Press, 2001.

Greenwood, D. 'Conflicts of Interest: The Genesis of Synthetic Antimalarial Agents in Peace and War', *Journal of Antimicrobial Chemotherapy*, 36 (1995), 857–72.

Hauck Center for the Albert Sabin archives, http://sabin.uc.edu

Inman, B. *Don't Tell the Patient: Behind the Drug Safety Net*, Los Angeles and Bishops Waltham, Highland Park Productions, 1999.

James Lind Web site, http://www.jameslindlibrary.org/

Jones, E. *The Business of Medicine*, London, Profile, 2001.

Liebenau, J. 'The Rise of the British Pharmaceutical Industry', *British Medical Journal*, 301 (1990), 724–28.

Lindenmann, J. and Schleunig, W-D. (eds.) *Interferon: The Dawn of Recombinant Protein Drugs*, Berlin and London, Springer, 1999.

Marks, H. *The Progress of Experiment: Science and Therapeutic Reform in the United States 1900–1990*, Cambridge, Cambridge University Press, 1997.

Mauskopf, S. H. (ed.) *Chemical Sciences in the Modern World*, Philadelphia, University of Pennsylvania Press, 1993.

Slinn, J. *A History of May & Baker 1834–1984*, Cambridge, Hobsons, 1984.

Spear, H. B. (Mott, J., ed.) *Heroin Addiction Care and Control: The British System 1916–1984*, London, Drug Scope, 2002.

Swann, J. P. *Academic Scientists and the Pharmaceutical Industry: Cooperative Research in Twentieth-Century America*, Baltimore, Johns Hopkins University Press, 1988.

Swazey, J. P. *Chlorpromazine in Psychiatry: A Study of Therapeutic Innovation*, Cambridge, MA, MIT Press, 1974.

Thomas, L. G. *The Japanese Pharmaceutical Industry: The New Drug Lag and the Failure of Industrial Policy*, Cheltenham, Edward Elgar, 2001.

Vlassov, V. et al., 'Do Drug Advertisements in Russian Medical Journals Provide Essential Information for Safe Prescribing?' *Western Journal of Medicine*, 174 (2001), 391–4.

Vos, R. *Drugs Looking for Diseases: Innovative Drug Research and the Development of the Beta Blockers and the Calcium Antagonists*, Dordrecht and London, Kluwer Academic Publishers, 1991.

Weatherall, M. *In Search of a Cure: A History of Pharmaceutical Discovery*, Oxford and New York, Oxford University Press, 1990.

Williams, T. I. *Howard Florey, Penicillin and After*, Oxford, Oxford University Press, 1984.

POPULATION AND FERTILITY

Marks, L. *Sexual Chemistry*, New Haven and London, Yale University Press, 2002.

Watkins, E. *On the Pill. A Social History of Oral Contraceptives 1950–1970*, Baltimore and London, Johns Hopkins University Press, 1998.

HOSPITALS

Abel-Smith, B. *The Hospitals, 1800–1948: A Study in Social Administration in England and Wales*, London, Heinemann, 1964.

Granshaw, L. 'The Hospital'. In Bynum, W. F. and Porter, R. (eds). *The Companion Encyclopedia of the History of Medicine*, vol 2., London and New York, Routledge, 1993, pp. 1180–203.

Granshaw, L. and Porter, R. *The Hospital in History*, London, Routledge, 1989.

McKee, M. and Healy, J. (eds.) *Hospitals in a Changing Europe*, Buckingham, Open University Press, 2002.

Richardson, H. (ed.) *English Hospitals, 1660–1948: A Survey of Their Architecture and Design*, Swindon, Royal Commission on the Historical Monuments of England, 1998.

Risse, G. B. *Mending Bodies, Saving Souls*, New York, Oxford University Press, 1999.

Rivett, G. *The Development of the London Hospital System, 1823–1982*, London, King Edward's Hospital Fund for London, 1986.

Rosenberg, C. *The Care of Strangers: The Rise of America's Hospital System*, New York, Basic Books, 1987.

Stevens, R. *In Sickness and in Wealth. American Hospitals in the Twentieth Century*, Baltimore and London, Johns Hopkins University Press, 1999.

Thompson, J. D. and Goldin, G. *The Hospital: A Social and Architectural History*, New Haven, Yale University Press, 1975.

Waddington, I. 'The Role of the Hospital in the Development of Modern Medicine: A Sociological Analysis', *Sociology*, 7 (1973), 211–24.

Waddington, K. *Charity and the London Hospitals, 1850–1898*, Woodbridge, Royal Historical Society, 2000.

NURSING

Allan, P. and Jolley, M. (eds.) *Nursing, Midwifery and Health Visiting since 1900*, London, Faber & Faber, 1982.

Baly, M. *Florence Nightingale and the Nursing Legacy*, London, Routledge, 1986.

Brickman, J. P. 'Public Health, Midwives and Nurses, 1880–1930', in Lagemann, E. C. (ed.) Nursing History: New Perspectives, New Possibilities, New York, Teachers College Press, 1983, pp. 65–88.

Davies, C. (ed.) *Rewriting Nursing History*, London, Croom Helm, 1980.

Fulton, J. *An Evolving Profession*, Manchester, Open College, 1996.

Higonnet, M. R. (ed.) *Nurses at the Front: Writing the Wounds of the Great War*, Boston, Northeastern University Press, 2001.

MacDonald, L. *The Roses of No Man's Land*, London Penguin Books, 1983.

Maggs, C. (ed.) *Nursing History: The State of the Art*, London, Croom Helm, 1987.

Reverby, S. *Ordered to Care, The Dilemma of American Nursing 1850–1945*, Cambridge, Cambridge University Press, 1987.

Salvage, J. and Heijnen, S. (eds.) *Nursing in Europe. A Resource for Better Health*, Copenhagen, World Health Organization, 1997.

Stapleton, D. H. and Welch, C. A. (eds.) *Critical Issues in American Nursing in the Twentieth Century: Perspectives and Case studies*, Guilderland, NY, The Foundation, 1994.

Summers, A. *Angels and Citizens, British Women as Military Nurses, 1854–1914*, London, Routledge, 1988.

Woods, C. Q. 'From Individual Dedication to Social Activism: Historical Development of Nursing Professionalism', in Maggs, C. (ed.) Nursing History, The State of the Art, London, Croom Helm, 1987, pp. 153–75.

MIDWIFERY

DeClerq, E. 'The Transformation of American Midwifery, 1975 to 1998', *American Journal of Public Health*, 82 (1992), 680–4.

Devries, R. G. and Barroso, R. 'Midwives Among the Machines. Recreating Midwifery in the Late Twentieth Century', in Marland, H. and Rafferty, A. M. (eds.) Midwives, Society and Childbirth, London, Routledge, 1997.

Litoff, J. B. *American Midwives 1860 to the Present*, Westport, CT, Greenwood Press, 1978.

Oakley, A. and Houd, S. *Helpers in Childbirth: Midwifery Today*, New York and London, Hemisphere, 1990.

PALLIATIVE CARE

Clark, D. and Wright, M. *Facing Death. Transitions in End of Life Care. Hospice and Related Developments in Eastern Europe*, Buckingham, Open University Press, 2003.

ten Have, H. and Clark, D. (eds.) *The Ethics of Palliative Care: European Perspectives*, Buckingham, Open University Press, 2002.

MEDICAL EDUCATION

Anning, S. T. 'Provincial Medical Schools in the Nineteenth Century', in Poynter, F. N. L. *The Evolution of Medical Education in Britain*, London, Pitman, 1966.

Association of American Medical Colleges, *Physicians for the Twenty-First Century: Report of the Project Panel on the General Professional Education of the Physician and College Preparation for Medicine*, Washington, DC, Association of American Medical Colleges, 1984.

Bonner, T. N. *Becoming a Physician, Medical Education in Great Britain, France, Germany and the United States, 1750–1945*, New York, Oxford University Press, 1995.

Bonner, T. N. *To the Ends of the Earth: Women's Search for Education in Medicine*, Cambridge, MA, Harvard University Press, 1992.

Bowers, J. Z. et al. (eds,) *Science and Medicine in Twentieth Century China: Research and Education*, Ann Arbor, Center for Chinese Studies, the University of Michigan, 1988.

Brockliss, L. 'Before the Clinic: French Medical Teaching in the Eighteenth Century', in C. Hannaway and A. La Berge, Constructing Paris Medicine, Amsterdam, Rodopi, 1998, pp. 71–115.

Cocks, G. and Jarausch, K. H. (eds.) *German Professions, 1800–1950*, New York, Oxford University Press, 1990.

Commission on Medical Education. *Final Report of the Commission on Medical Education*, New York, Office of the Director of Study, 1932.

Cope, Z. 'The Private Medical Schools of London', in Poynter, F. N. L., The Evolution of Medical Education in Britain, London, Pitman Medical Publising, 1966, pp. 89–109.

Flexner, A. *Medical Education: A Comparative Study*, New York, Macmillan, 1925.

575

Flexner, A. *Medical Education in Europe*, New York, Carnegie Foundation, 1912.

Flexner, A. *Medical Education in the United States and Canada*, New York, Carnegie Foundation, 1910.

Ford, J. M. T. (ed.) *A Medical Student at St. Thomas's Hospital, 1801–1802: The Weekes Family Letters*, London, Wellcome Institute for the History of Medicine, 1987.

General Medical Council. *Tomorrow's Doctors: Recommendations on Undergraduate Medical Education*, London, General Medical Council, 1993.

Graham, G. 'The Formation of the Medical and Surgical Professorial Units in the London Teaching Hospitals', *Annals of Science*, 26 (1970), 1–22.

Lesky, E. *The Vienna Medical School of the 19th Century*, Baltimore, Johns Hopkins University Press, 1976.

Ludmerer, K. M. *Learning to Heal, The Development of American Medical Education*, New York, Basic Books, 1985.

McClelland, C. E. *The German Experience of Professionalization*, Cambridge, Cambridge University Press, 1991.

Numbers, R. L. *The Education of American Physicians*, Berkeley, University of California Press, 1980.

Paul, H. *From Knowledge to Power: The Rise of the Science Empire in France, 1860–1939*, Cambridge, Cambridge University Press, 1985.

Richardson, R. *Death, Dissection and the Destitute*, London, Routledge & Kegan Paul, 1988.

Rothstein, W. G. *American Medical Schools and the Practice of Medicine*, New York, Oxford University Press, 1987.

Tuchman, A. M. *Science, Medicine and the State in Germany, The Case of Baden, 1815–1871*, New York, Oxford University Press, 1993.

Weisz, G. *The Emergence of Modern Universities in France, 1863–1914*, Princeton, Princeton University Press, 1983.

PUBLIC HEALTH AND PREVENTIVE MEDICINE

Baldwin, P. *Contagion and the State in Europe, 1830–1930*, Cambridge, Cambridge University Press, 1999.

Bashford, A. *Purity and Pollution: Gender, Embodiment, and Victorian Medicine*, New York, St. Martin's Press; Basingstoke, Macmillan, 1998.

Berg, M. and Cocks, G. *Medicine and Modernity, Public Health and Medical Care in the Nineteenth- and Twentieth-Century Germany*, New York, Syndicate of the University of Cambridge, 1997.

Birn, A-E. 'Wa(i)ves of Influence: Rockefeller Public Health in Mexico, 1920–50', *Studies in History and Philosophy of Biological and Biomedical Sciences*, 31 (2000), 381–95.

Blaupain, J. et al., *National Health Insurance and Health Resources: The European Experience*, Cambridge, MA, Harvard University Press, 1978.

Bynum, W. F. 'Policing Hearts of Darkness: Aspects of the International Sanitary Conferences', *History and Philosophy of the Life Sciences*, 15 (1993), 421–34.

Christiansen, N. F. and Petersen, K. 'The Nordic Welfare States: A Historical Reappraisal', *Scandinavian Journal of History*, Special issue, 26 (2001), 153–6.

Coleman, W. *Death Is a Social Disease: Public Health and Political Economy in Early Industrial France*, Madison, University of Wisconsin Press, 1982.

Dixon, A. and Mossialos, E. *Health Care Systems in Eight Countries: Trends and Challenges*, London, European Observatory on Health Care Systems, 2002.

Douglas-Wilson, I. and McLachlan, G. (eds.) *Health Service Prospects. An International Survey*, London, Lancet, Nuffield Provincial Hospitals Trust, 1973.

Duffy, J. *The Sanitarians, A History of American Public Health*, Urbana, University of Illinois Press, 1990.

Ellis, J. D. *The Physician-Legislators of France: Medicine and Politics in the Early Third Republic, 1870–1914*, Cambridge, Cambridge University Press, 1990.

Goubert, J-P. *The Conquest of Water, The Advent of Health in the Industrial Age*, trans. Wilson, A., Princeton, Princeton University Press, 1989.

Hamlin, C. *Public Health and Social Justice in the Age of Chadwick: Britain, 1800–1854*, Cambridge, Cambridge University Press, 1998.

Hardy, A. *The Epidemic Streets, Infectious Disease and the Rise of Preventive Medicine 1856–1900*, Oxford, Clarendon Press, 1993.

Heidenheimer, A. J. and Elvander, N. (eds.) *The Shaping of the Swedish Health System*, London, Croom Helm, 1980.

Hennock, E. P. *British Social Reform and German Precedents. The Case of Social Insurance, 1880–1914*, Oxford, Clarendon Press, 1987.

Hildreth, M. L. *Doctors, Bureaucrats, and the Public Health in France, 1888–1902*, New York, Garland, 1987.

Hollingsworth, J. R. et al., *State Intervention in Medical Care*, Ithaca and London, Cornell University Press, 1990.

Immergut, E. *Health Politics. Interests and Institutions in Western Europe*, Cambridge, Cambridge University Press, 1992.

Jones, N. H. *The Scientific Background of the International Sanitary Conferences, 1851–1938*, Geneva, World Health Organization, 1975.

Kraut, A. M. *Silent Travellers, Germs, Gene, and the 'Immigrant Menace'*, New York, Basic Books, 1994.

La Berge, A. F. *Mission and Method: The Early Nineteenth-Century French Public Health Movement*, Cambridge, Cambridge University Press, 1992.

Markel, H. *Quarantine! East European Jewish Immigrants and the New York City Epidemics of 1892*, Baltimore, Johns Hopkins University Press, 1997.

Mossialos, E. and Le Grand, J. (eds.) *Health Care and Cost Containment in the European Union*, Aldershot, Hampshire, Ashgate, 1999.

Porter, D. *Health, Civilization, and the State: A History of Public health from Ancient to Modern Times*, London, Routledge, 1999.

Poovey, M. *Making a Social Body: British Cultural Formation, 1830–1864*, Chicago, University of Chicago Press, 1995.

Porter, D. *The History of Public Health and the Modern State*, Amsterdam, Rodopi, 1994.

Prausnitz, C. *The Teaching of Preventive Medicine in Europe*, London, Oxford University Press, 1933.

Raffel, M. W. (ed.) *Comparative Health Systems: Descriptive Analyses of Fourteen National Health Systems*, University Park, Pennsylvania State University Press, 1984.

Raffel, M. W. and Raffel, N. K. *The US Health System. Origins and Functions*, New York, Wiley, 3rd ed., 1989.

Rivett, G. *From Cradle to Grave: Fifty Years of the National Health Service*, London, King's Fund, 1998. Also, www.nhshistory.com

Rosen, G. *A History of Public Health*, New York, MD Publications, 1958.

Warren, M. 'A Chronology of State Medicine, Public Health, Welfare and Related Services in Britain: 1066–1999', www.chronology.org.uk(

Webster, C. *The National Health Services since the War, vol. 1*, London, HMSO, 1994; vol. 2, HMSO, 1996.

OCCUPATIONAL HEALTH AND MEDICAL INSURANCE

Rabinbach, A. *The Human Motor: Energy, Fatigue and the Origins of Modernity*, Berkeley, University of California Press, 1992.

Sellers, C. C. *Hazards of the Job: From Industrial Disease to Environmental Health Science*, Chapel Hill and London, University of North Carolina Press, 1997.

Smith, T. B. 'The Social Transformation of Hospitals and the Rise of Medical Insurance in France, 1914–1943', *The Historical Journal*, 41 (1998), 1055–87.

Weindling, P. (ed.) *The Social History of Occupational Health*, London, Croom Helm, 1985.

PARIS MEDICINE

Ackerknecht, E. H. *Medicine at the Paris Hospital, 1794–1848*, Baltimore, Johns Hopkins University Press, 1967.

Ackerknecht, E. H. 'Broussais, or a Forgotten Medical Revolution', *Bulletin of the History of Medicine*, 27 (1953), 320–43.

Gelfand, T. *Professionalizing Modern Medicine: Paris Surgeons and Medical Science and Institutions in the 18th Century*, Westport, CT, Greenwood Press, 1980.

Haigh, E. 'The Roots of the Vitalism of Xavier Bichat', *Bulletin of the History of Medicine*, 49 (1975), 72–86.

Haigh, E. *Xavier Bichat and the Medical Theory of the Eighteenth Century*, London, Wellcome Institute for the History of Medicine, 1984.

Hannaway, C. and La Berge, A. (eds.) *Constructing Paris Medicine*, Amsterdam, Rodopi, 1998.

Jones, C. 'The Great Chain of Buying: Medical Advertisement, the Bourgeois Public Sphere, and the Origins of the French Revolution', *American Historical Review*, 101 (1996), 13–40.

La Berge, A. 'Medical Microscopy in Paris, 1830–1855', in La Berge, A. and Feingold, M. (eds.) French Medical Culture in the Nineteenth Century, Amsterdam: Rodopi, 1994, pp. 296–326.

Vess, D. M. *Medical Revolution in France 1789–1796*, Gainesville, University Presses of Florida, 1975.

Warner, J. H. 'Remembering Paris: Memory and the American Disciples of French Medicine in the Nineteenth Century', *Bulletin of the History of Medicine*, 65 (1991), 301–25.

SOVIET MEDICINE

Field, M. G. *Doctor and Patient in Soviet Russia*, Cambridge, MA, Harvard University Press, 1957.

Hyde, G. *The Soviet Health Service. A Historical and Comparative Study*, London, Lawrence and Wishart, 1974.

Krementsov, N. *Stalinist Science*, Princeton, Princeton University Press, 1997.

Newsholme, A. and Kingbury, J. A. *Red Medicine, Socialized Health in Soviet Russia*, London, William Heinemann, 1934.

Sigerist, H. E. *Socialised Medicine in the Soviet Union*, London, Victor Gollancz Ltd, 1937.

Solomon, S. G. and Hutchinson, J. F. (eds.) *Health and Society in Soviet Russia*, Bloomington, Indiana University Press, 1990.

Weissmann, N. B. 'Origins of Soviet Health Administration Narkomzdrav, 1918–1928', in Solomon, S. G. and Hutchinson, J. F. (eds.) *Health and Society in Soviet Russia*, Bloomington, Indiana University Press, 1990, pp. 97–120.

UNITED STATES MEDICINE

Warner, J. H. *The Therapeutic Perspective: Medical Knowledge, Practice, and Professional Identity in America, 1820–1885*, Cambridge, MA, Harvard University Press, 1984.

NAZI MEDICINE

Kater, M. *Doctors under Hitler*, Chapel Hill, University of North Carolina Press, 1989.

Light, D. W. and Schuller, A. (eds.) *Political Values and Health Care: The German Experience*, Cambridge MA, The MIT Press, 1976.

Proctor, R. N. 'Nazi Biomedicine Policies' in Caplan, A. L. (ed.) When Medicine Went Mad: Bioethics and the Holocaust, Totowa, NJ, Humana Press, 1992, pp. 23–42.

Proctor, R. N. *Racial Hygiene: Medicine under the Nazis*, Cambridge MA, Harvard University Press, 1988.

Seidelman, W. E. '"Medspeak" for Murder: The Nazi Experience and the Culture of Medicine' in Caplan, A. L. (ed.) When Medicine Went Mad: Bioethics and the Holocaust, Totowa, NJ, Humana Press, 1992, pp. 271–80.

Timmermann, C. 'Constitutional Medicine, Neoromanticism, and the Politics of Antimechanism in Interwar Germany', *Bulletin of the History of Medicine*, 75 (2001), 717–39.

Weindling, P. *Health, Race and German Politics between National Unification and Nazism 1870–1945*, Cambridge, Cambridge University Press, 1989.

TROPICAL AND IMPERIAL MEDICINE

Arnold, D. *Science, Technology and Medicine in Colonial India*, Cambridge, Cambridge University Press, 2000.

Arnold, D. (ed.) *Warm Climates and Western Medicine*, Amsterdam, Rodopi, 1996.

Arnold, D. (ed.) *Imperial Medicine and Indigenous Societies*, Manchester, Manchester University Press, 1988.

Bynum, W. F. and Overy, C. (eds.) *The Beast in the Mosquito: The Correspondence of Ronald Ross and Patrick Manson*, Amsterdam, Rodopi, 1998.

Curtin, P. *Disease and Empire: The Health of European Troops in the Conquest of Africa*, Cambridge, Cambridge University Press, 1998.

Harrison, M. *Public Health in British India, Anglo-Indian Preventive Medicine, 1859–1914*, Cambridge, Cambridge University Press, 1994.

Headrick, D. *The Tools of Empire, Technology and European Imperialism in the Nineteenth Century*, New York, Oxford University Press, 1981.

Macleod, R. and Lewis, M. (eds.) *Disease, Medicine and Empire*, London, Routledge, 1988.

Osborne, M. A. *Nature, the Exotic and the Science of French Colonialism*, Bloomington, Indiana University Press, 1994.

INTERNATIONAL ORGANIZATIONS AND THE DEVELOPING WORLD

Bhattacharya, S. et al. 'A Very Peculiar Triumph': The Control and Eradication of Smallpox in India (in press).

Brockington, F. The Health of the Developing World, Lewes, Sussex, Book Guild, 1985.

Broms, B. The United Nations, United Nations, Helsinki, 1990.

Caulfield, C. Masters of Illusion: The World Bank and the Poverty of Nations, London, Macmillan, 1997.

Dobbing, J. Infant Feeding. Anatomy of a Controversy 1973–1984, Berlin and London, Leiden, Springer-Verlag, 1988.

Fenner, F. et al. Smallpox and Its Eradication, Geneva, World Health Organization, 1988.

Goodman, N. M. International Health Organisations and Their Work, Edinburgh, Churchill Livinstone, 2nd ed., 1971.

League of Nations, Health Organisation, Geneva, Information Section, 1931.

Lee, S. 'WHO and the Developing World: The Contest for Ideology,' in Cunningham, A. and Andrews, B. (eds.) Western Medicine as Contested Knowledge, Manchester and New York, Manchester University Press, 1997, pp. 24–45.

Litsios, S. 'Malaria Control, the Cold War, and the Post-war Reorganisation of International Assistance' Medical Anthropology, 17 (1997), 255–78.

Melrose, D. Bitter Pills: Medicines and the Third World, Oxford, Oxfam, 1982.

Muraskin, W. The Politics of International Health: The Children's Vaccine Initiative, Albany, State University New York Press, 1998.

Packard, R. 'Malaria Dreams: Post-war Visions of Health and Development in the Third World', Medical Anthropology, 17 (1997), 279–96.

Phillips, D. R. Health and Health Care in the Third World, Harlow, Herts., Longman Scientific and Technical, 1990.

Power, J. (ed.) Vision of Hope: The Fiftieth Anniversary of the United Nations, London, Regency Corporation Ltd, 1995.

Weindling, P. (ed.) International Health Organisations and Movements, 1918–1939, Cambridge, Cambridge University Press, 1995.

THE ROCKEFELLER FOUNDATION

Corner, G. A History of the Rockefeller Institute, 1901–1953, New York, Rockefeller Institute Press, 1964.

Fisher, D. 'The Rockefeller Foundation and the Development of Scientific Medicine in Britain', Minerva, 16 (1978), 20–41.

Fosdick, R. B. The Story of the Rockefeller Foundation, New York, Harper and Brothers, 1952.

Hanson, E. The Rockefeller University Achievements: A Century of Science for the Benefit of Humankind 1901–2001, New York, Rockefeller University Press, 2000.

Löwy, I. and Zylberman, P. 'Medicine as a Social Instrument: Rockefeller Foundation, 1913–45', Studies in History and Philosophy of Biological and Biomedical Sciences, 31 (2000), 365–79.

MEDICINE, EUGENICS, AND RACE

Burleigh, M. Death and Deliverance: "Euthanasia" in Germany c. 1900–1945, Cambridge, Cambridge University Press, 1994.

Gaudillère, J-P. and Löwy, I. (eds.) *Heredity and Infection: The History of Disease Transmission*, London and New York, Routledge, 2001.

Kevles, D. *In the Name of Eugenics: Genetics and the Uses of Human Heredity*, Harmondsworth, England, Penguin Books, 1986.

Larson, E. J. *Sex, Race, and Science: Eugenics in the Deep South*, Baltimore, John Hopkins University Press, 1995.

Proctor, R. N. *Racial Hygiene: Medicine under the Nazis*, Cambridge MA, Harvard University Press, 1988.

Reilly, P. R. *The Surgical Solution: A History of Involuntary Sterilization in the United States*, Johns Hopkins University Press, Baltimore, 1991.

MEDICINE AND ETHICS

Baker, R. (ed.) *The Codification of Medical Morality, Vol. Two: Anglo-American Medical Ethics and Medical Jurisprudence in the Nineteenth Century*, Dordrecht, Kluwer, 1995.

Smith, R. G. *Medical Discipline: The Professional Conduct Jurisdiction of the General Medical Council, 1858–1990*, Oxford, Clarendon Press, 1994.

MEDICINE AND WAR

Bourke, Joanna, 'Disciplining the Emotions: Fear, Psychiatry and the Second World War', in Cooter, R., Harrison, M., and Sturdy, S. (eds.) War, Medicine and Modernity, Stroud, Sutton, 1998, pp. 225–38.

Bristow, N. K. *Making Men Moral: Social Engineering during the Great War*, New York, New York University Press, 1996.

Caplan, A. L. (ed.) *When Medicine Went Mad: Bioethics and the Holocaust*, Totowa, NJ, Humana Press, 1992.

Cooter, R. and Sturdy, S. 'Of War, Medicine and Modernity: an Introduction', in Cooter, R., Harrison, M., and Sturdy, S. (eds.) War, Medicine and Modernity, Stroud, Sutton, 1998, pp. 1–21.

Eghigian, G. A. 'The German Welfare State as a Discourse of Trauma', in Micale, M. S. and Lerner, P. (eds.) *Traumatic Pasts: History, Psychiatry, and Trauma in the Modern Age, 1870–1930*, Cambridge, Cambridge University Press 2001, pp. 92–112.

Gerber, D. A. (ed.) *Disabled Veterans in History*, Anne Arbor, University of Michigan Press, 2000.

Harrison, M. *Medicine and Victory: British Military Medicine in the Second World War*, Oxford, Oxford University Press, 2004.

Harrison, M. 'Medicine and the Management of Modern Warfare: An Introduction', in Cooter, R., Harrison, M., and Sturdy, S. (eds.) Medicine and Modern Warfare, Amsterdam, Rodopi, 1999, pp. 1–27.

Howell, J. D. '"Soldier's Heart": The Redefinition of Heart Disease and Specialty Formation in Early Twentieth-Century Great Britain', in Cooter, R., Harrison, M., and Sturdy, S. (eds.) War, Medicine and Modernity, Stroud, Sutton, 1998, pp. 85–105.

Linton, D. S. 'The Obscure Object of Knowledge: German Military Medicine Confronts Gas Gangrene During World War 1', *Bulletin of the History of Medicine*, 74 (2000), 291–316.

Price, M. 'Bodies and Souls: The Rehabilitation of Maimed Soldiers in France and Germany during the First World War', Ph.D. thesis, Stanford University, 1998.

581

Prüll, C-R. 'Pathology at War 1914–1918: Germany and Britain in Comparison' in Cooter, R., Harrison, M., and Sturdy, S. (eds.) Medicine and Modern Warfare, Amsterdam, Rodopi, 1999, pp.131–61.

Roudebush, M. 'A Battle of Nerves: Hysteria and Its Treatments in France During World War 1', in Micale, M. S. and Lerner, P. (eds.) Traumatic Pasts: History, Psychiatry, and Trauma in the Modern Age, 1870–1930, Cambridge, Cambridge University Press 2001, pp. 253–79.

Salusbury, A. (Sir), and Mellor, W. F. *Medical Services in War: The Principal Medical Lessons of the Second World War, Based on the Official Medical Histories of the United Kingdom, Canada, Australia, New Zealand and India*, London, H.M.S.O., 1968.

Shephard, B. *A War of Nerves*, London, Jonathan Cape, 2000.

Sturdy, S. 'War as Experiment. Physiology, Innovation and Administration in Britain, 1914–1918: The Case of Chemical Warfare', in Cooter, R., Harrison, M., and Sturdy, S. (eds.) *War, Medicine and Modernity*, Stroud, Sutton, 1998, pp. 65–84.

Whitehead, Ian R., *Doctors in the Great War*, London, Leo Cooper 1999.

MEDICAL ORGANIZATION AND POLICY

Leichter, H. M. *A Comparative Approach to Policy Analysis. Health Care Policy in Four Nations*, Cambridge, Cambridge University Press, 1979.

Morone, J. A. and Goggin, J. M. 'Health Policies in Europe: Welfare States in a Market Era', *Journal of Health Politics, Policy and Law*, 20 (1995), 557–69.

Wilsford, D. 'States Facing Interests: Struggles over Health Care Policy in Advanced Industrial Democracies', *Journal of Health Politics, Policy and Law*, 20 (1995), 571–613.

MEDICINE AND THE MEDIA

Karpf, A. *Doctoring the Media*, London, Routledge, 1988.

Lederer, S. and Rogers, N. 'Media', in Cooter, R. and Pickstone, J. (eds.) *Medicine in the Twentieth Century*, Amsterdam, Harwood Academic; Abingdon, Marston, 2000, 487–502.

PHILOSOPHY AND HISTORY OF IDEAS

Armstrong, D. 'Bodies of Knowledge(Knowledge of Bodies', in C. Jones and Porter, R. (eds.) *Reassessing Foucault: Power, Medicine and the Body*, London, Routledge, 1994.

Baudrillard, J. *Simulations*, New York, Semiotext(e), Inc, 1983.

Berman, M. *All That Is Solid Melts into Air: The Experience of Modernity*, London, Verso, 1983.

Crary, J. *Techniques of the Observer: On Vision and Modernity in the Nineteenth Century*, Cambridge, MA, MIT Press, 1990.

Driver, F. 'Bodies in Space: Foucault's Account of Disciplinary Power', in Jones, C. and Porter, R. (eds.) Re-assessing Foucault: Power, Medicine and the Body, London, Routledge, 1994, pp. 113–31.

Foucault, M. *The Birth of the Clinic: An Archaeology of Medical Perception*, London, Tavistock, 1973.

Foucault, M. 'The Politics of Health in the Eighteenth Century,' in Colin Gordon (ed.) Power (Knowledge: Selected Interviews & Other Writings, New York, Pantheon Books, 1972, pp. 166–82.

Marcuse, H. *One Dimensional Man*, Boston, Beacon Press, 1964.

Rosen, G. 'The Philosophy of Ideology and the Emergence of Modern Medicine in France', *Bulletin of the History of Medicine*, 20 (1946), pp. 328–39.

Wilson, C. *The Invisible World: Early Modern Philosophy and the Invention of the Microscope*, Princeton, Princeton University Press, 1995.

HISTORY OF SCIENCE

Golinski, J. *Making Natural Knowledge: Constructivism and the History of Science*, Cambridge University Press, 1998.

Lawrence, C. and Shapin, S. (eds.) *Science Incarnate: Historical Embodiments of Natural Knowledge*, University of Chicago Press, 1998.

Secord, A. 'Botany on a Plate: Pleasure and the Power of Pictures in Promoting Early Nineteenth-Century Scientific Knowledge', *Isis*, 93 (2002), 28–57.

Shapin, S. *A Social History of Truth: Civility and Science in Seventeenth-Century England*, Chicago, University of Chicago Press, 1994.

Shapin, S. and Schaffer, S. *Leviathan and the Air-Pump: Hobbes, Boyle, and the Experimental Life*, Princeton, Princeton University Press, 1985.

BIOGRAPHY AND AUTOBIOGRAPHY

Ackerknecht, E. *Rudolf Virchow: Doctor, Statesman, Anthropologist*, Madison, University of Wisconsin Press, 1953.

Benison, S. A., Barger, C. and Wolfe, E. L. *Walter B. Cannon: The Life and Times of a Young Scientist*, Cambridge, MA, The Belknap Press, 1987.

Braunstein, J-F. *Broussais et le Matérialisme: Médecine et Philosophie au XIXe Siècle*, Paris, Méridiens Klincksieck, 1986.

Brock, T. D. *Robert Koch, A Life in Medicine and Bacteriology*, Madison, University of Wisconsin Press, 1988.

Clark, R. W. *The Life of Ernst Chain: Penicillin and Beyond*, London, Weidenfeld and Nicolson, 1985.

Debré, P. *Louis Pasteur*, trans. Forster, E., Baltimore, Johns Hopkins University Press, 1998.

Duffin, J. *To See with a Better Eye: A Life of R. T. H. Laennec*, Princeton, Princeton University Press, 1998.

Eyler, J. M. *Sir Arthur Newsholme and State Medicine, 1885–1935*, Cambridge, Cambridge University Press, 1997.

Fayrer, J. *Recollections of My Life*, Edinburgh, William Blackwood, 1900.

Fraenkel, G. J. *Hugh Cairns: First Nuffield Professor of Surgery University of Oxford*, Oxford, Oxford University Press, 1991.

Fulton, J. F. *Harvey Cushing: A Biography*, Springfield, IL, Charles C. Thomas, 1946.

Gay, P. *Freud: A Life for Our Times*, London, Dent, 1988.

Gosse, E. *Father and Son*, Harmondsworth, Penguin, 1986 (originally pub., 1907).

Gosse, E. *The Life of Philip Henry Gosse, F. R. S*, London, Kegan Paul, 1890.

Holmes, F. L. *Claude Bernard and Animal Chemistry*. Cambridge, MA, Harvard University Press, 1974.

Johansen, P. V. et al., *Cholera, Chloroform and the Science of Medicine, A Life of John Snow*, New York, Oxford University Press, 2003.

Kass, A. M. and Kass, E. H. *Perfecting the World: The Life and Times of Dr. Thomas Hodgkin 1798–1866*, Boston, Harcourt Brace Jovanovich, 1988.

Lambert, R. *Sir John Simon 1816–1904 and English Social Administration*, London, MacGibbon and Kee, 1963.

Olmsted, J. E. D. and Olmsted E. H. *Claude Bernard and the Experimental Method in Medicine*, New York, Schuman, 1952.

Schiller, F. *Paul Broca: Founder of French Anthropology, Explorer of the Brain*, Berkeley, University of California Press, 1979.

Silverstein, A. M. *Paul Ehrlich's Receptor Immunology. The Magnificent Obsession*, San Diego, Academic Press, 2002.

Sykes, A. H. *Sharpey's Fibres: The Life of William Sharpey, the Father of Modern Physiology in England*, York, William Sessions Ltd, Ebor Press, 2001.

Tauber, A. I. *Metchnikoff and the Origins of Immunology: From Metaphor to Theory*, New York, Oxford University Press, 1991.

Thwaite, A. *Glimpses of the Wonderful. The Life of Philip Henry Gosse*, London, Faber and Faber, 2002.

Wolfe, E. L., Barger, A. C. and Benison, S. *Walter B. Cannon: Science and Society*, Cambridge, MA, Boston Medical Library, 2000.

Index